BREAST CANCER:
Controversies in Management

edited by

Leslie Wise, M.D.

Chairman
Department of Surgery
The Methodist Hospital
Brooklyn, New York;
Professor of Surgery
Albert Einstein College of Medicine
Bronx, New York

and

Houston Johnson, Jr., M.D.

Medical Director
Breast Care Center
Flower Hospital
Sylvania, Ohio;
Medical Associate Professor of Surgery
Medical College of Ohio
Toledo, Ohio

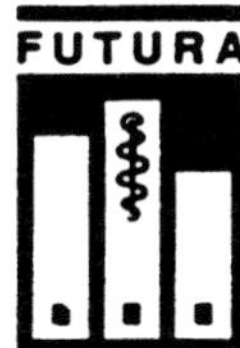

Futura Publishing Company, Inc.
Armonk, New York

Library of Congress Cataloging-in-Publication Data

Breast cancer : controversies in management / edited by Leslie Wise and
    Houston Johnson, Jr.
        p.   cm.
    Includes bibliographical references and index.
    ISBN 0-87993-562-6
    1. Breast—Cancer.   I. Wise, Leslie.   II. Johnson, Houston.
    [DNLM: 1. Breast Neoplasms—therapy.   2. Combined Modality
Therapy.   WP 870 B82337 1994]
    RC280.B8B668   1994
    616.99'44906—dc20
    DNLM/DLC
    for Library of Congress   93-31411
                                                                               CIP

Copyright 1994
Futura Publishing Company, Inc.

Published by
Futura Publishing Company, Inc.
135 Bedford Road
Armonk, New York 10504

LC #: 93-31411
ISBN #: 0-87993-562-6

Every effort has been made to ensure that the information in this book is as up to
date and as accurate as possible at the time of publication. However, due to the
constant developments in medicine, neither the author, nor the editor, nor the
publisher can accept any legal or any other responsibility for any errors or
omissions that may occur.

Printed in the United States of America on acid-free paper.

Contributors

Jeffrey S. Abrams, M.D.
Associate Professor of Medicine and Oncology; Head, Breast Evaluation Program, University of Maryland Cancer Center, Baltimore, Maryland

Roberto Agresti, M.D.
Department of Surgery, Istituto Nazionale per lo Studio e la Cura dei Tumori, Via G. Venezian 1, Milano, Italy

Joseph Aisner, M.D.
Chief of Medical Oncology; Director, University of Maryland Cancer Center, Baltimore, Maryland; Professor of Medicine and Oncology, University of Maryland School of Medicine, Baltimore, Maryland

Simon M. Allan, M.B.B.S., F.R.C.S.
Research Fellow, Department of Academic Surgery, The Royal Marsden Hospital, London, England

Salvatore Andreola, M.D.
Department of Pathologic Anatomy, Istituto Nazionale per lo Studio e la Cura dei Tumori, Via G. Venezian 1, Milano, Italy

Irving M. Ariel, M.D.
Professor of Clinical Surgery, New York Medical College, New York, New York, and Albert Einstein College of Medicine, Bronx, New York; Attending Surgeon, Cabrini Medical Center and Doctors Hospital, New York, New York; Consultant Surgeon, Long Island Jewish Medical Center, New Hyde Park, New York, and Hospital for Joint Diseases and Orthopedic Institute, New York, New York

Raj A. Badwe, M.S. (Bombay)
Research Fellow, Department of Academic Surgery, The Royal Marsden Hospital, London, England

Lester C. Barr, F.R.C.S.
Senior Registrar/Lecturer in Surgery, The Royal Marsden Hospital, London, England

Michael Baum, Ch.M., F.R.C.S., M.D.
Professor of Surgery, The Royal Marsden Hospital, London, England

Maurice M. Black, M.D.
Attending in Pathology at Westchester County Medical Center, Valhalla, New York; Clinical Professor of Pathology at New York Medical College, Valhalla, New York; Research Scientist, The Methodist Hospital, New York

Roger W. Blamey, M.D., F.R.C.S.
Professor of Surgical Science, Nottingham City Hospital, Nottingham, England
John Bostwick III, M.D., F.A.C.S.
Professor of Plastic, Reconstructive and Maxillo-facial Surgery, Emory University School of Medicine, Atlanta, Georgia
Murid A. Chaudary, Ch.M., F.R.C.S
Senior Lecturer and Honorary Consultant Surgeon, ICRF Clinic Oncology Unit, Guy's Hospital, London, England
Hiram S. Cody, III, M.D.
Assistant Professor of Clinical Surgery, Cornell University Medical College; Adjunct Professor of Clinical Surgery, Columbia University College of Physicians and Surgeons, New York, New York; Assistant Attending Surgeon, St. Luke's-Roosevelt Hospital, New York, New York
George Crile, Jr., M.D. (Deceased)
Emeritus Consultant; Department of General Surgery, Cleveland Clinic, Cleveland, Ohio
Stephen A. Feig, M.D.
Director, Breast Imaging Center, Department of Radiology, Thomas Jefferson University Hospital, Philadelphia, Pennsylvania; Professor of Radiology, Jefferson Medical College, Philadelphia, Pennsylvania
Sir Patrick M. Forrest, B.Sc., M.B., Ch.B., Ch.M., M.D.
Professor Emeritus, University of Edinburgh, Edinburgh, Scotland
Marcus H. Galea, D.M., F.R.C.S.
Lecturer, Department of Surgery, Nottingham City Hospital, Nottingham, England
Viviana Galimberti, M.D.
Department of Surgery, Istituto Nazionale per lo Studio e la Cura dei Tumori, Via G. Venezian 1, Milano, Italy
Paul A.C. Greenberg, M.D.
Attending, Beth Israel Hospital North, New York, New York
Marco Greco, M.D.
Department of Surgery, Istituto Nazionale per lo Studio e la Cura dei Tumori, Via G. Venezian 1, Milano, Italy
Frank E. Gump, M.D.
Chief, Surgical Service, Veterans Administration Medical Center, East Orange, New Jersey; Professor of Surgery, University of Medicine and Dentistry of New Jersey, New Jersey Medical School, Newark, New Jersey
John L. Hayward, F.R.C.S.
Consultant Surgeon, Emblem House, London Bridge Hospital, London, England
Vernon J. Henderson, M.D.
Assistant Professor of Surgery, University of California, Davis, East Bay, Oakland, California
James F. Holland, M.D.
Chairman, Department of Neoplastic Diseases and Director of The Derald H. Ruttenberg Cancer Center, The Mount Sinai Medical Center, New York, New York; Jane B. and Jack R. Aron Professor of Neoplastic Diseases, Mount Sinai School of Medicine, New York, New York

Gabriel N. Hortobagyi, M.D.
Chief, Breast Medical Oncology, Department of Medical Oncology, M.D. Anderson Cancer Center, Texas Medical Center, Houston, Texas; Professor of Medicine, University of Texas Medical School at Houston, Houston, Texas

Mary Jane Houlihan, M.D.
Instructor in Surgery, Harvard Medical School, Boston, Massachusetts; Associate Surgeon, Beth Israel Hospital, Boston, Massachusetts

Houston Johnson, Jr., M.D.
Medical Director, Breast Care Center, Flower Hospital, Sylvania, Ohio; Clinical Associate Professor of Surgery, Toledo, Ohio

Alfred S. Ketcham, M.D.
The Sylvester Professor of Oncology, University of Miami School of Medicine, Miami, Florida; Chief, Division of Oncology, Department of Surgery, University of Miami School of Medicine, Miami, Florida

David W. Kinne, M.D.
Chief, Breast Service, Memorial Sloan-Kettering Cancer Center, New York, New York; Professor of Surgery, Cornell University Medical College, New York, New York

Charles L. Loprinzi, M.D.
Associate Professor of Oncology, Division of Medical Oncology, Mayo Medical School, Rochester, Minnesota

Alberto Luini, M.D.
Department of Surgery, Istituto Nazionale per lo Studio e la Cura dei Tumori, Via G. Venezian 1, Milano, Italy

Joel Lundy, M.D.
Professor of Surgery, State University of New York (Stonybrook); Director of Surgical Oncology, Winthrop University Hospital, Mineola, New York

William A. Maddox, M.D.
Chief, Surgical Oncology Service, Veterans Administration Hospital, Birmingham, Alabama; Clinical Professor of Surgery, University of Alabama School of Medicine, Birmingham, Alabama

Peter Maguire, M.D.
Director, CRC Psychological Medicine Group, Stanley House, Christie Hospital, Withington, Manchester, England

Richard Margolese, M.D.
Director, Department of Oncology, Jewish General Hospital, Montreal, Quebec, Canada; Herbert Black Professor of Surgery, McGill University, Montreal, Quebec, Canada

Mirella Merson, M.D.
Department of Surgery, Istituto Nazionale per lo Studio e la Cura dei Tumori, Via G. Venezian 1, Milano, Italy

Frederick L. Moffat, Jr., M.D., F.R.C.S. (C)
Assistant Professor of Surgery, University of Miami School of Medicine, Miami, Florida

C. Barber Mueller, M.D., F.A.C.S.
Professor Emeritus, Department of Surgery, McMaster University, Hamilton, Ontario, Canada

Eric Munoz, M.D., M.B.A., F.A.C.S.
Associate Professor of Surgery at University of Medicine and Dentistry of New Jersey, New Jersey Medical School, Newark, New Jersey; Medical Director and Associate Dean of Clinical Affairs, University of Medicine and Dentistry of New Jersey, University Hospital, Newark, New Jersey

Paul H. O'Brien, M.D., F.A.C.S.
Professor of Surgical Oncology, Medical University of South Carolina, Charleston, South Carolina

Claude H. Organ, Jr., M.D.
Professor of Surgery, University of California, Davis, California; Chairman, Surgery Residency Program, University of California at Davis–East Bay, Oakland, California

Benjamin Pace, M.D.
Assistant Professor of Surgery at Albert Einstein College of Medicine, Bronx, New York; Assistant Director of Surgery, Mount Sinai Services at Queens Hospital Center, Jamaica, New York

David L. Page, M.D.
Director of Anatomic Pathology, Department of Pathology, Vanderbilt University Hospital, Nashville, Tennessee; Professor of Pathology, Vanderbilt University School of Medicine, Nashville, Tennessee

William P. Peters, M.D.
Director, Bone Marrow Transplantation Program, Duke University Medical Center, Durham, North Carolina; Associate Professor of Medicine, Duke University School of Medicine, Durham, North Carolina

Benjamin F. Rush, Jr., M.D.
Distinguished Professor of Surgery at University of Medicine and Dentistry of New Jersey, New Jersey Medical School, Newark, New Jersey; Chairman, Department of Surgery, University of Medicine and Dentistry of New Jersey, New Jersey Medical School, Newark, New Jersey

Virgilio Sacchini, M.D.
Department of Surgery, Istituto Nazionale per lo Studio e la Cura dei Tumori, Via G. Venezian 1, Milano, Italy

Nigel P. M. Sacks, M.S., F.R.A.C.S.
Senior Lecturer, Department of Academic Surgery, The Royal Marsden Hospital, London, England

Gordon Francis Schwartz, M.D., M.B.A.
Professor of Surgery, Jefferson Medical College, Philadelphia, Pennsylvania; Attending Surgeon, Thomas Jefferson University Hospital, Philadelphia, Pennsylvania; Consultant Surgeon, Pennsylvania Hospital, Philadelphia, Pennsylvania; Consultant Surgeon, Chestnut Hill Hospital, Philadelphia, Pennsylvania; Consultant Surgeon, Bryn Mawr Hospital, Bryn Mawr, Pennsylvania

Stephen D. Scoggin, M.D.
Clinical Instructor, Department of Surgery, Texas A & M University Health Science Center, Temple, Texas; Chief Resident, Department of Surgery, Scott & White Memorial Hospital, Temple, Texas

Brenda Shank, M.D., Ph.D.

Chairman, Department of Radiation Oncology, Mount Sinai Hospital, New York, New York; Professor of Radiation Oncology, Mount Sinai School of Medicine, New York, New York

Henry R. Shibata, M.D.

Professor of Surgery, McGill University and Director of Surgical Oncology, Royal Victoria Hospital, Montreal, Quebec, Canada

William Silen, M.D.

Johnson & Johnson Professor of Surgery at Harvard Medical School, Boston, Massachusetts; Surgeon-in-Chief, Beth Israel Hospital, Boston, Massachusetts

Maria Soler, M.D.

3rd-year resident, Department of Surgery, University of California, Davis, East Bay, Oakland, California

Jerome A. Urban, M.D. (Deceased)

Consultant, Breast Service, Department of Surgery, Memorial Sloan-Kettering Hospital, New York, New York; Clinical Professor of Surgery, Cornell University Medical School; Attending Surgeon, Roosevelt Hospital and Doctors Hospital, New York, New York

Umberto Veronesi

Il Direttore Generale; Istituto Nazionale per lo Studio e la Cura dei Tumori, Milano, Italy

Marc M. Wallack, M.D.

Professor of Surgery, New York Medical College, Valhalla, New York; Chairman, Department of Surgery, St. Vincent's Hospital and Medical Center, New York, New York

Leslie Wise, M.D.

Chairman, Department of Surgery, The Methodist Hospital, Brooklyn, New York; Professor of Surgery, Albert Einstein College of Medicine, Bronx, New York

Charles J. Wright, M.B., M.Sc., F.R.C.S.

Vice President, Medical & Academic Affairs, Vancouver General Hospital, Bi Columbia's Health Science Center, Vancouver, British Columbia

Reinhard E. Zachrau, M.D.

Co-Director, Institute of Breast Diseases; Professor of Pathology, New York Medical College, Valhalla, New York; Attending in Pathology, Westchester County Medical Center, Valhalla, New York

Stefano Zurrida, M.D.

Department of Surgery, Istituto Nazionale per lo Studio e la Cura dei Tumori, Via G. Venezian 1, Milano, Italy

Preface

The management of breast cancer has been fairly well standardized from the 1890s to the 1940s. The method of treatment was essentially that of the Halsted type of radical mastectomy. Around the 1940s, the concept of modified radical mastectomy was introduced by Patey from London and simple mastectomy and radiotherapy was advocated by McWhirter from Edinburgh. Simultaneously, extended supraradical mastectomy was popularized by Caceres from South America and Urban from New York. Although local excision with radiotherapy was first practiced by Geoffrey Keynes in the late 1920s, this method of therapy has only been popularized in the United States during the last two decades. In spite of these variations in treatment, the overall mortality rates from breast cancer did not change. In the late 1950s, a randomized adjuvant chemotherapy trial was begun using thiotepa in the perioperative period. The survival difference between the placebo and thiotepa patients was significant only in those who were premenopausal and had more than four involved nodes. Since that period, there have been many other studies showing the potential benefit of chemotherapy, even in premenopausal and node-negative patients, involving multiple drugs with varying treatment duration.

There has been recent interest in adjuvant hormonal therapy for the treatment of potentially curable breast cancer. It has even been suggested that some of the benefits of adjuvant chemotherapy in premenopausal women are mediated through a chemically induced castration. There are some data available that strongly suggest that adjuvant tamoxifen causes a significant improvement in disease-free survival regardless of estrogen receptor and menopausal status. In spite of all these advances, however, many aspects of the biology and management of breast cancer remain controversial. It seems clear, however, that breast cancer does not spread in an orderly manner to the regional lymph nodes and from there to the blood stream. Its behavior is more dependent on complex host-tumor relationships which control the development of metastases and affect every facet of the disease. It was as early as 1953 that Black pointed out that "the clinical detection of a tumor in the breast is not synonymous with early carcinoma" and that "while some tumors may remain localized for appreciable periods of time, the majority are apparently disseminated before they are detectable."

In preparing this book, we have selected authors from multiple disciplines concerned with treating patients with breast cancer and challenged them with developing their thoughts on some of these unanswered or controversial topics. The authors were asked to use their personal experience and understanding of the literature to construct their contributions; they were also asked not to produce an all-comprehensive referenced text since there are already other works that have attempted to do this. We have requested them, however, to provide key references relevant to their thesis to allow the reader access to information supporting the writer's position. In this book, it was more important that each author create for the reader a cogent understanding of the rationale of his views and data to support the author's position rather than be encyclopedic on the topic. We think that these goals were accomplished. In many respects the management of patients with breast cancer is still controversial; consequently, we have felt that it was important to put into perspective many of the issues that have substantial elements of uncertainty.

In a work of this kind, it is sometimes helpful to have more than one individual write on a particular topic. Where this has occurred, we think that each author has presented some views that needed to be emphasized differently and the chapters are not repetitive. There are also many topics that do not lend themselves well to "pro or con," and in these cases, we have asked our contributors to critically examine the issues. We believe that this book will be of value to all practitioners who are involved in the management of patients with breast cancer.

Leslie Wise, M.D.

Houston Johnson, Jr., M.D.

Contents

III   The Role of Mammography

IV   Adjuvant Therapy For Breast Cancer

Section *I*

History and Biology

Editorial Commentary

Chapter 1

Dr. Irving Ariel has been a dominant figure in surgical oncology for over half a century. He and the late Dr. George Pack compiled one of the most comprehensive works in the management of cancer. Dr. Ariel's experience involves several decades at The Memorial Sloan-Kettering Cancer Center; he has literally lived through the evolution in the treatment of breast cancer from the advocacy of radical and supraradical mastectomies to our current views on minimal surgery as the principal way of the future. Dr. Ariel discusses the major changes in the management of breast cancer from the earliest times to the 1990s, from both a factual and a philosophical point of view, and we think that every student of breast disease will find this chapter to be informative.

Chapter 2

The late George Crile, Jr., was a major advocate of minimal surgery for breast cancer. He strongly believed that most cases of breast cancer metastasized long before the primary tumor was diagnosed. In his well-known book, *What Women Should Know About the Breast Cancer Controversy*, he emphasized the need to support women's rights to obtain all the facts and data that were available with regard to the various methods of treatment for cancer of the breast, and he believed that women should become active, informed participants with their surgeons in their choice regarding treatment. Some of Dr. Crile's views with regard to chemotherapy or hormonal therapy may well be criticized. We believe, however, that it will be of great interest for all of us to read what was probably one of the last articles of the late Dr. Crile.

Chapter 3

In this chapter, Dr. Mueller draws our attention with appropriate data to support three important conclusions. First, that for at least 30 years, following the diagnosis of palpable breast cancer, patients with stage I and stage II breast cancer die at a constant rate. These data suggest that at least for palpable tumors there is probably no real cure (i.e., complete elimination of the disease), and even if there is a cure, the cure involves only a small proportion of these patients. This of course does not mean that many of these patients are not *clinically* cured, because some of them may die from other causes. The second point Dr. Mueller brings to our attention is that the type of local therapy (i.e., lumpectomy with radiotherapy, simple mastectomy with radiotherapy, radical mastectomy, or supraradical mastectomy) does not have a significant effect on survival. And third, he suggests that node-positive tumors are fundamentally different from node-negative tumors and that node positivity implies a degree of aggressiveness of the tumor rather than being a chronological marker.

Chapter 4

We believe Dr. Mueller's follow-up to Chapter 3 is extremely significant for our understanding of the biology of breast cancer. He provides evidence against the currently accepted view that stage II breast cancer is merely a late phase of stage I breast cancer. The evidence from the NSABP B-04 trial and the Connecticut Tumor Registry are very suggestive that stage II breast cancer is not a progression of stage I breast cancer, but that it is a more severe form of breast cancer than stage I. In addition, Dr. Fox's data (JAMA 1979; 241:489) also support Dr. Mueller's thesis. He has shown that there are two subgroups of breast cancer patients: one subgroup had a yearly mortality rate of 2.5%, whereas the other had a mortality rate of 25% per year. This, Fox feels, is evidence for the existence of an entity which by histologic criteria is malignant, but is biologically relatively benign. Aggressive detection campaigns could be responsible for an increase in the diagnosis and treatment of such benign cases and so result in an apparent but not real improvement in the survival of breast cancer patients.

Chapter 5

This is a very thoughtful, if not the most thoughtful, report of the curability of breast cancer that we have seen and it emphasizes three important points. First, that lobular carcinoma in situ and ductal carcinoma in situ are not cancers with metastatic potential. Therefore, they are not true cancers but only markers of potentially developing cancers, and thus neither of them should be included in any study discussing the curability of breast cancer. The second point emphasized is that if one really looks at true cancers, the currently available data suggest that, if not all, then certainly the vast majority of them are not curable in the true sense. Although many patients may live for long periods of time and die from some other cause, patients with cancer of the breast will continue to die at a higher rate than those without cancer for an indefinite period of time. And finally, Dr. Mueller brings to our attention the fact that it has never been proven that adjuvant chemotherapy affects the curability of breast cancer, although there is evidence to suggest that it delays the mortality in 5% to 7% of women for a period of 12 to 18 months. Although a recent review of the results of 133 randomized trials (Lancet 1992; 339:71) indicated that adjuvant chemotherapy resulted in an 11% odds reduction for mortality, it has never been shown that chemotherapy affects the final mortality from breast cancer.

Chapter 6

Drs. Baum and Badwe give us a thoughtful dissertation on many aspects of the biology of breast cancer. However, they have been unable to answer the question as to whether surgery influences the natural history of breast cancer, although unquestionably surgery decreases the incidence of local disease and therefore improves the quality of life. They also reemphasize the important fact that leaving tumor behind in the axilla does not affect the survival and it is not a nidus for tertiary spread.

Chapter 7

In this chapter, Dr. David Kinne gives extensive consideration to the definitions of cure. He emphasizes the fact that although statistical cure from breast cancer may not be possible, many patients will experience a personal cure following treatment.

1

The Diagnosis and Treatment of Breast Cancer:

A Historic Review

Irving M. Ariel

Let us not cast aside things that belong to the past,
for only with the past can we weave the fabric of the future.
—Anatole France

Introduction

Cancer of the breast is as ancient as medical history can record. The two major forces that have dominated the development of treatment policies are: (1) the attitude of the women suffering from breast cancer toward their breasts, and (2) the development of medical science, spurred on by medical pioneers.

The Attitude of Women Toward Their Breasts

The attitude of women toward their breasts has been a dominant force through the ages. It determines the willingness or reluctance of women to lose their breasts and the repugnance of surgeons to do that which women accept with disdain.

The female breasts have been acclaimed universally through the centuries as symbols of beauty. In art, literature, theater, movies, television, and advertising, the female breast is glorified. These same modified sweat glands, however, are defined in a mundane manner in Gray's *Anatomy:*

From: Wise L, Johnson H Jr (eds): *Breast Cancer: Controversies in Management*. Futura Publishing Company, Inc., Armonk, NY, © 1994.

5

> The mammae secrete the milk and are the accessory glands of the generative system. . . . In the female they are two large hemispherical eminences lying within the superficial fascia and situated on the front and sides of the chest; each extends from the second rib above to the sixth rib below, and from the side of the sternum to the mid-axillary line. Their weight and dimensions differ at different periods of life and in different individuals.

These two hemispheric sacs of skin filled with adipose, glandular, and fibrous tissue, have been the objects of erotic desire by the male and the source of either self-gratification or, at times, self-loathing by the female. In *The Kinsey Report*, Dr. Kinsey observes that "American men are more aroused erotically by observing female breasts or touching them than they are by the site of, or contact with, female genitalia."

The poets, painters, and sculptors have, with artistic license, taken Gray's strict anatomical description and altered it to suit their conception of beauty. The breasts have thus been changed from organs originally designed for the benefit of the species to ones that glorify the woman. From the earliest paleolithic statues designed for fertility, breasts are portrayed as very large and filled with milk. The Cretan female statue showed huge breasts covering the entire chest, whereas early Egyptian iconography revealed the breasts to be of a virginal type, i.e., small, high, and immature. The early Greek sculptors took full artistic license and portrayed the breasts as either small and flat or huge, pendulous, and often asymmetric. Praxiteles (350 BC) apparently was one of the first to carve stone figures with graceful, somewhat voluptuous breasts, and on the Pompeian frescoes the female breasts are projected with licentious beauty.

The Breasts as the Seat of Fertility

The breasts were originally regarded by many primitive people as the "seat of fertility." Accordingly, multimammillary goddesses were created to epitomize fertility. A widespread belief prevailed that the seat of life enters the mother's body through the nipples. This led to the wearing of charms and amulets on the areola to insure a "good flowering." Spartan women wore diamonds on their breasts as a sign of strength, and metal discs over the areola to guard against the intrusion of evil spirits. A remote tribe in New Guinea still believes that conception takes place through the breasts. In early Roman mythology, when Jupiter placed Hercules to the breast of Juno, the infant suckling was so powerful that the milk gushed out, spilling into the heavens and creating the Milky Way. In fact, the Romans had breast-shaped wine cups, originally introduced by a Roman senator, and many of the Roman men had molds made of their mistresses' breasts.

In the early Greek and Hebrew history, women were modest regarding exposure of their breasts. There was no such person as a male gynecologist, and if the woman had a gynecologic or breast problem, she was examined by a female who then reported her findings to a male obstetrician.

The Chinese women in the olden days came to the doctor with an ivory doll called the "doctor's daughter." If the patient had symptoms referable to the breast, she pointed to the breast of the doll, from which the physician was to make a diagnosis.

In Afghanistan, as late as 1959, women came to the doctor's office wearing a chadeny (a form of clothing that covered the entire body except for a small part of the face), waited in the waiting room while their husband described their symptoms to the doctor in the consulting room, after which he related the proposed treatment to his wife.

Ancient Times

The breasts were held in such great esteem by the ancients that they believed that as soon as a woman became pregnant, her blood (the menses) would become muddy and turn to milk. Aristotle stated that: "The menses goes to the breasts and becomes milk." Avicenna believed that there was a direct connection between the uterus and the mammary glands, and some of the primitive people of that day forbade the woman who was suckling a baby to have sexual intercourse because they believed that the baby might imbibe sperm with the milk. The Old Testament further states that the child should suckle for about 2 years. The Law of Confucius has a 3-year time period for the suckling of an infant. These regulations had great practical significance because if the husband of a woman who was suckling her child died, she was not allowed to remarry for 24 months for fear that she might become pregnant and thereby stop the production of breast milk. The Old Testament further prohibits a widow from remarrying until 24 months have elapsed even if her suckling baby has died, because at one time a woman had killed her baby in order to be able to remarry.

Even in those days there existed women in whom the suckling of their own children would have been considered to be "denigration" of their position. It was believed that these women had totally disregarded the natural feelings of the mother's heart. As the Talmud states, "More than the calf wishes to suck does the cow desire to suckle" (*Genesis* 49:25). The mother who refuses her suckling breast to her babe—even if she is near death from hunger—is considered cruel and guilty of a heinous act. Wet nurses existed for some of the women in royal families who did not want to nurse or who were incapable of nursing (thus Rebecca had a wet nurse named Deborah). If a woman nursed a baby in public it was cause for divorce.

There is no mention in the Old Testament of babies suckling from bottles, although it is highly probable that they suckled from other animals' nipples if the mother could not produce milk. In ancient Roman mythology, the fable of Romulus and Remus, who were suckled by a she-wolf, and in Greek mythology the story of the goat of Amalthea, who was the wet nurse of Zeus, reflect the practice of nursing from animals.

The Influence of Fashion

Gradually, fashion dictated the appearance of the breasts as women discovered the powers of these organs. Accordingly, fashion has decreed that they become compressed, flattened, stretched, pointed upward or downward, or enlarged. As early as 3000 BC, primitive brassieres and corsets were in vogue among Minoans to emphasize the bosom and diminish the waist. Cretan women totally exposed their breasts and emphasized them with tight waistbands. The Greeks also used such devices to lift the breasts. Sacks, a modern psychologist, describes the supporting bandeau worn beneath the breasts by the Greeks (800 BC) as a more extensive combination of bands and cords which presaged the modern corselet. The nipples of the partially exposed breasts of Roman, Egyptian, and Minoan women were rouged and gilded. Corsets were introduced in the 13th century to raise and accentuate the breasts. By the 15th century, the breasts of growing girls were supported by heavy metallic plates. This unnatural practice persisted among such widely separated people as the Bavarians, the Cherokees, and various tribes in and around the Caucasus. Because of the almost total mutilation caused by these heavy bodices, lactation became virtually nonexistent.

By the 16th century, various types of corsets and bodices became prominent. A double standard existed for breasts during the Elizabethan period. The partly exposed breasts became a sign of virginity, while a concealing bodice symbolized a married woman. A gentleman, when he met a single girl, would greet her with a gentle pinch of her breast with his thumb and forefinger. After the French Revolution, a lowering of décolletage with transparent gowns, which were sometimes dampened to cling more tightly to the body and reveal rouged nipples, became prominent. The partial to complete exposure of the breast continued until the Victorian Age, which ushered in a new era of concealment that prevailed. In 1845, Sir Astley Cooper, the famous English surgeon, described the breasts as follows:

> The breasts, from their prominence, their roundness, the white color of their skin, and the red color of the nipples, by which they are surmounted, add great beauty to the female form. For prior to the age of puberty, the boy and the girl differ but little in the shape of the chest or in general appearance, but as the breast develops, the female figure is established in all its elegance.

During the Roaring Twenties, the female breast again became a less prominent force. Since women were engaging in masculine activities, including boyish clothing and the vote, the flat chest became stylish, often requiring strapping and binding of the breasts. Attention was focused away from the breasts to the lower parts of the body as evidenced by short skirts with many frills. Flat chestedness was soon passed over and the full breast became again prominent in the 1940s and exists today.

Today, the entertainment world and the advertising media have focused so much attention upon the breasts that every young girl is conscious of her breasts.

The 37-inch breast of Venus de Milo, long considered the ideal, has been topped by the 40-inch American breast. Some women, in an effort to be prominently endowed, have resorted to "falsies," of which eight million pairs are sold per year.

Breast Mutilation

In many of the early Christian sculptors' works, the breasts were shown to be mutilated by animals devouring them; this was common in French ecclesiastical architecture. French sculptors, dating from the 11th century, depict women guilty of the sin of lewdness, writhing in anguish while serpents, toads, and dragons "gnawed away at their breasts."

Another cause for mutilation of the breasts was necessity. Among the Basuto women, the breasts were manually elongated in order to enable working mothers who carried their infants on their backs to be able to nurse without interruption of their tasks.

The Code of Hammurabi (1950 BC), the first code to govern the practice of medicine in ancient Babylon, contained 282 clauses, and clause #194 referred to breast mutilation as a form of punishment. Because of the importance of the breast to women in India, punishment for adultery was amputation of the breasts.

The Greek historian Herodotus mentioned one warrior tribe beyond Scythian country that practiced breast amputation on all its female prisoners.

Removal of the breasts by the Amazons is referred to by many authors including Virgil, Ptolemy, and Hippocrates who stated:

> They have no right breast, for, while still at a tender age, their
> mothers heat strongly a copper instrument constructed for this
> very purpose and apply it to the right breast which is burnt off.

Breast amputation as a form of malicious punishment is depicted by several artists in their portrayals of the martyrdom of Saint Agatha, who is considered the saint of breasts. The Sicilian governor Quintianus fell madly in love with Agatha who was born of a noble family in the 3rd century, and he did his best to seduce her. She spurned his attention, and he then ordered her to the House of Aphrodisia to observe her possible future if she continued to reject him. After a month in that brothel, she still refused to accept his advances. He then ordered that she be bound to a pillar where her breasts would be torn off with iron shears. Myths had it that following the amputation of the breasts, she had such healing powers that they regrew in 4 days. Several other sufferers from breast mutilation listed in the Litany of the Saints were Saints Barbara, Foya, Apollina, and Christina. Schechter, after studying paintings of the tortured saints, came to the conclusion that the instruments used to "cut off" the breasts for penal reasons (2250 BC) were used as models for the development of instruments used in the treatment of breast diseases, including cancer, in the 16th and 17th centuries. Konig, a famous German surgeon, wrote in 1893:

> Before me I have fifteen . . . preserved breasts of women from the
> past ten years. Most of them were taken from women who feared
> they had carcinoma. These women failed to calm down even after
> they had been told that their breasts were not cancerous but due
> to an infection (mastitis). . . .

In these instances the women feared cancer more than they wanted to preserve their breasts, and were subjected to mastectomy at their insistence. The situation has now changed in that many women believe their breasts can be preserved in the presence of mammary cancer. Their attitude, plus certain developments in medical circles, have influenced physicians to seek a means of curing the patient of her cancer and preserving the afflicted breast.

The Development of Medical Science in The Treatment of Breast Cancer

Breast cancer in the female is a ubiquitous disease that has been present from time immemorial and has killed many women all over the world. Generations of surgeons have boldly attempted every conceivable method of combating the disease, and through the ages there has been a gradual evolution in both the understanding of this form of cancer and the methods to aid in the attack upon it.

Cancer, as such, has been with us from prehistoric times. Preserved relics, ancient bones, and paleopathological remnants reveal cancer to be worldwide and to afflict all life, both plant and animal. Dinosaurs of the Mesozoic period have shown signs of cancer in the bones. Cancer is found in such ancient treasures as mummies from the Egyptian pyramids and the Etruscan tombs. A historic review of this disease and methods to control it will help us to understand better the enigma that confronts us today regarding the best treatment of breast cancer, as well as help us prevent mistakes made in the past.

Ancient History

The Edwin Smith Surgical Papyrus

The very earliest medical record regarding medical history is the ancient Edwin Smith Surgical Papyrus, originally written during the Egyptian Pyramid Age (3000–2500 BC). Although we do not know who is the author, it is believed to represent teachings of the oldest known physician, Imhotep. J.H. Breasted, the late director of the Oriental Institute of the University of Chicago, who translated and made commentaries on this papyrus, stated that the papyrus describes eight cases concerned with tumors of the breast:

> If you examine a man having bulging tumors on his breast, and
> you find that they have spread over his breast; and you place your

> hand upon his breast tumors and you find them to be cool, there
> being no fever at all therein when your hand feels him; they have
> no granulations, contain no fluid, give rise to no liquid discharge,
> yet they feel protuberant to your touch, you should say concern-
> ing him: this is a case of bulging tumors I have to contend with.

As for treatment of these bulging tumors, a simple statement was made: "There is no treatment." These hard, cool tumors are thus separated from the inflammatory diseases or abscesses of the breast. Cauterization or "fire drill" was used for abscesses, and no treatment whatsoever was advocated for the cancers. Does this not sound similar to the teachings of some of today's surgeons regarding the treatment of primary tumor, which is a nihilistic approach?

The Ebers papyrus gives a great deal of insight regarding the status of the surgeon at that time. A surgeon had to make one of three decisions on seeing a patient. He could say, "I can cure this patient," and thereby he made a contract to do so. He could say, "I cannot cure this ailment," and he then had to refuse to treat it at all because no allowances were made for therapeutic results short of cure. Or he could say, "I must observe longer before I know whether I can cure." These notations gave rise to the Code of Hammurabi (1950 BC) regarding medical ethics.

We learn from the Code of Hammurabi that the medical profession in Babylon had advanced far enough in public esteem to be rewarded with adequate fees, carefully described and regulated by law. Thus, 10 shekels in silver was the statutory fee for treating a wound or a tumor, or opening an abscess of the eye with a bronze lancet, if the patient happened to be a gentleman. For a poor man or a servant, the fee was 5 or 2 shekels, respectively. If the doctor caused the patient to lose his life or his eyes, he had his hands cut off, in the case of the gentleman, or had to render a value for a value in the case of a slave. Their fees were relatively high when one considers that yearly rent was 5 shekels for a middle-class dwelling, or 1/50 of a shekel for daily pay for an ordinary craftsman. Modern malpractice seems mild in comparison to those days.

The Greek historian Herodotus who lived just prior to Hippocrates, relates a story of Princess Atossa, who had a tumor of her breast which, after a time, ulcerated and spread. False modesty prevented her from complaining about this tumor while it was small. But when it grew larger and gave trouble, she sent for the famous physician Democedes (525 BC), and he cured her from the disease from which she suffered. The type of treatment is not mentioned. The fact that she was cured is presumptive evidence that she did not have cancer. The case does demonstrate the vanity of women regarding their breasts, even during this very early period.

We now jump ahead to the famous physician Hippocrates (400 BC), the father of medicine. All physicians today take an oath regarding their duties as physicians, "The Hippocratic Oath." Hippocrates made little mention of breast cancer. He did state that it was better to give no treatment for deep-seated cancers because treatment accelerated the dying process, but if one omitted treatment, one might prolong life. The average life span at the time of Christ was about 18 years, hence it is not surprising that breast cancer is mentioned so infrequently. Hippocrates established three precepts, namely, those diseases that are curable by medicine are best; those that are not curable by medicine are curable by the knife, and those that are not curable by the knife are curable by fire. Those that fire cannot cure are incurable. It is doubtful that he ever recommended surgery for breast cancer.

The Early Christian Era

A great scholar who lived between 30 BC and 38 AD was Aulus Cornelius Celsus. Although not a doctor, he wrote extensively on agriculture, common medicine, military science, law, and philosophy. He divided the Greek practitioners into three groups: those who attempted to cure by diet (the dietitians), those who employed medicaments (the pharmaceutists), and those who resorted to manipulations (the chirurgeons). Celsus had specific recommendations for the treatment of breast cancer. He was opposed to surgery and cautery for advanced cancer and recommended local application of caustics. If improvement occurred, one could proceed to surgery or cautery. If the disease worsened, one should conclude that it is a cancer and withhold treatment so as not to hasten the demise of the patient. He established the first classification of breast cancer. The early surgically curable pre-cancers were classified as the *cacoethes*. "First there is the cacoethes, then carcinoma without ulceration, then the fungating ulcer."

Medical treatment consisted of venesection and purgatives. Local treatment consisted of applications of the juice of strichnos for the early cancers:

> None of these can be removed but the cacoethes; the rest are irritated by every method of cure. The more violent the operations the more angry they grow. Some use caustics, some burning irons, others remove the growth with the scalpel. After excision, even though a cicatrix is formed, it recurs, bringing with it the cause of death, whereas at the same time, most people, by using no violent methods to attempt the extirpation of the disease but only applying mild medications to soothe it, protract their lives, notwithstanding the disorder, to an extreme old age.

We next jump ahead about 200 years to Galen of Pergamum (131–203 AD), who was probably responsible for the first surgical treatment of breast cancer and coined the term "crab" to describe cancer:

> Just as a crab has legs on both sides of his body, so in this disease the veins extending out from the unnatural growth take the shape of crab's legs.

He further goes on to say:

> We have often cured this disease in the early stages, but after it has grown to a noticeable size no one has cured it with surgery. In

> all surgery we attempt to excise a pathologic tumor in a circle in
> the region where it borders on the healing tissue.

Ligatures, used today to tie blood vessels, were frowned upon in Galen's day for it was believed that they caused extension of the cancer. Galen introduced the concept of "humors" being responsible for cancer, a theory that dominated medicine for over 1,000 years. Cancer was due to an excess of black bile (humor). Shortly after this time (372 AD), the Roman Empire had fallen, the Barbarians had invaded Europe, and the Byzantine Empire was at its height (550 AD). Aetius of Ameda lived in the 6th century and was physician to the Byzantine Emperor Justinian. He described local excision of the cancer followed by cautery and stated: "The first burns are for the sake of bleeding and the last for the intention of eradicating the disease." Although most of the doctors of the time adhered to a nihilistic attitude toward cancer, Leonides, in Egypt, performed courageous surgery, being careful not to operate on advanced cases. He was the first to describe nipple retraction as a clinical sign of breast cancer.

Paulus Aegineta, a 7th-century Greek surgeon, agreed with the principle of Galen that disease was caused by humors. He believed that cancers were formed from black bile and

> . . . if overheated it is attended with ulceration, and owing to the
> thickness of the humor, cancer of the breast is an incurable
> disease, for it can neither be repelled nor discussed; not yielding
> to purging of the whole body, resisting the milder applications
> and being exasperated by the stronger ones. The only chance for
> a radical cure consisted in making a complete excision of the part.

Rhazes (841–926 AD), a great Arabic physician, warned that those who incise a breast cancer would merely produce an ulceration, and that only if the breast could be completely removed and the parts burned, should an excision be done. If ulceration had taken place, he approved of using cooling applications.

Haly Ben-Abbas, a Persian who died in 994 AD, recommended excision of the breast, allowing bleeding to rid the body of melancholic humors. He disapproved of tying arteries. It is assumed he used pressure for hemostasis.

Albucasis, during the first half of the 11th century, concerning breast cancer stated: "As for me, I have never been able to cure a case nor have I known one who has." Lanfrank (1300) is considered the father of French surgery and was still using the method of Leonides despite the lapse of more than 1,000 years.

Guy de Chaulaac, a 14th-century surgeon and the patron saint of the American College of Surgeons, recommended conservative treatment primarily, but he stated that if one could excise the entire mass, surgery might be done. He devised various unique instruments for the rapid amputation of the breast, designed after instruments used for mutilation.

A unique practice was performed by the Spanish surgeon Francisco Arceo (1493–1571). He divided the cancerous breast lengthwise and dissolved the tumor by means of a ligature. Fuchs (1501–1566), a German, compressed cancers of the breast by means of a lead plate.

The Influence of Religion and Mysticism

Religion played a role, and after the Council of Tours in 1162, religious fervor frowned on surgery and put a ban on the barbarous practice of surgery for breast cancer. This ban on surgery lasted well into the 15th century. It was believed that faith could cure.

The practice of exorcism dates back to time immemorial, as does the laying on of hands and other mystic practices. William Clowes (1516–1584), physician to Queen Elizabeth, practiced exorcism for breast cancer. The simple ritual of laying on of royal hands was the Queen's couterpart of curing the King's evil. The "royal touch" was said to have originated with Edward the Confessor, but served several of his successors who were somewhat skeptical of their own divine power of faith healing. William III possessed no self-delusion when he told his ailing subjects, "May God give you better health and better sense." When he discontinued the practice, he was accused of cruelty. Queen Elizabeth had a blessed ring that she wore suspended between her breasts. The ring had the virtue of expelling infected air and preventing disease. Similar amulets of asafedita were worn until recently as protection against occult or evil influences, including breast cancer.

An important contributor to the development of the treatment of breast cancer was Ambrose Paré (1510–1590), a French surgeon who stated: "If the cancer was small, nonulcerated, and situated in a region where it could be easily removed, the tumor should be excised, but one should go well beyond its boundaries." Large and ulcerated lesions were treated with sweet milk, vinegar, and ointments. Paré called attention to the fact that the primary breast cancer and the axillary extension of the breast were related. This was the first time that the spread of cancer to regional sites was described. It would dictate methods of treatment until today. Its significance from a prognostic standpoint is currently being debated vociferously, 450 years after the relationship was recognized.

The Age of Anatomy

Vaselius (1514–1564) was one of the first who vigorously opposed Galen's doctrines of humors and discarded the old anatomy. His anatomy book, published in 1543, marks the beginning of modern anatomy. Vaselius treated cancer by wide surgical excision, and controlled bleeding by means of ligatures. Previous to Vaselius' description of anatomy, there was no way of understanding the manner of the spread of cancer. His description of the anatomy of the breast paved the way for future surgical techniques aimed at eradicating breast cancer.

Informed Consent

Fabricius Ab Aquapendente (1537–1619), teacher of William Harvey, who was the first to describe the circulation of blood, performed radical surgery for cancer only at the patient's request, and decried partial excision as worthless. This is an example of the role of the patient with cancer being involved in the decision-making of her treatment practices.

Nicholaes Tulp (1594–1674), a Dutch anatomist who commissioned Rembrandt to paint the now famous "Anatomy Lesson," showing Dr. Tulp doing an anatomy demonstration, believed that breast cancer was contagious and described a case in which the disease was passed presumably from his mistress to her servant girl. History has proved that cancer is not an infection by bacteria. Whether viruses play a role has not been determined to date.

Scultetus (1595–1645), a Greek, described the operation in which heavy ligatures were passed through the breast, traction was then applied as the breast was rapidly amputated, and bleeding from the operative area was quickly scarred with a hot iron.

The Renaissance

Henry LeDran (1684–1770), a French surgeon, once and for all put to sleep Galen's humoral theory which had dominated all medical thinking for over 1,500 years. He stressed the fact that cancer was a local lesion in its earlier stages and spread by way of lymphatics. This was not universally accepted, as the prevailing thought was that breast cancer was a systemic disease and the lesion of the breast was but a local expression of the constitutional malady. LeDran stressed early treatment, which consisted of local excision with lymph node dissection. He called attention to the fact that hope for cure was decidedly less when the axillary nodes were involved.

Jean Louis Petit (1674–1750), another Frenchman, believed in wide surgical excision and stated that although the breast tumor should be carefully avoided during the operation, as little skin as possible was to be removed, with preservation of the nipple. He is noted for his wide excision, careful removal of the axillary nodes, and appreciation of dissection in continuity,at a time when major surgical procedures so often resulted in widespread infection and death. He further called attention to evaluating the pectoralis major muscle at a time before microscopic examination became available. Whether or not the pectoralis should be removed became a bone of contention.

Gloom and Pessimism Regarding Breast Cancer

The latter part of the 19th century and the first half of the 20th century are characterized by pessimism and gloom regarding breast cancer. Alexander Monro (1773–1859), of England, stated that of 60 cases treated, only four were free of disease at the end of 2 years. The unscientific approach is emphasized by Velpeau, a Frenchman, in a lecture he presented before the Syddenham Society in 1856. Among the various methods used for treating breast cancer by internal measures, largely influenced by Galen's teachings of the humors, were the use of repeated bleedings, leeches, purgatives, and emetics. There were various drugs used to accomplish the destruction of the humors. These included, as outlined by Velpeau, hemlock, iron, arsenic, mercury solutions, and alkaline substances including the water from Vichy. Regarding surgery he stated:

> To destroy a cancerous tumor by surgical means is usually an easy
> matter and but little dangerous in itself; but the question arises,
> whether such a procedure affords a chance of radically curing the
> patient. This proposition remains undecided.

He continued: "The disease always returns after removal, and operation only accelerates its growth and fatal termination."

The pessimism is reflected by others of that time. Mayo spoke of 95 cases of recurrences in 100 operations, and MacFarlane did not know of a single positive cure after performing 118 operations.

James Syme (1799–1870), a Scotsman, condemned the practice of palliative procedures including purging, bleeding, the application of ointments, and limited surgery in the treatment of cancer. He stated: "The only proceeding that deserves at all to be considered a remedy for cancer is removal of the morbid structure."

It is to be recalled that all of this was done without the availability of microscopic anatomy. Further, all surgery was performed without anesthesia. (Nitrous oxide was described in 1842 and ether was first demonstrated in 1846.) Local anesthesia (cocaine) was first described in 1884. Halsted, a surgeon at the Johns Hopkins Medical School in Baltimore, who first described the radical mastectomy, became addicted to cocaine while researching the drug upon himself.

Surgery at the time was performed without a knowledge of sepsis and was often complicated by local and systemic infection. Louis Pasteur advocated heat to destroy bacteria, and Joseph Lister, in 1867, advocated carbolic acid spray to prevent infection. Not everyone accepted the theory and practice of preventing infection. Samuel Gross, a great surgeon of that time in Philadelphia, stated: "Little if any faith is placed by an enlightened or experienced surgeon on this side of the Atlantic in the so-called carbolic acid treatment of Professor Lister."

Halsted was the first surgeon to use gloves in the operating room. He was also the first to describe the use of gloves by a nurse in the operating room. Transfusions were delayed until 1901, when Landsteiner described the different types of blood so necessary for compatible transfusions to be given. Is it any wonder that surgeons of the time were limited in their surgical attack on breast cancer?

Schleiden (1838), a German, was among the first to appreciate the significance of the cell as a unit in plant structure, and Virchow, another German, considered to be the father of pathology, epitomized the matter by saying: "Omnis cellula e cellula." He advanced the concept that any normal cell can become a cancer cell as a result of irritation.

Sir James Paget (1814–1899), without the availability of anesthesia or asepsis, stated: "We have to ask ourselves whether it is probable that the operation will add to the length or comfort of life enough to justify incurring the risk of its own consequences." He had an operative mortality rate of 10% in 235 cases of breast cancer. He believed the disease to be hopeless and stated:

> In deciding for or against removal of the cancerous breast, in any single case, we may, I think, dismiss all hope that the operation will be a final remedy for the disease. I would not say that such a thing is impossible; but it is so highly improbable that a hope of its occurring in any single case cannot be reasonably entertained.

This pessimistic attitude was also voiced by Robert Liston (1794–1847): "No one can now be found so rash or so cruel as to attempt the removal of the glands thus affected whether primary or secondary."

In this pessimistic atmosphere, Velpeau (1856) favored thorough excision in preference to complete amputation. He stated:

> If the disease requires, the pectoralis muscle should not arrest us. The smallest shade of the disease must be taken away, if we are determined not to lose any chance of success. However, should there appear to be any necessity of interfering with the bones or resecting the ribs we must not deceive ourselves. The return of the disease is then inevitable and it would have been better not to have undertaken the operation at all.

His basic operation consisted of complete excision of the tumor with its overlying skin, with preservation of the nipple when possible, and only in certain cases amputation of the entire breast.

Hayes Agnew (1818–1892), of the United States, resorted to surgery solely for its moral effect. He believed that surgery actually shortened the life of the patient. He was most pessimistic and stated: "I do not despair of carcinoma being cured somewhere in the future, but this blessed achievement will, I believe, never be wrought by the knife of the surgeon."

The Lymphatic Spread of Cancer

The intellectual basis for the modern mastectomy operation depends upon an understanding of the lymphatic spread of cancer. Aselius (1627) was the first to demonstrate lacteals, which he found in a recently fed dog. Mascagni (1787) and Sappey (1885), using mercury injections, clearly outlined the lymphatics of the breast. Heidenhain (1888) demonstrated microscopically that delicate extensions of breast parenchyma follow the pectoral fascia down into the muscle and that foci of carcinoma are often found in the same deep plane within the lymphatics. It was an anatomical concept based on the belief that the extent of the mastectomy operation must be such as to prevent recurrence. He suspected that such an operation would have to include excision of part of the pectoralis major muscle. He stated that the pectoralis was involved in most cancers and should be excised. Previously, in 1869, Richard Sweeting, from England, advocated complete removal of the pectoralis major muscle. He espoused it as a routine part of the mastectomy.

The attitude toward the surgical treatment of breast cancer at the time is exemplified by the practices of three surgeons from Jefferson Medical School in Philadelphia. Pancoast (1805–1882) emphasized the importance of excising the axillary nodes with the breast in continuity. Previously, a large amount of skin was excised and the wound left open to granulate until it healed. Pancoast's successor was Samuel D. Gross (1859), who advocated amputation of the breast but who sacrificed thoroughness for conservation of the skin and preservation of the axilla. His distinguished son, Samuel W. Gross, wrote a classic book in 1880, *Tumors of the Mammary Gland,* in which he advocated amputation of the breast and the axillary nodes in continuity with excision of the pectoral fascia. He believed that breast cancer could be cured "before it has disseminated itself extensively locally or has tainted the general system."

Charles H. Moore of England, in 1867, acknowledged that surgery was being performed earlier than before but asserted that it was not nearly so radical as required. A century before, wide excision was the rule, but now the skin, undermined by dissection and after removal of the tumor, was reapplied. At times even the nipple and areola were preserved. Moore espoused the following major points: (1) during the operation the tumor should not be cut into, nor even seen; (2) recurrence was determined by centrifugal dispersion from the primary site and not by any independent organic origin; (3) the entire mammary gland must be removed; (4) the removal of the breast is most likely to be incomplete at the sternal margin; (5) unsound tissue adjacent to the lesion, such as skin, ought to be removed in continuity with the whole; the skin and the nipple should be removed or the results may be disastrous. He did not remove the pectoral muscles. Three years later, Lister described his technique of dividing but not removing the pectoral muscles. In 1877, Banks wrote regarding the axillary lymph nodes: "As you cannot tell whether the glands are affected or not till you see them in your hand, let them be always removed and so increase the patient's chances of future immunity." Through the ages one can trace a constant ongoing extension of the surgical treatment of breast cancer as new techniques were developed. These techniques included: (1) safer surgery with the understanding of the anatomy and control of infection and transfusions; (2) the development of anesthesia; (3) a better understanding of the biology of cancer, especially that cancer starts as a single entity and spreads by direct extension, lymphatic spread, and vascular dissemination.

No Treatment At All

No treatment at all was the approach of the first records of breast cancer in the world history. Some form of treatment must have been tried and found unsuccessful because it is unlikely that no attempt at treatment would ever have been made. In the 1500s, Ambrose Paré advised wide excision, but if the cancers were large, advanced, and ulcerated, he advised no surgery but only treatment with sweet milk, vinegar, and ointment. Robert Liston (1794–1847), in England, advised against surgery if the axillary nodes were involved. The extension to the nodes was considered a contraindication for the operation. Much confusion existed regarding the origin of cancer. Was it related to the humors of Galen? Was it a manifestation of a constitutional disease, an infection, or a parasite? Could it be transmitted?

Keen, in 1894, made the following statement:

> There is no question at all in the present day that cancer is of local origin. In my earlier professional life, it was one of the disputed points constantly coming up in medical society as to whether it was local or from the first a constitutional disease, and if the latter, it was said that no good could come from operating upon the breast. But this question of local origin is no longer confronting us. It is a thing settled. And women must be taught that this brings help to them. Don't wait, I beg of you, gentlemen and ladies, don't wait for that old classic symptom, retraction of the nipple, for in nearly one half of the cases it will not exist. I take no account of it. I make an incision into the tumor, and if it is malignant or suspicious, I amputate the entire breast.

The same problem exists today regarding the treatment of the locoregional cancer, but for an entirely different reason. Instead of believing that the cancer is a local manifestation of a systemic disease, some claim that when the patient is seen by the doctor, although the disease began locally it has already disseminated and local control is meaningless.

The Axillary Nodes

The axillary nodes have always posed a problem regarding treatment. Cervinius (1580) was one of the first to call attention to them and to remove them. It is unlikely that any of the previous surgeons tackled the nodes. Aetus (1542) first mentioned axillary swelling, which may have represented metastases. Henry LeDran (1685–1770), a Frenchman, stressed the need for early surgery and was the first to remove the axillary lymph nodes routinely. It took this period of time in order to repudiate Galen's humors. LeDran stressed the fact that cancer was a local lesion when early and spread by way of the lymphatics. He was the one who stressed a poor prognosis if the axillary nodes were involved. Benjamin Bell (1749–1886), a Scotsman, stated that the small cancers should be treated by total mastectomy and axillary dissection.

Bryant (1887) stated:

> When a cancer or carcinomatous growth ceases to be a local disease, it spreads by three methods: by continuous or local infection, by lymphatic infection, or by secondary vascular infection. One form may be more marked than another or all forms may coexist together.

Charles Moore (1867), an Englishman, was the one who advised amputation of the breast with axillary dissection in continuity. Samuel D. Gross advocated amputation of the breast but sacrificed thoroughness by preserving the skin and the axilla. His son, Samuel W. Gross, corrected the omissions of his father and brought to America the Moore operation. The great German surgeons, Volkman, Billroth, and Heidenhain, advised routine removal of the lymph nodes in the late 1800s.

The Skin

Until the mid-1700s, a large mass of skin was usually removed. However, Benjamin Bell was one of the first to state that unless the cancer had invaded the skin, thin skin flaps could be developed and thus facilitate closure, which is the technique followed today. The question of skin flaps has been debated for many years. Some, such as Haagensen, advise very thin skin flaps; others say it does not matter. But at present, the development of skin flaps is mandatory in order to facilitate closure and as a precursor for adequate cosmetic reconstructive surgery at a later date.

Wide Excision or Amputation

The question of whether a wide excision or an amputation of the breast should be performed has dominated surgical thought throughout the ages. Aetus, Guy de Chaulaac, Ambrose Paré, Vaselius, and Velpeau advocated a wide excision, whereas Leonides, Aquapendente, Scaltetus, Bell, and, of course, the surgeons of the later 19th century, all advised amputation, even for the smallest cancer. It is doubtful, however, that they ever saw a small cancer inasmuch as the combination of modesty of the women and ignorance of the profession usually caused the cancers to become rather large and widespread before attempts at their eradication were made.

The Pectoralis Muscle

The pectoralis muscle is now receiving a great deal of attention, with the frequent performance of the modified radical mastectomy in order to preserve the form and function of the patient. There have been arguments both for and against its removal throughout the ages. Even when an amputation was done in those early days, the pectoral muscle was not removed. Jean Louis Petit (1674–1750) removed the pectoral fascia and some of the fibers if they were involved. He believed that the roots of the cancer were the enlarged lymph nodes and removed them. He preserved the skin and sutured it to prevent hemorrhage. The earlier surgeons left the wound open. Concerned with aesthetics, Petit preserved the nipple.

At first, only the fascia was removed, but gradually more and more of the muscles were resected. Samuel D. Gross removed only the fascia; Volkman, in

1875, carried the incision down to the pectoral muscle: "Carrying the knife parallel with the fibers of the muscle and penetrating into their interstices, the pectoral fascia is thus entirely removed." He stated that he adopted this procedure because on microscopic examination he found the fascia "carcinomatous" where he least expected it. He described the resection of the pectoralis major muscle and, at times, the pectoralis minor in 38 patients with far advanced cases, with a 3-year survival rate of 14%.

Heidenheim (1889) stated that "a tumor, however freely moveable on the underlying parts, has almost certainly advanced as far as the surface of the muscle." He believed that cancer cells were propagated through the lymphatics by muscular action. He described 18 cases examined microscopically in which the superficial layer of the pectoralis major was involved. Bryant (1887) stated: "When the pectoral muscle is infiltrated, it must be freely excised."

The Radical Mastectomy

Degenshein and Caccarelli give credit to a Frenchman, Bartoleny Cabrol, who in 1590 performed the first radical mastectomy, similar to how it is done today (with the excision of the pectoral muscle). Charles Hewlitt Moore, in 1867, presented a paper on "The Influence of Inadequate Operations on the Theory of Cancer," in which he actually described the radical mastectomy. He thus championed a new cause in the relatively futile era of surgery of the breast. Three years later, Lister supported and extended Moore's teachings. He cut the pectoralis muscle to expose the axilla and performed a meticulous axillary dissection. His aseptic technique, using carbolic spray, probably played a major role in the outcome of his patients. The availability of the microscope caused Speese, who studied the involvement of the muscle in 100 consecutive operative cases and found involvement of the muscle in 25 of those cases and in the fascia in 18 cases, to advocate its routine removal.

The stage was thus set for William Halsted (1852–1923), at the Johns Hopkins Hospital, to construct out of this sizeable background of details a practical solution to the problem, and in 1894 he published his paper on the classic radical mastectomy as we know it today.

Ten days after Halsted's paper was published, Willy Meyer presented before the New York Academy of Medicine a similar operation in which he transected the pectoralis minor muscle, thus making the radical mastectomy complete.

Thus the development of the radical mastectomy was a laborious and tedious process that actually began with Petit in 1739 (although occasionally it had been performed earlier, as early as 1590) and ended with Halsted in 1894.

> The story is not one of ordinary progression, but fraught with retrogressions that are prominent even today. The horror of sepsis, the need for anesthesia, and the wide acceptance of the incurability of cancer were prominent in delaying the development of surgery of the breast.

An Englishman conceived the operation (Charles H. Moore), the Germans began to practice the operation as conceived by Moore (Volkman, Billroth, Heidenheim), and two Americans independently implemented the completed procedure (Halsted and Meyer).

Since the advent of the radical mastectomy, the operation has been extended in every direction. It has been extended proximally to include the neck dissection, associated with the radical mastectomy by Dahl Iverson, et al., with no improved survival rate. It has been extended to include the internal mammary nodes. Wangensteen extended it to remove the entire chest plastron with a dissection of the mediastinal lymph nodes, and Prudente extended it to combine an interscapulo-mammothoracic amputation in selected situations.

Now, 100 years after the development of the radical mastectomy, many are advocating less and less surgery, in a 180-degree turnabout to performing surgical procedures practiced many years ago. Lewison labels it an example of an historic piroutte. Is the change warranted?

Development of Radiation Therapy for Breast Cancer

Irradiation, using orthovoltage generators (250 kV) as the sole means of treating breast cancer, had been tried, but the results in the past had been poor. Microscopic studies of the irradiated tissues did not reveal any changes from orthovoltage radiation therapy in four-fifths of the cases, and cancer-bearing lymph nodes seemed unaffected by the irradiation. Preoperative irradiation had been largely abandoned, but it is now receiving a resurgence. Simple mastectomy, or lumpectomy, with postoperative irradiation is being strongly advocated, using supervoltage irradiation and/or interstitial irradiation. Grace, from the United States, treated 40 patients by simple mastectomy with postoperative orthovoltage irradiation and reported a 44% 5-year "cure." McWhirter, after simple mastectomy and postoperative orthovoltage radiation therapy, reported a 42% 5-year survival and a 25% 10-year survival for 1,345 patients treated between 1941 and 1962. Modern radiation equipment and more reliable methods of radiation techniques are largely responsible for the increased use of radiation therapy and the improved results.

The advent of supervoltage X-ray therapy was first inaugurated in 1932. In 1935, Stone, Livingston, Sloane, and Chaffe built a million-volt generator, and reports regarding its initial use were encouraging. In 1941, Kerst built the first betatron, which generated 20 million electron volts and was utilized by Roger Harvey in the treatment of cancer. Ernest Orlando Lawrence built the first cyclotron in 1932, which contributed greatly to the development of radioactive isotopes. Two of these isotopes, cobalt-60 and radioactive cesium, are used for supervoltage therapy. Now, over 50 years since the supervoltage treatment units were first described, there are observations that better results for breast cancer are being obtained. Most of the results presented have a relatively short-term follow-up, with only a few 10-year follow-up studies. If continued good results are obtained for prolonged periods, mastectomy (both simple and radical) may be abandoned.

Cancer Chemotherapy

Every form of chemical measure for treating cancer has been attempted, from the earliest times until the present. Some of these measures include purgatives, blood letting, weird diets, reptile venom, heavy metals, and thousands of others. It is lamentable that certain charlatans, both in and out of the medical profession, still practice some of these measures, thereby depriving patients of methods which can be curative. Paul Ehrlich (1854–1950) coined the term cancer chemotherapy after his brilliant discovery of arsphenamine for the treatment of syphilis. He started research in cancer, which he soon abandoned, stating: "Cancer is abnormal life and nothing will be discovered about cancer until something is learned about life itself."

Some of the earliest chemicals used were arsenic as administered in Fowler's solution, stilbamidine, and urethane. The advent of modern chemotherapy occurred on June 12, 1917, when the Germans bombed the British during World War I with sulfur mustard. In addition to other symptoms, leukopenia, due to bone marrow depression, was described by Krumbhaars in 1919. After one of our liberty ships, during World War II, was hit by a bomb in the Italian harbor of Barato and leukopenia occurred in the survivors, Gilman and Philips started using nitrogen mustard for the treatment of cancer of the lymphoid system. Sidney Farber, pathologist at Harvard, developed rectal cancer and gave up formal pathology. In 1948 he introduced an antifolic agent, aminopterin, which then gave rise to the current drug methotrexate (N Engl J Med 238; 787–793,1948). Heidelberger, using knowledge from sulfanilamide destruction of bacteria, devised an anticancer drug by placing a fluoride atom in the 5 position of the uracil molecule, and developed 5-fluoro-urethol. Then followed a list of antibiotics and miscellaneous drugs, so that in the 1970s, thousands of potential anticancer drugs were tested at the National Cancer Institute. This rapid influx of new drugs has slowed, so that now concentration is being focused upon logistics, which include methods of drug administration, dosages, combination drug therapy, bone-marrow transplants, treatment of drug-induced infection, etc. Although chemotherapy seems to be effective in preventing metastases and prolonging life, it nevertheless leaves much to be desired. I am reminded of a statement attributed to Ochsner who is reputed to have said, "I must rush to use these drugs while they are still effective."

Hormone Manipulation

Hormone manipulation has been used for treating breast cancer and received its impetus from the studies of Huggins, which opened the road for hormone therapy. Before Huggins' observation, cancer cells were considered wild cells that did not adhere to body controls. His observation demonstrated a varied response of the cancer cell to a given hormonal environment.

In 1889, Freyberg advocated oophorectomy in the treatment of breast cancer. It had been noted by Beatson (1896) that improvement occurred after oophorectomy. At present, the beneficial effects of oophorectomy have been established. Many types of hormone manipulation have been advocated, from the administration of testosterone to the current use of nolvodex, which appear promising.

Miscellaneous

The current population of scientists and clinicians cooperating in the learning about the natural history and methods of coping with breast cancer is innumerable. The development of the National Cancer Institute (1971) has resulted in thousands of randomized trials being conducted in the United States. While considering these advances, it must be recalled that cancer facilities were not available as recently as 100 years ago. In 1884 the Womens's Hospital in New York denied admission to patients with cancer. It was considered a venereal disease and thought to be contagious. Accordingly, the Memorial Hospital for cancer was founded with Dr. William Coley as one of the medical directors, and Dr. James Ewing, pathologist at Cornell Medical Center, was hired in 1909 as the medical administrator. Dr. Ewing published a book, "Neoplastic Diseases," in 1918 after 10 years of intensive research, which contained 2,500 references. This was the first attempt to classify the different causes of cancer, and thus started the effort to divide and conquer this disease.

Broders, in 1926, called attention to the histologic grading and since then the advances in pathology and biology have been great. These include ploidy determination, oncogenes, tumor markers, monoclonal antibodies, and growth factors, to mention a few. Diagnosis by means of mammography permits the very early detection of breast cancer, and public education had made every woman aware of the problem.

Summary

Despite the tremendous effort to understand and treat breast cancer, there has been no significant increase in the survival rate. We must admit our humility in the face of this enemy. Maryls Witte teaches a course at the University of Arizona, entitled: "Medical Ignorance." Ignorance has been modified by Charles Kettering (after whom the Sloan-Kettering Hospital has been named, which has developed from the Memorial Hospital), who has enlarged on the term, which he defined as "educated ignorance." This I interpret to mean that as we become educated in a given field, we lose track of our ignorance. We must further recall "that tomorrow is not a projection of today." By continued and intense perseverance in the quest for newer knowledge, we may some day control this dread disease.

The Evolution of the Treatment of Breast Cancer

George Crile, Jr.

Introduction

When I entered Harvard Medical School in 1929, there were no arguments in Boston about the treatment of breast cancer: the Halsted radical mastectomy was the only option. But in the midwest, a Cleveland Clinic surgeon named George W. Crile never did a radical mastectomy. He treated breast cancer with a cosmetically excellent, modified radical operation, saying, and I quote, "Halsted is an obsessional fuddy-duddy who takes all day to do an operation that should never be done at all."

But when did a son ever heed what his father told him? I had fallen under the spell of Dr. Tom Jones—the best technical surgeon I have ever known—who was also on the Cleveland Clinic staff. Jones' radical mastectomies were of the Mayo Clinic variety with a cosmetically suitable semitransverse incision, not the thin-flapped, graft-ridden Halsted type.

In the early 1940s Dr. Allen Graham, head of the Cleveland Clinic Department of Pathology, made a study of Crile's patients, treated with modified radical mastectomies, and Jones' patients, treated in the same period with radical mastectomies. He found no differences in local recurrence or survival. But I was young and stubborn, and thought bigger must be better. I started to do the newly introduced ultraradical operation and to dissect out the internal mammary nodes. Then came World War II, when there was little concern about the treatment of breast cancer.

Doubts About Radical Mastectomies

Around this time, Sir Reginald Murley had published a paper that compared the results of Sir Geoffrey Keynes' breast surgery performed in the 1930s with

From: Wise L, Johnson H Jr (eds): *Breast Cancer: Controversies in Management.* Futura Publishing Company, Inc., Armonk, NY, © 1994.

those of Keynes' colleagues at the same hospital. Keynes' treatment was partial mastectomy and radiation; the controls had radical mastectomies. The difference in survival favored the patients treated by partial mastectomy.

At about the same time, Dr. Dinsmore, then head of the Cleveland Clinic Department of Surgery, returned from a visit with Dr. McWhirter in Scotland. There, Dinsmore found patients were being treated successfully with simple mastectomy and radiation. I also remembered a patient who 10 years before had an excisional biopsy and had refused mastectomy. She was still alive and well. It was not hard for Murley and Dinsmore to persuade me. I did my last radical mastectomy in 1954.

At the same time, Smith and Myer in Rockford, Illinois, published their account of more than 400 cases of breast cancer treated at three community hospitals. Of these patients, 334 had radical mastectomies, 97 had simple mastectomies, and 11 had local excision. At both 5 and 10 years, there was no difference in the survival rate of those treated by radical as compared to conservative operations. Furthermore, the survival rates of those treated by skilled and qualified surgeons were comparable to those achieved by occasional operators.

In the early 1960s I published my first report of the survival of patients treated by modified radical, simple, or partial mastectomy; fewer than 20% of the latter had been irradiated. The survival was comparable to that of a group treated by radical mastectomy, a higher proportion of whom received radiation.

Today's Issues

Today there is no debate about the place for the Halsted radical mastectomy. There is no place for it. But irradiation after a partial mastectomy is an issue today. If cases are unselected and randomized, the incidence of local recurrence is high in the absence of radiation. With proper patient selection, however, and the cooperation of experienced surgeons and pathologists, the incidence of local recurrence after partial mastectomy can be acceptably low.

Chemotherapy also remains debatable. The head of the National Cancer Institute advocated chemotherapy for everyone who has ever had a favorable stage I cancer, so we may be overdoing chemotherapy just as years ago our surgery was too radical and, later, we added radiation too often. There is no question that chemotherapy delays the appearance of recurrence, but there is no hard evidence that it is better than endocrine therapy. Indeed, many believe that chemotherapy exerts its effect through the endocrine system by making the patient so sick that she cannot produce estrogens.

Both radiation and chemotherapy, given as adjuvants to patients who have favorable cancers, not only have unpleasant side effects but also may increase the risk of contracting leukemia, lymphoma, and other cancers. Endocrine therapy (e.g., tamoxifen), on the other hand, has no serious side effects. We should not rush into universal chemotherapy for patients with breast cancer, but should wait until we have the long-term results of randomized studies. We do well to remember past mistakes: the "value" of the low-residue diet in the prevention and treatment of diverticulitis, the "necessity" of circumcision and tonsillectomy, and the myth of radical mastectomy. We should not always believe everything that we are taught!

Now For the Current Issues

Should stage I breast cancer be treated by chemotherapy? The February 1989 issue of the *New England Journal of Medicine* contained the results of four studies on the administration of long-term systemic adjuvant chemotherapy to node-negative breast cancer patients. In all of them, there was a prolongation of the disease-free survival time, but this was followed by a shorter period of survival between recurrence and death, so that there was no difference in the overall length of survival.

Dr. C. Barber Mueller, reviewing these and other studies, concluded with the following question: "Does it seem to be in the classic tradition of ethical medical practice to recommend to any woman a drug or a treatment that can never be seen to be to her benefit? It strains ethical credibility to recommend such treatment, particularly when the gain is a delay in recurrence and less time between recurrence and death."

I think all patients with breast cancer should have a short course of perioperative chemotherapy and also treatment with tamoxifen. Many studies have shown that a short course of perioperative chemotherapy that hits the cancer cells in the blood and lymph streams before they have had an opportunity to establish themselves as metastases is as effective as a long course, yet it gives no side effects. In most patients with favorable stage I cancers, the tamoxifen could be given for only a few months, but in those with more advanced cancers, it should be given for 5 years or perhaps longer. The optimum duration has not yet been established. I also think that premenopausal women should be sterilized either by oophorectomy or radiation.

In patients more than 70 years of age, and perhaps in all postmenopausal patients, there is mounting evidence that a prolonged course of tamoxifen, with or without radiation, may be curative. The tumor is removed only when it fails to disappear or continues to enlarge. R.S. Margolese and Roger Foster, Jr., treated 30 elderly patients in this way, followed them for 3 years, and had to operate on or radiate only nine of them. Twenty patients were still alive after 33 months, and only one patient died of breast cancer. There were no inoperable local recurrences. Although this study is not long enough to be highly significant, I predict that short perioperative courses of chemotherapy will supplant the long ones, and it has already been proven that 1 year is as good as 2 years and that 6 months is as good as a year. We must remember Burkett's lymphoma, in which he proved that a single short course of chemotherapy was much more effective than prolonged treatment. Burkett reasoned that the unexpected result was because prolonged therapy destroyed the immune system which is highly effective in controlling this kind of tumor. Nissen Meyer's observations on the results of a short perioperative course of chemotherapy in controlling breast cancer may be explicable by the same principle.

This history of the treatment of breast cancer can be summarized by saying that (1) we operated too much, (2) we radiated too much, (3) we gave chemotherapy for too long, and (4) that, to date, we have underused and underestimated the value of a long, 5-year period of treatment with tamoxifen, perhaps in all patients regardless of the status of the estrogen receptors.

Thirty years ago, Sir Hedley Atkins said what summarizes the situation today: "Our recent knowledge of breast cancer has progressed so fast that now no one knows how to treat it."

3

The Natural History of Breast Cancer

C. Barber Mueller

Introduction

The natural history of breast cancer may be described from several viewpoints: molecular/genetic, cellular/pathological, statistical/epidemiologic, or clinical/patient. This chapter deals with patients with breast cancer and approaches its natural history from a clinical viewpoint. The basic question is not who or why does a woman get it, but what happens to women who develop it. Is all breast cancer the same merely because pathological descriptions are similar, are there clinical variances in manifestation, is anything other than the breast capable of being treated, and does treatment of any sort have any effect on the ultimate outcome-survival? This chapter deals with attack rates and survival data. It pays considerable attention to the methods whereby these outcomes are reported and how they are displayed.

Almost every manuscript looking at the overall effects of breast cancer begins with a statement that in the current year 150,000 women will develop it and 50,000 will die of it. By implication, the remaining 100,000 do *not* die of breast cancer. Statements such as this must reflect an author's concept of the magnitude of the problem for similar numbers have been passed from manuscript to manuscript. The second figure is always one-third of the initial figure and the initial figure has been rising over the past 10 years from approximately 90,000 10 years ago to close to 160,000 currently. The SEER (Surveillance, Epidemiology and End Results) reports and American Cancer Society (ACS) data have always held to two such figures. Cancer survival statistics are reported by SEER and ACS as 5-year *relative* survival rates. This is the ratio of the observed survival rate for the patient group to the expected survival rate for persons in the general population similar to the patient group.

From: Wise L, Johnson H Jr (eds): *Breast Cancer: Controversies in Management.* Futura Publishing Company, Inc., Armonk, NY, © 1994.

Age is the most significant risk factor and the development of breast canc
increases with age to the point where it is approximately 400 times as prevale
in the octogenarian as it is in the 20-year old. The age distribution of patients w
present with breast cancer extends from 20 to 90 and presents with a peak in t
fifth and sixth decades of life (Figs. 1, 2).

A generally cited statistic is the fact that breast cancer will affect one out
nine women—a 12% attack rate. This is the anticipated attack rate at time
birth. Following the 50 to 60 year age range, this number decreases despite t
increasing incidence with age.

Direct Analysis and Survival

There are two general ways in which survival data are presented: the dire
method and the indirect (life table analysis) method. The direct method (1)
retrospective, (2) gives actual survival, (3) does not use cases treated within t
time period, (4) is always out of date, (5) has difficulty dealing with "lost
follow-up," and (6) may or may not ignore deaths due to other causes. T
indirect method, on the other hand, (1) is progressive, (2) gives probabilities
survival, (3) requires an annual status of every entrant, (4) utilizes informati

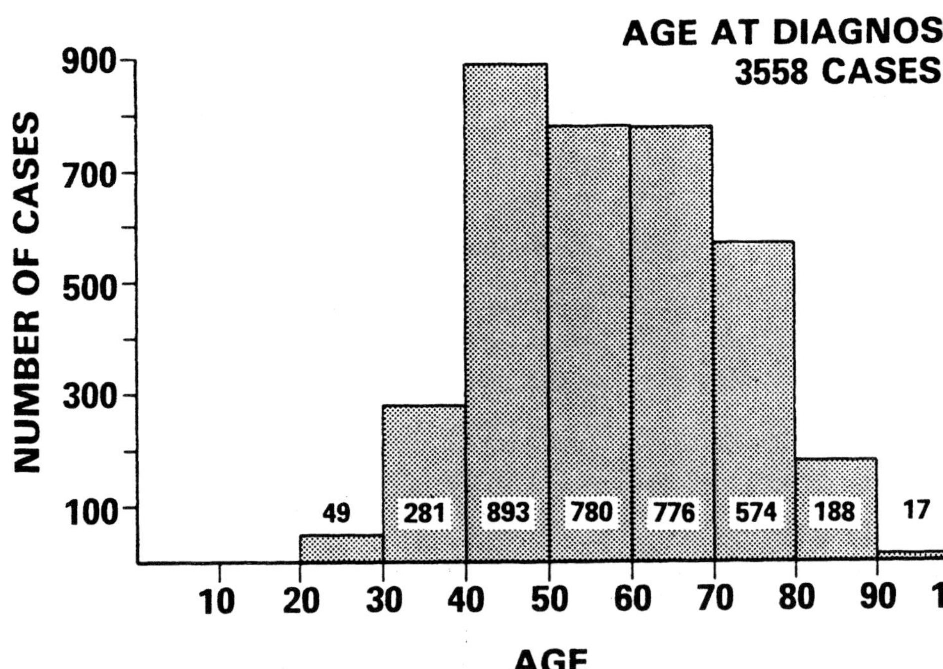

Figure 1: *Age at diagnosis in 3,558 patients. From Mueller et al.[3]*

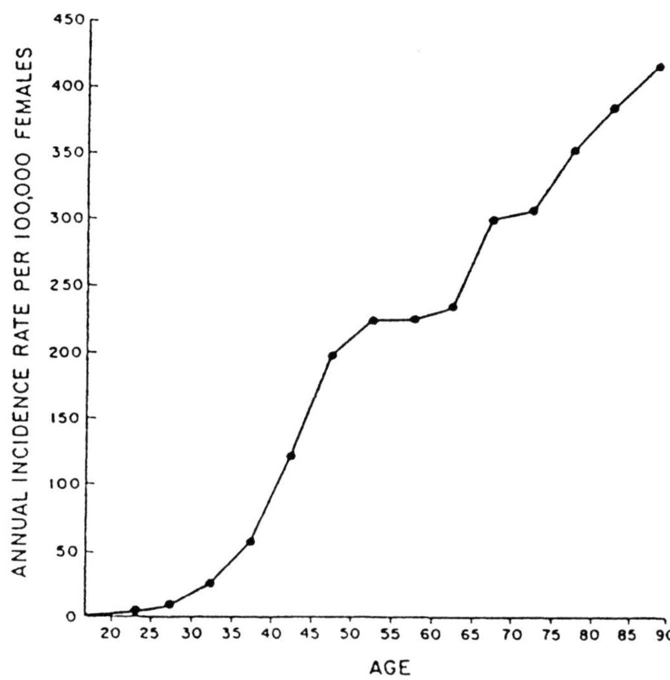

Figure 2: *Average annual age specific incidence of breast carcinoma in Connecticut, 1971–1975. From Feig SA: Breast carcinoma, current diagnosis and treatment. Am Coll Radiol 1983.*

for all patients at all times, (5) is always up to date, (6) is easy to manage "lost to follow-up," and (7) may or may not ignore deaths due to other causes.

When looking at survival data by the direct method, crude rates for mortality at 5 years are generally somewhere in the neighborhood of 50% and diminish progressively with each 5-year period (Tables 1, 2).[1]

Survival rates following operations, which do not include all of the women with breast cancer, give a 65% survival rate at 5 years, implying a 35% death rate at 5 years. This number is always better in node-negative women than in node-positive women, but much of the older data are presented with a mix of the two (Table 3).

All long-term studies show continuing reduction in survival over 5, 10, and 15 years. These numbers may be improved by (1) improving therapy or (2) advancing the diagnostic time without changing the time of death. Currently, the effectiveness of "salvage" chemotherapy and endocrine therapy visible by improvement in the symptoms of many women with metastatic disease suggests that the time between diagnosis and death will likely be lengthened, perhaps by 1 or 2 years, without a change in the cause of death. This should be reflected in slightly improved percentages at any fixed time.

Table 1
Five-Year Survival Rates*

Aberdeen (1,335 patients)	40.1%
Dundee (1,700 patients)	44%
Southeast England (16,516 patients)	42%
Southwest England (1,045 patients)	43%

*Crude survival rates for all patients with breast cancer. From Bruce J.[1]

Table 2
Overall Crude Survival Rates*

Length of Follow-up (years)	No. Cases "Eligible"	No. of Survivors	% Survival Rates
5	876	371	42
10	876	247	28
15	487	106	22

*Crude survival rates showing that deaths continue after five years. From Bruce J.[1]

Table 3
Percentage 5-Year Survival, Operable Cancer of Breast*

Author	Method	Result
Williams and Curwen	Radical	66
Watson	Radical	63
Butcher	Radical	60
Dahl-Iversen	Extended radical	66
Handley and Thackray	Conservative radical	67
Kaae and Johansen	Simple + radiotherapy	67
Bruce et al.	Simple + radiotherapy	63
Kennedy and Millar	Simple + radiotherapy	57
Philip	Various	55
Porritt	Tumor excision + radiotherapy	65

*Crude survival rates of selected "operable" cases of breast cancer as reported from various sources with various methods of therapy. From Bruce J.[1]

Life Table Analysis and Survival

The reports stemming from SEER and utilized by ACS report survival as measured by the direct method, a standard way of reporting outcome. Currently, however, life table analysis, the indirect or actuarial method, is in vogue for reporting clinical trials and presenting data from comprehensive registries. This method permits the display of (1) the percentage of those at risk who die during any year, (2) the time at which half are dead, and (3) the percentage surviving at 5, 10, 15, or 20 years. When displayed with a logarithmic ordinate (log-normal), it becomes a dynamic expression of rate of loss rather than amount. This may be expressed with confidence limits, which are essential when two life table curves are compared.[4]

Few registries are truly demographic, for hospital-based registries have been emphasized. A demographic, comprehensive registry enrolls all women in an area, follows them annually, and records both time of death and cause of death. When this is done, it appears that at 20 years post diagnosis approximately 80% of the women will be dead and most of them will have died of breast cancer. A survey of the Syracuse Cancer Registry, which registered all women with breast cancer, not just operative cases, showed a 20-year survival curve of approximately 20% with 88% of the deaths being due to breast cancer (Fig. 3).[3]

This study also acknowledged that all deaths are not necessarily due to breast cancer. It generated three age categories—under 50, 50–70, over 70—and found that the oldest group had a more rapid rate of dying. This group contained most of the deaths due to competing causes. These differences in rates of dying were seen even when node-negative deaths (stage I) were plotted using only deaths due to breast cancer. The oldest group still had the more rapid rate of dying, and it was concluded that cancer is a more virulent disease in the aged. In looking at those 1,750 women who had died, approximately 88% had died of their breast cancer and only 12% had died of competing risks (other causes). Recognizing that "cause of death data" comes only from those who have already died, it is inappropriate to make the assumption that the documented causes of death can be transferred in prognostic fashion to the upcoming cause of death of those who are still alive.

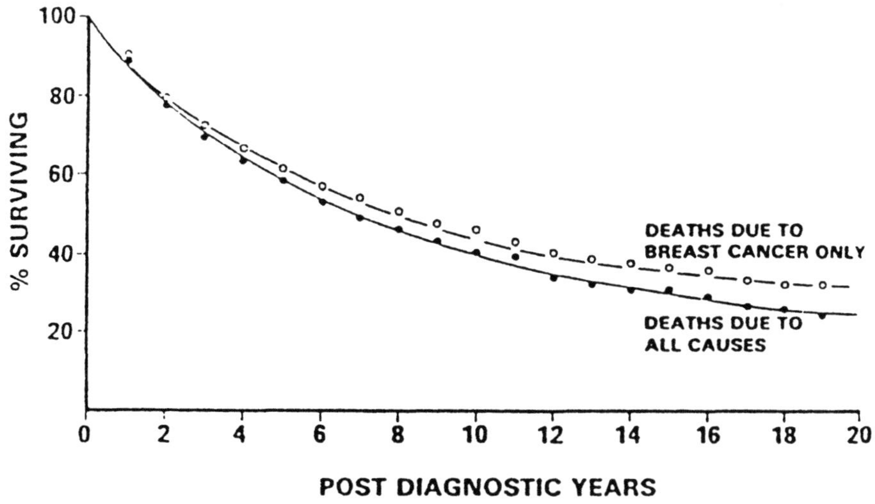

Figure 3: *Life table analysis of 3,558 women showing depletion of the group by deaths due to all causes as well as deaths due to cancer of the breast. Mueller et al.[3]*

Presenting the Data

Life table data may be presented as a curve on an arithmetic plot; this shows the *amount* of change each year. It can also be presented on a semilogarithmic plot in which the ordinate (y axis) is a logarithmic scale and time (the x axis) is arithmetic. This permits the calculation of the *rate* of change each year. When survival curves of demographic registries or specific groups are presented in logarithmic fashion, the curve becomes a straight line, signifying that the rate is constant. This was found clearly in one of the clinical trials—National Surgical Adjuvant Breast Project (NSABP) B-04;[5] it has been seen in Syracuse, in the Connecticut Tumor Registry material, and in the National Cancer Institute Registry (Fig. 4A, B).

These latter two registries extend for 20 to 40 years, and the annual rate of death is constant throughout this time. It must thus be concluded that breast cancer operates as a force of mortality for at least 25 or 30 years. Frequently these mortality rates are reported as "relative," which is an attempt to take the crude specific death rate and relate it to the death rates of the population at large which contains deaths due to all other causes. It is statistically acceptable to assume that when the two rates become parallel, there is a "statistical cure" even though this does not necessarily represent a "clinical cure." It assumes that breast cancer no longer operates as a force of mortality in excess of the forces due to other

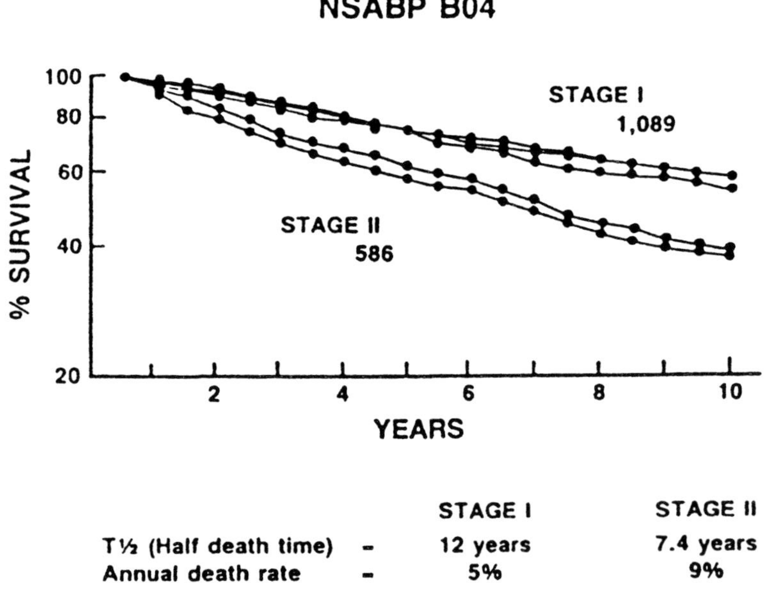

Figure 4A: *Survival results in stage I and stage II women as reported by NSABP B-04. Redrawn with additional derived data. From Mueller.[8]*

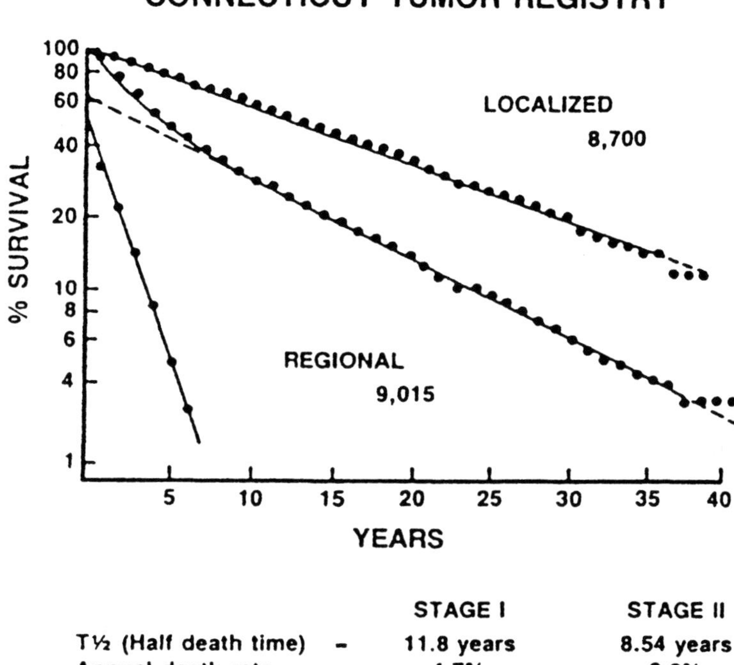

Figure 4B: *Survival results reported by Connecticut Tumor Registry. Redrawn with additional derived data. From Mueller.[8]*

diseases. This may occur by one of two means: either the breast cancer rate slows (and there is no evidence that this happens) or deaths due to other causes increase. A study from Cambridge first reported[6] that the rate of dying in the groups of women with breast cancer became the same as the expected rate of the normal population between 20 and 25 years post diagnosis. Ten years later, with continued follow-up, it was recognized that breast cancer death rates were still in excess of those seen in the expected population.[7] This later analysis is presented in Figure 5A, which is presented on a logarithmic plot (Fig. 5A, B).

The conversion of this figure to an arithmetic plot shows a continuous decay and that approximately 3% of the women with breast cancer are alive 35 years after diagnosis (Fig. 5B). The difference between the death curves for the breast cancer group and the expected normal population, the stippled area, constitutes the force of mortality of breast cancer. This study also reported that one-fourth of the women dying in the 20- to 25-year period were node-positive at the time of diagnosis. At the 35-year point, more than 20% of the women dying were still dying of their breast cancer. These numbers are so small that confidence in such percentages must be very wide. They do show, however, the continuous operation of the force of mortality of breast cancer.

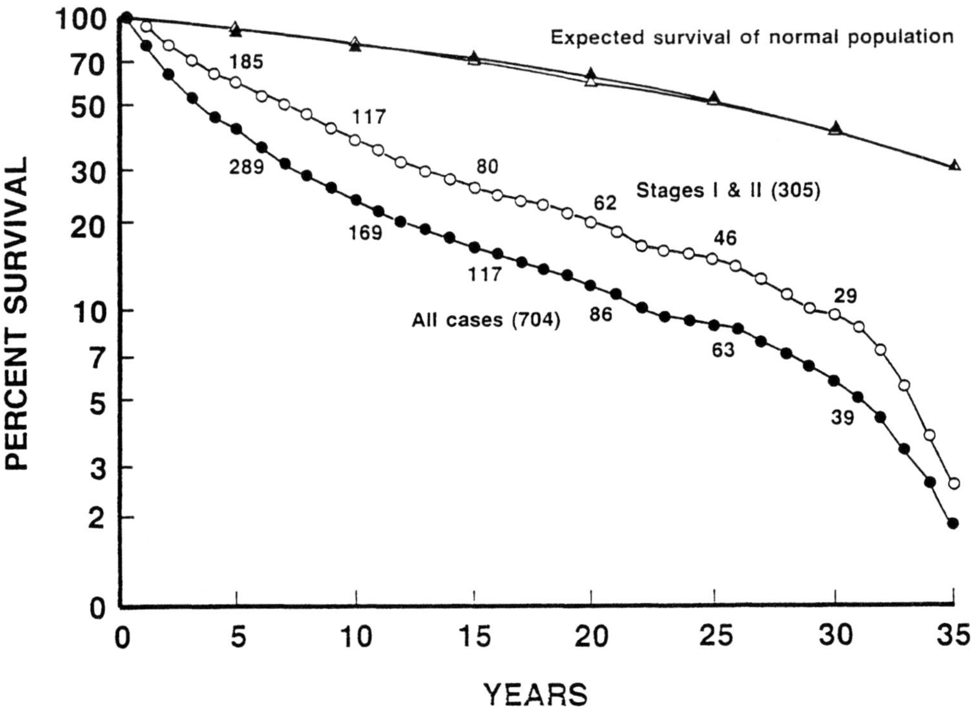

Figure 5A: *Survival curves for all patients and for stages I and II only. Expected survival curves from a normal population of the same age distribution also shown. Redrawn from Brinkley and Haybittle.[7]*

Stage I and Stage II Rates are Different

The NSABP B-04 study probably contains the most precise data showing that the rates of dying for stage I and stage II breast cancer patients are different. The input criteria were quite tightly fixed and death measurements were precise. The Connecticut Tumor Registry shows two rates that are quite similar to those of B-04. For stage I, half of the women are dead at 12 years and for stage II, half of the women are dead at 8 years.[8] If breast cancer were the same disease and stage II was merely a delay in diagnosis, the rates should be the same and the starting time different. This is not what the data show. Histologic features also suggest differences. The stage II group contains lymphatic and venous invasion, a worse nuclear grade and lesser cell differentiation. The conclusion is unavoidable that the presence of positive nodes at diagnosis marks a fundamentally different tumor in the breast. Positive lymph nodes in the axilla are markers of the degree of aggressiveness of the breast tumor, not a step in progression, a biological marker, not a chronological marker.

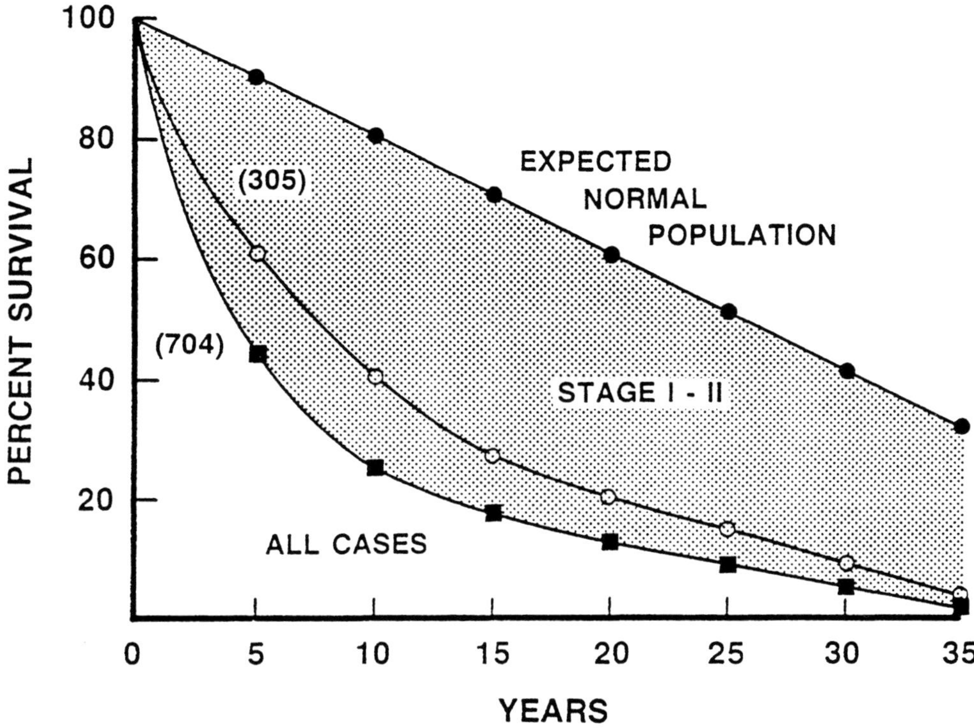

Figure 5B: *Survival curves from Figure 5A. Redrawn on arithmetic scale. The stippled area represents the force of mortality of breast cancer.*

The Operative Choices

All of the patients in reported clinical studies have been operated upon and an important question has become "Does the type of operation make a difference?" There are several clinical trials and many reports about this problem. The most powerful observations are randomized clinical trials. Less powerful are cohort studies, case control, and case series. The randomized clinical trials began with a 1976 report by Lacour et al. on the findings of a cooperative study of 1,580 cases comparing radical mastectomy to extended radical mastectomy. No significant difference was found in 5-year survival rates. A Copenhagen trial started in 1951, enrolled 355 patients to compare the McWhirter simple mastectomy and radiation to standard radical mastectomy. There was no difference in survival at 5 and 10 years. A trial at Guy's Hospital started in 1961 accrued 370 patients, testing radical mastectomy against lumpectomy with x-ray therapy. In stage I women, the recurrence rate was higher in the lumpectomy group but both groups had the same survival. In stage II women, there was a shorter survival and more local recurrences in the lumpectomy group.

A Hammersmith trial with 195 patients compared simple mastectomy with radical mastectomy. This trial ran for 8 years and there was no statistical difference in survival at either 5 or 8 years. The Milan group under Veronesi randomized 701 patients with small breast cancer and clinically negative axilla to compare radical mastectomy against quadrantectomy with axillary dissection. There were no differences in survival at 7 years.

A Southeast Scotland trial ran from 1964 to 1974, enrolling 498 patients randomized between radical mastectomy and simple mastectomy with x-ray therapy. At 5 years, there was no difference in survival rate although a markedly worse survival rate was noted in the postmenopausal patients when compared with the premenopausal patients. In the United States, NSABP B-04 was begun in 1971. It compared radical mastectomy to simple mastectomy in stage I and stage II women. A 10-year report shows that the survival curves comparing the two operative procedures in stage II women were identical. This study confirmed other trials and many reports that permitted the conclusion that "depending upon stage, there was no 10-year survival difference resulting from the operation itself." In a recent report, NSABP B-06 compared simple mastectomy to lumpectomy with or without radiation. At 5 and 8 years, there was no difference in survival among the three groups.

All of these trials show that survival is no different among patients with extended radical mastectomy, simple mastectomy, or lumpectomy whenever any two are compared "within a trial."[9] Although it is probably fallacious to make intertrial comparisons because patient selection, staging, and other forms of bias creep into every trial, a recent report from England attempted a meta-analysis statistical treatment to coalesce information between many trials.[10] No significant differences in survival that could be ascribed to the operation were shown. A delay in recurrence and possibly a survival benefit associated with adjuvant cytotoxic chemotherapy or antiestrogen therapy was acknowledged.

Within these several trials, the evidence seems sufficiently strong to make the following conclusions. When measured by survival, no operation is superior to any other and the selection of one procedure over another must be made with other outcomes in mind. The lesser procedures have a greater incidence of local recurrence than the greater procedures, but this has not been shown to have an effect on survival.

Conclusion

1. The incidence of breast carcinoma increases with increasing age.

2. Breast cancer is the cause of death in 80% to 85% of all women who develop it.

3. As a force of mortality, it operates continuously for at least 30 to 35 years.

4. Younger women with breast carcinoma have a better prognosis regarding length of life than do older women.

5. There are inherent differences between node-negative and node-positive groups of women that can be seen in the rates of dying, the local recurrences, and the histopathology.

6. If the cancer is completely removed, no operation is superior to any other when measured by survival.

7. The use of adjuvant chemotherapy or hormonal therapy produces minimal if any significant change in the rates of dying.

8. Skin or chest wall recurrences follow mastectomy in 10% to 15% of women.

References

1. Bruce J: The enigma of breast cancer. Cancer 1969; 24:1314–1320.
2. Mueller CB: Perspectives on primary treatment, local recurrence and ultimate outcome: statistics on breast carcinoma. In: Gant TD, Vanconez LO (eds). Postmastectomy Reconstruction. Williams and Wilkins, Baltimore, 1988.
3. Mueller CB, Ames F, Anderson G: Breast cancer in 3,558 women: age as a significant determinant in rate of dying and cause of death. Surgery 1978; 83:123–132.
4. Beahrs O, Hensen DE, Hutten RV, Myers M: Manual for Staging of Cancer. Lippincott, Philadelphia, 1988.
5. Fisher B, Redmond C, Fisher ER, et al: Ten-year results of a randomized clinical trial comparing radical mastectomy to simple mastectomy with or without radiation. NEJM 1985; 312:674–681.
6. Brinkley D, Haybittle JL: The curability of breast cancer. Lancet 1975; ii:95–101.
7. Brinkley D, Haybittle JL: Long term survival of women with breast cancer. Lancet 1984; ii:1118.
8. Mueller CB: Stage II breast cancer is not simply a late stage I. Surgery 1988; 104:631–638.
9. Mueller CB: Valid alternatives in the management of early breast cancer. Adv Surg 1987; 20:183–216.
10. Early Breast Cancer Trialists Collaborative Group: Effect of tamoxifen and of cytotoxic therapy on mortality in early breast cancer. NEJM 1988; 319:1681–1692.

Stage II Breast Cancer Is Not Necessarily a Progression of Stage I Disease

C. Barber Mueller

Introduction

Conventional wisdom holds that breast cancer originates in one or more cells, grows to the point where a diagnosis in the breast is possible, either mammographically or clinically (stage I), following which it spreads to axillary nodes (stage II), then to distant sites (stage III and IV), and finally results in death. The basic and simple staging system, the Manchester System,[1] relates the primary tumor to axillary nodes and then to distant sites. The Tumor Node Metastasis System (TNM)[2] has refined this by including size of the primary tumor and the creation of subsets within each stage, resulting in a minimum of 14 subsets. All staging classifications (I, II, III, IV) reinforce the idea that there is a sequential or a chronological relationship between the stages. The early dissections of Sampson Handley,[3] which demonstrated a contigual relationship between primary tumor and axillary metastases, were important in establishing the concept of and need for en bloc resections. Interest in "early diagnosis" is supported by this concept and has led to a general belief that *early* treatment might result in a "cure" since the local tumor might possibly be removed before distant spread occurs.

When measured by "direct" or "fixed-time" analysis, a superior 5- or 10-year survivorship is always found when stage I patients are compared to stage II patients. This has led to what seems to be an obvious assumption that stage II women arrive at diagnosis closer to their time of death, and although earlier diagnosis would improve their postdiagnostic survival, no one has yet shown whether or not earlier diagnosis would change the *cause* of death rather than the time of death. When life table analysis—the indirect method—is used to report survival, the concept that stage I and stage II breast cancer are chronologically related must be reconsidered, for this postulate does not fit observations that come either from survival data, local recurrence rates, or the histopathology plus other features of the primary tumors. The observations display two major subsets of breast cancer, divided according to the presence or absence of positive axillary nodes at the time of diagnosis, and these two variants probably represent biological and not chronological differences between stage I and stage II.

Two decades ago, Bross and Blumensen created a mathematical model of breast cancer to fit some of the early studies of the National Surgical Adjuvant Breast Project (NSABP) and felt that a two-disease model best represented data that had been generated in NSABP B-03 and NSABP B-04.[4-7] It is well known that the incidence of breast cancer rises progressively with age and that this rising rate has a plateau or slight dip at the 45- to 60-year period, sometimes called Clemmensen's hook. Attempts have been made to interpret this as a demonstration of two types of breast cancer—pre- and postmenopausal—which overlap at this midlife period. The premenopausal tumors were thought to be related to ovarian estrogens and the postmenopausal tumors to adrenal estrogens, obesity, hypertension, and hyperglycemia.[8,9] Neither of these studies considered nodal status as a significant determinant. Twenty-five years ago, Devitt, in a very prescient article, concluded that stage I and stage II represented two different diseases presenting with similar histologic appearances. In looking at the significance of lymph node metastases, he concluded that the poorer prognosis was not due to the metastases but to the biological potential of the tumor.[10,11]

This chapter attempts to collect data that not only support the concept but lead to the conclusion that node-negative breast cancer (stage I) is different in many of its features from node-positive breast cancer (stage II).

Survival Evidence

Life table analysis requires an annual assessment of the status of all patients and develops an arithmetic projection of the probability of survival by post-diagnostic year.[12] This creates a decay curve that describes attrition in a selected group of patients. When such curves are drawn on semilog plots (log-normal), this attrition is displayed as a straight line—a constant rate—that can be represented either by the half-death time (T½, the length of time required for 50% to die) or an annual death rate (the percent of women who die each year as a fraction of those who were alive at the beginning of the year).[13] The relationship between stage I and stage II is universally dealt with as though the two stages are different because of a delay in diagnosis (Fig. 1), but if so, such a delay should cause a "zero time shift" or "lead-time bias."[14] If this delay were to constitute the difference between stage I and stage II, the survival curves created by life table analysis should start at different times and *should be parallel*. The delay should be seen at the start (Fig. 2). Observed data do not fit this construct.

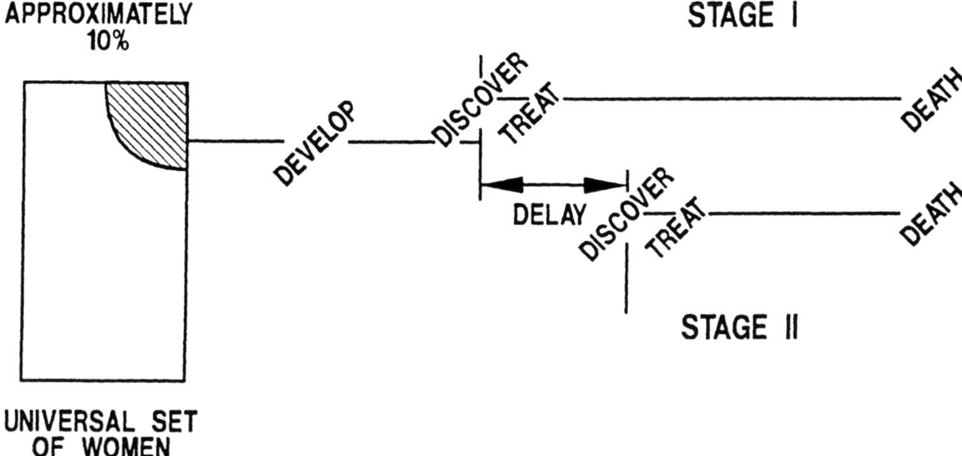

Figure 1: *Schematic representation of the concept that the difference between stage I and stage II breast cancer is a delay in diagnosis that provides less postdiagnostic treatment time before death for those women who present as stage II. From Mueller.*[38]

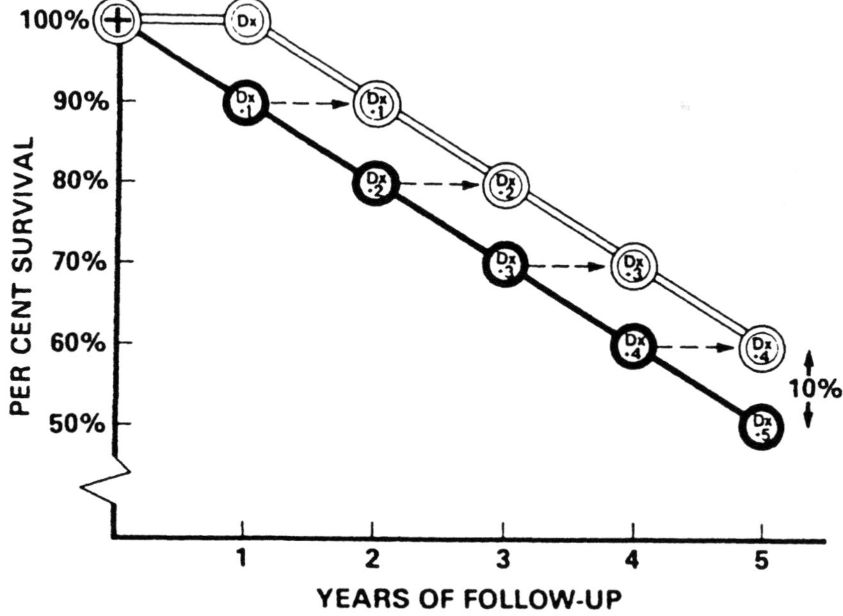

Failure to correct for "zero-time shift" in assessing the value of early diagnosis.

Figure 2: *This shows the "expected" survival curves if a delay in diagnosis were the element that created the difference between stage I and stage II women. From Sackett et al.*[14]

National Surgical Adjuvant Breast Project (NSABP) B-04 is a clinical trial that tested radical mastectomy against simple mastectomy, with or without x-ray treatment.[15] For reasons not explained in the text, the survival data were presented on a semilog plot. Figure 3 shows the 10-year survival curves of three treated groups of stage I women and two treated groups of stage II women. No difference that could be related to the treatment was found within either of the two stages. Both stages show decay as a straight line function, but the *lines are not parallel*. Deaths occurred in the first year in all groups and continued with a steady annual rate for the entire 10 years. The half-death times (T½) and annual death rates were different between the two stages but remarkably uniform between the groups. This study probably has the most precise separation of stage I and stage II patients currently available, since observations on the treatment were contingent upon precise separation and were made in institutions of authority. Since the entrance criteria excluded women with associated life-threatening illnesses and the study was conducted with reasonable rigor throughout all participating institutions, this is probably the most precise display of survival rate differences between stage I and stage II currently available.

The Connecticut Tumor Registry records its cases at time of diagnosis as

NSABP B04

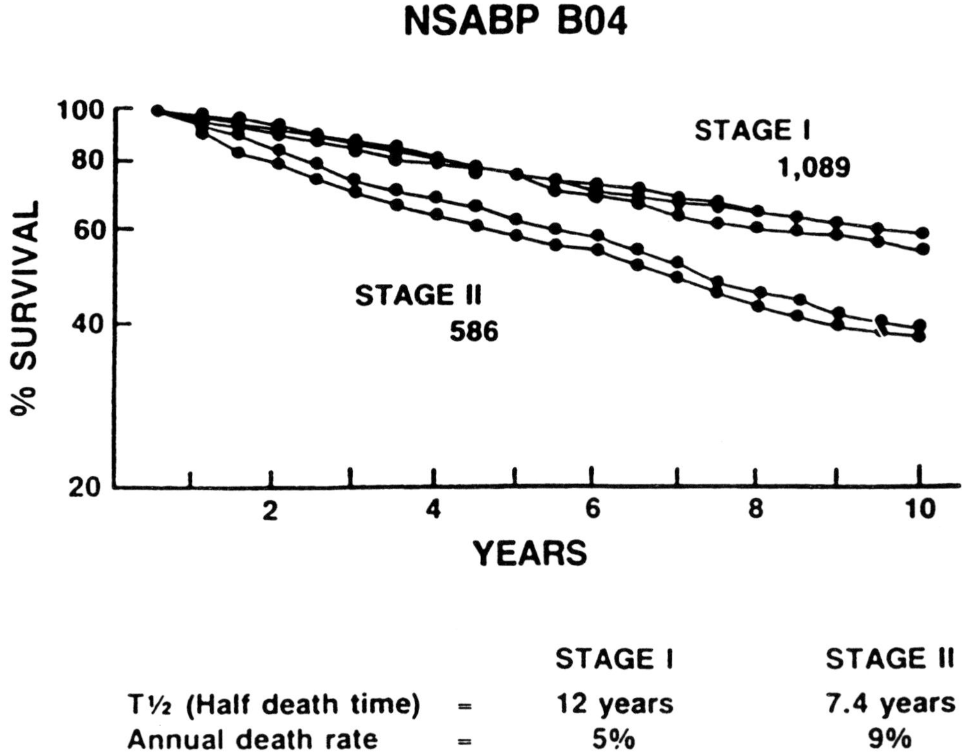

	STAGE I	STAGE II
T½ (Half death time) =	12 years	7.4 years
Annual death rate =	5%	9%

Figure 3: *Survival results, determined by life table analysis as reported by NASBP - B04. Redrawn with additional derived data from Fisher et al.[15] Stage I represents three treatment groups: radical mastectomy, simple mastectomy alone, and simple mastectomy with radiotherapy. Stage II represents two treatment groups: radical mastectomy and simple mastectomy with radiotherapy.*

local versus regional, and for purposes of this chapter these have been converted to stage I/stage II. When these data are presented by life table analysis on a semilog plot, once again the survival curves of stage I and stage II women constitute straight lines, but the *lines are not parallel*[16] (Fig. 4). The half-death times and the annual death rates are remarkably similar to those seen in the B-04 report. In Connecticut, as in B-04, deaths occur in both groups in the early years and continue in a steady fashion for 40 years.

The survival data in both reports show that the rates of dying in the two stages are different, and there is no evidence to suggest that they are different because of therapy. The significant difference is the presence or absence of metastases in the axilla at the time of diagnosis. This suggests that tumors that progress to the lymph nodes are different from tumors that do not, and this difference may be seen in the rates of dying.

It might be considered that these survival differences are due to errors in staging. There is extensive evidence to indicate that clinical examination of the

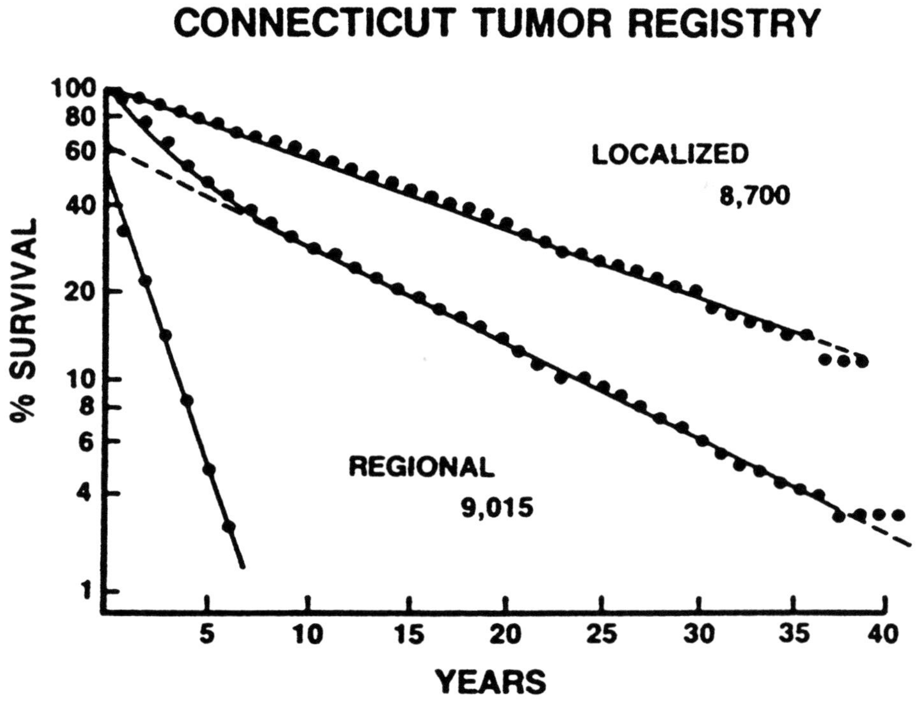

CONNECTICUT TUMOR REGISTRY

	STAGE I	STAGE II
T½ (Half death time) —	11.8 years	8.54 years
Annual death rate —	4.7%	8.0%

Figure 4. *Survival results as reported by Connecticut Tumor Registry. Redrawn with additional derived data from Metcalfe.*[16]

axilla has a 20% to 30% error rate in both directions.[17] Since pathological examination of the resected axillary specimens may miss nodal metastases, any pathological staging errors that occur will always be in one direction—a false stage I. It is very unlikely that a pathologist would erroneously record the presence of carcinoma in negative axillary nodes and a false stage II would occur. Thus, it is possible that the stage I groups contain *true* stage II women. If these were to be removed from the stage I group and placed into the stage II group, the stage II death rate would be unchanged. The stage I curve, however, would be less steep, and differences between the two would be even greater than shown.

Local Recurrence Evidence

Local recurrences of breast cancer, post mastectomy, occur in two principal sites: (1) in the scar/grafted area and/or the adjacent skin flaps, or (2) in regional nodal areas: axillary, internal mammary, or supraclavicular. Such recurrences are reported in approximately 10% of stage I women and 20% of stage II women at 5 years. The definition of and the reporting of local recurrences are not uniform throughout the literature, ranging from the persistence or enlargement of axillary nodes, a recurrence in the skin flaps, enlargement of supraclavicular or internal mammary nodes, down to merely local recurrences within the operative site, i.e., the breast, the chest wall, or the axilla.[18]

To this author, *local recurrence* is the reappearance of carcinoma in the soft tissues of the surgically treated or irradiated area. Its clinical significance remains unclear, but its biological significance is related to the issues discussed in this chapter. *Regional recurrence* is the appearance of carcinoma in regional nodes—supraclavicular, internal mammary, or axillary nodes if the axilla has not been dissected—and represents nodal extension of the tumor process, probably not a *true* local recurrence.

Regardless of definition, however, there is consistency in the reporting of local recurrences when any author compares the local-regional recurrences in stage I patients to those in stage II. The percentages may vary from author to author, depending on what is considered to be local or regional and how they are measured, i.e., direct versus indirect methods, but everyone reports significantly more local recurrences in patients with initially involved lymph nodes than in those without.[18-21]

There are five possible explanations for the appearance of local recurrences:

1. incomplete removal of the local lesion with residual tumor at the margins of the specimen;
2. surgical carelessness, or transection of vessels or lymphatics in the en bloc resection, leading to implantation of tumor from lymphatics or from the primary tumor;
3. retrograde lymphatic spread from regional nodes;

4. the first manifestation of distant disease, made more obvious because of the scar deformity on the chest wall;

5. cancer occurring in residual breast tissue—a second primary.

These possibilities are not mutually exclusive, nor has any single one been found specifically to be the cause of local recurrence.[22] With the increased use of lumpectomy, local recurrence rates have increased, probably indicating that incomplete removal is the basic problem.[23] When radical mastectomy was the standard procedure and was utilized independent of axillary involvement, giving a maximally wide excision of breast, chest wall, and axilla, the local recurrence rates were always different between node-negative and node-positive women. Forrest reported the Manchester trial at 10 years as 16% for stage I and 41.5% for stage II.[24] The Sheffield 10-year experience reported 9.1% for stage I and 20% for stage II.[25] Donegan reported the Ellis Fischel Hospital experience as 10.2% for stage I and 20.5% for stage II at 5 years.[26] White, surveying five hospitals, found 6% to 10% for stage I and 20% to 30% for stage II at 5 years.[27] Table 1 shows the experience of several institutions, again confirming that the local recurrence rates are different between the two stages. These differences could possibly represent technical problems (item 1 above), but when en bloc radical mastectomy was utilized almost universally, regardless of stage, technical differences are probably at the minimal achievable level and differences in local recurrence must represent differences in the biology of the tumor rather than operative consequences. Such differences would be suspect with breast conservation procedures and therefore can be found only in the older radical and modified radical mastectomy literature.

In today's world, local recurrence rates are higher than those previously reported. They may be modified to some extent by local X-ray treatment or chemotherapy as an adjunct to the operative procedure,[28] and are probably more related to the extent of the procedure and the tumor left behind than they are to phenomena associated with the biological characteristics of the tumor. The conclusion must be drawn that the disease that shows itself at the time of diagnosis in a woman with positive nodes has different properties than the disease that shows itself in a woman with negative nodes, and one manifestation of this difference is the recurrence rate of breast cancer on the chest wall.

Evidence from the Primary Tumor

McDivitt[29] and Hellman[30] have stated that the most useful parameter for predicting probability of breast cancer relapse is the presence or absence and extent of axillary lymph node metastases. Both have indicated it would be useful to extend our ability to predict the probability of relapse to patients of the same nodal status if a parameter that is reproducible and easily obtained could be found. A few studies have attempted to relate histopathological or other findings within the primary tumor to the presence or absence of lymph node metastases.

Table 1
The 10-Year Local Recurrence Rates from a Group of Major Extirpative Studies*

Columbia Clinical Classification	Method of Treatment	No. of Patients	Recurrence at 10 years (%)			Totals of Local Recurrences (%)
			Parasternal	Chest Wall	Axilla	
A	Total mastectomy plus axillary dissection plus irradiation (Williams and Stone)	68	0 (0)	8 (12)	7 (10)	15 (22)
	Conservative radical mastectomy (Handley and Thackray)	77	4 (5)	9 (12)	2 (2)	15 (16)
	McWhirter method (Kaae and Johansen)	159	1 (1)	16 (10)	13 (8)	30 (19)
	Extended radical mastectomy (Dahl-Iversen and Tobiassen)	134	3 (2)	14 (10)	10 (8)	27 (20)
	Radical mastectomy (Haagensen and Cooley)	344	13 (4)	12 (3)	0 (0)	25 (7)
B	Total mastectomy plus axillary dissection plus irradiation	57	0 (0)	7 (12)	8 (14)	15 (26)
	Conservative radical mastectomy	58	3 (0)	13 (22)	0 (0)	16 (26)
	McWhirter method	28	0 (0)	3 (11)	5 (18)	8 (29)
	Extended radical mastectomy	32	0 (0)	5 (16)	5 (16)	10 (32)
	Radical mastectomy	138	7 (5)	18 (13)	1 (1)	25 (18)

*Compiled from Kaae and Johansen (1969).

*This table relates local recurrences to the stage of disease rather than to the operative procedures. Reproduced courtesy of Mosby, Year Book.

A monumental study of the pathology of breast cancers removed in the NSABP B-04 study attempted to identify a pathological and clinical profile with prognostic and therapeutic implications. In this study, Fisher[31] found that lymph node metastases were highly correlated with "bad" nuclear grade and "bad" histologic grade. Fisher stated: "nodal status does appear related to tumor differentiation—a relationship that in subsequent observations leads me to consider it almost axiomatic."[32] McDivitt[33] and Meyer[34] have reported extensive studies of the primary tumor with reference to ploidy, S-phase fractions (SpF), border contour, thymidine labeling index and flow cytometry. They attempted to correlate these with steroid receptors as well as a pathological review, which included size, number of nodes, histologic type, border contour, amount of invasive tumor necrosis, histologic and cytologic grades, presence or absence of lymphatic invasion, and number of mitoses per 10 high-powered fields. They observed a "high degree of correlation between lymphatic invasion and the presence of axillary node metastases (chi square 28.6)" and felt that "if confirmed it could prove useful in estimating pathologic stage from biopsy specimens." There was no correlation with any other element. A small study by Frank[35] found lymphatic invasion in 4 of 22 stage I tumors and 9 of 14 stage II tumors when tissue specimens were reviewed without knowledge of the axillary status. These differences are significant at the $P = 0.005$ level. He failed to find differences in tumor margin, mitoses, lymphocytic infiltration, degree of cellular differentiation, nuclear atypia, associated fibroplasia, or intraductal/invasive ratio. Kim[36] proposed that the "lymph node homing" property of carcinoma cells might be acquired by incorporating lymphocyte genomes through somatic hybridization. His group tested this in rats with mammary tumor cell lines and concluded that the acquisition of lymphotrophicism by the rat tumor cells had been achieved. Similar chimerism was found in other rat mammary cell lines. Perhaps most significantly they also noted this to be present in all stage II human breast cancer cells, whereas some stage I cancer cells had the T-cell markers and others did not.

The capability to invade lymphatics and/or blood vessels may be related to properties within the tumor cell itself, e.g., ameboid motion, lymphocyte homing genomes, metalloproteinases or others, or possibly to the vascular or lymphatic endothelium, and it may be these properties that determine the presence and extent of axillary nodal metastases as opposed to disseminated disease that has not traversed the axillary nodes. Further studies in this area will almost certainly yield fruit in terms of the invasive properties possessed by breast cancer cells and their display in terms of survival or local recurrence.[37]

The Clinical Evidence

In an earlier report on this subject,[38] this author suggested that there was sufficient evidence to state that the response to tamoxifen in stage II postmenopausal women was different than in stage I postmenopausal women.[39,40] Evidence for these observations is difficult to obtain because few trials separate patients in a node-negative/node-positive fashion within any trial and relate differences in response to treatment to those stages. Thus, I now believe that evidence regarding the response to tamoxifen between cancer stages is too vague to rely upon. There is little evidence to suggest that response to treatment, either adjuvant or salvage, is different between the two stages.

Conclusions

From the Data

1. Staging of breast cancer by axillary node involvement constitutes a separation into two groups that die at steady but different rates.

2. Stage II patients probably do not "come later" but have a different type of tumor than stage I.

3. Stage II is probably not simply a later consequence of stage I and does not represent a delay in diagnosis.

The Significance of It All

If one accepts that the above data are correct, then the significance of these data must be determined.

Statistical

Statistical significance of differences between the stages has been demonstrated and it is this that leads to the conclusion that stage I and stage II represent two variants of the breast cancer problem.

Biological

At present, the biological significance is fairly minimal or unclear. If it is accepted that the two stages are biologically different, then perhaps this may lead to an exploration of and final explanation of the nature of the invasive and metastatic potential of one set of cells versus another.

Clinical

The significance of these observations on clinical practice is probably not very great. Already the two stages are looked upon as being chronologically different, and generally speaking, stage II is credited with having early relapses whereas stage I has later relapses. These ideas derive from direct (fixed-time) measurements rather than life-table analysis. Regardless of stage, however, everyone seems to attempt to identify women who die early as opposed to those who will die later. As currently used, staging does *not* do this, for in both stages there are women who die early and in both stages there are women who die later. Staging creates two groups of patients who die at different rates, not earlier and later.

Legal

The legal significance of these observations is probably the most important, for they cast doubt upon implicit or self-evident allegations regarding "delay in diagnosis," allegations that lead to extensive litigation with the expenditure of money and time in legal action.

References

1. Langlands AO, Kerr GR: Prognosis in breast cancer: the relevance of clinical staging. Clin Radiol 1978; 29:598–606.
2. Reporting of cancer survival and end results. In: Beahrs OH, Hensen DE, et al. (eds) Manual for Staging of Cancer. JP Lippincott, Philadelphia, pp 11–23, 1988.
3. Handley WS: Cancer of the Breast and its Treatment. 2nd Ed. John Murray, London, 1922.
4. Bross IDJ, Blumensen LE: Statistical testing of a deep mathematical model for human breast cancer. J Chron Dis 1968; 21:493–506.
5. Blumensen LE, Bross IDJ: A mathematical analysis of the growth and spread of breast cancer. Biometrics 1969; 25:95–109.
6. Slack NH, Blumensen LE, Bross IDJ: Therapeutic implications from a mathematical model characterizing the course of breast cancer. Cancer 1969; 24:960–971.
7. Bross IDJ, Blumensen LE, Slack NH, Prioro RL: A two-disease model for breast cancer. In: Forrest APM, Kunkler PB (eds). Prognostic Factors in Breast Cancer. E & S Livingstone, Edinburgh, pp 288–300, 1967.
8. Hakama M: The peculiar age-specific incidence for cancer of the breast: Clemmensen's hook. Acta Path Microbiol Scand 1969; 75:370–374.
9. de Waard F, Baanders-van Halewijn EA, Huizinga J: The biomodal age distribution of patients with mammary carcinoma. Cancer 1964; 17:141–150.
10. Devitt JE: The clinical stages of breast cancer: what do they mean? Can Med Assoc J 1967; 97:1257–1261.
11. Devitt JE: The enigmatic behavior of breast cancer. Cancer 1971; 27:13–17.
12. Colton T: Longitudinal studies and use of life tables. In: Statistics in Medicine. Little Brown & Co, Boston, Chap. 9, 1974.
13. Metcalfe W: Analysis of cancer survival as an exponential phenomenon. Surg Gyn Obst 1974; 138:730–738.
14. Sackett DL, Haynes RB, Tugwell P: Clinical Epidemiology: A Basic Science for Medicine. Little Brown and Co, Boston/Toronto, pp 146–148, 1985.
15. Fisher B, Redmond C, Fisher ER, et al: Ten-year results of a randomized clinical trial comparing radical mastectomy and total mastectomy with or without irradiation. N Engl J Med 1985; 312:674–681.
16. Metcalfe W: Accurate representations, comparisons and predictions for operable breast cancer. Albert Einstein College of Medicine NY, 1981.
17. Fisher B, Wolmark N, Bauer M, et al: The accuracy of clinical node staging and of limited axillary dissection as a determinant of histologic nodal status in carcinoma of the breast. Surg Obstet Gynecol 1981; 152:765–772.
18. Donegan WL, Perez-Mesa CM, Watson FR: A biostatistical study of locally recurrent breast carcinoma. Surg Gynecol Obstet 1966; 112:529–539.
19. Dao RH, Nemoto T: The clinical significance of skin recurrence after radical mastectomy in women with cancer of the breast. Surg Gynecol Obstet 1963; 117:447–453.
20. Spratt JS: Locally recurrent cancer after mastectomy. Cancer 1967; 20:1051–1053.

21. Carter RL: Significance of local recurrence. In: Stoll BA (ed). Secondary Spread of Breast Cancer. London, William Heineman Medical Books, 1977.
22. Clark GM, Sledge GW Jr, Osborne CK, McGuire WL: Survival from first recurrence: relative importance of the prognostic factors in 1015 breast cancer patients. J Clin Oncol 1987; 5(1):55–61.
23. Gump F, Habif DV, Logerfo P, et al: The extent and distribution of cancer in breasts with palpable primary tumors. Ann Surg 1986; 204:384–390.
24. Forrest APM: Conservative local treatment of breast cancer. Cancer 1977; 39:2813–2821.
25. Brooman P, Taylor I, Rouling ST: Results of an aggressive treatment policy towards carcinoma of the breast. Br J Clin Pract 1977; 31:102–104.
26. Donegan WL: Local and regional recurrence. In: Donegan WL, Spratt JS (eds). Cancer of the Breast. WB Saunders Co, Philadelphia, 1979.
27. White WC: The problem of local recurrence after radical mastectomy for carcinoma. Surgery 1946; 19:149–153.
28. Fisher B, Bauer M, Margolese R: Five-year results of a randomized clinical trial comparing total mastectomy and segmental mastectomy with or without radiation in the treatment of breast cancer. N Engl J Med 1985; 312:665–673.
29. McDivitt RW, Stewart FS, Berg JJ: Breast tumor pathology. In: Atlas of Tumor Pathology, Series 2. Armed Forces Institute of Pathology, Washington, DC, pp 52, 1967.
30. Hellman S, Harris JR, Canellos GP, Fisher B: Cancer of the breast. In: De Vita, VT Jr, Hellman S, Rosenberg SA (eds). Cancer: Principles and Practice of Oncology. JP Lippincott, Philadelphia, pp 915, 1982.
31. Fisher ER, Gergorio RM, Fisher B, et al: The pathology of invasive breast cancer. Cancer 1975; 36:1–85.
32. Fisher E: Personal communication.
33. McDivitt RW, Stone KR, Craig RB, et al: A proposed classification of breast cancer based on kinetic information. Cancer 1986; 57:269–276.
34. Meyer JS, Lee JY: Relationships of S-phase fraction of breast carcinoma in relapse to duration of remission, estrogen receptor content, therapeutic responsiveness, and duration of survival. Cancer Research 1980; 40:1890–1896.
35. Frank G: Personal communication.
36. Kim U, Kadohama N, Srivastara S, et al: T-cell chimerism in lymphotrophic mammary cancer cells. Breast Cancer Res Treat 1988; 12:144.
37. Liotta LA: Cancer cell invasion and metastasis. Sci Am 1992; 266:54–63.
38. Mueller CB: Stage II breast cancer is not simply a late stage I. Surgery 1988; 104:631–638.
39. Breast Cancer Trials Committee: Adjuvant tamoxifen in the management of operable breast cancer: the Scottish Trial. Lancet 1987; 11:171–173.
40. Nolvadex Adjuvant Trial Organisation: Controlled trial of tamoxifen as single adjuvant agent in management of early breast cancer. Lancet 1985; 1:837–839.

5

Is Breast Cancer "Curable"?

C. Barber Mueller

That "cancer is curable" is an unquestioned belief of many physicians, as well as a basic hope of the lay public, particularly those whose lives have been touched by it. As a rallying cry of the American Cancer Society, it carries the caveat that cancer is curable only *if* it is treated *early* enough. "If" is an uncertain possibility that does not lend itself to measurement and "early" has not been defined, even though it is generally felt to be related to size rather than to a biological potential for growth and metastasis. Thus the caveat renders the initial premise an act of faith not a statement of fact; it is unable to be measured. "Cure" has never been defined as a measurable outcome and it certainly is not a 5-year survival statistic. Everyone having contact with this disease must have developed some general concept of it and all concepts are not necessarily the same since they may be framed in DNA, cell, metastasis, sick people, or epidemiologic terms. Conventional wisdom holds that breast cancer is a disease of epithelial cells that have developed the ability to invade the basement membrane, be transported to distant sites, and ultimately cause death of the host. No conventional concept of "cure" has been formulated and probably the word should not be applied to this disease. The Random House Dictionary states cure is "to relieve or rid of something detrimental," and if this definition were to apply to breast cancer, cure would become "the provision of a state in which no cells from the primary breast cancer reside in any location in the host." Although such a state may be imagined, it cannot be measured and is not useful either as a scientific concept or as a measurable outcome, though it remains a very useful emotional, political, and financial concept.

Other definitions of cure have been stated. Plotkin[1] writes that cure is the "elimination of hazard of death due to breast cancer." Haybittle[2] believes that a personal cure will occur when "a significant proportion of patients will . . . live without overt signs of their breast cancer until they die from some other cause."

From: Wise L, Johnson H Jr (eds): *Breast Cancer: Controversies in Management.* Futura Publishing Company, Inc., Armonk, NY, © 1994.

53

Brinkley and Haybittle[3] state that it ". . . may be uncertain whether treatment can "cure" in the absolute sense . . . a portion of patients remain symptom-free until their death from other causes . . . and would personally consider themselves to have been cured." As a statistical definition, cure is achieved when the death rate of the group of women with breast cancer is identical to the death rate of a comparable group of women who have never had breast cancer and are dying of other causes. Statistical cure may be achieved even though some of the deaths are still caused by breast cancer since the subject group has attained a normal mortality risk. This is yet to be demonstrated in breast cancer.

Cure, if it were to happen, must be the consequence of an act of commission that alters a preordained lethality. If so, it should be seen only if the natural history is modified by some therapeutic intervention and would be described only in group terms, for it could never be seen in an individual since an individual's future is unknown and unmeasurable. It is both possible and probable to imagine that there are many women with breast cancer in whom no known therapeutic intervention would have an effect on survival. It is also possible, however improbable, to imagine that a small subgroup exists in which some therapeutic intervention would produce a "cure." Cure, then, will require at least two basic assumptions. First, if untreated, death will result and second, if treated, there will be a measurable modification of the expected natural history, either in an individual (impossible to measure) or in a group.

This leads to a consideration of what can be measured. Following the development of breast cancer and some type of intervention, there are five things that lend themselves to measurement. They may be reported on an individual basis, or by using statistical techniques, they may be dealt with as a group. They are:
1. survival;
2. disease-free interval;
3. cause of death;
4. local recurrence;
5. quality of life.

In Chapter 3 of this volume, the natural history of breast cancer is described,[4] and 5-, 10-, and 15-year survivorship of "all comers" is displayed, utilizing the direct measure of survival. If direct measurements are utilized, cure should be reflected by an improvement in the 5-, 10-, or 15-year survival percentage. Crude postdiagnostic 5-year survival rates are reported in the neighborhood of 40% to 50% and may be improved by the selection of more favorable groups, ages, or stages and likewise may be worsened by the selection or inclusion of less favorable groups, ages, or stages. Fixed-term survival has many co-variants that influence this temporal outcome but do not represent a basic change in the issue of "curability." If there exists a subgroup of women that has a greater percentage alive at 5 years, then the diagnostic identification of this subgroup becomes more important than the therapeutic intervention. This survival problem is further confounded since it may be accomplished by (1) changing the starting time, (2) introducing less aggressive stages, or (3) including different ages. Table 2 in Chapter 3 demonstrates the effect of stage at the time of diagnosis, and the influence of age as well as stage has been addressed by Mueller.[4,5]

When life-table analysis is used as the statistical technique, a modification of survival will be seen in a change in the death rate, something that requires the comparison of the death rate in two groups. The benefits may be only a delay in death, not the elimination of death. Data from Syracuse indicate that at 20 years approximately 80% of the women who developed breast cancer had died. This is in keeping with the information that comes from fixed-time survival (Fig. 1).[4]

"Cure" must also be addressed by looking at "cause of death" data, acknowledging that cure is related not only to time of death but also to its cause. "Cause of death" information can be based only on those who have died. When the Syracuse registry of 3,558 women was examined, 1,660 had died, and approximately 88% did so because of their breast cancer.[5] Although these percentages cannot be used to conclude that the 1,898 women still alive at the time of that report would die with similar causes of death, it does emphasize the lethality of the disease. If "cure" is achievable, it should probably require that the cause of death be changed as well as the time of death, i.e., there should be an increase in the percentage of deaths due to other causes. To do this, consideration must be given to age at diagnosis since our population is aging and older women are more likely to develop breast cancer but die of other causes. Consideration must also be given to stage at diagnosis, for new breast cancers now produced by refined imaging techniques are increasingly likely to be ductal carcinoma in situ (DCIS) or lobular carcinoma in situ (LCIS).[6] Inclusion of these women will prolong postdiagnostic survival time as well as provide an increase in deaths due to other causes since both of these states appear to be markers of upcoming cancer, not lethal disease per se.

The Cambridge Study of 704 women found that at 35 years, approximately 3% to 3½% of the women with a prior diagnosis of breast cancer were alive. Of those who had died during the 20–25 year interval, 25% were node-positive at the time of diagnosis. During the 30–35 year period, approximately 40% of the women who died had done so because of their breast cancer (Figs. 2A, B).[3,7]

Adjuvant chemotherapy or hormonal therapy given postoperatively became popular in clinical trials during the 1970s to 1990s. Many of these trials claim that such therapy reduces the mortality rates of breast cancer by 10% to 25%. Such claims occur when two groups are compared using a fixed (specific) time such as 5 to 10 years as the end-point. This statistical maneuver uses the "relative risk reduction" ratio rather than "actual" benefits. These studies calculate "relative risk" by using the control survival figure as the denominator and the difference between it and the experimental figure as the numerator. "Actual" benefits utilize 100% as the denominator and the percentage difference between the two as the numerator (Fig. 3).

Whenever measurements are made at a specific or fixed time, they do not take into account the fact that both groups *always* achieve the same percent survival but do so at different times. In reviewing the multitude of graphic presentations that portray a percent reduction in mortality at a fixed time, it appears equally explicit to expand this observation and state that the results of an

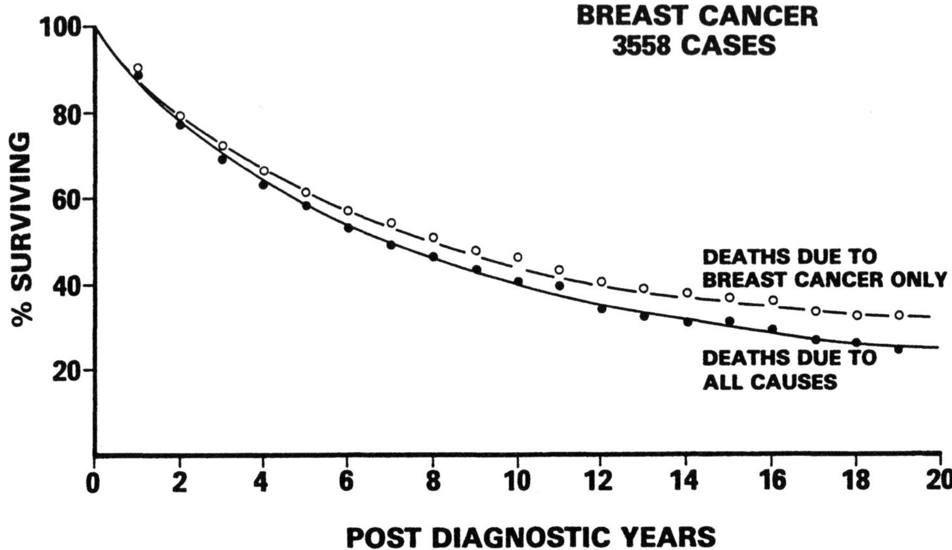

Figure 1: *Life-table analysis of 3,558 women showing decreasing survival by deaths due to all causes as well as deaths due to breast cancer. From Mueller CB, et al.*[5]

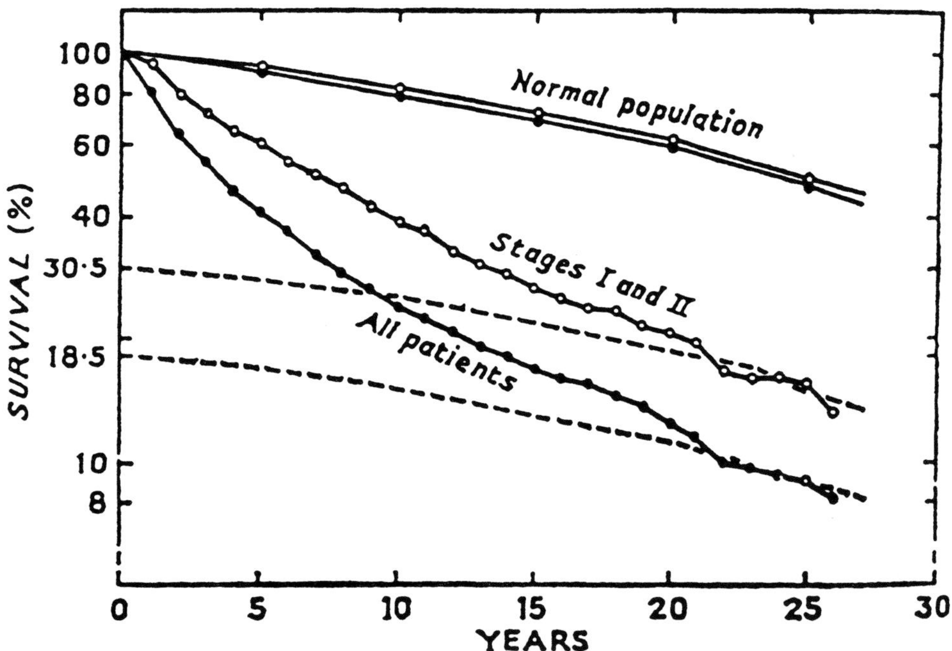

Figure 2A: *Survival rates after treatment in 704 cases of cancer of the breast compared with the expected survival of the normal populations of the same age group. The interrupted lines show extrapolation back to zero time of the portion of the curves which are approximately parallel to those of the corresponding normal populations. This represents "statistical cure." The intercepts on the vertical axis show the size of the "cured" group. From Brinkley D, et al.*[7]

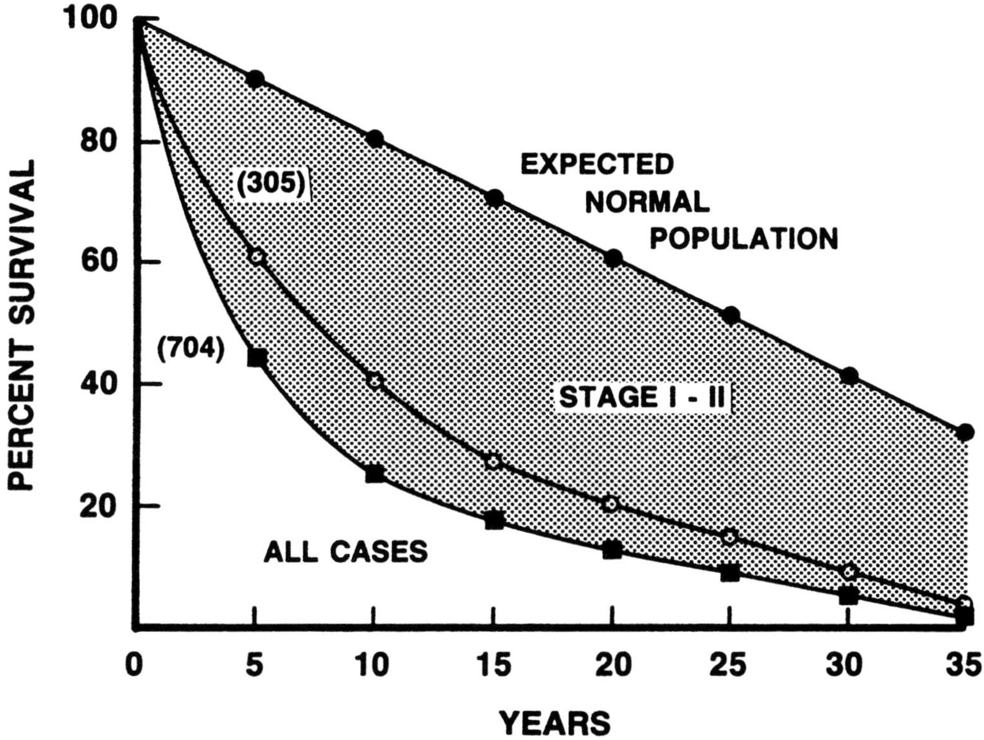

Figure 2B: *The survival rates after treatment in 704 cases of breast cancer compared with the expected survival of the normal populations of the same age groups. This figure is drawn to an arithmetic ordinate rather than logarithmic and contains the same data as shown in Figure 2A, with an extension for a further 10 years. Redrawn from Brinkley D, et al.[3]*

intervention such as adjuvant chemotherapy may give 5% to 7% of the women a delay in death of 12–14 months. This then represents not a reduction in mortality rate but a delay in death—not a "cure" (Fig. 4).

Delay in death is an admirable therapeutic objective, but only if the delay is longer in duration than the illness that is occasioned by adjuvant chemotherapy. In the meta-analyses conducted by Peto and his group, the 5-year benefits generally showed that 5% to 7% of the women achieved a delay of 12–18 months in mortality.[8] At present, adjuvant chemotherapy is proposed to be of benefit chiefly in one small subgroup—premenopausal stage II women, a group estimated to be no more than 20% of the total number of women who develop breast cancer. A marginal benefit in this group will not be seen in overall mortality figures. The results of adjuvant chemotherapy to node-negative women are even more marginal.[9]

The General Accounting Office was asked by a committee of Congress to review the benefits of chemotherapy to the premenopausal stage II subgroup of patients.[10] The report describes an 8-year period during which adjuvant chemo-

RELATIVE/ACTUAL

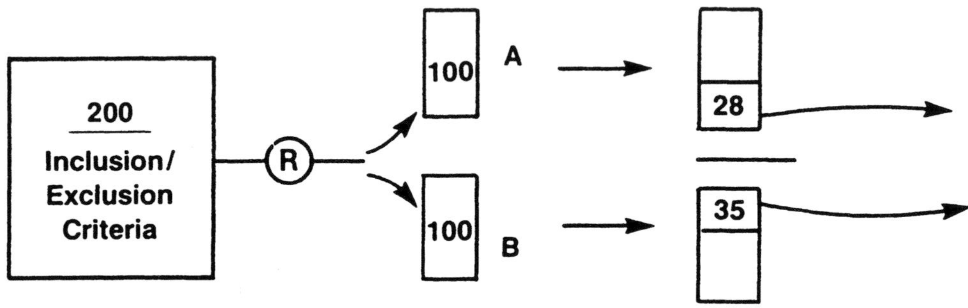

RELATIVE   **35 : 28 = 20% reduction**

ACTUAL   **7/100 = 7% benefit /100 treated (93 no benefit)**

Figure 3: *A schema to show the two methods of reporting results of a clinical trial. Here, 200 women are randomized to treatments A or B. Upon subsequent analysis, treatment A shows 28 women with recurrence and B shows 35. "Actual" reports the percent benefitted—here 7%. "Relative" describes the percent improvement as 7/35 or 20%. Relative reporting constructs a ratio between the two outcomes, whereas actual is the difference between them. Even though both are correct, they convey a different message.*

therapy administered to stage II premenopausal women increased from approximately 20% to 70%; no improvement in survival was found at 3, 5, or 7 years. This study utilized SEER data and was sufficiently powerful to pick up the claimed 20% to 25% relative survival benefit, but acknowledged that it might be unable to detect a benefit as small as 6% to 7%. At present, evidence suggests that adjuvant chemotherapy has had only marginal, immeasurable impact on the survivability (curability?) of breast cancer even in the premenopausal node-positive group.

Plotkin wrote "available evidence leads to the conclusion that . . . cure of invasive breast cancer is not possible. Death due to metastatic disease is postponable at times, but never avoidable unless competing fatal illness intervenes."[1] There is little evidence that any intervention other than complete removal of the primary tumor has benefits that can be seen either in survival time or in cause of death.[11]

In an attempt to answer the initial question—Is breast cancer curable?—it may be stated unequivocally that some women do survive for 20, 30, or 40 years following mastectomy for breast cancer to die of other causes. If this constitutes a personal cure then, "yes," breast cancer is occasionally curable. This group must represent perhaps 15%, certainly no more than 20%, of those who develop

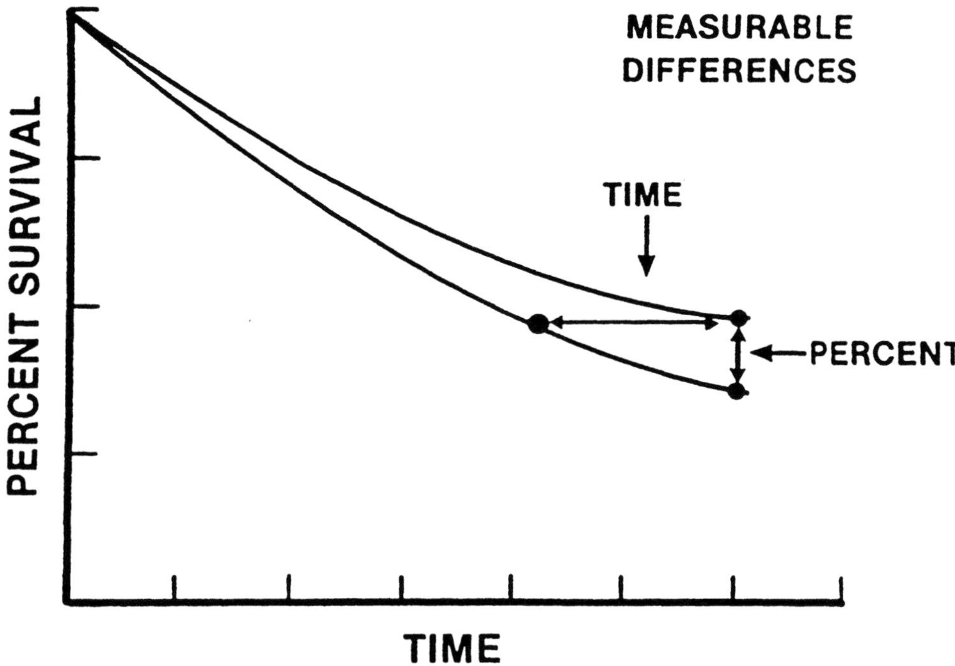

Figure 4: *Theoretical life-table analyses showing the decreasing survival rates of two groups under study. The curves may be compared at a fixed time, producing percentage differences, or at a fixed percent, producing time differences. The use of both indices is the complete way in which to express differences between two groups being compared. From Mueller CB: Adjuvant chemotherapy for breast cancer: ethical considerations. Bull Am Coll Surgeons.*

the disease. It does acknowledge the fact that young women on reasonably rare occasions, following the removal of their breast for cancer, are free of the clinical metastatic manifestations of breast cancer until they die of other causes many years later.

References

1. Plotkin D, Blankenberg F: Breast cancer: biology and malpractice. Am J Clin Oncol 1991; 14:254–266.
2. Haybittle JL: The evidence for cure in female breast cancer. In: Bulbrook RD, Taylor DJ (eds). Commentaries on Research on Breast Disease, Vol III. Alan Liss, New York, pp 181, 1983.
3. Brinkley D, Haybittle JL: Long-term survival of women with breast cancer. Lancet 1984; i:1118.
4. Mueller CB: The natural history of breast cancer. In: Wise L, Johnson H (eds). Breast Cancer: Controversies in Management. Futura Publishing Co, Inc, Mt. Kisco, NY, Chapter 3, 1993.

  5. Mueller CB, Ames F, Anderson G: Breast cancer in 3558 women: age as a significant determinant in the rate of dying and causes of death. Surgery 1978; 83:123–134.
  6. Kelly PT: Risk of breast cancer: some genetic and epidemiologic factors. In: Postmastectomy Reconstruction, 2nd Ed. Gant TD, Vasconez LO (eds). Williams and Wilkins, Baltimore, pp 18–27, 1988.
  7. Brinkley D, Haybittle JL: The curability of breast cancer. Lancet 1975; ii:95–101.
  8. Early Breast Cancer Trialists Collaborative Group: *The Treatment of Early Breast Cancer, Vol I. Worldwide Evidence, 1985–1990.* Oxford University Press, New York, 1990.
  9. Mueller CB: The disease-free interval in breast cancer trials: scientific or spurious? Surgery 1991; 110:629–635.
 10. Breast cancer, patients' survival. GAO/PEMD 89-9. U.S. General Accounting Office, Washington, D.C.
 11. Mueller CB: Valid alternatives in the management of early breast cancer. In: Advances in Surgery. Year Book Medical Publisher, Chicago, pp 183–216, 1987.

6

Does Surgery Influence the Natural History of Breast Cancer?

Michael Baum, Raj A. Badwe

Introduction

Surgery has been the primary treatment for breast cancer for over 100 years. Such a prolonged "affair" needs to be examined in the light of contemporary biological theory and clinical experience.

Pre-Halstedian Era

The unfortunate victim of breast cancer in the pre-Halstedian era would suffer from uncontrolled, malodorous, fungating disease with or without excruciating pain, culminating in the patient being shunned by her relatives and society. Such poor quality of life was not always mercifully short. The 5-year survival from diagnosis ranged from 11–18%.[1-3] Gross reported 97 untreated patients where skin infiltration appeared 14 months after detection of the primary, skin ulceration followed 6 months later, and 5% were alive at the end of 7 years.[1] Greenwood found 10% of 651 patients alive at the end of 6 years without treatment.[2] Bloom in his classic study reported 18%, 3.6%, and 0.8% survivors at the end of 5, 10, and 15 years, respectively, in 250 untreated breast cancer patients.[3] It must be noted that these data speak of stage III and IV disease at the time of diagnosis. After the development of anesthesia and antisepsis more and more patients with breast cancer were subjected to total mastectomy with or without removal of clinically obvious lymph nodes. These early years following the introduction of surgery were paradoxically associated with a rise in breast cancer mortality in England and Wales.[4]

From: Wise L, Johnson H Jr (eds): *Breast Cancer: Controversies in Management*. Futura Publishing Company, Inc., Armonk, NY, © 1994.

61

The Halstedian Era

The approach to breast cancer was revolutionized by the description of the Halsted-Handley hypothesis based on the pathological teachings of Virchow. This was an anatomical model derived from meticulous postmortem examination of the breast, axilla, and contiguous structures (pectoralis major and minor). It postulated growth of primary tumor within its organ of origin with subsequent invasion of lymph nodes by either permeation or embolization, followed by a third step of distant metastasis. It was then logical to subject patients to en bloc excision of the tumor-bearing organ with its lymphatic drainage.[5] Lewis and Rinehoff reporting results of this strategy from Johns Hopkins Hospital[6] found only 36% survival at 5 years and 12% at 10 years, which in comparison to the historical controls was a very modest gain. The scientific rationale was weak and the gains small, yet radical mastectomy evolved as an irrefutable dogma for the next the 50 years. There is no doubt that the widespread acceptance of this treatment can be attributed to its remarkable success in reducing the incidence of uncontrolled local disease and improvement in the quality of life. It was an era of an encounter between the enthusiastic surgeon armed with newly acquired techiniques, such as asepsis and anesthesia, attacking a chronologically old and advanced tumor. With the advent of staging systems to document the primary and metastatic tumor burden (Columbia Clinical Classification[7] and Manchester staging system[8]) the futility of such an exercise in increasing the length of life for locally advanced or metastatic disease was well documented. Radical surgery was then confined to early stage (A, B or I, II) disease.

The Deterministic Era

The deterministic era was marked by two important events. The first was Fisher's contribution to the biological model and the second was appreciation of the possible benefit of early detection.

The conceptual revolution was encouraged by the inescapable fact that a plateau in survival was observed, with about 45% dying of distant metastasis within 10 years despite radical surgical treatment of operable breast cancer. Fisher postulated that occult micrometastases existed prior to the diagnosis of clinically evident breast cancer. He considered the presence of lymph node metastasis to be a reliable sign of existence of micrometastases and not a source for tertiary spread.[9]

Randomized trials conducted by the National Surgical Adjuvant Breast Project (NSABP) in the United States[10] and the CRC in the United Kingdom[11] further paved the way for the resurrection of the deterministic model, which was first expressed in the writings of James Symes.[12] MacDonald[13] described this belief as "biological predeterminism," whereas Park and Lee[14] drew the same conclusion, that there was no time margin between the point of diagnosis and dissemination. This model provided justification for systemic therapy to suppress or eradicate micrometastasis. We now have mature data on adjuvant systemic therapy showing moderate gains in disease-free survival rates and modest increments in overall survival[15] that provide some objective evidence to support the deterministic model. This assumes that the dates of recurrence and death are relatively fixed points in the natural history of breast cancer, unaffected by diagnostic and therapeutic surgery in patients who are predetermined to relapse after primary treatment. The only determinant of survival is thought to be the existence and extent of occult micrometastases at the time of diagnosis and treatment. The reduction in case fatality rates following treatment for stage I tumor compared to stage II tumor is attributed to a "lead time bias."[16] The dominant role played by the surgeon in the Halstedian era is now reduced to that of a mere technician in this era of biological predeterminism where the medical oncologist rules the roost!

The second important consequence of the deterministic era was the development of mammographic screening for the early detection of breast cancer. This initiative followed the logical deduction that the case fatality rates following treatment of patients with smaller primary tumor burden would be reduced. The dictum then was "to catch when green." A number of trials of screening for breast cancer were instituted in the '70s and '80s. All the trials showed a significant reduction in cause-specific mortality over a follow-up of 7 years or more for women above the age of 50 years, but failed to show such benefit in women below the age of 50 years.[17–21] This implied that the outcome of interaction between surgery and reduction in tumor size at presentation was different in premenopausal and postmenopausal women. This is also evident in the national mortality statistics from 1950 to 1985. Figures 1A and 1B present the scenario from 1950 to 1985 as regards the incidence, mortality, average tumor size and hazard rates for death in pre- and postmenopausal women with breast cancer. In *postmenopausal* women, the age-adjusted incidence in 1950 was 160/100,000, rising gradually to 330/100,000 in 1985 (100% increase). The mortality increased by about 10% despite the fact that the average tumor size had fallen from 5 cm to less than 3 cm in the same period. In 1950 we were treating a smaller number of patients with larger tumors with greater hazard rates compared to 1985 when we treated a larger number of patients with smaller tumors with lesser hazard rates. In *premenopausal* women, the incidence increased by about 40% over the same years (compared to 100% in postmenopausal women). In spite of a reduction in the tumor size of the same magnitude, the mortality has shown a marginal reduction of less than 10%. This further confirms a differential impact of surgical intervention with reducing tumor burden on survival in pre- and postmenopausal women.

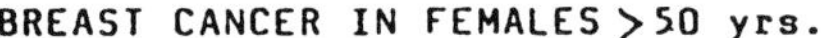

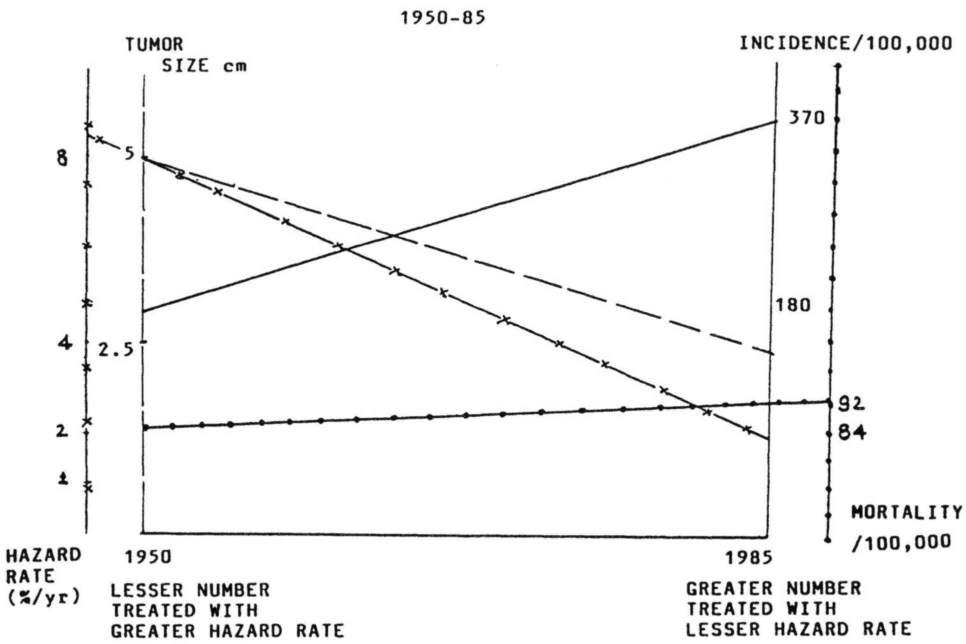

Figure 1A: *The negative impact of surgery is related to the degree of perturbation produced by surgical intervention. This is related to the levels of circulating unopposed estrogens and primary tumor burden at the time of treatment. The random event of surgery during the unopposed estrogen in women less than 50 years varies from 35% to 50%, depending on the number of perturbation related to surgery in reducing primary tumor surgical interventions carried out during the diagnosis and treatment of breast cancer. Hence, the reduction in the chance of burden is evident in only 35% to 50% of the total number of women less than 50 years of age. Unopposed estrogen of varying concentration is present in all postmenopausal women and hence the impact of the reduction in the perturbation-related surgery as the primary tumor burden reduces is evident in almost 100% of postmenopausal women. Figure 1A shows almost no change in mortality in women >50 years old in spite of >100% increase in the incidence of breast cancer. -x- = average annual hazard rate (5) for death; --- = mean tumor size (cm) at presentation; solid line = annual incidence of breast cancer (per 100,000); -•- = annual mortality for breast cancer (per 100,000). Cancer statistics review 1987, NCI, Division of Cancer Prevention and Control Surveillance Program.*

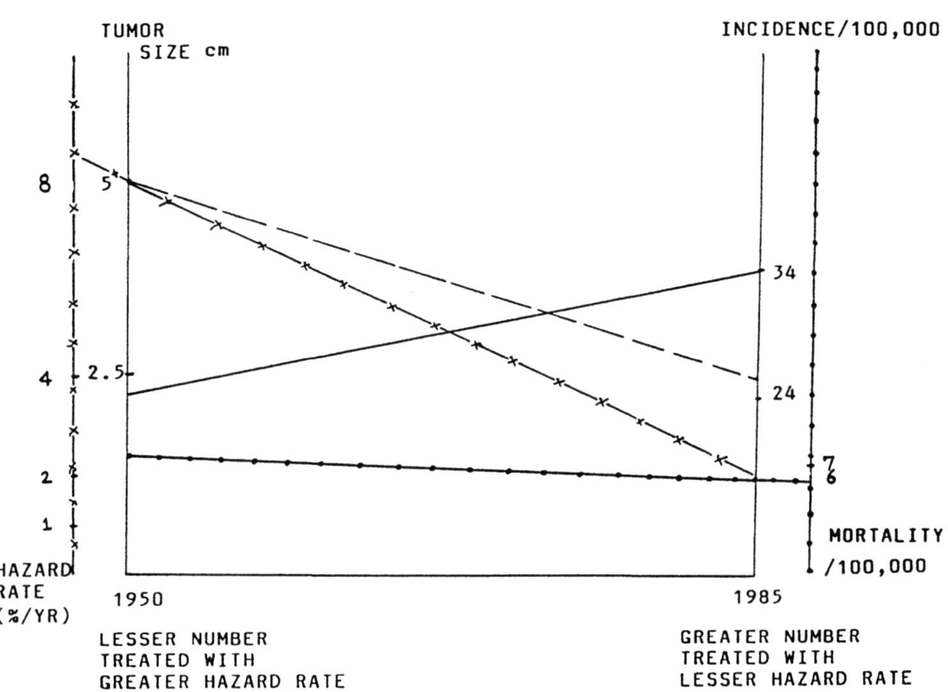

Figure 1B: *The graph shows a marginal reduction in mortality (<10%) in women <50 years in light of <40% rise in the incidence of breast cancer. As predicted by the argument put forth above, the gains related to reducing tumor burden in premenopausal women should be 35% to 50% of the gains in the postmenopausal women, which is evident in the figures. See Figure 1A legend for further explanation.*

The Role of Surgery Revisited: A Middle Pathway

If we examine the wealth of data from the randomized trials of the past we can refine our conclusions and probably shed new light on the biology of breast cancer.

The NSABP B-04[22] and the King's/Cambridge trial[11] proved that lesser procedures were as good as the radical mastectomy even if occult metastasis in the axillary nodes were left untreated. This should be interpreted to suggest that leaving tumor behind in the axilla does not affect the survival as a nidus for tertiary spread. Unfortunately, there has been no trial comparing surgery against untreated controls (the true natural history of breast cancer) to prove that surgery reduces cause-specific mortality.

A reexamination of the King's/Cambridge trial and Guy's Hospital database (in press) have yielded some interesting insights on the interaction between surgery and the natural history of breast cancer. The lifetable analysis demonstrates the expected differences in survival between T1 (<2 cm) and T2 (2–5 cm) tumors. The annual hazard rates for the same subgroups failed to reveal a lead time. The hazard for relapse for both groups began in the first year, albeit at a different magnitude (Fig. 2). The findings were similar for subgroups according to the number of lymph nodes with metastasis (Fig. 3). It was not that the smaller tumors recurred late and the larger tumors recurred early, but the smaller tumors recurred at a lesser rate compared to the larger tumors. The conventional theory teaches that the seeding of micrometastases occurs prior to the diagnosis and treatment of clinically detectable tumors and that the volume of these micrometastases is directly proportional to the primary tumor burden at the time of treatment. Existence of a lead time is pivotal in this theory, whereas the evidence from these large databases is contrary to this prediction.[23,24]

Studies on tumor doubling time estimate an average duration of 2 years for transition from stage I to II.[25,26] In the absence of a lead time, a patient with a stage I tumor may have an 11–17% chance of relapse and a 4–8% chance of death in 2 years following treatment, during which time in the estimated natural course

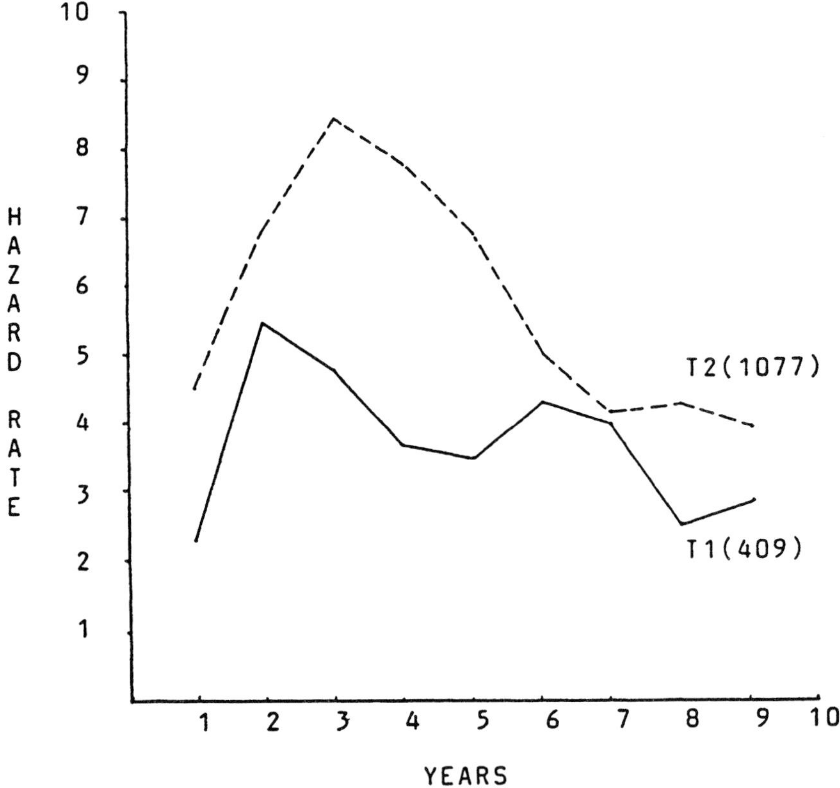

Figure 2: *Annual hazard rates for death by tumor size at presentation: King's/Cambridge trial. Hazard rate = % dying per year of those alive at the beginning of the year.*

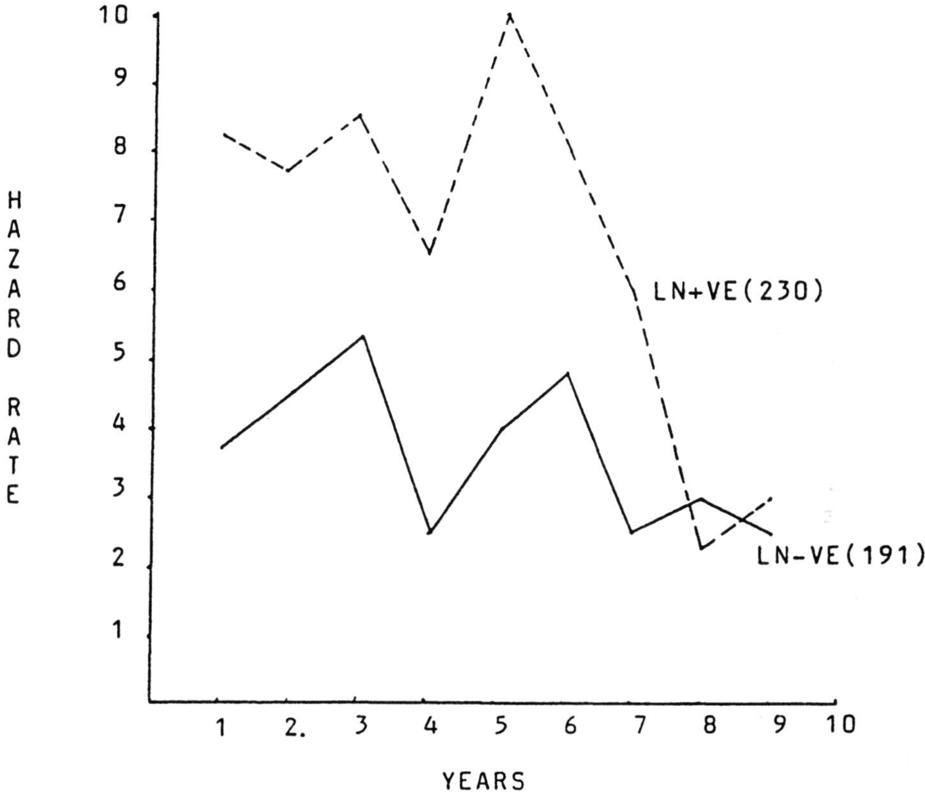

Figure 3: *Annual hazard rates for death by presence or absence of lymph node metastasis: King's/Cambridge trial.*

the tumor would progress to stage II. The incidence of metastatic disease at stage II is less than 3%,[27] and death prior to diagnosis of stage II is almost unknown. It is important to note that the outcome of surgery measured in terms of the proportion of long-term survivors is at least 20% better for stage I as compared to stage II. Thus, there appears to be a trade-off between accelerated relapse (8–14%) and death(4–8%) and a long-term gain in survival (20%).

Thus, in patients with operable breast cancer, the interaction between surgery and natural history of breast cancer appears to be biphasic. The proportion in whom this interaction is deleterious is determined by the primary tumor burden at the time of treatment. These findings can be explained by two hypotheses. The conventional explanation would suggest that the removal of the primary tumor bestows autonomy on the micrometastases resulting in acceleration of their growth and death of the host. This could be related to a complex interplay of stimulatory and inhibitory factors elaborated by the primary tumor.[28] The second possibility is that surgery itself disseminates tumor cells. This was postulated by Tyzzer[29] and later revived by Nissen-Myer[30] who used it as a justification for perioperative chemotherapy.

Recent publications related to the menstrual phase at the time of diagnostic and therapeutic surgery suggest that surgical handling of tumor during the unopposed estrogenic milieu is associated with a significantly worse survival. This effect was seen mainly in patients with lymph node metastasis. The events at the time of surgery seem to segregate tumors into metastasizing and non-metastasizing groups,[31-33] and if these results are true, the event of metastasis may be preventable by appropriate timing of surgery in premenopausal women and by replication of a favorable endocrine milieu in peri- and postmenopausal women with operable breast cancer.

The theoretical basis of understanding breast cancer and its interaction with treatment modalities has swung from an entirely anatomical (Halsted) view to the other extreme of biological determinism (Fisher). Both these theories fall short of explaining the available data from randomized trials and national incidence/mortality statistics.

References

1. Gross SW: A Practical Treatise of Tumors of the Mammary Gland. Appleton, New York, 1880.
2. Greenwood M: A report on the natural duration of cancer. Report on public health and medical subjects, London HMSO, No. 33, 1926.
3. Bloom HJG, Richardson WW, Harries EJ: Natural history of untreated breast cancer (1805–1933). Br Med J 1962; i:213–221.
4. Churchill JF: A letter to the Registrar General on the increase of cancer in England and its cause. D. Scott, London, 1888.
5. Halsted WS: The radical operation for the cure of cancer of the breast. Johns Hopkins Hosp Reports 1898; 28:557.
6. Lewis D, Rinehoff WF: A study of results of operations for cure of cancer of the breast performed at the Johns Hopkins Hospital for 1889–1931. Ann Surg 1932; 95:336.
7. Haagensen CD: Diseases of the Breast. WB Saunders, Philadelphia, 1986.
8. Patterson R: The Treatment of Malignant Diseases by Radium and X-rays. Edward Arnold, London, 1948.
9. Fisher B: Biology and clinical considerations regarding the use of surgery and chemotherapy in treatment of primary breast cancer. Cancer 1977; 40:574–587.
10. Fisher B, Slack NH, Cavanagh PJ, et al: Post-operative radiotherapy in treatment of breast cancer: results of NSABP trial. Ann Surg 1970; 172:711.
11. CRC working party CRC (King's/Cambridge) trial for early breast cancer: a detailed update at the tenth year. Lancet 1980; ii:55–60.
12. Symes J: Principles of surgery. Bailliere Tindall, London, 1842.
13. MacDonald I: Biological predeterminism in human cancer. Surg Gynecol Obstet 1951; 92:443.
14. Park WS, Lee JC: The absolute curability of cancer of the breast. Surg Gynecol Obstet 1951; 93:129.
15. Early breast cancer trialist collaborative group: systemic treatment of early breast cancer by hormonal, cytotoxic or immunotherapy. Lancet 1992; 339:1–15 & 71–85.
16. Shapiro S, Goldberg J, Hutchison G: Lead time in breast cancer detection and implication for periodicity of screening. Am J Epidemiol 1974; 100:357–366.
17. Shapiro S: Evidence on screening for breast cancer from a randomized trial. Cancer 1977; 39:2772–2782.

18. Tabar L, Gad A, Holmberg LH, et al: Reduction in mortality from breast cancer after mass screening with mammography. Lancet 1985; i:829–832.
19. UK trial of early detection of breast cancer group: the first results of mortality reduction. Lancet 1988; ii:411–416.
20. Verbeek AC, Hendricks JH, Holland R, et al: Reduction of breast cancer mortality through mass screening with modern mammography: Nijmegan Project. Lancet 1984; i:1222–1224.
21. Andersson I, Aspergren K, Janzon L, et al: Mammography screening and mortality in breast cancer: the Malmo Trial. Br Med J 1988; 297:944–948.
22. Fisher B, Redmond C, Fisher ER, et al: Ten-year results of a randomized trial comparing radical mastectomy and total mastectomy with/without radiotherapy. N Engl J Med 1985; 312:674–681.
23. Mueller CB: Stage II breast cancer is not simply late stage I. Surgery 1988; 104:631–638.
24. Gore S, Pocock SJ, Kerr GR: Regression models and non-proportional hazards in analysis of breast cancer survival. Appl Statist 1984; 33:176–195.
25. Tubiana M, Koscielny S: Natural history of breast cancer: recent data and clinical implications. Breast Cancer Research Treatment 1991; 18:125–140.
26. Gershon-Cohen J, Berger SM, Klickstein HS: Roentgenography of breast cancer moderating concept of "biological predeterminism." Cancer 1963; 16:961–964.
27. Coleman RE, Rubens RD, Fogleman I: Reppraisal of baseline bone scan in breast cancer. J Nucl Med 1988; 29:1045–1049.
28. Fisher B, Gunduz N, Coyle J, et al: Presence of growth stimulating factor in the serum following primary tumor removal in mice. Cancer Res 1989; 49:1996–2001.
29. Tyzzer EE: Factors in production and growth of tumor metastasis. J Med Res 1913: 28:309–332.
30. Nissen-Myer R: Adjuvant cytotoxic and endocrine therapy: increased cure rates or delayed manifest disease. Comment Res Breast Dis 1979;1:95–109.
31. Badwe RA, Gregory WM, Chaudary MA, et al: Timing of surgery during the menstrual cycle and survival of premenopausal women with operable breast cancer. Lancet 1991; 337:1261–1264.
32. Badwe RA, Fentiman IS, Richards MA, et al: Surgical procedures, menstrual cycle phase and prognosis in breast cancer (letter). Lancet 1991; 338:815–816.
33. Senie RT, Rosen PP, Rhodes P, Lesser ML: Timing of breast cancer excision during the menstrual cycle influences duration of disease-free survival. Ann Int Med 1991; 115:337–342.

Clinically Localized Breast Cancer Is Usually Curable

David W. Kinne

Introduction

Patients with breast cancer require a long term of follow-up after adequate local-regional and systemic therapy before assessing results. Complicating the assessment of curability are the relatively few series with 20 or more years of follow-up and some uncertainty about causes of death. Nevertheless, one would surmise that among the solid tumors we treat, breast cancer is far more curable than many, such as pancreatic or esophageal cancers.

What do we mean by cure? If we accept definitions listed in Webster's Unabridged Dictionary,[1] they are listed as:

1. a healing; the act of healing; restoration to health;
2. a remedy; that which makes one well; "Cold, hunger, prisons: ills without a cure." Dryden;
3. a system or method of medical treatment.

Using these definitions, clearly most breast cancers are curable. A more stringent definition, probably used in medical terms and implied in this controversy, means that patients treated for breast cancer remain free of disease for their lifetimes and die of other causes with no evidence of recurrence or spread of breast cancer. By this definition, proof is difficult, principally because of few long-term follow-up studies of breast cancer patients, and little evidence from autopsy studies as to actual causes of death is available. As Sir Thomas Browne (1605–1682) said, "We all labour against our own cure, for death is the cure of all diseases."

From: Wise L, Johnson H Jr (eds): *Breast Cancer: Controversies in Management.* Futura Publishing Company, Inc., Armonk, NY, © 1994.

Results

The natural history of breast cancer is characterized by a long duration and marked heterogeneity within and between patients. Breast cancer is among the more slowly growing tumors, and as a result, both the preclinical period (before diagnosis) and the clinical phases after initial treatment and metastases are measured in years and decades. Nevertheless, some patients have a very aggressive form of the disease and do poorly. An equal number have such an indolent form of the disease that it is difficult to demonstrate that therapy has any effect at all on survival. During the long clinical phase, there is ample opportunity for clonal mutation and evolution, and it seems probable that almost all breast cancer patients have multiple tumor clones, each with its own growth requirements, growth rates, propensity to metastasize, and sensitivity to drugs.[2]

The long natural history of breast cancer has been emphasized in about a half-dozen studies of patients with untreated breast cancer. Most of the patients in these studies were identified in the late nineteenth and early twentieth century, and then, as now, such patients were self-selected. Therefore, it cannot be assumed that they are truly representative of the full spectrum of breast cancer patients. All of these series include some patients who lived for two or three decades without any treatment at all.

By documenting the natural history of untreated breast cancer, one can establish a baseline by which to judge the effects of treatment. Since breast cancer has been considered a treatable disease for at least the last several hundred years, series of untreated but well-documented patients are not generally available. One such series is from Middlesex Hospital in England, where the first cancer wards were established in 1792.[3] They reported a group of 250 patients seen at Middlesex Hospital between 1805 and 1933. Patients were generally admitted to the hospital with advanced disease. Seventy-four percent were in stage IV, 23% in stage III, and only 2% in stage II. There were no stage I cases. Sixty-eight percent had ulceration when first seen in the hospital. No patient was treated with any form of surgery, radiotherapy, or hormone therapy. It is important to note that patients were not admitted to the hospital at the clinical onset of the disease but for terminal care. In all cases, a postmortem examination was performed. Because of the meticulous medical records kept, it was possible to determine the alleged onset of the disease with a fair degree of accuracy. Only 7% of the patients presented within 6 months of the initial symptom of the disease and only 29% within 1 year. The median survival time from the alleged onset of symptoms was 2.7 years. Eighteen percent of untreated patients survived 5 years, and 4% survived 10 years. These figures are comparable with those seen from other series and indicate that survival of breast cancer patients can be lengthy, even if the disease is untreated.

Much can be learned by plotting survival curves semilogarithmically for the Middlesex Hospital experience. This is approximately a straight line, indicating that the annual hazard or force of mortality (i.e., the percentage of remaining patients who die each year) is constant. In this group of patients, about 25% of the patients at the start of any year died by the end of that year.

Seen in modern times, results collected by the End Results Section of the Biometry Branch of the National Cancer Institute on a large group of patients treated for histologically confirmed breast cancer apply to patients who are treated for their cancer, and they are corrected for causes of death other than breast cancer.[4] This survival curve has been interpreted as showing that there are two subgroups of patients. One subgroup is manifested by the curve past 10 years and represents patients who have a force mortality of 2.5% per year. By backward extrapolation of this portion of the curve to time zero, one can estimate that this subgroup represents approximately 60% of the total group. The other subgroup has more aggressive disease with a force mortality of 25% per year, similar to that observed for untreated patients seen at Middlesex Hospital. These results suggest that breast cancer is not a homogeneous disease and that its natural history is even more protracted than was apparent in the Middlesex series. It is possible that there are clinically definable subsets of patients with a very high annual hazard of death (>25%) and other subsets with very low hazards of death (<2%). An alternative explanation is that breast disease is a single, but heterogeneous disease, in which patients fall along a continuum of biological aggressiveness.

An understanding of the survival curve for breast cancer patients is important in assessing new therapies, as Harris and Hellman have pointed out.[5] For most populations, the slope of the survival curve of treated breast cancer patients becomes considerably more shallow at 10 years (called the "inflection point"). The demonstration of a "cured" subgroup, therefore, requires follow-up of longer than 10 years. Improvements in the early portion of the survival curve by new therapies do not always result in an improvement in the survival curve past the inflection point. Conversely, in some cases, an early detrimental effect may obscure a benefit in long-term outcome. These considerations emphasize that effects seen on the early portion of survival curves may not only be premature but also may be misleading.

Henderson and Canellos[6] plotted the survival curve of patients treated by radical mastectomy at Johns Hopkins Hospital between 1889 and 1933 against the Middlesex series, and it is not much different from that of untreated patients. The percentages of patients who ultimately died as a direct result of breast cancer are almost identical in the two series. This comparison undermines the claim that the radical mastectomy is the proven therapy for breast cancer.

In all likelihood, these differences shown by Fox[4] may explain the observation of Mueller and Jeffries[7] that 80% to 85% of patients examined in their series died of breast cancer.

The heterogeneity of this disease can also be illustrated by the wide variability in growth rates as measured with labeling indices. The labeling index is a measure of the percentage of cells in a tumor that are undergoing cell division at a single point in time. Patients with high labeling indices are therefore more likely to have rapidly growing cancer than are those with low labeling indices.

About 60% of breast cancer patients have labeling indices less than 4%. The remaining 40% have indices that range from 4% to 41%.[8]

Our understanding of the preclinical behavior of breast cancer is dependent on either extrapolation backward from clinical observation or the use of tumor models. Both of these approaches have important limitations. Tumors large enough to be detected and measured in the clinic are likely to have a slower growth rate than microscopic preclinical lesions. Animal model tumors are usually selected because of a high growth fraction, which facilitates laboratory study. However, many human breast cancers have low growth fractions.

The relative growth rates of human tumors can be determined from clinical measurements, and these studies suggest that, on average, breast cancer has a lower labeling index, a longer doubling time, and a lower growth fraction than most other human tumors.[9] For example, the mean labeling index for adenocarcinomas consisting predominantly of breast cancer has been estimated to be 2.1%, compared with 29% for lymphomas. The doubling time for breast cancer is estimated to be about 83 days, compared with 27 days for embryonal tumors, and the growth fraction of breast cancer is about 6%, compared with 90% for embryonal tumors and lymphomas. These differences in growth fraction may be a factor in the greater success obtained in curing testicular cancers and lymphomas with chemotherapy.

The doubling time of breast cancer in its earliest clinical phases has been determined from measurements of lesions present but not initially appreciated as cancer in serial mammograms.[10–13] The observed doubling time in these studies averaged between 115 and 325 days, but the range of doubling times in individual patients extended from 23 days to more than 940 days.

It is usually assumed that the preclinical growth of breast cancer is logarithmic and continuous. Tumors can usually be palpated within the breast at a size of about 1 cm, and a sphere of this size could contain approximately 10^9 cells. Assuming origin of the cancer in a single-cell mutation, it would take 30 doublings for a malignant cell to produce 10^9 cells, assuming no cell loss during that interval. If all of these assumptions are true, and if one accepts a preclinical doubling time of about 100 days (a value substantially lower than all the mean values obtained in doubling-time measurements of clinically measurable lesions), then the preclinical phase of breast cancer should, on average, exceed 10 years. Even if breast cancer doubling times are actually one-half to one-fourth of that assumed in this illustration, the preclinical phase of breast cancer would still range from 2.5 to 5 years. Of course, these assumptions are all subject to challenge and may seriously underestimate differences in the growth rate of preclinical lesions growing logarithmically compared with clinically detectable lesions in a plateau phase of growth (i.e., Gompertzian growth). It is also possible that the preclinical growth of breast cancer is less than logarithmic or even discontinuous, in which case the preclinical phase would be even longer.

It has recently been suggested that the assumption that preclinical breast cancer growth is logarithmic is inconsistent with observations from large clinical studies. Utilizing data on the interval from initial diagnosis of breast cancer to the appearance of clinically detectable metastases, it has been concluded by mathematical modeling that preclinical breast cancer might be better characterized as having short spurts of logarithmic growth alternating with quiescent periods of little or no growth.[14] To further complicate the issue, it is plausible that growth at various metastatic sites within each patient is asynchronous.

The protracted nature of the above described survival curves raises the question of whether a patient with breast cancer is ever truly cured of the disease. There are several reasons why it is difficult to answer this question. Breast cancer has a relatively late age of onset and an extremely long natural history, with death from the disease occurring long after diagnosis. As a result, a large group of patients must be followed a very long time to begin to address this question. Furthermore, the definition of "cure" is not straightforward. It is possible to describe cure in a number of different ways. Haybittle has summarized these ways and the evidence for cure of the disease.[15] These various definitions of cure have not yet been found useful in an assessment of the impact of treatment. Given the heterogeneity of breast cancer as described earlier, it is possible that long-term survival after treatment may relate principally to the inherent biology of the patient's disease rather than to the treatment.

The most common concept of cure is referred to as *statistical* cure. A group of treated patients can be considered statistically cured if their subsequent death rate from all causes is similar to that of a normal population group with the same age and sex distribution. *Clinical* cure for an individual refers to the complete eradication of the disease. Clinical cure for a group occurs when long-term follow-up of the causes of death reveals that the risk of dying from breast cancer is the same as for women of the same age in the general population. An assessment of the likelihood of clinical cure involves determining the cause of death for treated patients. The unreliability of the information recorded on death certificates, however, greatly limits the usefulness of this definition of cure. *Personal* cure for an individual refers to a patient living symptom-free from breast cancer and dying of other causes.

Statistical cure is the usual method for assessing outcome in cancer treatment. Attempts to assess statistical cure in breast cancer patients have all indicated a persistent excess risk of mortality. Brinkley and Haybittle reported on a group of 704 breast cancer patients from the Cambridge, England, area, in whom the first diagnosis was made between 1947 and 1950. The minimum follow-up period for survivors was 31 years.[16] They calculated the survival curves by the lifetable method and compared them to the expected curves for the normal population of the region with the same age distribution. The survival curves for breast cancer patients never became parallel with those for the normal population. There were eight deaths from breast cancer more than 25 years after treatment, which is 15 times the number that would be expected. Hibberd et al. followed 2,019 cases for 30 years and found a small excess of observed over expected deaths even between 25 and 30 years.[17] Rutquist and Wallgren presented follow-up on 458 patients 40 years of age or younger at diagnosis and found an excess mortality that persisted for at least 40 years.[18] These studies all indicate a persistent excess risk of mortality after treatment for breast cancer.

Despite the lack of evidence for a statistical cure, a considerable percentage of patients will experience a personal cure, as defined earlier. In the Brinkley and Haybittle report, 176 (26%) of the 683 patients fell into this category.[16] In the experience from Memorial Sloan-Kettering Cancer Center reported by Adair et al., 300 of the 1,458 patients (21%) with operable breast cancer had a personal cure of their disease.[19] In a more recent report from Memorial Sloan-Kettering Cancer Center, Rosen et al.[20] reported on 382 patients with breast cancers 2 cm or smaller and negative axillary nodes treated with radical mastectomy and followed for a median of 18.2 years. Although recurrences were observed during the entire 20-year follow-up period, it was estimated that 80% of patients with tumors 1.0 cm or smaller would have personal cures, and 70% of patients with tumors 1.1 to 2.0 cm would have personal cures. This means that many patients treated for breast cancer will live out their normal life expectancy free of further evidence of the disease.

A similar long-term analysis of patients with T2NOMO has been reported by Rosen also.[21] In a study of prognosis in node-negative breast carcinoma, he investigated 293 T2NOMO patients treated by mastectomy and axillary dissection with a median follow-up of 19.8 years. The probability of surviving 20 years considering *all* causes of death was 41.3%. Recurrence-free survival (Kaplan-Meier estimate) was 68.6% at 10 years and 63.2% at 20 years. The estimated probability of cure determined by the method of Brinkley and Haybittle was 63%. Prognosis was related to primary tumor size with the best separation (P = .06) when tumors from 2.1 to 3.0 cm (33% chance of recurrence at 20 years) and from 3.1 to 5.0 cm (44% chance of recurrence at 20 years) were compared. All causes of death may, in other series, be ascribed to breast cancer, complicating accurate analysis of causes of death. The histologic tumor type was prognostically important. Recurrence at 20 years was not significantly different for patients with invasive duct (34%) and lobular (42%) carcinoma. Women with special types (medullary, mucinous, papillary, etc.) of carcinoma had a 25% chance of recurrence.

Summary

Although difficult to prove, and subject to complex statistical analyses, when the heterogeneity of breast cancer is taken into account, long-term follow-up suggests that a significant percentage of patients with local-regional breast cancer can be cured.

References

1. Webster's Unabridged Dictionary. Simon and Schuster, NY, 1983.
2. Henderson IC, Harris JR, Kinne DW, Hellman S: Cancer of the Breast. In: DeVita VT, Hellman S, et al. (eds). Principles and Practice of Oncology, 3rd Ed. JB Lippincott, Philadelphia, pp 1197–1202, 1989.
3. Bloom HJG, Richardson WW, Harrier EJ: Natural history of untreated breast cancer (1805–1933). Br Med J 1962; 2:213–221.

4. Fox MS: On the diagnosis and treatment of breast cancer. JAMA 1979; 241:489–494.
5. Harris JR, Hellman S: Observations on survival curve analysis with particular reference to breast cancer treatment. Cancer 1986; 57:925–928.
6. Henderson IC, Canellos GP: Cancer of the breast: the past decade. N Engl J Med 1980; 302:17–30.
7. Mueller CB, Jeffries W: Cancer of the breast: its outcome as measured by the rate of dying and causes of death. Ann Surg 1975; 182:334–341.
8. Silvestrini R, Daidone MG, Gentili C: Biologic characteristics of breast cancer and their clinical relevance. In: Bulbrook RD (ed): Commentaries on Research in Breast Disease, Vol 2. Alan R Liss, NY, pp 1–40, 1981.
9. Malaise EP, Chevaudra N, Tublana M: The relationship between growth rate, labelling index and histological type of human solid tumors. Eur J Cancer 1973; 9:305–312.
10. von Fournier D, Weber E, Hoeffken W, et al: Growth rate of 147 mammary carcinomas. Cancer 1980; 45:2198–2207.
11. Heuser L, Spratt JS, Polk HC: Growth rates of primary breast cancers. Cancer 1979; 43:1888–1894.
12. Lundgren B: Observations on growth rate of breast carcinomas and its possible implications for lead time. Cancer 1977; 40:1722–1725.
13. Gershon-Cohen J, Berger SM, Klickstein HS: Roentgenography of breast cancer moderating concept of "biologic determinism." Cancer 1963; 16:961–964.
14. Speer JF, Petrosky VE, Retsky MW, Wardwell RH: A stochastic numeral model of breast cancer growth that simulates clinical data. Cancer Res 1984; 44:4124–4230.
15. Haybittle JL: The evidence for cure in female breast cancer. Comment Res Breast Dis 1983; 3:181–194.
16. Brinkley D, Haybittle JL: Long-term survival of women with breast cancer. Lancet 1984; 1:1118.
17. Hibberd AD, Harwood IJ, Wells JE: Long-term prognosis of women with breast cancer in New Zealand: study of survival to 30 years. Br Med J 1983; 286:1777–1779.
18. Rutquist LE, Wallgren A: Long-term survival of 458 young breast cancer patients. Cancer 1985; 55:658–665.
19. Adair F, Berg J, Joubert L: Long-term follow-up of breast cancer patients: The thirty-year report. Cancer 1974; 33:1145—1150.
20. Rosen PP, Groshen S, Saigo PE, et al: A long-term follow-up study of survival in stage I (TINOMO) and stage II (TINIMO) breast carcinoma. J Clin Oncol 1989; 7:355–366.
21. Rosen PP, Groshen S, Kinne DW: Prognosis in T2NOMO stage I breast carcinoma: a 20-year follow-up study. J Clin Oncol 1991; 9:1650–1661.

The Management of Clinically Curable Breast Cancer

Editorial Commentary

Chapter 8

Dr. Maddox's chapter is important because it emphasizes a now not very popular thesis: namely that radical mastectomy may still have some role in the management of breast cancer. At a 15-year follow-up of a randomized trial comparing radical mastectomy with modified radical mastectomy, the local recurrence rate was higher ($P = 0.04$) in the modified radical mastectomy group and the overall survival was higher ($P = 0.05$) in the radical mastectomy group. We do not agree with Dr. Maddox's conclusion that radical mastectomy is a viable option for patients who do not want to undergo chemotherapy, since the main purpose of chemotherapy is to deal with distant metastases and this does not seem to be affected by the type of local therapy.

Chapter 9

Although Dr. Kinne agrees that the overall results of mastectomy are not different from that of lumpectomy, axillary clearance, and radiotherapy, he feels that there are four possible problems with lumpectomy:
1. High local recurrence rate.
2. Low survival following local recurrence and salvage mastectomy.
3. Cost.
4. No psychological advantage of lumpectomy over mastectomy.

Although Dr. Kinne quotes a high local recurrence rate following lumpectomy, most studies show an approximately 8% recurrence rate at 5 years and a 12% recurrence rate at 10 years. Additionally, most of the local recurrences

From: Wise L, Johnson H Jr (eds): *Breast Cancer: Controversies in Management.* Futura Publishing Company, Inc., Armonk, NY, © 1994.

following lumpectomy seem to be due to inadequate resections with positive margins. In fact, about 75% of the recurrences following conservative surgery and radiation are true recurrences occurring in the vicinity of the original primary tumor, and many of these are probably due to incomplete excision and failure to give a boost dose of radiation. Only 25% of the recurrences following lumpectomy occur in a separate quadrant from the original primary and these are the ones that probably represent a new primary tumor. Dr. Kinne suggests that the 5-year survival rate following salvage mastectomy is 20%. Most studies, however, indicate a far higher 5-year survival rate; indeed the average 5-year survival following salvage mastectomy for an isolated breast recurrence is approximately 75%. There are at least two series (Calle et al: Int J Rad Oncol Biol Phys 1986; 12:873 and Clark et al: Int J Rad Oncol Biol Phys 1982; 8:967) that have demonstrated no difference in the 10-year survival rates among patients who developed an isolated breast recurrence and underwent salvage mastectomy and those who did not develop such a recurrence. It should also be mentioned that the incidence of locoregional recurrence following mastectomy in some studies such as that of Turner et al. was over 20%. Although Dr. Kinne and some other workers claim that mastectomy does not have more severe psychological sequelae than lumpectomy, our own study (Am J Psychol 1985; 142:34) did show a significantly better psychological outcome for lumpectomy patients than for mastectomy patients. We agree with Dr. Kinne that the cost of lumpectomy with radiotherapy is higher than that of modified radical mastectomy, but we do not believe that this should be a primary consideration in our choice of therapy.

Chapter 10

This chapter provides evidence to support lumpectomy as the treatment of choice for most patients with potentially curable breast cancer.

Chapter 11

In this chapter, Dr. Margolese reemphasizes some important biological principles:

1. Leaving clinically negative nodes untreated or leaving the breast untreated following lumpectomy has no effect on survival or distant metastases (i.e., these do not serve as a nidus for further metastases).

2. Following lumpectomy, a combination of chemotherapy and radiotherapy results in a synergistically improved rate of local control.

3. The larger the clear margin following lumpectomy, the lower the incidence of local recurrence.

Chapter 12

We believe that Professor Veronesi has provided the major stimulus for the acceptance of conservative treatment in the management of breast cancer. In this chapter, he and his coauthors summarize the results of the most significant trials of his group, including the new and exciting studies of the possible use of preoperative chemotherapy for the management of large primary tumors.

Chapter 13

Drs. Chaudary and Hayward, in their thoughtful chapter, discuss 11 factors to potentially support modified radical mastectomy versus lumpectomy plus radiation therapy.

1. Local recurrence: In many, but not all studies, this is higher with lumpectomy. Although most studies do not support it, this could still theoretically have a small effect on survival.

2. Long-term complications from radiation therapy: Increased incidence of other cancers (chest wall sarcoma and leukemia), coronary artery disease, brachial neuropathy, rib fractures, lung fibrosis, some degree of breast fibrosis and edema, and potentially an increased incidence of contralateral breast cancer.

3. Psychological morbidity: Patients with lumpectomy may worry about the lack of effectiveness of eradicating local disease.

4. Influence of delay from lumpectomy to radiation therapy: Delay may increase incidence of local recurrence.

5. Tumor size: This probably has no effect as long as the excision is complete. Incomplete excision, however, may lead to increased local recurrence.

6. Age: Some studies suggest increased local recurrence in younger (under 35 years) versus older (over 55 years) patients.

7. Tumor histology: There is a relatively high local recurrence rate with extensive DCIS (probably due to residual DCIS)

8. Cosmesis: Lumpectomy is not suitable for large tumors versus small breasts. Also, consider mastectomy with immediate reconstruction.

9. Multiple cancers: Patients with macroscopically multiple breast cancers have a high risk of local recurrence.

10. Elderly: Six weeks of radiation therapy may be a severe burden for many old patients.

11. Pregnancy: This is a contraindication to radiation therapy.

Overall, this is an excellent chapter pointing out some of the potential dangers of conservative surgery with radiotherapy. Although we feel that most cases of breast cancer are suitable for conservative therapy, we agree with the authors that there may be some subsets of women for whom this approach may not be the best.

Chapter 14

Professor Veronesi and co-workers bring to our attention a number of important points:

1. The number of cancer foci decreases progressively with the distance from the tumor edge and so the wider the local excision, the less chance for local recurrence.

2. An invaded margin may escape observation by the pathologist.

3. In 80% of patients with microscopically positive margins, radiotherapy will eradicate the residual disease.

Chapters 15, 16, and 17

Dr. Urban, for many years, was one of the leaders in the field of breast surgery and a strong advocate for radical surgery. In Chapter 15, co-authored with Dr. Cody, he makes the case for full axillary dissection for all patients with invasive carcinomas. We were fortunate to have obtained this chapter before Dr. Urban's untimely death.

Dr. Shibata, on the other hand, provides a good case for limited axillary dissection only. He reminds us that axillary dissection does not affect survival, but that a limited axillary dissection is necessary for staging and prognosis.

Professor Baum and co-workers provide us with a superb overview for the pros and cons of axillary dissection and conclude that the only reasons for axillary dissection would be local regional control and staging for adjuvant therapy. For local control, they advocate removal of all palpable axillary nodes.

Almost everybody would agree that patients with pure intraductal tumors and nonpalpable axillary nodes do not require axillary dissection. The major controversy involves infiltrating cancers without palpable axillary nodes. Most surgeons in the United States would still advise routine axillary dissection for all these patients, but we do not believe that this is necessarily logical. The routine practice in the United States is to give chemotherapy to all premenopausal patients with infiltrating cancers that are more than 1 cm in diameter. Therefore, it could be argued that axillary dissection in these patients is not indicated.

Professor Baum and his group feel that adjuvant tamoxifen is indicated for all postmenopausal patients regardless of nodal or estrogen receptor status; in the United States, many would question the use of tamoxifen in the estrogen receptor negative patient. If one agrees with Professor Baum, then in the absence of palpable nodes, axillary dissection would not be indicated in any of the postmenopausal patients.

Chapter 18

It was Drs. DuPont and Page (NEJM 1985; 312:146) who first drew our attention to the relative malignant potential of some of the benign breast lesions. They emphasized that the absolute risk was the most useful index for clinicians rather than the relative risk. They found that during a 15-year period the absolute risk of developing invasive breast cancer in a group of women in the age group 30–60 years who presented with a benign breast lesion was as follows:

atypia with family history 20%

atypia with no family history 8%

hyperplasia without atypia 4%

nonproliferative lesions 2%

It should be noted that the invasive cancer will develop with equal frequency in the ipsilateral and contralateral breasts.

Dr. Page draws our attention to the difficulties with definitions of multicentricity; i.e., is the lesion truly multicentric or is the multicentricity only an artifact because one is looking at only the two-dimensional rather than the three-dimensional picture. Another definitional problem is whether under multicentricity we include only the invasive forms of cancer or whether we include the in-situ forms also.

Reported prevalences of multicentricity range from 5% to 75%. This major disparity between prevalence rates can be explained by many variables including (1) definition of multicentricity, (2) method of examining the mastectomy specimens, including the number of quadrants sampled and the number of sections from each quadrant examined, and (3) whether the primary lesions were detected clinically or mammographically. There are some other associated factors that seem to affect multicentricity: central (subareolar) lesions have an increased incidence of multicentricity compared to peripheral lesions.

The relationship of tumor size to multicentricity is controversial. Most authors have reported an increased risk of multicentricity with larger lesions. Some have also shown an increased risk of multicentricity in patients with positive family history for breast carcinoma, but other studies did not confirm this. The incidence of multicentricity is higher with the noninvasive varieties of breast cancer, being roughly 30% with DCIS and 50% or more with lobular carcinoma in situ. The incidence of multicentricity with invasive ductal cancer is approximately 20% and with invasive lobular cancer it is 30%. Concurrent bilaterality has been demonstrated with lobular carcinoma in situ in approximately 90% of cases, whereas with DCIS it is only noted in about 10%.

Chapter 19

We feel the term *lobular carcinoma in situ* (LCIS) is an unfortunate one and we much prefer Haagensen's term of *lobular neoplasia*, since LCIS is not really a cancer but is primarily a marker of increased risk. The absolute risk of developing an invasive cancer is approximately 25% during the patient's lifetime and the risk is equal in each breast. The incidence of multicentricity in the ipsilateral breast is approximately 50%, and the incidence of concurrent LCIS in the opposite breast, if extensively biopsied, is also approximately 50%. It is also worth mentioning that LCIS itself never manifests in the clinical or mammographic setting. It is a microscopic entity that is found incidentally in biopsied specimens that were obtained for clinically or mammographically suspicious lesions.

Further evidence that lobular carcinoma in situ is only an index for the future development of invasive cancer and is not what one would expect to be from the transition theory is that when an invasive cancer develops, then the histology in approximately 50% of cases is an invasive ductal carcinoma and not an invasive lobular carcinoma.

Since the chance of developing an invasive breast cancer is equal on each side, there are only two logical treatments for this disease: either bilateral total mastectomy or just observation. Since 75% of these patients will never develop the invasive form of cancer, and even if they develop it, in the majority of cases lumpectomy with radiotherapy will suffice as treatment, we advise only observation for this disease with lifelong surveillance, which means six monthly clinical evaluations and yearly mammograms.

In our view, prophylactic bilateral mastectomy is indicated only in the very unusual case of a woman with an extremely high level of anxiety and a full understanding of the disease and the alternative management.

Chapters 20 and 21

Drs. Gump and Schwartz are the two major investigators involved in the study of the modern management of ductal carcinoma in situ (DCIS). We agree with them that gross disease should be treated as an invasive cancer because many of these might contain an invasive element. Approximately 20% of mammographically detected cancers are ductal carcinoma in situ.

The three treatment options for microscopic intraductal carcinoma are simple mastectomy, wide excision and radiation, and wide excision alone. The rationale for mastectomy for DCIS is related to the observed frequency of multicentric foci. The average incidence of ipsilateral multicentricity with DCIS is approximately 30%. The incidence of residual intraductal carcinoma following a wide excision with negative margins has been reported in the NSABP B-06 protocol; 40% of patients in this protocol with negative inked margins were found to have residual intraductal carcinoma. Breast recurrence rates following wide excision with negative margins of resection are approximately 15%. The lowest recurrence rates were reported by Lagios; he, however, evaluated the completeness of excision not only by negative margins but also by a negative postbiopsy mammogram. Almost all the recurrences following wide excision occur in the vicinity of the original tumor and approximately 50% recur as an invasive cancer. The ability of postoperative radiotherapy to decrease the incidence of breast cancer recurrence following wide excision for DCIS was demonstrated by the NSABP B-06 trial.

The treatment that we favor for microscopic DCIS is lumpectomy followed by radiation. However, we also feel that the surgical excision should have negative margins and the completeness of resection should be demonstrated by a negative postbiopsy mammogram revealing no residual calcifications.

The incidence of positive axillary nodes for microscopic DCIS is less than 1% and therefore we do not advise axillary clearance for these patients. The indications for simple mastectomy in our view include the presence of diffuse microcalcifications, gross multicentric disease, multiple or diffuse positive margins following reexcision, and cases in which the patient does not desire postoperative radiotherapy. Consideration for wide excision alone (without radiotherapy) should probably be restricted to elderly patients whose lesions are detected by mammography alone and where complete excision is confirmed by negative margins of resection with postbiopsy mammograms demonstrating no residual microcalcifications. The risk for the development of contralateral DCIS is approximately 10% during a woman's lifetime following the development of DCIS in the ipsilateral breast.

Chapter 22

This controversial subject is well summarized by Professor Forrest. Many of the articles published do not distinguish between in situ and invasive cancers, whereas Professor Forrest carefully evaluates and differentiates between these two entities. It needs special emphasis to note that the incidence of clinical cancer developing in a woman's lifetime in the contralateral breast is significantly less than the incidence of histologic contralateral breast cancer, which implies that many of these cancers are biologically relatively inactive.

Chapter 23

Dr. Loprinzi provides a good discussion of the topic and emphasizes that pregnancy does not portend a bad prognosis for patients with breast cancer. And since there is no modern series suggesting that abortion benefits the course of patients with breast cancer during pregnancy, we feel that termination of pregnancy has very little role in the management of patients with Stages I and II breast cancer.

Chemotherapy can be given during pregnancy. However, the risk of teratogenesis with chemotherapy is about 12% during the first trimester; there is no clear evidence of teratogenesis from chemotherapy during the second and third trimesters of pregnancy, but we would still not advise it.

There is no good evidence to indicate that following the treatment of breast cancer, subsequent pregnancy would have a deleterious effect on prognosis.

Similarly, there are no good studies available on the effect of a combined estrogen/progesterone replacement therapy for menopausal symptoms in patients with a prior history of breast cancer. In general, however, until more data become available, we do not favor the use of these agents.

Chapter 24

Dr. Bostwick is a leading authority on breast reconstruction and provides us with a good overview of the subject.

Chapters 25 and 26

Drs. Houlihan and Silen and Dr. Lundy provide an excellent discussion of the factors influencing their decision to perform prophylactic mastectomy and define the situations where the procedure may be justified. We agree with them that prophylactic mastectomy is only very rarely indicated. There is no study available that shows any benefit in survival for patients subjected to prophylactic mastectomy, although the incidence of this is so low that it would be very difficult indeed to show scientifically such a benefit.

Radical Mastectomy Still Has a Role

William A. Maddox

Introduction

Breast cancer is the most common cancer afflicting women. Radical mastectomy (RM) was/is the most effective, single treatment modality for cure and was the most commonly recommended therapeutic procedure until the last two decades. Earlier detection and better understanding of prognostic factors related to the primary tumor along with improved adjunctive therapies have allowed less extensive surgical intervention with improved psychological (functional) and cosmetic results, without compromise of cure rates for certain patients.

Patey[1] introduced the modified radical mastectomy (MRM) and published his results with its use for 146 women. Surgeons in Alabama were concerned that cure rates with the MRM would be less than with RM. They were willing, however, to compare the two methods in a prospective randomized clinical trial. Three hundred and eleven patients were entered into the study between 1975 and 1978. Patients with histologically positive axillary lymph nodes were randomized after operation to receive melphalan or intermittent intravenous cyclophosphamide, methotrexate, and 5-fluorouracil for one year. This is a report of the trial after a median follow-up of 15 years.

Materials and Methods

A detailed description of this study has been published.[2] After giving consent, patients were randomized by the operating surgeon by year of birth. Those born on even-numbered years were treated with radical mastectomy, and

From: Wise L, Johnson H Jr (eds): *Breast Cancer: Controversies in Management.* Futura Publishing Company, Inc., Armonk, NY, © 1994.

those born in odd-numbered years were treated with modified radical mastectomy. Patients with histologically positive axillary lymph nodes were further randomized to receive either melphalan (L-PAM) or an intermittent, intravenous combination of cyclophosphamide, methotrexate, and 5-fluorouracil (I-CMF).

Patient Eligibility

Female patients with histologically documented ductal or lobular carcinoma of the breast were eligible for inclusion in this study. The international classification for staging (Union Internationale Contre le Cancer) was used. All patients with T1a, T2a, T3a, N1a, and N1b classifications were eligible for this study. Categories Tis, T0, T1 <0.5 cm, T1b, T2b, T3b, N2, N3, and M1 were excluded. No patient older than 70 years was included.

Preoperative Assessment

Preoperative workup included a careful history and physical examination, chest roentgenogram, complete blood count, liver chemistries, and roentgenogram of any bone suspected of metastatic involvement. Optional measurements included mammography of the opposite breast and bone scan.

Surgical Technique and Quality Control

Operative procedures were detailed in a series of monographs published in the *Journal of the Medical Association of the State of Alabama*[3] and distributed to all participating surgeons. The RM included both pectoralis muscles and axillary contents as described by Haagensen,[4] Zollinger and Cutler,[5] and others. The modified radical mastectomy preserved the pectoralis muscles using the technique described by Madden,[6] Maddox,[3] and others.

Ninety-one surgeons participated in this study. All surgeons were certified by the American Board of Surgery and were members of the Alabama Chapter of the American College of Surgeons. The qualifications of each participating surgeon were examined and approved by the 19-member Quality Control Advisory Committee of the Alabama Breast Cancer Project.

Pathological Examination

The pathological diagnosis was established at each hospital where patients were treated. Representative slides were then reviewed by one pathologist (Tariq Murad, MD) at the University of Alabama in Birmingham. If there was any discrepancy in the pathological interpretation of the slides, they were automatically sent to a referee (Paul Peter Rosen, MD, Memorial Sloan-Kettering Cancer

Center, NY). Axillary nodes were examined by each pathologist for the presence or absence of nodal metastases. Hormone receptor assays were not usually performed.

Chemotherapy

Patients with histologically positive axillary lymph nodes and no evidence of distant metastases were randomized to receive adjuvant chemotherapy for approximately one year. Chemotherapy was initiated as soon as feasible, usually within 14 to 21 days after surgery. Patients randomized to L-PAM (melphalan) received 7 mg/m^2/d orally for 5 days (maximum, 70 mg). This was repeated in 6-week cycles for eight courses. Patients randomized to CMF received pulse intravenous doses of cyclophosphamide (300 mg/m^2), methotrexate (30 mg/m^2), and 5-fluorouracil (300 mg/m^2). These drugs were administered in 2-week cycles for a total of 24 courses. The survival results of the two adjuvant chemotherapy regimens were essentially the same throughout the study.

Statistical Methods

We used X^2 tests to evaluate the comparability of the two surgical treatment groups with respect to race, age, menopausal status, clinical stage, pathological stage, number of positive nodes, and chemotherapy. Survival curves were calculated based on the Kaplan-Meier method, and the log-rank test was used to determine if significant differences existed between the curves. A proportional hazard regression model was used to determine an odds ratio for comparing the surgical treatments.

Patient Characteristics

A total of 311 patients with documented infiltrating ductal or infiltrating lobular carcinomas of the breast were entered into the surgical part of the trial. All patients received adjuvant chemotherapy if they had histologically positive nodal metastases. The patients were entered into the study by 91 surgeons. Only 15% of the patients were entered from the University of Alabama at Birmingham Medical Center. Twenty-six surgeons (29%) entered 1 patient each, 39 (43%) entered 2 to 5 patients, 10 (11%) entered 6 to 10 patients, 7 (8%) entered 11 to 20 patients, 7 (8%) entered 21 to 29 patients.

Radical mastectomy was performed on 136 women, and 175 women underwent a modified radical mastectomy. Comparison of these two treatments, subdivided by major prognostic factors, is shown in Figure 1. The two treatment methods were well matched with respect to race, age, menopausal status, clinical stage, number of nodes involved, type of chemotherapy employed, and pathological stage.

Patient Characteristics*			
	Procedure		
	Modified Radical Mastectomy	**Radical Mastectomy**	**P**
No. (%) of patients	175 (56)	136 (44)	...
Race, % of patients			
B	22	21	
W	77	79	.66
Other	1	0	
Age, % of patients			
<50 y	40	36	
≥50 y	60	64	.42
Menopause, % of patients			
Before	35	30	
After	65	70	.39
Pathologic stage, % of patients			
I	25	27	
II	64	61	.37
III	11	12	
Nodes involved, % of patients			
0	55	57	
1-3	26	27	
≥4	18	16	.72
Unknown	1	0	
Chemotherapy, % of patients			
None	57	57	
Cyclophosphamide, methotrexate, and fluorouracil	14	13	
Melphalan	20	24	.29
Switched	1	2	
Other	8	2	

Figure 1: *Characteristics of the patients in the two groups.*

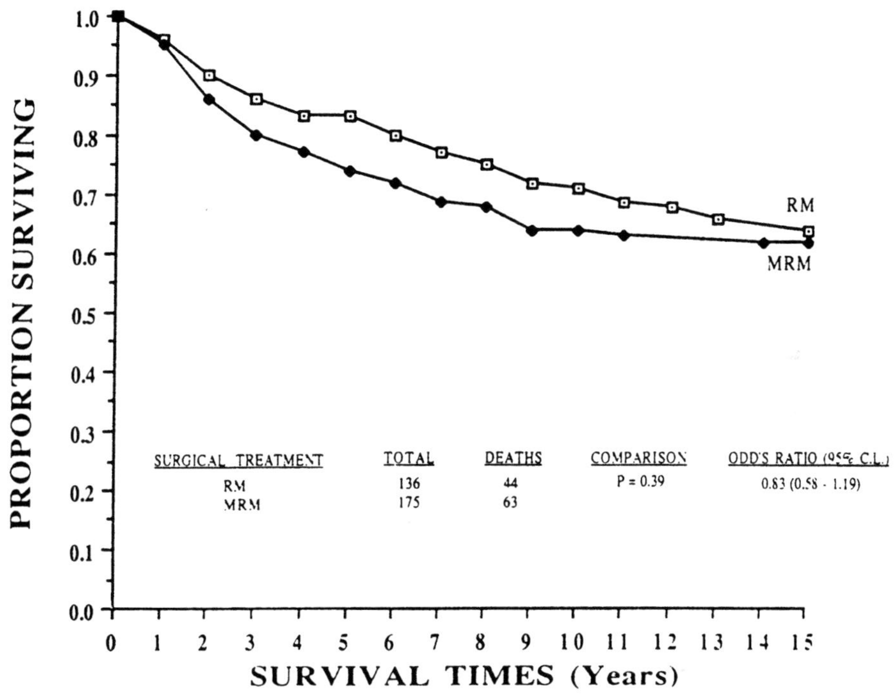

Figure 2: *The Alabama Breast Cancer Project survival curves.*

Results

The median duration of follow-up for all patients was 15 years. The overall survival was not significantly different for patients treated with RM or MRM (65% and 63%, respectively; P = 0.39, odds ratio 0.83) (Fig. 2).

Local recurrence was defined as recurrence in the dissected wound of the chest wall and axilla. A total of 33 patients had local recurrences with or without other metastases. Twenty-four had local recurrence in the MRM group, and nine in the radical mastectomy group. The 15-year local recurrence rate was 14% for the MRM group and 7% for the RM group (P = 0.04, odds ratio 0.47) (Fig. 3). Although the local recurrence rate was higher in the MRM group, there was no statistically significant difference in survival between the two groups.

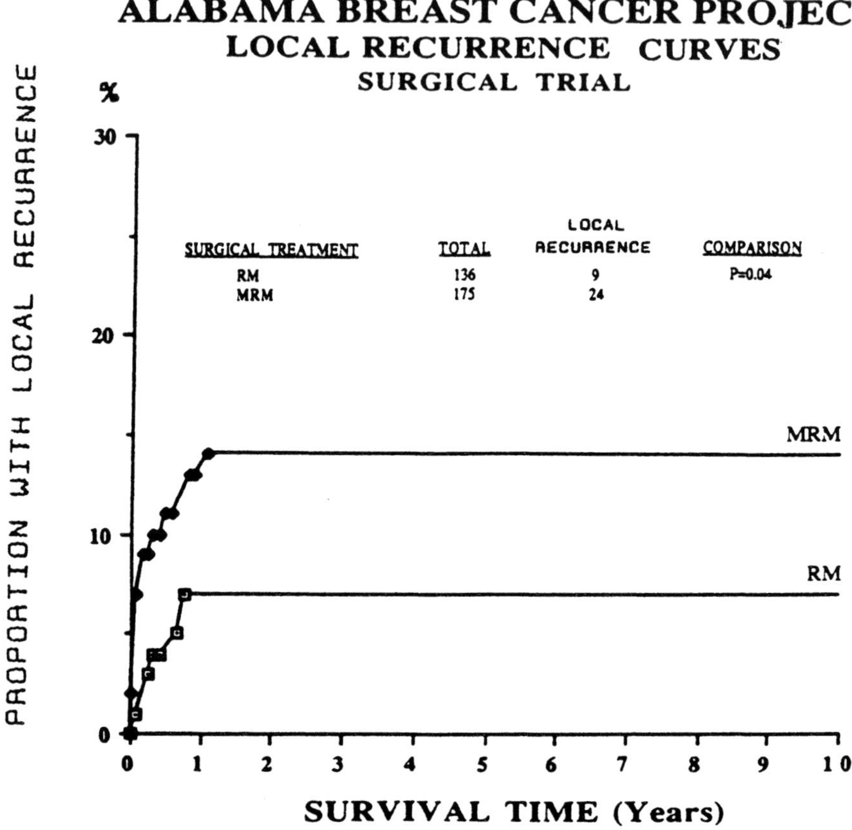

Figure 3:   *The Alabama Breast Cancer Project local recurrence curves.*

The patients with more advanced local disease, i.e., T2a with clinically positive axillary lymph node metastases N1b and all T3a tumors, were analyzed separately for survival after RM or MRM. The 15-year survival rate was higher for the RM versus the MRM group (52% vs. 38%, P = 0.13, odds ratio = 0.58–odds of survival almost double) (Fig. 4).

In addition, patients found to have microscopically positive axillary lymph node metastases, regardless of primary tumor size, were analyzed separately for survival. The 15-year survival was higher for the RM versus the MRM group (63% vs. 46%, P = 0.05, odds ratio 0.61) (Fig. 5).

Comment

The results of this prospective randomized trial demonstrate no significant difference in overall survival rates for patients who underwent a Halsted RM

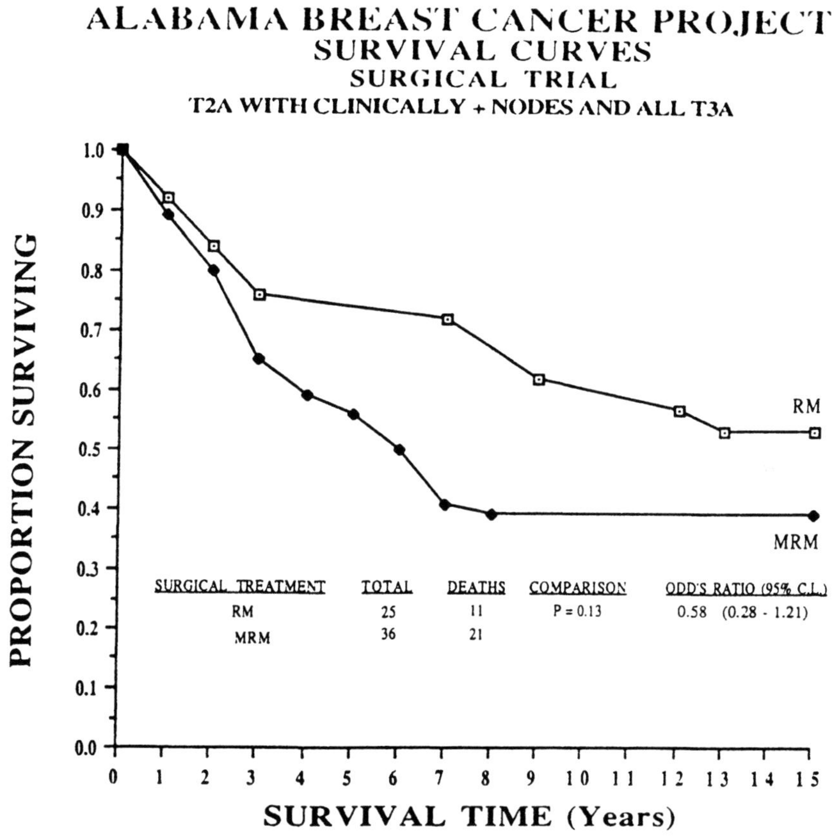

ALABAMA BREAST CANCER PROJECT
SURVIVAL CURVES
SURGICAL TRIAL
T2A WITH CLINICALLY + NODES AND ALL T3A

Figure 4: *The Alabama Breast Cancer Project survival curves.*

compared with an MRM. However, there was a trend for increased survival for those who underwent RM. The odds of death due to breast cancer for patients treated with RM is 83% that of MRM. This is not a very impressive statistic. There is also a slightly higher local recurrence rate for patients who underwent an MRM. These results are very nearly the same as those reported by Turner et al.[7] for a randomized trial involving 534 patients who underwent RM or MRM. There is good evidence that the larger the primary breast cancer, the more frequently axillary lymph nodes are involved. These factors led to analysis of the results of treatment by RM or MRM in patients with T2a lesions with clinically involved axillary nodes and T3a tumors with or without clinically palpable axillary lymph nodes. In addition, another subset of patients with microscopically positive axillary lymph nodes, regardless of primary tumor size, was analyzed. These findings suggest that patients with more advanced local disease substantially benefit from a more comprehensive surgical procedure. These results gain credibility by their consistency throughout the trial.

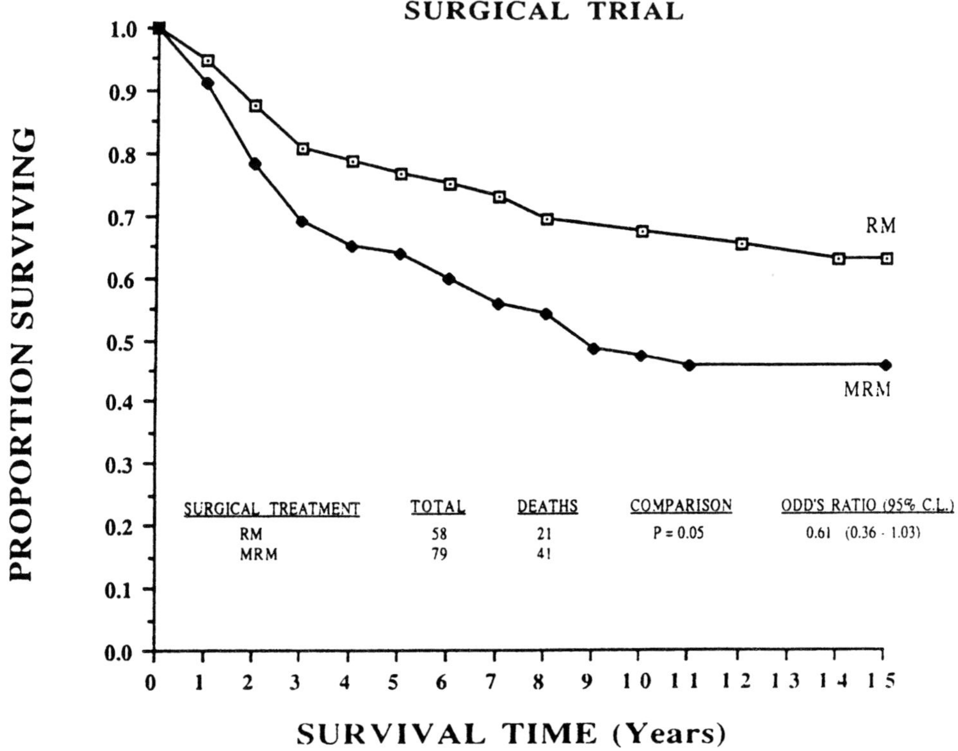

Figure 5: *The Alabama Breast Cancer Project survival curves for node-positive patients.*

Summary

The surgical management of primary breast cancer is still evolving. There are three goals of the operation (cure, local disease control, and staging) and three components of the disease that require treatment (primary tumor, multifocal carcinoma within the breast, and axillary node metastasis). A node sampling procedure of the lower axilla underestimates the incidence of nodal metastases by 10% or more.[8] The results of this study indicate that although overall survival was similar for patients treated by RM or MRM, there may be subsets of patients with more advanced local disease whose survival can be favorably influenced by RM.

Radical mastectomy is a viable option for patients with primary operable carcinoma of the breast who do not desire to undergo adjunctive radiotherapy or chemotherapy.

References

1. Patey DH: A review of 146 cases of carcinoma of the breast operated on between 1930 and 1943. Br J Cancer 1967; 21:260.
2. Maddox WA, Laws HL, Carpenter JT Jr: Breast cancer management: Parts I and II. J Med Assoc State Ala 1974; 44:1–20.
3. Carpenter JT Jr, Laws HL, Maddox WA: Breast cancer management: Part III. J Med Assoc State Ala 1975; 45:37–46.
4. Haagensen CD: Diseases of the Breast. WB Saunders Co, Philadelphia, pp 676–702, 1971.
5. Zollinger RM, Cutler EC: Atlas of Surgical Operations, ed 2. Macmillan Publishing Co Inc, NY, pp 30–37, 1961.
6. Madden JL: Modified radical mastectomy. Surg Gynecol Obstet 1965; 121:1221.
7. Turner L, Swindell R, Bell WGT, et al: Radical versus modified radical mastectomy for breast cancer. Ann R Coll Surg Engl 1981; 63:239–243.
8. Pigott J, Nichols R, Maddox WA, Balch CM: Metastases to the upper levels of the axillary nodes in carcinoma of the breast and its implications for nodal sampling procedures. Surg Gynecol Obstet 1984; 158:255–259.

9

Modified Radical Mastectomy Is the "Gold Standard"

David W. Kinne

Introduction

There is no doubt that patients with potentially curable breast cancer have equal overall survival rates, whether managed by modified radical mastectomy or lumpectomy with axillary dissection and breast irradiation.

What is the definition of "gold standard"? According to Webster's Unabridged Dictionary,[1] it is defined as a monetary standard solely in terms of gold, in which the basic currency unit is made equal to and redeemable by a specified quantity of gold. This definition is not pertinent to medical practices, and yet the term is used commonly when comparing therapies. An appropriate definition of gold standard as it pertains to medicine is a proven, accepted, widely applicable procedure (or test) leading to equal or better results than other procedures at equal or less morbidity and cost.

Results

A few decades ago, virtually every patient with primary operable breast cancer underwent a radical mastectomy. Postoperatively, therapy consisted of irradiation (usually for patients with pathologically involved axillary lymph nodes) or no treatment at all. No systemic therapy was given. This approach to treatment of breast cancer has since evolved to include more than 20 different local-regional therapeutic approaches (with some of these differences in treatment being semantic). Many systemic treatment regimens are now also available, with or without radiation therapy, resulting in more than 100 possible treatment programs for breast cancer patients.

From: Wise L, Johnson H Jr (eds): *Breast Cancer: Controversies in Management.* Futura Publishing Company, Inc., Armonk, NY, © 1994.

97

To put these many choices in perspective, it is helpful to note the frequency with which they are used. A large survey conducted in 1982 by the American College of Surgeons includes data from several hundred hospitals in the United States, and reports about one-fifth of the incident cases of breast cancer for that year.[2] When the results of this survey are compared with those of similar surveys conducted in 1972 and 1977, significant differences between 1977 and 1981 are evident. The frequency of modified radical mastectomy increased from 55.6% to 78.2%, whereas the frequency of radical mastectomy decreased from 27.5% to only 3.4%. Use of partial mastectomy procedures increased from 2.8% to 7.2%. The 1972 data indicate that modified radical mastectomy became the standard operation in the mid-1970s. It must be recognized that a certain lag time is reflected in these figures, and it is likely that the percentage of breast-sparing procedures being done in many parts of the country today has increased. At Memorial Sloan-Kettering Cancer Center, 914 patients with breast cancer were treated by the Breast Service staff in 1989 (Table 1). Modified radical mastectomy was done in 516 patients (56%), and breast conservation in 264 (29%). Radical mastectomy was done in 1% of patients, for bulky breast disease involving pectoralis muscle and/or bulky axillary nodes including interpectoral (Rotter's) nodes not possible to remove without radical mastectomy.

Of recent interest is a report from the United Kingdom.[3] In September of 1983, Gazet and associates conducted a survey by mail of 766 consultant surgeons who were Fellows of the Association of Surgeons of Great Britain and Ireland. Questionnaires were completed by 454 surgeons who had an interest in or who treated breast diseases in a total of 17,000 new patients per year. Eighty-four percent of these surgeons treated most of their patients with breast cancer by mastectomy (usually, total mastectomy followed in frequency by modified radical mastectomy). Only 16% of the surgeons who practiced breast preservation techniques performed a biopsy of the axillary nodes. In a more recent survey in England, 287 surgeons reported a preference for conservative surgery in 64% of cases, and mastectomy in 36%.[4]

Table 2 shows our experience in the last 2 years, indicating an increase in breast preservation in 350 cases in 1991 (36% of cases). Modified radical mastectomy was done in 443 patients, or 45% of total breast cancer cases numbering 974. Total mastectomy, often with immediate reconstruction, is one option for the increasing number of patients with duct carcinoma in situ (DCIS).

Table 1
Surgical Procedures Performed by the Memorial Sloan-Kettering
Cancer Center Breast Service: 1989

Operation	No. of Patients (%)
Modified radical mastectomy	516 (56)
Limited resection, axillary dissection and radiotherapy	264 (29)
Total mastectomy	125 (14)
Radical mastectomy	9 (1)
Total	914 (100)

Table 2
Surgical Procedures Performed by the Memorial Sloan-Kettering
Cancer Center Breast Service: 1990 and 1991

	No. of Patients (%)	
Operation	1990	1991
Modified radical mastectomy	456 (51)	443 (45)
Limited resection, axillary dissection and radiotherapy	270 (30)	350 (36)
Total mastectomy	156 (18)	167 (17)
Radical mastectomy	10 (1)	7 (1)
Total	892 (100)	974 (100)

In comparing modified radical to breast preservation, the two procedures carried out for most patients in 1991 (793), mastectomy was done in 56% and breast preservation in 44% of cases.

The nationwide experience with breast preservation is difficult to estimate, but recently Osteen et al.[5] analyzed over 40,000 lumpectomy cases nationwide by region. It was carried out most often in New England (40%) as noted in Table 3, but for the country as a whole, only about 25% of patients underwent breast preservation.

An individual surgeon's experience has been reported by Wolberg.[6] As listed in Table 4, of 424 patients with potentially curable breast cancer, 50% of these considered suitable for breast preservation elected to undergo mastectomy. Another 20% had intraoperative findings necessitating mastectomy (frozen section demonstration of positive histologic margins). Therefore, approximately 25% had breast preservation, a number exactly like that shown in the nationwide analysis by Osteen et al.[5] cited above.

Why would patients eligible for breast preservation according to accepted selection criteria opt to have mastectomy instead? In our experience, there are several possible reasons. A truly well-informed patient, given details of both options, understands the extra time and effort needed in a breast preservation approach, and will verbalize that saving the breast is not that important. This is often seen in older patients. Another subset do not want the 5 to 6 weeks of breast irradiation, or live too far away from a radiation facility to make this option feasible. Some of these patients are too busy in their family or professional lives to spend the required time for this treatment. Another, and perhaps the most important, factor is the awareness that a new or persistent breast cancer can develop in the preserved breast, necessitating periodic physical exam and mammography, and perhaps salvage mastectomy, often years after primary therapy. These are individual, personal assessments made by informed patients choosing between two different local-regional approaches offering equal results in terms of overall survival. Although there are philosophical differences, I believe it is inappropriate for surgeons to pressure patients toward either option in the absence of objective selection criteria or verbalization by patients of their

Table 3
Percent of Breast Cancer Patients with Partial Mastectomy by Region, 1988

Region	Total
New England	40.2
Middle Atlantic	28.1
South Atlantic	21.0
East North Central	23.8
East South Central	11.5
West North Central	13.6
West South Central	20.9
Mountain	27.9
Pacific	29.8
Total Percent	25.5
Total Cases	41,680

From Osteen et al.[5]

Table 4
Surgical Options in 424 Patients

50% considered suitable for breast preservation elected to have mastectomy
20% had intraoperative findings dictating mastectomy
25% (approximate) had breast preservation

Wolberg WH: Arch Surg 1991; 126:817.

preferences. This pertains to either option. Inappropriate recommendations for breast conservation might include these examples: "You have stage I disease and therefore should save your breast," or "Because you have such a small cancer, the NCI has advised that you save your breast." Perhaps heard most often from surgeons is inappropriate pressure for patients to have mastectomy, such as misunderstanding selection criteria, or the commonly expressed "choose either approach, but if you were my wife (mother, sister), I'd advise mastectomy" in the absence of objective evidence.

There is no suggestion in this chapter that the overall results of mastectomy versus breast preservation (lumpectomy, axillary dissection, and breast irradiation) are different. Randomized studies comparing the two show no differences. The two principal trials, Milan quadrantectomy, axillary dissection, and breast irradiation compared to radical mastectomy[7-9] and the three-arm National Surgical Adjuvant Breast Project (NSABP) trial B-06[10,11] have shown no significant differences in long-term survival, and are not a subject of contention in this discussion.

The problem of salvage mastectomy for persistent or new cancer in preserved breasts presents problems for patients and physicians following them. Although chest wall recurrence after mastectomy carries a worse prognosis than breast recurrence, it happens less often in anecdotal and randomized series, develops within a shorter time frame, and is easier to detect.[12]

Harris and co-workers analyzed long-term risk for recurrence and results of salvage mastectomy.[13] Two series in France, and one in Canada, in which the pathology of the specimens could be confirmed and survival assessed, were combined in this study. The risk of developing recurrence persisted for 14 years, although it was greatest during the first 5 years after treatment. In 22% of the patients included in the study, breast cancer developed in the irradiated breast. Salvage mastectomy resulted in a survival rate of 50%.

These findings have led other groups to report salvage mastectomy survival rates in patients with documented viable cancer in the mastectomy specimens. Osborne and colleagues, reporting 20-year results after performing breast preservation procedures with irradiation, found that 5-year results after salvage mastectomy correlated with the original axillary status.[14] The survival rate was 42% for patients with a clinically negative axilla, and zero if the axilla was clinically positive initially. Local excision resulted in a decreased survival rate, and another subgroup of patients was considered to be inoperable as a result of the local extent of disease or distant metastases.

These results, and the recent finding regarding ipsilateral breast tumor recurrence in NSABP B-06,[15] indicate that the prognostic implication after salvage mastectomy should lead to the recommendation that systemic therapy be added to the management of these patients. The initial impression that this development was relatively unimportant in affecting prognosis is being reconsidered, indicating the need for continued follow-up to assess accurately, in modern series, the true incidence and prognostic implications.

Perhaps the most persuasive arguments favoring modified radical mastectomy over breast conservation involve assessment and application of selection criteria. It is far easier for surgeons and other specialists to choose breast cancer patients suitable for mastectomy. Contraindications for breast conservation, most relative rather than absolute, are principally (1) size of tumor to size and location in the breast, suggesting that lumpectomy would lead to disfigurement, and (2) multicentric disease to physical examination and/or by mammography. Many other relative contraindications have been discussed elsewhere[16] and are changing with growing experience with breast conservation. Although newer approaches may increase the pool of patients for breast conservation, especially through so-called primary chemotherapy to shrink tumors presurgery, as proposed by Bonadonna et al.,[17] these experiments require widespread application and longer follow-up.

A final consideration is cost. In a climate where the cost of delivering health care is being scrutinized and questioned, it is apparent that breast preservation is one and one-half to two times as expensive as mastectomy. Wise and associates documented this in their institution,[18] where physician charges alone were 50% higher in lumpectomy with axillary dissection and breast irradiation versus mastectomy.

Furthermore, several psychological studies have shown no significant differences in breast preservation patients, and in some, even greater concern for recurrence than in mastectomy patients.[19]

In making the case for mastectomy, several points are pertinent. It is the most cosmetically acceptable local-regional approach uniformly applicable to all patients with potentially curable breast cancer. Patients with large tumors or multicentric disease clinically, or those on mammography are not candidates for breast preservation. These selection criteria are not standardized nor well understood and require extra effort for pathologists to assess margins (also not standardized and somewhat random) and for radiologists. Mastectomy, on the other hand, is easier, faster, done better by most surgeons, carries no increased morbidity, and is a less expensive treatment to deliver.

Summary

Therefore, there are several reasons why modified radical mastectomy is the "gold standard" for potentially curable breast cancer patients. They are listed as follows:

1. Mastectomy is easier to do in standard fashion by more surgeons than breast preservation.

2. Mastectomy is more widely applicable, with less selection criteria.

3. Mastectomy is less expensive and time-consuming.

4. There is no need for specialized radiation therapy.

5. Mastectomy requires less work (cost) for pathology, mammography.

6. Mastectomy requires no subsequent mammograms, and no possible salvage mastectomy requiring systemic treatment after surgery.

References

1. Webster's Unabridged Dictionary, Simon and Schuster, NY, 1983.
2. Wilson RE, Donegan WL, Mettlin C, et al: The 1982 survey of carcinoma of the breast in the United States by the American College of Surgeons. Surg Gynecol Obstet 1984; 159:309.
3. Gazet J-C, Rainsbury RM, Ford HT, et al: Survey of treatment of primary breast cancer in Great Britain. Br Med J 1985; 290:1793.
4. Morris J, Royle GT, Taylor I: Changes in the surgical management of early breast cancer in Great Britain. J R Soc Med 1989; 82:12–14.
5. Osteen RT, Steele GD, Menck HR, Winchester DP: Regional differences in surgical management of breast cancer. CA 1992; 41:39–43.
6. Wolberg WH: Surgical options in 424 patients with primary breast cancer without systemic metastases. Arch Surg 1991; 126:817.
7. Veronesi U, Saccozzi R, Del Vecchio M, et al: Comparing radical mastectomy with quadrantectomy, axillary dissection and radiotherapy in patients with small cancers of the breast. N Engl J Med 1981; 305:6.
8. Veronesi U, Banfi A, Del Vecchio M, et al: Comparison of Halsted mastectomy with quadrantectomy, axillary dissection, and radiotherapy in early breast cancer: long-term results. Eur J Cancer Clin Oncol 1986; 22:1085–1089.
9. Veronesi U, Salvadori B, Luini A, et al: Conservative treatment of early breast cancer: long-term results of 1232 cases treated with quadrantectomy, axillary dissection, and radiotherapy. Ann Surg 1990; 211:250–259.
10. Fisher B, Bauer M, Margolese R, et al: Five-year results of a randomized clinical trial comparing total mastectomy and segmental mastectomy with or without radiation in the treatment of breast cancer. N Engl J Med 1985; 312:665.
11. Fisher B, Redmond C, Poisson R, et al: Eight-year results of a randomized clinical trial

comparing total mastectomy and lumpectomy with or without irradiation in the treatment of breast cancer. N Engl J Med 1989; 320:822–828.
12. Kinne DW: Primary treatment of breast cancer. In: Harris JR, Hellman S, et al. (eds). Breast Diseases, 2nd Ed. JB Lippincott, Philadelphia, pp 347–1373, 1992.
13. Harris JR, Recht A, Amalric R, et al: Time course and prognosis of local recurrence following primary radiation therapy for early breast cancer. J Clin Oncol 1984; 2:37.
14. Osborne MP, Ormiston N, Harmer C, et al: Breast conservation in the treatment of early breast cancer: a 20-year follow-up. Cancer 1984; 53:349.
15. Fisher B, Anderson S, Fisher ER, et al: Significance of ipsilateral breast tumour recurrence after lumpectomy. Lancet 1991; 338:327–331.
16. Harris HR, Hellman S, Kinne DW: Limited surgery and radiotherapy for early breast cancer. N Engl J Med 1985; 313:1365.
17. Bonadonna G, Veronesi U, Brambilla C, et al: Primary chemotherapy to avoid mastectomy in tumors with diameters larger than 3 cm. JNCI 1990; 82:1539–1545.
18. Munoz E, Shamash F, Friedman M, Teicher E, Wise L: Lumpectomy vs mastectomy: the costs of breast preservation for cancer. Arch Surg 1986; 121:1297–1301.
19. Kiebert GM, DeHaes JCJM, van de Velde CJH: The impact of breast-conserving treatment and mastectomy on the quality of life of early-stage breast cancer patients: a review. J Clin Oncol 1991; 9:1059–1070.

10

The Role for Mastectomy Is Very Limited:

Lumpectomy Is the Usual Choice

Leslie Wise

Introduction

In the United States, carcinoma of the breast is the most common cancer in females and it kills more women than any other form of cancer. The average probability of a woman eventually developing breast cancer is approximately 8%.

The objective of this chapter is to show that the role for mastectomy in the management of potentially curable breast cancer is very limited and that lumpectomy is the usual choice.

Historical Survey

It was in 1894 that William Halsted published his first paper on radical mastectomy.[1] In this article, he reported his results on 50 patients with radical mastectomies who were operated on between June 1889 and January 1894. The follow-up varied from zero time to 5 years. Four of eight patients with a 3-year follow-up were alive and well. Halsted stated that "the prognosis at the time of operation was hopeless and unfavorable in 27 of the 50 cases. In every one of the 50 cases, some or all of the axillary glands were cancerous." He quoted Volkmann, the well-known German surgeon, as to what he regarded as a "radical cure." Volkman stated the following: "I unhesitatingly make this statement for all cancers, that when a whole year has passed and the most careful examination can detect neither a local recurrence nor swollen glands, nor

From: Wise L, Johnson H Jr (eds): *Breast Cancer: Controversies in Management.* Futura Publishing Company, Inc., Armonk, NY, © 1994.

any symptoms of internal disease, one may begin to hope that a permanent cure may be effected; but after 2 years usually, and after 3 years almost without exception, one may feel sure of the result." Halsted also quoted Billroth who felt that Volkmann was too cautious and he said "I think that one may express himself more boldly, and may declare that if the careful examination of an experienced surgeon detects no recurrence when 1 year has passed since the operation, one may be sure that there will be neither a local or glandular recurrence, and may pronounce the patient as radically cured." At any rate, in a further article published in 1907, Halsted[2] reported his results with 232 radical mastectomies. His operative mortality rate was 1.7% and his 3-year survival rate was 42%. Historically, it is interesting to note that in 1914, Halsted published another paper describing what he thought were the advantages of skin grafting.[3] His final paper regarding radical mastectomy was published in 1922, where he expressed the view that edema of the arm following radical mastectomy was due to a faulty technique in the closure of the wound.[4] It should be noted that in 1894 when Halsted's first article on radical mastectomy appeared in print, William Meyer also described a form of mastectomy that was essentially similar to that described by Halsted.[5] In fact, the first radical mastectomy apparently was carried out by Joseph Lister in 1867 on his own sister.[6]

It was as early as 1928 that Geoffrey Keynes[7] reported his results on 42 patients with biopsy-proven breast carcinoma (only 22 of whom were considered to have operable lesions), by implantation of radium needles. Thirty-four patients were alive at a follow-up of 4 years; 13 of these had no evidence of recurrence. In 1937 Keynes[8] again reported his data on breast cancer with radiotherapy; 85 patients with clinical stage I disease had a 71.4% 5-year survival rate and 91 patients with stage II disease had a 29.3% 5-year survival rate. These results compared favorably with patients treated during the same period with radical mastectomy at the University College Hospital, where the 5-year survival rate was 89% for stage I and 30% for stage II lesions.[9] There are numerous other retrospective reports on lumpectomy and radiotherapy, which we have summarized in a previous report.[10]

In the 1930s, Patey began performing modified radical mastectomies in order to reduce postsurgical deformities. In 1948 Patey, during a 3- to 16-year follow-up, reported a 37% survival rate with 49 radical mastectomies versus a 33% survival with 69 modified radical mastectomies.[11] He re-reviewed his cases in 1967 again, and could find no significant difference in the survival rate following these two procedures.[12] The three other major advocates of modified radical mastectomy were Handley,[13] Madden,[14] and Auchincloss.[15,16]

The next major advance came from McWhirter.[17] He suggested that simple mastectomy combined with radiotherapy gave just as satisfactory survival results as radical mastectomy. The bases for this suggestion were the results at the Royal Infirmary in Edinburgh with stage I and stage II breast cancers. Those treated with radical mastectomy and postoperative radiotherapy during the period from 1935 to 1940 (411 operable cases) had a 50.1% 5-year survival rate. During the period from 1941 to 1945, 757 similar patients were treated with simple mastectomy and radiotherapy with a 5-year survival rate of 62.1%.

McWhirter's results were reviewed by Ackerman, who made some constructive criticisms but found little that would have changed the overall conclusions.[18]

In 1952 Urban described his experience with supraradical mastectomies (radical mastectomy in continuity with en bloc resection of the internal mammary lymph node chain); in 40 patients he had zero operative mortality.[19] The lesions were located mainly in the medial segment (38/40); 52% had positive internal mammary nodes, 65% had positive axillary nodes, and in 30% all nodes were clear. As far as the results are concerned, he stated that: "adequate follow-up in these patients is impossible, since all operations were performed during the last 15 months." In 1986 Urban re-reviewed his results.[20] During the period from 1965 to 1970, he performed 351 radical mastectomies and 105 extended radical mastectomies. The 5-year survival was 80% in each group. The 10-year survival was 70% for radical mastectomy and 67% for extended radical mastectomy (Table 1).

Prospective Randomized Trials Between the Various Forms of Mastectomy

Supraradical Mastectomy versus Simple Mastectomy with Radiotherapy

Kaae and Johansen in 1969 published their results of a prospective randomized study comparing simple mastectomy with postoperative radiotherapy versus extended radical mastectomy.[21] In the simple mastectomy group, no axillary dissection was carried out. Postoperative radiation fields included the axilla, the supraclavicular region, the internal mammary chain, and the chest wall. There was no statistically significant difference in the overall or the disease-free survival rate between the two groups at 5 or 10 years (Table 2). The 10-year local recurrence rates were also similar (Table 3).

Table 1*
Radical Mastectomy Versus Extended Radical Mastectomy—Primary Operable Breast Cancer, 1965–1970

		No.	5-Year %		10-Year %	
			Alive	*NED*	*Alive*	*NED*
RM						
	Axilla -	176	89	82	83	75
	Axilla +	175	70	62	57	50
	TOTAL	351	80	72	70	63
ERM						
	Axilla -	64	82	75	73	66
	Axilla +	41	78	61	59	49
	TOTAL	105	80	69	67	60

*From reference 20.
RM = radical mastectomy; ERM = extended radical mastectomy; NED = no evidence of disease.

Table 2*
Extended Radical Mastectomy Versus Simple Mastectomy + RT—Survival Data

Clinical Stage	5-Year Survival		10-Year Survival	
	SM & RT	ERM	SM & RT	ERM
I	70%	74%	50%	55%
II	50%	47%	32%	34%

*From reference 19.
SM = simple mastectomy; RT = radiation therapy.

Table 3*
Extended Radical Mastectomy Versus Simple Mastectomy + RT—10-Year Local
Recurrence Rate (Parasternal, Chest Wall, Axillary)

Clinical Stage	SM & RT	ERM
I	19%	20%
II	29%	32%

*From reference 19.
SM = simple mastectomy; RT = radiation therapy; ERM = extended radical mastectomy.

Radical Mastectomy versus Supraradical Mastectomy

There are two studies to be considered, one by Lacour et al.[22–24] and the other by Veronesi and Valagussa.[25] The Lacour study,[24] after a 20-year follow-up, showed no significant difference for overall or disease-free survival between the two treatment groups (classic radical mastectomy versus extended radical mastectomy, i.e., radical mastectomy plus internal mammary dissection). However, when compared to radical mastectomy, extended radical mastectomy significantly (P = 0.05) decreased the risk of death in the subgroup of patients with medial tumor and positive axillary nodes. No beneficial effect of extended mastectomy was observed for any of the other patients; on the contrary, extended radical mastectomy seemed to increase the risk of death for patients with lateral tumor and negative axillary nodes (P = 0.07). This 1987 report from Lacour et al.[24] included 243 patients, all of whom were observed in the French Center, the Institut Gustave Roussy. The results are summarized in Tables 4, 5, and 6.

The first paper from the Lacour group was published in 1976.[22] At that stage, five cancer centers were involved in the study: Lima, Milan, Villejuif, Warsaw, and Rome. From 1963 to 1968, 1,580 cases were collected and randomized into two therapeutic groups: radical mastectomy versus extended radical mastectomy. No significant difference was observed between the two groups in the overall 5-year survival rate. However, on more detailed analysis, a significant improvement in survival was noted in the extended mastectomy group, 71% versus 52%, when the subgroup of cancers of the medial quadrant with positive axillary nodes was considered. The conclusion of this study was that there was

Table 4*
Extended Radical Mastectomy Versus Radical Mastectomy—Overall Survival

	5-Years	10-Years	15-Years
RM	69%	60%	51%
ERM	75%	60%	51%

*From reference 22.
RM = radical mastectomy; ERM = extended radical mastectomy.

Table 5*
Extended Radical Mastectomy Versus Radical Mastectomy—Survival at 15 Years

Treatment	15-Year Survival	
	Overall	Disease-Free
RM	51%	49%
ERM	51%	47%

*From reference 22.
RM = radical mastectomy; ERM = extended radical mastectomy.

Table 6*
15-Year Survival Rates by Nodal Status, Site of Tumor
and Type of Mastectomy—15-Year Survival Rate

Nodal Status	Site of Tumor	Treatment	Overall	Disease-Free
N-	Lateral	RM	82%	76%
			>p = 0.07	
		ERM	58%	58%
N+	Medial	RM	28%	25%
			>p = 0.02	
		ERM	53%	44%

*From reference 22.
RM = radical mastectomy; ERM = extended radical mastectomy.

no indication for supraradical mastectomy in any of the cancers of the outer quadrant, but that there may be a limited indication for extended radical mastectomy for cancers of the medial quadrants with axillary involvement.

In 1983, a 10-year follow-up of the above cases was presented and here again no difference in overall or disease-free survival was noted between the two groups.[23] The center from Rome apparently did not follow their patients and therefore they were excluded from the analysis. The authors in this article noted that there was a significant variation between the number of axillary nodes resected in the centers involved in the study, the mean number ranging from 8.3 to 22.2. A similar variation between the various centers was found for internal mammary nodes, the mean number of nodes resected varying from 1.9 to 4.1. Therefore, no evaluation was made with regard to subgroups in this study.

Veronesi and Vallagusa in 1981 reported their results with 737 breast cancer patients who were randomized in Milan to undergo either radical mastectomy or radical mastectomy with internal mammary node dissection.[25] The two groups were comparable with regard to age, menopausal status, quadrant distribution, and frequency of axillary metastases. No patients received postoperative radiotherapy or adjuvant treatment. At 10 years, no difference was found between the two groups with regard to either the disease-free or overall survival rates. The overall 10-year survival was 60.7% with Halsted mastectomy and 57.0% with extended radical mastectomy. In no subgroup was a statistically significant difference found between the two groups. In the series treated by extended radical mastectomy, the incidence of internal mammary node metastases was 20.5% (24.6% in cases with tumor in the medial or central quadrants and 17.7% in cases with tumor in the lateral quadrants).

Radical Mastectomy versus Modified Radical Mastectomy

Modified radical mastectomy has been practiced for a long period of time. It was not until 1981, however, that Turner and his colleagues from Manchester, England, published their results of the first prospective randomized trial comparing radical mastectomy with modified radical mastectomy.[26] Their data showed no statistically significant 5-year overall or disease-free survival difference between the radical and modified radical mastectomy groups, both for clinical stage I and stage II breast cancers (Table 7).

A similar study was carried out in the United States by Maddox et al.[27–31] who compared radical mastectomy with modified radical mastectomy. After a median follow-up of 10 years, there was no significant difference in the overall survival between the two groups (radical mastectomy 71%, modified radical mastectomy 64%). The 10-year local recurrence rate, however, was significantly (P = 0.04) higher after modified radical mastectomy (11%) than after radical mastectomy (6%). In addition, a subset of patients with more advanced cancers (T3 and T2 with clinically positive axillary nodes) experienced significantly better 10-year survival following radical mastectomy compared with modified radical mastectomy (59% versus 38%). Maddox and his colleagues concluded that although the overall survival is similar for patients treated by either radical mastectomy or modified radical mastectomy, in the subset of patients discussed above with more advanced cancers, the ultimate survival can be favorably influenced by radical mastectomy.

Table 7*
Radical Mastectomy Versus Modified Radical Mastectomy—5-Year Survival

Treatment	Overall	Disease-Free
RM	70%	58%
MRM	70%	58%

From reference 28.
RM = radical mastectomy; MRM = modified radical mastectomy.

Their 15-year results, which are presented in Chapter 8, still show an advantage for radical mastectomy in this subgroup of patients.

Radical Mastectomy versus Simple Mastectomy with or without Radiotherapy (NSABP B-04 Protocol)[32]

Patients in this study were divided into two subgroups: i.e., those with clinically negative nodes (stage I) and those with clinically positive nodes (stage II). Patients with *clinically negative nodes* were treated by one of three ways: radical mastectomy versus simple mastectomy versus simple mastectomy plus radiotherapy. At 10 years, the disease-free and overall survival rates were the same (Table 8). It should be noted, however, that in this study, patients with clinically negative nodes who were treated by simple mastectomy and who subsequently developed clinically positive nodes requiring an axillary dissection were not deemed to have had a treatment failure at that time unless the nodes could not be completely removed. In fact, 17.8% of the 365 patients with clinically negative nodes who underwent simple mastectomy without radiation subsequently developed histologically confirmed positive ipsilateral axillary nodes that were removed by delayed axillary dissection. The median time from mastectomy to axillary dissection was 14.7 months. Seventy-eight percent of such dissections occurred within 24 months following the mastectomy; only 4.6% occurred during the second 5 years of follow-up.

Patients with *clinically positive nodes* (stage II disease) were randomized between radical mastectomy and simple mastectomy with irradiation. There was no significant difference in the 10-year overall or disease-free survival rates between the two groups (Table 8). During the follow-up, 4.4% of all the patients

Table 8*
Radical Mastectomy Versus Simple Mastectomy ± RT—10-Year Survival and
Locoregional Recurrence Rates

Clinical Stage I	Overall Survival	Disease-Free Survival	Local [Chest Wall, Scar] Recurrence	Axillary Recurrence
RM Alone	58%	47%	4.4%	1.4%
SM & RT	59%	48%	1.1%	3.1%
SM Alone	54%	42%	7.7%	1.1%**

Clinical Stage II	Overall Survival	Disease-Free Survival	Local [Chest Wall, Scar] Recurrence	Axillary Recurrence
RM	38%	29%	7.2%	1.0%
SM & RT	39%	25%	1.7%	11.9%

*From reference 29.
**17.8% of patients with delayed axillary clearance were not deemed to have had a treatment failure.
RM = radical mastectomy; SM = simple mastectomy; RT = radiation therapy.

(i.e., stages I and II combined) developed tumors (metastases or second primary) in the opposite breast.

Retrospective Reports of Local Excision Plus Radiotherapy versus Mastectomy

Given a choice, women with breast cancer will opt for a surgical procedure that would preserve their breasts with acceptable cosmesis without jeopardizing the chances for survival.

There have been six major retrospective reports comparing local excision with radiation therapy versus mastectomy with or without radiation therapy. In 1964, Sir Arthur Porritt[33] reported his personal experience with local excision and postoperative radiotherapy versus radical mastectomy and selective radiotherapy. Porritt classified the tumors as "early" and "late"; it is not clear from his report as to how many patients in each treatment group had stage I or stage II disease. The 5-year overall survival rate for the local excision group was 65% and for the radical mastectomy group 50%; the 10-year survival rates were 45% and 34%, respectively (Table 9). Porritt concluded that "one can fairly say that, without decreasing survival rate, a simple method of treatment has been employed which has eliminated deformity and reduced morbidity."

Another series was reported by Vera Peters.[34, 35] In her 1977 publication, she compared 203 patients with clinical stage I and II disease who had local excision with or without radiotherapy versus 609 patients (again with clinical stage I and II disease) who had radical mastectomy (with or without radiotherapy). The 10-year overall survival for the local excision group was 75% and for the radical mastectomy group it was 70%. The local recurrence rate at 10 years was 8% for the local excision group and 5% for the radical mastectomy group; i.e., both overall and disease-free survival rates were similar.

Table 9*
Results in a Series of 263 Cases

	Local Excision and RT		Radical Mastectomy and Selective RT	
	No. of Patients	Survivors	No. of Patients	Survivors
5-Year Survivals				
Early	30	26 (85%)	50	30 (60%)
Late	44	22 (50%)	59	26 (42.5%)
TOTAL	74	48 (65%)	109	56 (50%)
10-Year Survivals				
Early	13	9 (70%)	18	7 (38%)
Late	20	6 (30%)	29	9 (31%)
TOTAL	33	15 (45%)	47	16 (34%)

*From reference 33.

Rissanen in 1969 compared 415 patients with local excision plus radiotherapy versus 593 patients with radical mastectomy plus radiotherapy.[36] All of these patients had clinical stage I disease. The 5-year overall survival was 79% for the local excision and 82% for the radical mastectomy group. The 10-year overall survival was 71% for each therapy. In 1974 Rissanen re-reviewed his results and subdivided them into two clinical substages.[37] For $T_1N_0M_0$, the 10-year survival was 89% for local excision plus radiotherapy versus 92% for radical mastectomy plus radiotherapy. For $T_2N_0M_0$, the 10-year survival was 67% for local excision plus radiotherapy versus 76% for radical mastectomy plus radiotherapy. These differences do not appear to be statistically significant.

It was in 1971 when Wise et al. first published their data comparing 207 patients treated with radical mastectomy with or without radiotherapy depending on the histologic positivity of the axillary nodes versus local excision and radiotherapy.[38] Although this was a retrospective nonrandomized series, there was no significant difference in the age distribution, duration of symptoms, size of tumor, and histopathological appearance among the patients in the alternative methods of therapy. At 5 and 10 years, there was no significant difference between the survival rates of the two groups (Table 10). We concluded that "the present study, together with previous publications on the subject, would suggest that local excision with modern irradiation may be a suitable alternative to radical mastectomy for early breast cancer."

In 1976, Maisin and Wambersie[39] from the Cancer Institute in Louvain, reported on 377 patients with stage I and stage II breast cancers treated with various methods of surgical and radiation therapy. Between 1955 and 1959, radical mastectomy plus radiotherapy were compared with local excision plus radioimplants and radiotherapy. At both 5 and 10 years of follow-up, the patients with stage II disease had a better survival rate following local excision than those with mastectomy; 70% versus 34% at 5 years and 55% versus 23% at 10 years (Table 11). In the second time period considered, 1965 to 1969, local excision with radioneedles and cobalt therapy was compared with radical mastectomy with cobalt therapy and with simple mastectomy with cobalt therapy. At 5 years, no difference in survival rate was noted (61%, 64%, and 61%, respectively). Patients treated with local excision, ^{198}Au seeds and cobalt between 1958 and 1971 had a 62% 5-year and 48% 10-year survival rate. About 10% of the patients in each group had local regional recurrences.

Table 10
Survival Rates

Stage	Five Years		Ten Years	
	Local Excision +RT	Radical Mastectomy ±RT	Local Excision +RT	Radical Mastectomy ±RT
I	96%	81%	68%	69%
II	74%	70%	53%	59%

*From reference 38.

Table 11*
Survival as a Function of the Type of Treatment
and of the Stage in Breast Cancer

Period	Types of Treatment	No. of Treated Pts.	Stages	Survival 5 Yrs.	Survival 10 Yrs.	Mean Survival in Months	Median Survival in Months
1955	Radical mastectomy	44	I	68%	59%	114	151
	+ 200 KV	44	II	34%	23%	62	40
to							
1959	Radium + 200 KV	38	I	71%	55%	109	139
		33	II	70%	55%	100	112

*From reference 39.
Pts = patients.

Montague et al., from the M.D. Anderson Hospital, compared the results of 728 patients treated with radical or modified radical mastectomy alone with 345 patients treated with conservation surgery and radiation.[40]

The 5- and 10-year survival rates are shown in Table 12. There was no difference in the 5- and 10-year survival rates between the two groups. During the period of analysis, the local recurrence rate (Table 13) was slightly higher (5.6%) in the mastectomy group than in the conservation surgery group (4.9%).

Prospective Randomized Trials of Local Excision with Radiotherapy versus Radical Mastectomy: Eight Trials

Guy's Hospital Trial: First Series[41–43]

Three hundred seventy patients, older than 50 years of age with stage I and stage II breast cancers were entered into this trial. Both the local excision group and the radical mastectomy group patients were given postoperative radiotherapy. Those who had radical mastectomies were given radiotherapy to the axilla, supraclavicular triangle, and internal mammary chain. The supraclavicular and axillary fields were directed to cross at the apex of the axilla, giving a tumor dose at this point of between 2,500 and 2,700 rads. Patients were treated 5 days a week for 18 days. Those patients having a local excision were given the same course as the radical mastectomy patients except that in addition, the breast was treated at a tumor dose of 3,500 to 3,800 rads in 3 weeks. The survival of these patients is depicted in Figure 1. The results of the Atkins trial were reanalyzed by Hayward in 1977[42] and in 1983.[43] As shown in Table 14, the reanalyzed data have shown that there was no significant difference in the 5- and 10-year overall survival rates between the two groups. Table 15 shows, however, that both for stage I and stage II disease, the local recurrence rate was higher in the patients treated by wide excision than those treated by radical mastectomy. Even Hayward admit-

Table 12*
Five- and Ten-Year Disease-Free Survival Rates, 1955–1980

	Conservation Surgery + RT		Radical or Modified Radical Mastectomy Alone	
	5-yr.	10-yr.	5-yr.	10-yr.
Minimal Breast Cancer	97 %	92 %	97 %	95 %
Stage I T_1N_0	85 %	78 %	88 %	80 %
Stage II T_1N_1 $T_2N_0N_1$	78 %	73 %	77 %	65 %

*From reference 40.

Table 13*
Sites of Local Recurrences

	Conservation Surgery + RT			Radical or Modified Radical Mastectomy		
	No.	Breast	Nodes	No.	Chest Wall	Nodes
Minimal Breast Cancer	54		1	134		1
Stage I T_1N_0	134	8	1	224	6	6
Stage II T_1N_1 $T_2N_0N_1$	157	8	1	370	19	14
No. of Patients With Recurrence	17/345 = 4.9%			41/728 = 5.6%		

*From reference 40.

Table 14*
Survival Rates (Guy's Hospital 1st Trial)

	Percent Survival				
	Stage I		Stage II		
Years after Operation	Wide Excision	Radical Mastectomy	Wide Excision	Radical Mastectomy
5	71	72	60	65
10	52	58	30	43

*From reference 42.

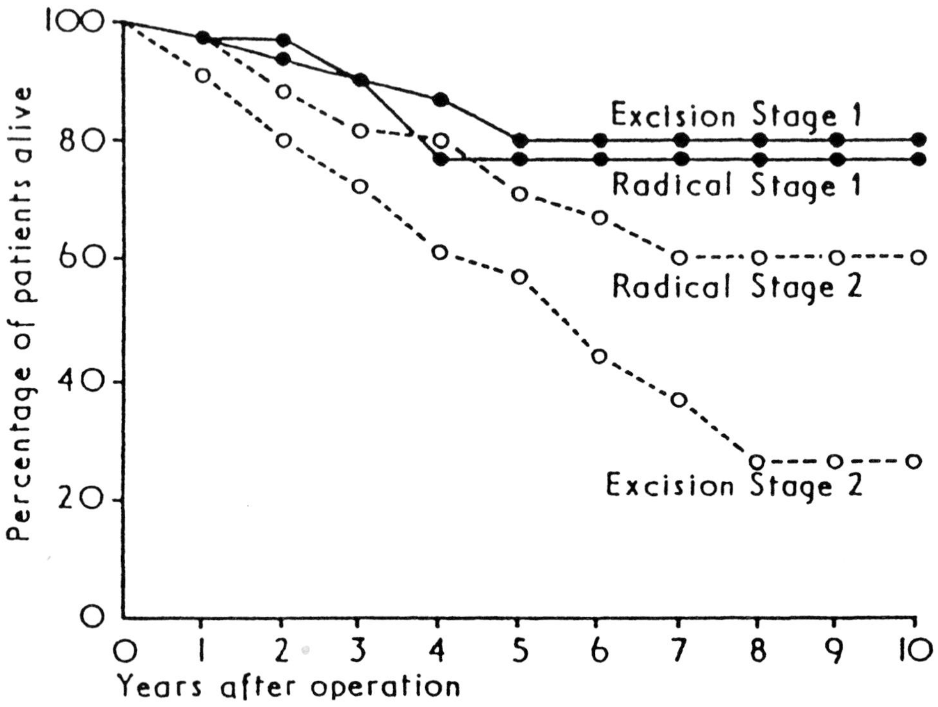

Figure 1: *Survival proportions according to stage. From Atkins et al.[41]*

Table 15*
Local Recurrence Rates (Guy's Hospital 1st Trial)

| | Percent Local Recurrence | | | |
| | Stage I | | Stage II | |
Years after Operation	Wide Excision	Radical Mastectomy	Wide Excision	Radical Mastectomy
5	25	11	48	21
10	37	15	57	35

*From reference 42.

ted, however, that "the course of radiotherapy applied in this trial would nowadays be considered less than optimal."

When Hayward reanalyzed the data again in 1983, he found that for clinical stage I disease, there was no significant difference in the 5- and 10-year survival rates between radical mastectomy and wide excision (Fig. 2); the local recurrence rate, however, at 10 years was higher in the local excision group than in the mastectomy group. As seen in Figure 3 for stage II cases, radical mastectomy patients had a significantly better survival rate at 10 years than the lumpectomy

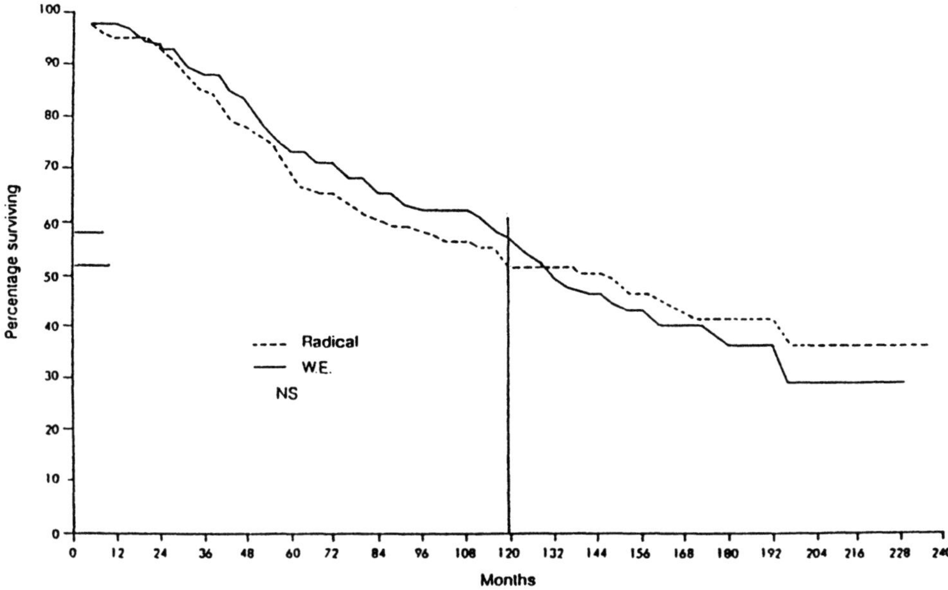

Figure 2: *Comparison of survival in patients with stage I disease (Guy's Hospital 1st Trial). From Hayward.[43]*

patients. The local recurrence for clinical stage II patients was again higher in the local excision group than in the mastectomy group (57% vs. 24%).

Guy's Hospital Trial: Second Series[43]

The second series included 252 patients, some younger than 50 years, all with clinically *uninvolved* axilla, i.e., all clinical stage I patients. One hundred twenty-two patients had wide excision and 130 underwent radical mastectomy. Again, both groups received postoperative radiotherapy, the dosage being the same as in the first series. Unlike in the original Atkins analysis in the first series, in the second series, the mastectomy group had a significantly better 10-year survival rate than the lumpectomy group (Fig. 4). Part of the explanation for the significant improvement in survival of the mastectomy group versus the lumpectomy group in the second series, compared to the first series, is that in the second series, the mastectomy group had a much better survival rate than in the first series (Fig. 5). It is difficult to explain the difference in survival rates between these two mastectomy groups. Hayward, in an unconvincing argument, stated that "those in the first series were admitted to the general wards and in many cases were operated on by junior surgeons in training. Patients in the second series were admitted to the breast unit and their operations were always carried out by full-time surgeons working at the unit."

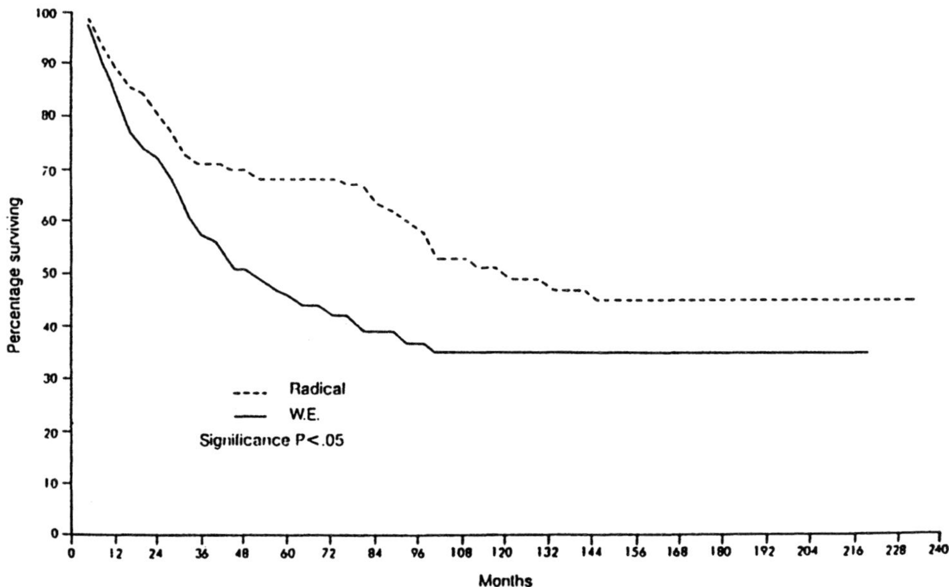

Figure 3: *Comparison of survival in patients with Stage II disease (Guy's Hospital 1st Trial). From Hayward.*[43]

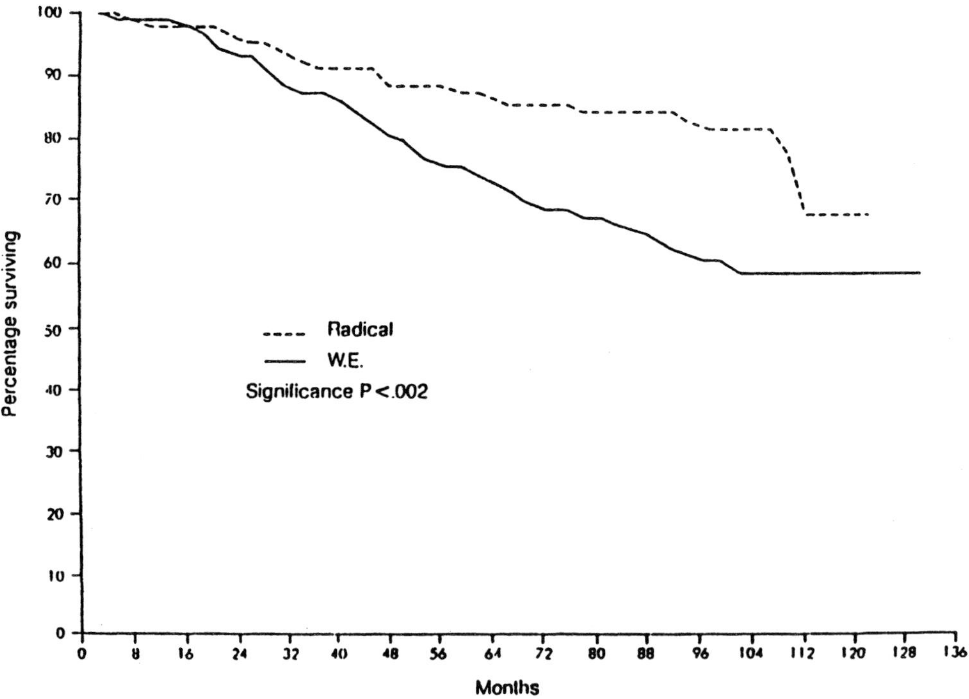

Figure 4: *Comparison of survival in patients with Stage I disease (Guy's Hospital 2nd Trial). From Hayward.*[43]

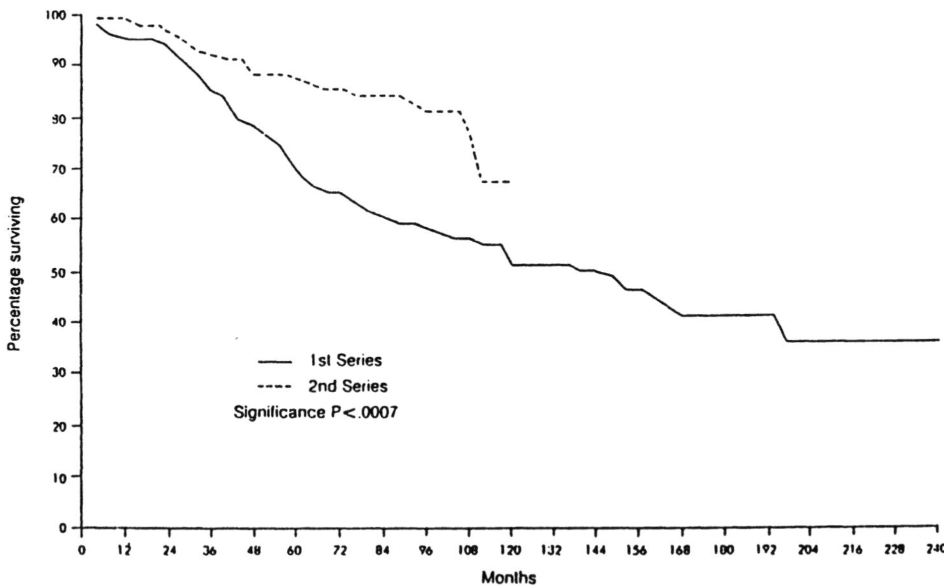

Figure 5: *Comparison of survival in patients with Stage I disease having a radical mastectomy in the first and second series. From Hayward.[42]*

Veronesi (Milan I) Trial[44–49]

It was in 1981 when Professor Veronesi first published the results of what is now called The Milan One Trial where he compared in a prospective, randomized fashion radical mastectomy versus quadrantectomy with axillary dissection, and radiotherapy in patients with tumors less than 2 cm in diameter and with no palpable axillary lymph nodes. He treated 349 patients with Halsted mastectomy and 352 with quadrantectomy. The two groups were comparable with regard to age, size and site of primary tumor, menopausal status, and frequency of pathological axillary metastases. At the 5-year follow-up, there was no difference between the two groups in disease-free or overall survival; there were three local recurrences in the mastectomy group and one in the quadrantectomy group. From these results, Veronesi and his coworkers concluded that mastectomy involves unnecessary mutilation in patients with breast cancer of less than 2 cm in diameter and no palpable axillary nodes. By 1986, Veronesi et al. had an average follow-up of 103 months and thus he was able to report a meaningful 8-year follow-up. At 8 years, the disease-free survival rate was 77% for the mastectomy and 80% for the quadrantectomy group; the overall survivals were 83% and 85%, respectively. Veronesi et al. concluded that "small breast cancers may be safely treated with the conservative treatment described. In our opinion, total ablative operations are not justified."[46] The results were updated in 1990,[48] when Veronesi et al. were able to report on the results of 1,232 women with quadrantectomy, axillary dissections, and radiotherapy for invasive breast cancer lesions measuring less than 2 cm in diameter and clinically negative nodes. Pathological evidence of lymph node metastases in fact was found in 32% of these patients. The overall 5- and 10-year survival rates were 91% and 78%, respectively. No difference was found between the patients without node metastases versus patients with only one node involved, whereas patients with more than one node showed a lower probability of survival. The survival curves of 352 cases treated inside a randomized trial and that of 800 cases routinely treated outside the trial appeared to be superimposable.

Local recurrences and new primary ipsilateral tumors are found, respectively, in 35 (2.8%) and 19 (1.6%) patients. Even when considering all the ipsilateral recurrences and second tumors, this would account for only 4.4%, which is a lower rate than those reported from two similar controlled studies: Sarrazin[50] reporting a 6% and Fisher[54] reporting a 7.7% recurrence rate at 5 years. In the contralateral breast, 45 carcinomas (3.6%) were recorded by Veronesi at a median follow-up of 72 months. Veronesi suggests that since the oncogenic effect of radiation is proportional to the dosage, one would expect an increase in the number of new primary breast carcinomas in the heavily irradiated primary breasts compared to the number of primary carcinomas appearing in the contralateral breasts. However, in this series, the contrary was noted; i.e., 19 primary carcinomas appeared in the ipsilateral irradiated breasts, while 45 carcinomas occurred in the contralateral breasts. In addition, the distribution by quadrant of the 45 contralateral cases did not show an increased incidence at the inner quadrants.

Sarrazin Trial[50–53]

In 1983, Sarrazin, from the Institut Gustave-Roussy in Villejuif, France, reported on 179 patients with breast cancer tumors of 2.0 cm or less and no palpable axillary nodes who entered into a prospective randomized trial comparing lumpectomy, lower axillary dissection, and radiation therapy versus modified radical mastectomy. At 5 years, there was no significant difference between the two types of treatment as far as overall or disease-free survival rates were concerned. The overall and disease-free survival rates at 5 years were 95% and 84% for the lumpectomy group and 91% and 72% for the modified radical mastectomy group. The results have been further reviewed in 1984, 1989, and 1991. There was no sig nificant difference at 10 years in the overall survival, relapse-free survival, and the incidence of distant metastases and contralateral breast cancers between the two groups.

NSABP B-06 Trial[54,55]

In 1985, Fisher published the data from the National Surgical Adjuvant Breast Project (NSABP) Protocol B-06. In this randomized trial, women were assigned to local excision plus axillary dissection versus local excision plus axillary dissection, plus radiotherapy versus modified radical mastectomy. The purpose of this randomized trial was to evaluate breast conservation by local excision in the treatment of stage I and stage II breast tumors less than 4 cm in size. The operation removed only sufficient tissue to ensure that the margins of the resected specimens were free of tumor. All the patients had an axillary dissection; patients with positive nodes also received postoperative chemotherapy. The data were analyzed when the mean duration of follow-up was 39 months (5 to 99 months). Life-table analysis at that stage indicated that treatment by local excision, with or without breast irradiation resulted in disease-free and overall survival at 5 years that was no worse than after modified radical mastectomy.

The incidence of positive specimen margin in the local excision group was 10% and all these patients according to the protocol had a mastectomy. In addition to these patients, the patients with segmental mastectomy whose specimen margins were free of tumor and who subsequently developed a tumor in the ipsilateral breast and underwent a total mastectomy were considered a cosmetic failure instead of a local recurrence. In these cases, patients continued to participate in the study remaining in the original group to which they have been assigned. In my opinion, a recurrence in the ipsilateral breast is obviously a local treatment failure and should be classified as such.

The addition of radiation therapy to the lumpectomy significantly decreased the possibility that the tumor would recur (P<0.001). At 5 years, 7.7% of patients receiving local excision with radiotherapy had a recurrence of the tumor in the ipsilateral breast compared to 27.9% of those treated by local excision without radiation. These findings clearly indicate the value of breast radiation for reducing the incidence of "recurrent" tumor in the ipsilateral breast after local excision.

These data were reanalyzed in 1991; life-table estimates at 8 years of follow-up did not indicate a significant difference in disease-free or overall survival rates among the three groups: i.e., modified radical mastectomy, lumpectomy with axillary clearance, and lumpectomy, axillary clearance plus postoperative radiotherapy. The incidence of recurrence in the ipsilateral breast was 10% following lumpectomy with radiotherapy and 39% following lumpectomy without radiotherapy.

NCI Trial[56,57,82]

In 1979, the National Cancer Institute (NCI) orginated a randomized prospective trial of modified radical mastectomy versus lumpectomy (with axillary resection and postoperative radiotherapy for the treatment of invasive breast cancer, clinical stage T_{1-2}, N_{0-1}, M_0. Between 1979 and 1987, 237 patients entered the trial; all patients with pathologically positive lymph nodes received adjuvant chemotherapy consisting of adriamycin and cytoxan. At a median follow-up of 67.7 months, there were no significant differences in the 5-year

EORTC Trial

The European Organization for Research on Treatment of Cancer (EORTC) Trial was reported by Van Dongen et al. and it included 903 patients with clinical stage I and stage II cancers who entered the study between 1980 and 1986.[58] Lumpectomy, axillary dissection, and radiotherapy was compared with modified radical mastectomy. At a follow-up in 1992, the survival curves and local recurrence rates were identical for both groups. Measurements of quality of life showed a clear benefit for the breast-conserving therapy group.

DBCG Trial[83]

The Danish Breast Cancer Cooperative Group (DBCG) conducted a randomized trial comparing lumpectomy (grossly free margins), axillary dissection, and radiotherapy versus modified radical mastectomy. Between 1983 and 1989, 657 patients were randomly assigned to one of these two groups. At 6 years of life-table analysis, the overall survival rates were 79% lumpectomy arm versus 82% mastectomy arm; the recurrence-free survival rates were 70% versus 66%, respectively.

Local Recurrence and Development of a New Primary Tumor in the Ipsilateral Breast[72,73]

Overall, recurrence in the ipsilateral breast following lumpectomy and radiation occurs in approximately 5% to 10% at 5 years and 10% to 15% at 10 years.[59–61] The risk of ipsilateral breast recurrence has been estimated to be 2%/year for the first 5 years, diminishing to less than 1%/year after 10 years. Patients with *grossly* positive margins at the resection line have an increased risk of recurrence.[62] Patients with only *microscopically* positive margins, on the other hand, do *not* have an increased risk of recurrence if a boost dose of radiotherapy is given.[63–65] Long delay in the initiation of radiotherapy also seems to be associated with an increased risk of breast recurrence.[66]

About 80% of the recurrences following lumpectomy and irradiation occur in the vicinity of the original tumor (true or marginal recurrences), whereas in 20% the recurrences occur in a separate quadrant from the original primary (new primary).

The average interval for true breast cancer recurrence following lumpectomy and radiotherapy is 3 years, whereas most new primary tumors (located in different quadrants from the original tumor) tend to occur after 5 years.

The development of a local recurrence after radical mastectomy or modified radical mastectomy usually coincides with the appearance of systemic metastases and heralds the rapid demise of the patient. The 5-year survival of patients treated for local recurrence following mastectomy is in the range of 30%. In contradistinction, the appearance of local recurrence following conservative operation and radiation therapy does not carry the same grave prognosis. Local recurrence under these circumstances implies local failure and not necessarily systemic failure, and the 5-year survival following salvage surgery for an isolated breast recurrence in these cases is in the 70% range.[67]

Bartelink et al. found no decrease in local control with microscopically positive margins when patients were treated with 5,000 c GY to the breast and 2,500 c GY boost to the primary site.[63] After gross excisional biopsy, patients with extensive *intraductal* marginal involvement have higher local recurrence rates than patients with infiltrating ductal carcinoma. It is possible that the high rate of local recurrence in patients with an extensive intraductal component is due to a large residual burden following gross excisional biopsy.[68] Schmitt et al. found the 5-year local recurrence rate after lumpectomy plus radiation to be 5% for infiltrating ductal carcinoma, 23% for intraductal, and 12% for lobular carcinoma. Lumpectomy consisted only of gross excision in this series.[69]

Some representative examples of the incidence of local recurrence are shown below:

1. Veronesi[48]

With QART:
Cumulative probability of ipsilateral local recurrence   7.5%
Cumulative probability of second ipsilateral tumor   2.8%
Cumulative probability of contralateral tumor   5.0%

At 5 years, Veronesi did not find a significant difference in the local recurrence rate between QART and radical mastectomy.

2. NSABP/Protocol B-06[54]

At 5 years (LE = local excision; RT = radiation therapy):
Ipsilateral recurrence [LE + axilla + RT]   7.7%
                  [LE + axilla]   27.9%

3. Sarrazin[52]

At 10 years:
Ipsilateral local recurrence - with mastectomy   9%
                - with [LE + axilla + RT]   7%
Contralateral tumor - with mastectomy   9%
                - with [LE + axilla + RT]   9%

Salvage After Local Recurrence

Kurtz et al. found an 11% local recurrence with a median follow-up of 11 years following macroscopic local excision and radiotherapy.[70] These recurrences were treated with mastectomy or with further local excision. No additional radiation was administered and hormone therapy or chemotherapy was used on an individualized basis. The overall survival rate after such salvage therapy was 69% at 5 years and 57% at 10 years. Prognosis was not affected by the extent of the salvage operation (mastectomy versus lumpectomy).

Contralateral Breast Malignancies

The risk of contralateral breast malignancies following radiation therapy and local excision appears to be similar to the risk following surgery alone. Kurtz found the incidence of contralateral breast cancer to be 4.5% at 5 years, 7.9% at 10 years and 11% at 20 years following local excision plus radiation therapy.[71]

Cosmetic Results[73,74]

The majority of patients with lumpectomy plus radiation therapy attain excellent or good cosmetic results, which are related to the tumor size/breast size relationship and the irradiation technique. Furthermore, the patients tend to be less critical of their cosmetic results than their surgeons.

Psychological Sequelae[76–81]

Women delay seeking therapy for breast cancer due both to fear of mastectomy and fear of being told that they have cancer. Both Maguire and Morris found high levels of anxiety, depression, and sexual dysfunction among mastectomy-treated women. When lumpectomy patients were compared to mastectomy patients, both Schain and De Haes found less negative body image in the lumpectomy group. In another study, it was also found that lumpectomy patients did much better than those undergoing mastectomies. Studies in our own patients[81] also indicated that the lumpectomy patients had significantly less loss of feelings of attractiveness and femininity. Additionally, lumpectomy patients rated their husband's sexual behavior as having been enhanced after surgery, whereas the mastectomy patients felt that their husband's sexual behavior showed a decline. The two treatment groups were also compared on the frequency of severe sexual dysfunction after surgery; these were almost three times as common in the mastectomy than in the lumpectomy group.

Conclusions

The overall data indicate that for patients with potentially curable breast cancer, variations in local therapy (e.g., supraradical mastectomy, radical mastectomy, modified radical mastectomy, simple mastectomy with radiotherapy, or lumpectomy with radiotherapy) do not significantly affect survival. If survival is not affected, then the least mutilating procedure, which is local excision with radiotherapy, should clearly be the usual choice.

References

1. Halsted WS: The results of operations for the cure of cancer of the breast performed at Johns Hopkins Hospital from June 1889 to January 1894. Ann Surg 1894; 20:497.
2. Halsted WS: The results of radical operations for the cure of cancer. Ann Surg 1907; 46:1.
3. Halsted WS: Developments in the skin grafting operations for cancer of the breast. JAMA 1913; 60:416.
4. Halsted WS: The swelling of the arm after operations for cancer of the breast–elephantiasis chirurgica–its cause and prevention. Johns Hopkins Hosp Bull 1921; 32:309.
5. Meyer W: An improved method of the radical operation for carcinoma of the breast. M Rec 1894; 46:746.
6. Forrest P Sir: Personal communication. 1992.
7. Keynes G: Radium treatment of primary carcinoma of the breast. Lancet 1928; 2:108.
8. Keynes G: Conservative treatment of cancer of the breast. Br Med J 1937; 2:643.
9. Jessop WHG: Results of operative treatment of cancer of the breast. Lancet 1936; 2:424.
10. Tinker MA, Wise L: The conservative management of breast cancer. Surg Ann 1987; 19:279.
11. Patey DH, Dyson WH: Prognosis of carcinoma of the breast in relation to the type of operation performed. Br J Cancer 1948; 2:7.
12. Patey DH: A review of 146 cases of carcinoma of the breast operated on between 1930 and 1943. Br J Cancer 1967; 21:260.
13. Handley RS: The technic and results of conservative radical mastectomy (Patey's operation). Prog Clin Cancer 1965; 1:462.
14. Madden JL: Modified radical mastectomy. Surg Gynecol Obstet 1965; 121:1221.
15. Auchincloss H Jr: Significance of location and number of axillary metastases in carcinoma of the breast: A justification for conservative operation. Ann Surg 1963; 158:37.
16. Pickren JW, Rube J, Auchincloss H Jr: Modification of conventional radical mastectomy. Cancer 1965; 18:942.
17. McWhirter R: Simple mastectomy and radiotherapy in the treatment of breast cancer. Br J Radiol 1955; 28:128.
18. Ackerman LV: Evaluation of treatment of cancer of the breast at the University of Edinburgh (Scotland) under the direction of Dr. Robert McWhirter. Cancer 1955; 8:883.
19. Urban JA, Baker HW: Radical mastectomy in continuity with en bloc resection of the internal mammary lymph node chain. Cancer 1952; 5:992.
20. Cody HS III, Urban JA: Adequate surgery including radical mastectomy. In: Ariel IM, Cleary JB (eds). Breast Cancer. McGraw Hill, NY, p. 261, 1986.

21. Kaae S, Johansen H: Simple mastectomy plus postoperative irradiation by the method of McWhirter for mammary carcinoma. Ann Surg 1969; 170:895.
22. Lacour J, Bucalossi P, Caceres E, Jacobelli G, et al: Radical mastectomy versus radical mastectomy plus internal mammary dissection. Five-year results of an International Cooperative Study. Cancer 1976; 37:206.
23. Lacour J, Le MG, Caceres E, Koszarowski T, et al: Radical mastectomy versus radical mastectomy plus internal mammary dissection. Ten-year results of an International Cooperative Trial in Breast Cancer. Cancer 1983; 51:1941.
24. Lacour J, Le MG, Hill C, Kramer A, et al: Is it useful to remove internal mammary nodes in operable breast cancer? Eur J Surg Oncol 1987; 13:309.
25. Veronesi U, Valagussa P: Inefficacy of internal mammary node dissection in breast cancer surgery. Cancer 1981; 47:170.
26. Turner L, Swindell R, Bell WGT, et al: Radical versus modified radical mastectomy for breast cancer. Ann Royal Coll Surg (Engl) 1981; 63:239.
27. Maddox WA, Laws HL, Carpenter JT Jr: Breast cancer management - Part I. J Med Assoc Ala 1974; 44:293.
28. Laws HL, Carpenter JT Jr, Maddox WA: Breast cancer management - Part II. J Med Assoc Ala 1975; 44:481.
29. Maddox WA, Carpenter JT, Laws HL, et al: A randomized prospective trial of radical (Halsted) mastectomy versus modified radical mastectomy in 311 breast cancer patients. Ann Surg 1983; 198:207.
30. Maddox WA, Carpenter JT, Laws HT, et al: Does radical mastectomy still have a place in the treatment of primary operable breast cancer? Arch Surg 1987; 122:1317.
31. Maddox WA: Personal communication. 1992.
32. Fisher B, Redmond C, Fisher ER, et al: Ten-year results of a randomized clinical trial comparing radical mastectomy and total mastectomy with or without radiation. N Engl J Med 1985; 312:674.
33. Porritt A: Early carcinoma of the breast. Br J Surg 1964; 51:214.
34. Peters MV: Wedge resection and irradiation: An effective treatment in early breast cancer. JAMA 1967; 200:144.
35. Peters MV: Wedge resection with or without radiation in early breast cancer. Int J Radiation Oncol Biol Phys 1977; 3:1151.
36. Rissanen PM: A comparison of conservative and radical surgery combined with radiotherapy in the treatment of stage I carcinoma of the breast. Br J Radiol 1969; 42:423.
37. Rissanen PM, Holsti P: Vergleich Zwischen Ronservatiner und radicaler Chirurgie, Kombiniert mit Strahlentherapie, bei oher Benandlung des BrustKrebses in Stadium I. Strohlentherapie 1974; 147:370.
38. Wise L, Mason AY, Ackerman LV: Local excision and irradiation: an alternative method for the treatment of early mammary cancer. Ann Surg 1971; 174:392.
39. Maisin H, Wambersie A: Curietherapy in breast cancer of stages I and II by radium implant or 198 Au seeds. Panminerva Medica 1976; 18:50.
40. Montague ED, Ames FC, Schell SR, Romsdahl MM: Conservative surgery and irradiation as an alternative to mastectomy in the treatment of clinically favorable breast cancer. Cancer 1984; 54:2668.
41. Atkins H, Hayward JL, Klugman DJ, Wayte AG: Treatment of early breast cancer: a report after ten years of a clinical trial. Br Med J 1972; 2:423.
42. Hayward JL: The Guy's Trial of treatments of "early" breast cancer. World J Surg 1977; 1:314.
43. Hayward JL: The Guy's Hospital Trials on breast conservation. In: Harris JR, Hellman S, Silen W (eds). Conservative Management of Breast Cancer. J.B. Lippincott, Philadelphia, 1983.
44. Veronesi U, Saccozzi R, Del Vecchio M, et al: Comparing radical mastectomy with quadrantectomy, axillary dissection and radiotherapy in patients with small cancers of the breast. New Engl J Med 1981; 305:6.

45. Veronesi U, Zuculo R, Vecchio MD: Conservative treatment of breast cancer with the QUART technique. World J Surg 1985; 9:676.
46. Veronesi U, Banfi A, Vecchio MD, et al: Comparison of Halsted mastectomy with quadrantectomy, axillary dissection and radiotherapy in early breast cancer: long-term results. J Cancer Clin Oncol 1986; 22:1085.
47. Veronesi U: Rationale and indications for limited surgery in breast cancer: current data. World J Surg 1987; 11:493.
48. Veronesi U, Salvadovi B, Luini A, et al: Conservative treatment of early breast cancer: long-term results of 1232 cases treated with quadrantectomy, axillary dissection and radiotherapy. Ann Surgery 1990; 211:250.
49. Veronesi U: Conservative surgery and irradiation in stages I & II disease at the Institute Nazionale Tumori (Milan) In: Bland KI, Copeland EM (eds). The Breast. W. B. Saunders, Philadelphia, 1991.
50. Sarrazin D, Le M, Fontaine MF, Arriagada R: Conservative treatment versus mastectomy in T_1 or small T_2 breast cancer: a randomized clinical trial. In: Harris JR, Hellman S, Silen W (eds). Conservative Management of Breast Cancer. J.B. Lippincott, Philadelphia, 1983.
51. Sarrazin E, Le M, Rouess E, et al: Conservative treatment versus mastectomy in breast cancer: tumors with macroscopic diameter of 20 millimeters or less. Cancer 1984; 53:1209.
52. Sarrazin D, Le MG, Arriagada R, et al: Ten-year results of a randomized trial comparing conservative treatment to mastectomy in early breast cancer. Radiother Oncol 1989; 14:177.
53. Sarrazin D, Le MG, Contesso G, et al: Randomized trial comparing conservative treatment of early breast cancers to mastectomy at the Institut Gustave-Roussy. In: Bland KI, Copeland EM (eds). The Breast. W. B. Saunders, Philadelphia, 1991.
54. Fisher B, Bauer M, Margolese R: Five-year results of a randomized clinical trial comparing total mastectomy and segmental mastectomy with or without radiation in the treatment of breast cancer. N Engl J Med 1985; 312:665.
55. Fisher B: Lumpectomy (segmental mastectomy) and axillary dissection. In: Bland KI, Copeland EM (eds). The Breast. W. B. Saunders, Philadelphia, 1991.
56. Findlay PA, Lippman ME, Danforth D, et al: Mastectomy versus radiotherapy as treatment for Stage I–II breast cancer: a prospective randomized trial at the National Cancer Institute. World J Surg 1985; 9:671.
57. Findlay P, Lippman M, Danforth D, et al: A randomized trial comparing mastectomy to radiotherapy in the treatment of Stage I–II breast cancer: a preliminary report. Proc of ASCO 1986; 5:63.
58. Van Dongen JA, Bartelink H, Fentiman IS, Lerut T, et al: Randomized clinical trial to assess the value of breast-conserving therapy in Stage I & II breast cancer, EORTC 10801 trial. J Natl Cancer Inst 1992; 11:15.
59. Clark RM, Wilkinson, RH, Miceli RU, MacDonald WD: Breast cancer: experiences with conservation therapy. Am J Clin Oncol 1987; 10:461.
60. Greco M, Sacchini V, Herson M, Galimberti V: Risk of local failure in conservative treatment of breast cancer. Breast Cancer Res Treat 1988; 12:116.
61. Kurtz JM, AmaPric R, Brandone H, et al: Local recurrence after breast conserving surgery and radiotherapy. Cancer 1989; 63:1912.
62. Zafrani B, Vielk P, Fourquet A, et al: Conservative treatment of early breast cancer: prognostic value of ductal in situ component and other pathologic variables on local control and survival. Eur J Cancer Clin Oncol 1989; 25:1645.
63. Bartelink H, Border JH, Van Dongen JA, Peterse JL: The impact of tumor size and histology on local control after breast conserving therapy. Radiother Oncol 1988; 11:297.
64. Ryoo ME, Kagan AR, Wollir M, et al: Prognostic factors for recurrence and cosmesis in 393 patients after radiation therapy for early mammary carcinoma. Radiology 1989; 172:555.

65. Schmidt-Ullrich R, Wazer DE, Tercilla O, et al: Tumor margin assessment as a guide to optimal conservation surgery and irradiation in early stage breast cancer. Int J Radiat Oncol Bio Phys 1989; 17:733.
66. Stomper PC, Recht A, Berenberg AL, et al: Mammographic detection of the recurrent cancer in the irradiated breast. AJR 1987; 148:39.
67. Fowble B, Schwaibold F: Local-regional recurrence following definitive treatment for operable breast cancer. In: Fowble B, Goodman RL, Glick JH, et al (eds). Breast Cancer Treatment. Mosby Year Book, St. Louis, 1991.
68. Kurtz JM, Almaric R, Brandone H: Local recurrence after breast conserving surgery and radiotherapy. Cancer 1989; 63:1912.
69. Schmitt SJ, Connolly JL, Khettry V, et al: Pathologic findings on re-excision of the primary site in breast cancer patients considered for treatment by primary radiation therapy. Cancer 1987; 59:675.
70. Kurtz JM, Spitalier JM, Almaric R, et al: Results of wide excision of local recurrence after breast conserving therapy. Cancer 1989; 61:1969.
71. Kurtz JM, Almaric R, Brandone H, et al: Contralateral breast cancer and other second malignancies in patients treated by breast conserving therapy with radiation. Int J Radiat Oncol Biol Phys 1988; 15:277.
72. Kurtz JM, Almaric R, Delonche G, et al: The second ten years: long-term risks of breast conservation in early breast cancer. Int J Radiat Oncol Biol Phys 1987; 13:1327.
73. Recht A, Sileu W, Schmitt SJ, et al: Time-course of local recurrence following conservative surgery and radiotherapy for early stage breast cancer. Int J Radiat Oncol Bio Phys 1988; 15:255.
74. Beadle GF, Silver B, Botnick L, et al: Cosmetic results following primary radiation therapy for early breast cancer. Cancer 1984; 54:2911.
75. Clarke D, Martinez A, Cox RS: Analysis of cosmetic results in Stages I–II breast cancer treated by biopsy and irradiation. Int J Radiat Oncol Biol Phys 1983; 9:1807.
76. Green HS: Psychological aspects: delay in the treatment of breast cancer. Proc Phys Soc Ded 1974; 67:470.
77. Maguire GP, Lee EG, Berington DJ, et al: Psychiatric problems in the first year after mastectomy. Br Med J 1978; 1:963.
78. Morris T, Green HB, White P: Psychological and social adjustment to mastectomy. Cancer 1977; 40:2381.
79. Schain W: Psychosocial and physical outcomes of Stage I breast cancer therapy: mastectomy versus excisional biopsy and irradiation. Br Cancer Res Treat 1983; 3:377.
80. De Haes JC, Welvaart K: Quality of life after breast cancer surgery. J Surg Oncol 1985; 28:123.
81. Steinberg MD, Juliano MA, Wise L: Psychological outcome of lumpectomy versus mastectomy in the treatment of breast cancer. Am J Psychiatr 1985; 142:34.
82. Straus K, Lichter A, Lippman M, Danforth D, et al: Results of the National Cancer Institute Early Breast Cancer Trial. J Natl Cancer Instit 1992; 11:27.
83. Blichert-Toft M, Rose C, Andersen JA, Overgaard M, et al: Danish randomized trial comparing breast conservation therapy with mastectomy: six years of life-table analysis. J Natl Cancer Inst 1992; 11:19.

11

Lumpectomy and Radiotherapy as the Procedure of Choice in Primary Breast Cancer

Richard Margolese

Introduction

In considering the choice of procedure for primary breast cancer treatment, a full understanding of the biological significance of local recurrence (LR) is necessary. If LR represents a lost opportunity to cure a patient, then local control becomes of paramount importance. If ultimate cure is independent of local manifestations, a less stringent policy makes sense, and cosmetic factors should be more strongly considered.

Of course, tumor recurrence occurs in the scar or chest wall even following radical mastectomy (Fig. 1), so it becomes important to understand the difference between this event and local failure following lumpectomy. Published reviews indicate a low rate of long-term survival following treatment for appearance of cancer at the operative site following Halsted mastectomy.[1,2] Spratt[3] demonstrated that, in most of these cases, distant metastases appear simultaneously, indicating that the LR is part of the widespread metastatic pattern. Thus, local-regional malignancy after radical mastectomy is, with rare exceptions, not curable, and the term "local recurrence" is a misnomer.

Clinical trials have clearly demonstrated that total or radical mastectomies offer no advantage in disease-free survival (DFS) or overall survival as compared to breast-conserving surgery.[4,5] While variations of local therapy have no apparent effect on distant disease outcome, there may be differences in LR itself depending on the extent of surgery performed and the use of radiotherapy, so technical factors are worth considering in this context. In choosing between lumpectomy and quadrantectomy for conservative breast surgery there is an

From: Wise L, Johnson H Jr (eds): *Breast Cancer: Controversies in Management.* Futura Publishing Company, Inc., Armonk, NY, © 1994.

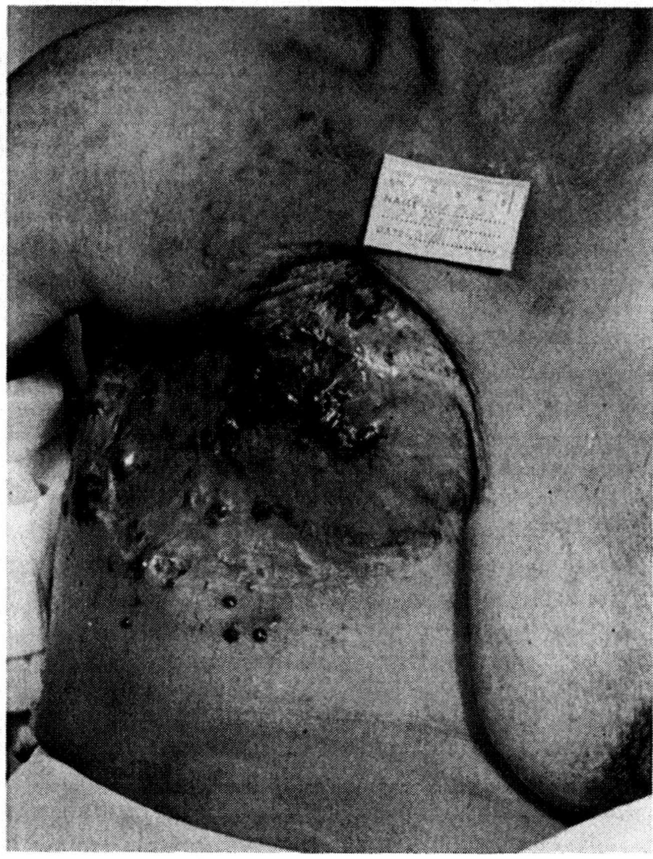

Figure 1: *"Local recurrence" following Halsted type radical mastectomy.*

implied trade-off between freedom from recurrence on the one hand and cosmetic outcome on the other.

Patterns of Local Recurrences

Local recurrence can be categorized into two types (Fig. 2):

Type I: A nodular recurrence at or close to the site of the original tumor site, which usually represents residual disease arising from microscopic remnants not adequately removed at the initial operation. This category is amenable to further local surgery, either repeat lumpectomy or mastectomy, and is associated with a high survival rate. Five-year disease-free survivals are similar to those for the original stage I and II primary cancers.[6,7]

Type II: A more widespread pattern, which may often involve skin and lymphatics, and may extend beyond the breast onto the adjacent chest wall (Fig.

A.   Patterns of Local Recurrence

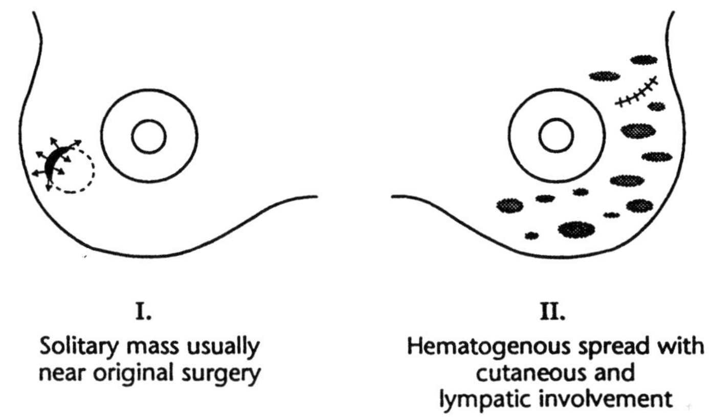

B.   Mechanisms of Local Recurrence

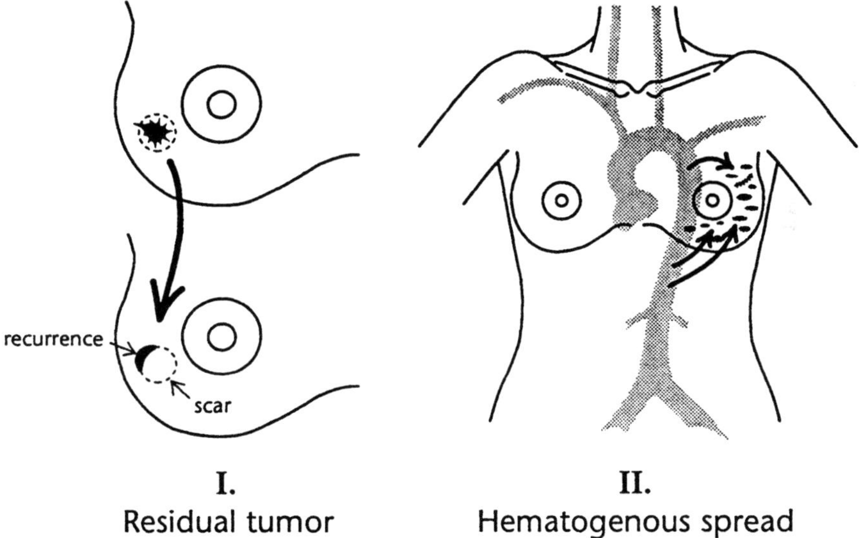

Figure 2: *Patterns and suggested mechanism of local recurrence in lumpectomy patients.*

3). This form usually appears at the same time as distant metastases and has very low 5-year disease-free survivals. This is similar to the type of recurrence seen after Halsted or total mastectomy and clearly represents local manifestation of widespread metastases.

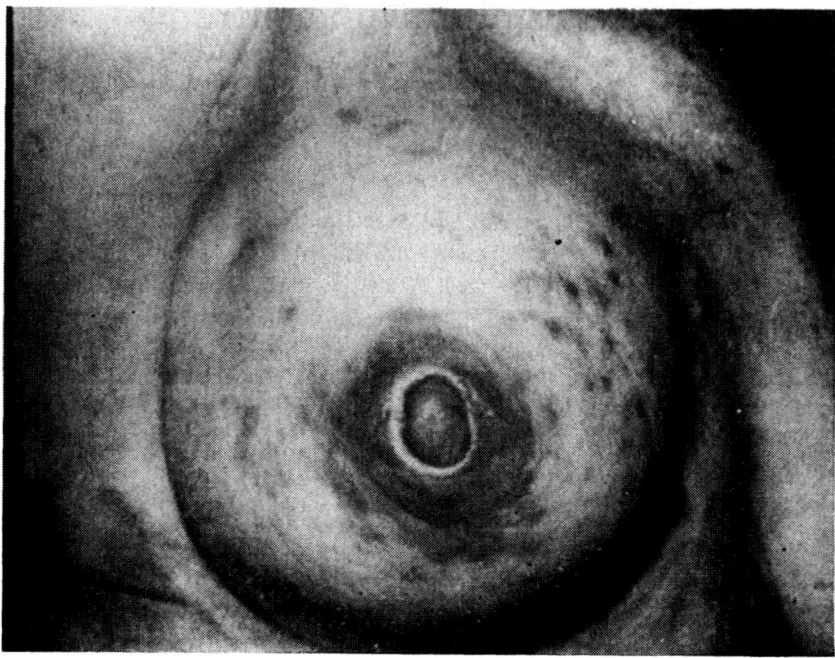

Figure 3: *Examples of type II "local recurrence" following lumpectomy and radiation therapy. The process is diffuse throughout the breast with multiple skin satellites and extends away from the breast onto the chest wall.*

NSABP Protocols

The NSABP protocol B-06 evaluated breast removal versus breast-conserving surgery. Patients were treated by total mastectomy or lumpectomy with or without postoperative radiotherapy (axillary dissections were done in all cases and N+ patients received chemotherapy). Patients with tumor size up to 4 cm were eligible for this protocol. Those not treated by irradiation following lumpectomy had a high incidence of local recurrence, but during 9 years of follow-up there was no difference in the overall incidence of distant metastases or overall survival between the three groups[4] (Fig. 4). Thus, while local recurrence may often be part of a disseminated process, it is not by itself an event that leads to an increased number of treatment failures, and it can be considered simply with respect to the problems it creates for local control.

The NSABP protocol B-04 is usually viewed as a comparison of radical versus modified mastectomy and protocol B-06 as a comparison of modified mastectomy versus breast-conserving surgery, but these studies are more properly viewed as evaluations of biological properties. In protocol B-04, it is the lymph nodes, and in B-06, it is the grossly normal breast parenchyma which is being studied. Since leaving the nodes untreated (B-04) and the remaining breast untreated (B-06) have no deleterious effect on metastases or survival, the

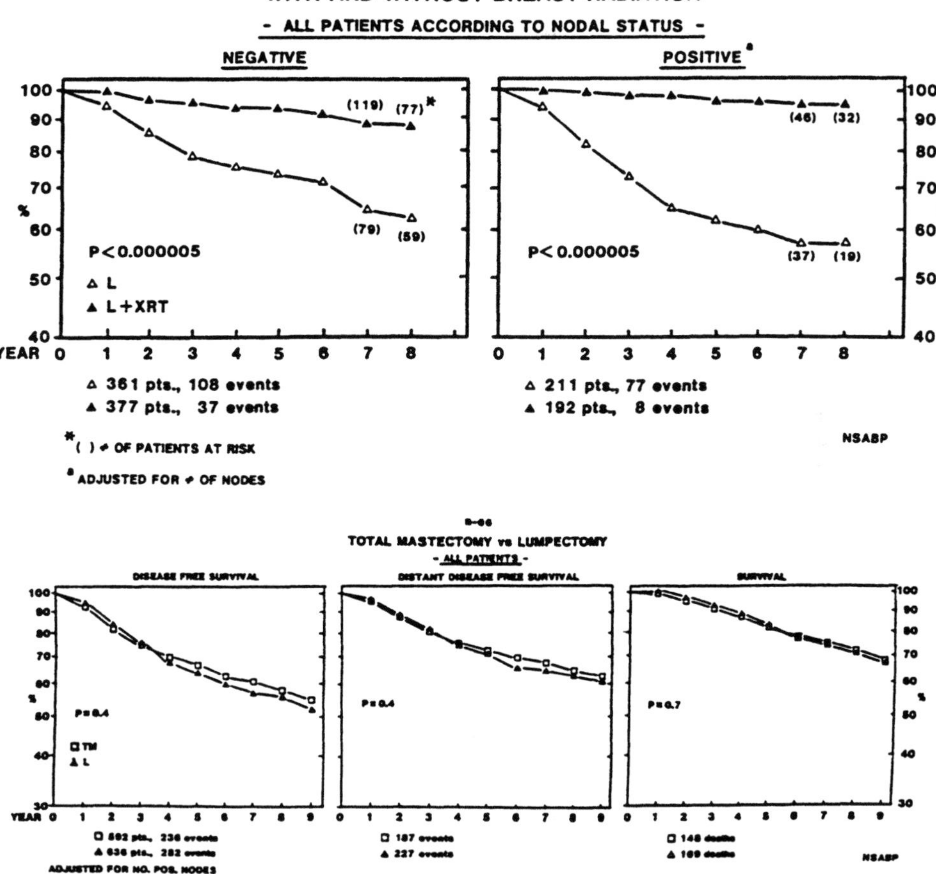

Figure 4: *Top: Local recurrence rates for lumpectomy patients with (L + RT) and without (L) radiation therapy. Bottom: Long-term disease-free survival and survival rates for total mastectomy (TM) and lumpectomy (L) patients.*

problem of local recurrence can be viewed as one of local importance only. The issue of overall treatment failure and survival is not affected by the choice of primary surgery.[4,5,8] The most recent review of local recurrences in protocol B-06[9] provides the view that many LRs can be considered as markers for the existence of distant disease and confirms the evidence that LR is not the source of nor the pathway for that disease or those metastases to disseminate. When local recurrences in B-06 are analyzed according to the size of the original tumor, it is clear that those less than 1 cm in diameter have a favorable rate of local control, but those tumors in the 2-, 3-, or 4-cm range all have substantially similar but higher levels of local recurrence, according to the use of radiation (Fig. 5), suggesting that all but the smallest tumors have similar features that contribute to LR.

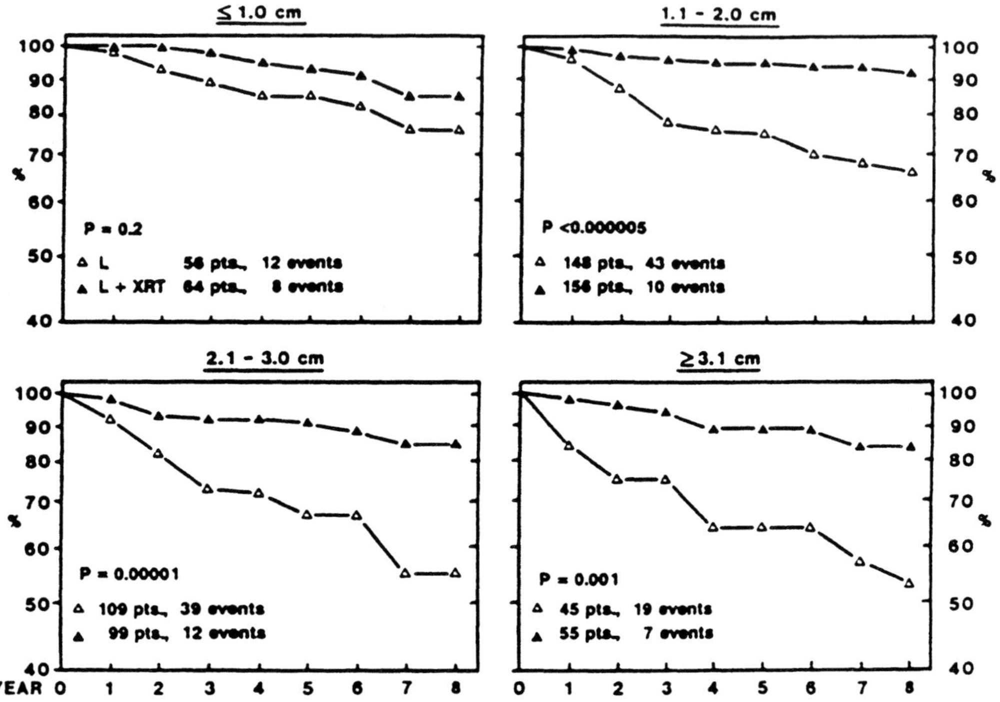

Figure 5: *Protocol B-06. Local recurrence rates according to clinical size of original tumor.*

In this protocol (B-06), careful attention to pathological evaluation of margins including India ink technique was universally employed. All patients followed in the lumpectomy group for risk of local recurrence had pathologically free margins. With the finding that 4% to 5% of these had local recurrence if they were not treated with X-ray therapy,[10] it is clear that this pathological assessment is a false reassurance and that a significant sampling error must exist. In other words, cancer cells at the margins are often left behind, but still there is no apparent change in long-term survival compared to total mastectomy patients (Fig. 4). Radiological and pathological correlations as performed by Holland[11] demonstrate that the histologic extent of the tumor is usually larger than implied by the gross appearance of the tumor. These anatomical findings explain the rather high rate of local recurrence following surgery alone and also explain why smaller tumors will have a lesser incidence of local recurrence. Clinical studies have demonstrated that radiation therapy diminishes this recurrence rate dramatically.[4] The remaining consideration to lessen LR would be wider local surgery such as quadrantectomy, but the gains in terms of local control must be balanced against the necessary increased effects of more tissue removal. In other words, what are the risks of local recurrence and can LR be diminished by any other means?

In subsequent NSABP protocols, patients in adjuvant chemotherapy programs who were treated by lumpectomy and radiation had local recurrence rates that were lower than those seen in protocol B-06 (Table 1). This confirms a speculation derived from an observation in protocol B-06: patients receiving chemotherapy and radiotherapy have an improved rate of local control, possibly due to the additive or synergistic effects of the two modalities. With the demonstration that stage I patients also benefit from adjuvant therapies in terms of disease-free and overall survival rates,[12,13] it appears likely that more patients will receive adjuvant therapy and that local recurrence rates will improve beyond those seen in the original surgical trial.

Since local recurrence will sometimes result in the need for mastectomy in order to achieve local control, successful control at the initial operation is a desirable goal. On the other hand, initial mastectomy will always achieve local control, but of course this does not result in acceptable breast cosmesis. One could not sensibly propose a mastectomy in order to prevent the possible future need for mastectomy in the case of local recurrence, but a cavalier approach with insufficient surgery would cause unnecessary local failures, so a reasonable compromise between inadequate and excessive surgery is required. Patients may be advised to accept mastectomy (or quadrantectomy) in order to avoid the anxiety and fear engendered by a breast cancer recurrence. In reality, this possibility should be evaluated against the daily distress of seeing a distorted breast, especially if this is unnecessary.

Veronesi reports a much lower rate of LR following quadrantectomy compared to lumpectomy.[14] In this study, margins were not studied in all cases, adjuvant therapy was not given to node-negative women, no revision surgery was done for possible margin involvement in lumpectomy (TART) cases, and the method of RT was not the same for the two groups (although the theoretical total dose was calculated to be the same). It is unclear how much effect these

Table 1
Ipsilateral Breast Recurrence—NSABP Lumpectomy Patients

Trial	No. of Patients	No. of Events	Average Annual Failure Rate
B-06			
L + RT	568	47	1.38
B-13			
Operation only	121	9	2.78
MTX + FU-5	117	2	0.57
B-14			
Placebo	537	19	1.24
Tamoxifen	537	0	0.50

Note that patients were selected for inclusion in different protocols according to differing prognostic features; therefore, direct comparisions between protocols are not valid. The overall trend towards fewer LR is, however, apparent.
LR = local recurrence; L = lumpectomy; RT = radiation therapy; MTX = methotrexate; FU-5 = fluorouracil.

differences would have on ultimate LR, but it is reasonable to speculate that the NSABP standard practice of surgical revision for positive margins might be a way of selecting those patients who need extra surgery but still do not require quadrantectomy or even, perhaps, mastectomy.

The quadrantectomy may be a useful compromise between mastectomy and excisional biopsy but is associated with a more noticeable cosmetic defect than lumpectomy, especially if the tumor lies in the inner or lower quadrants. The quadrantectomy approach is a severe solution, and such wider operations may be appropriate for selected larger, or diffuse tumors, but there should first be an attempt at lumpectomy with evaluation of margins. Figure 6 illustrates three broad categories requiring surgical decisions. Three typical patterns of mammographic presentation with microcalcifications are shown. The first, a small cluster, is easily removed by a small operation. The third type may need a quadrantectomy approach and may, in some cases, require mastectomy if all calcifications represent malignancy, but this does not mean that quadrantectomy should be a general first choice. The intermediate type requires careful planning and evaluation. I favor tailoring the operation to the specific situation.

The average clinical tumor size at presentation is 2 cm and may be easily circumscribed with a healthy cuff of normal tissue in virtually all cases. (See the NSABP Workshops publication on technique for details.[15]) If gross or frozen examination suggests involved margin(s), then additional tissue can be taken immediately. Indeed, quadrantectomy-type operations may sometimes be necessary, but the better cosmesis of lumpectomies is appropriate for the vast majority of cases. The Milan quadrantectomy studies accepted patients with tumor sizes up to 2 cm, but the NSABP protocols allow for tumor sizes up to 4 (and later 5 cm) and the recurrence figures cited are valid even for these larger

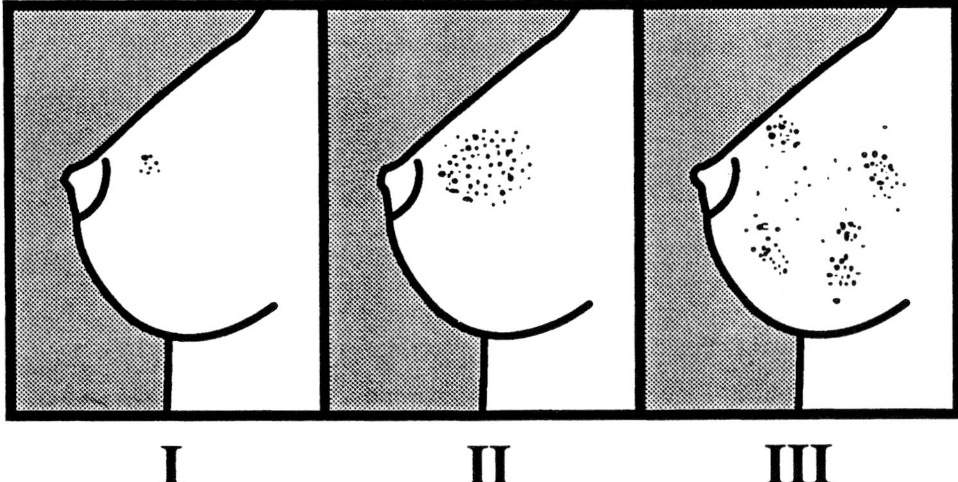

Figure 6: *Patterns of microcalcifications. Type I: Local cluster. Type II: "Cloud burst." Type III: Widespread "galaxy."*

tumors. Local recurrences vary significantly between tumors smaller than 1 cm and those of larger sizes, but no significant differences exist between any of the other sizes (Fig. 5). The techniques of lumpectomy, adequate local excision with grossly and microscopically clear margins, and the use of postoperative radiation and adjuvant systemic therapies produce average annual recurrence rates of well under 1%. The combination of this low rate of local recurrence and the associated better cosmesis makes the lumpectomy operation the preferred approach, especially for all small and medium size tumors that are typical of the presentation for the majority of today's patients.

References

1. Gilliland MD, Barton RM, Copeland EM: The implications of local recurrence of breast cancer as the first site of the therapeutic failure. Ann Surg 1983; 197:284-287.
2. Auchincloss H: The nature of local recurrence following radical mastectomy, Cancer 1958; 11:611–619.
3. Spratt JS: Locally recurrent cancer after radical mastectomy. Cancer 1967; 20:1051–1053.
4. Fisher B, Bauer M, Margolese R, Poisson R, et al: Five-year results of a randomized clinical trial comparing total mastectomy and segmental with or without radiation in the treatment of breast cancer. N Engl J Med 1985; 312:665–673.
5. Veronesi U, Salvadori B, Lun A, et al: Conservative treatment of early breast cancer (long-term results of 1232 cases treated with quadrantectomy, axillary dissection, and radiotherapy). Ann Surg 1990; 211:250–259.
6. Kurtz JM, Amalric R, Brandone H, Ayme Y, et al: Results of wide excision for mammary recurrence after breast-conserving therapy. Cancer 1988; 61:1969–1972.
7. Clarke DH, Lé MG, Sarrazin D, Lacombe MJ, et al: Analysis of local-regional relapses in patients with early breast cancers treated by excision and radiotherapy: experience of the Institut Gustave-Roussy. J Radiation Oncology 1985; II:137–145.
8. Fisher B, Redmond C, Fisher E, Bauer M, et al: Ten-year results of a randomized clinical trial comparing radical mastectomy and total mastectomy with or without radiation. N Engl J Med 1985; 312:674–681.
9. Fisher B, Anderson S, Fisher ER, Redmond C, et al: Significance of ipsilateral breast tumour recurrence after lumpectomy. Lancet 1991; 338:327–331.
10. Fisher B, Redmond C, Poisson R, Margolese R, et al: Eight-year results of a randomized clinical trial comparing total mastectomy and lumpectomy with or without irradiation in the treatment of breast cancer. N Engl J Med 1989; 320:822–828.
11. Holland R, Solke H, Veling J, et al: Histologic multifocality of T1, 1–2 breast carcinomas: implications for clinical trials of breast-conserving surgery. Cancer 1985; 979–990.
12. Fisher B, Constantino J, Redmond C, Poisson R, et al: Randomized clinical trial evaluating tamoxifen in the treatment of patients with node-negative breast cancer who have estrogen-receptor-positive tumors. N Engl J Med 1989; 320:479–484.
13. Fisher B, Redmond C, Dimitrov N, Bowman D, et al: A randomized clinical trial evaluating sequential methotrexate and fluorouracil in the treatment of patients with node-negative breast cancer who have estrogen-receptor-negative tumors. N Engl J Med 1989; 320:473–478.
14. Veronesi U, Volterrani F, Luini V, Saccozzi R, et al: Quadrantectomy versus lumpectomy for small size breast cancer. Eur J Cancer 1990; 26:671–673.
15. Margolese R, Poisson R, Shibata H, Pilch Y, et al: The technique of segmental mastectomy (lumpectomy) and axillary dissection: a syllabus from National Surgical Adjuvant Breast Project workshops. Surgery 1987; 102:828–834.

12

Conservative Treatment of Breast Cancer:
The Milan Experience

Umberto Veronesi, Marco Greco, Alberto Luini, Mirella Merson, Virgilio Sacchini, Stefano Zurrida

History

The idea of preserving the breast in patients with small breast carcinomas was developed at the Milan Cancer Institute in 1968. The reasons for the interest of Milan surgeons for this course were: (1) new information available on the natural history of breast cancer, (2) progressive reduction in size of the tumors in the breast cancer patients thanks to the widespread use of mammography, and (3) the dramatic failure of aggressive local-regional surgical treatments in improving the prognosis of breast cancer patients. Regarding the latter point, it must be remembered that the Milan Institute was the main contributor to the international group that conducted a randomized trial comparing the traditional Halsted mastectomy with the Halsted mastectomy and dissection of the internal mammary nodes. It was just at the end of the 1960s that this trial yielded preliminary results that showed no advantage of the internal mammary dissection over the traditional mastectomy.

The principles of the breast conservation procedure developed at the Milan Cancer Institute were, however, very cautious, and the main objectives were good cosmetic results together with good local control. A high rate of local recurrences was considered unacceptable both because a recurrence might be the source of new metastases and because a local reappearance of the disease creates a condition of anxiety and often depression in the patient. We therefore developed a procedure based on an extensive surgical excision which we defined

From: Wise L, Johnson H Jr (eds): *Breast Cancer: Controversies in Management*. Futura Publishing Company, Inc., Armonk, NY, © 1994.

"quadrantectomy," the main characteristic of which was the radial direction of the incision so that the resection would encompass the whole ductal tree, from the retroareolar region to the periphery. We were convinced that one of the ways in which breast cancer spreads is via the intraductal permeation and that all the ductal branches connected with the involved duct should be removed. This entity (the main duct and the entire ductal tree) is often defined as a breast lobe. Our operation could have been defined as a "lobectomy," but we thought that for the surgeons, the quadrant concept is easier to be defined and understood. Moreover, the breast lobes are not separated into anatomical entities. After the quadrantectomy, we planned aggressive radiotherapy consisting of 50 Gy administered through two tangential opposing fields with high-energy apparatus plus a boost of 10 Gy on the scar with orthovoltage equipment. A total axillary dissection was also part of the procedure. This operation, which later we abbreviated to QUART, was then a somewhat radical operation, but we considered it prudent anyway to apply it to very early cases, and only patients with T1 tumors (less than 2 cm) were considered candidates for this conservative procedure. The first objective was then to organize a trial (possibly multicentric and international) to compare the new procedure with the traditional mastectomy. The occasion occurred in December 1968 at the "Meeting of Investigators on Diagnosis and Treatment of Breast Cancer" called by the WHO in Geneva. At this meeting, chaired by the late Pierre Denoix, some 12 experts (including one of us, UV) were invited from all over the world. The plan for an international trial on breast conservation was presented by the Milan Institute, but was not considered possible, being defined as "premature." One year later, the same group of experts who were at the last meeting, after a long discussion of the Milan renewed proposal, finally accepted the idea of testing the conservative procedure in a randomized trial.

Since one of the most important recommendations was setting up a multicentric trial comparing the Halsted mastectomy with modified radical mastectomy, it was stated in the proposed protocol that each participating center could consider also the third option of the conservative procedure. The minutes of that meeting report that "after discussion of Professor Veronesi's paper which was concerned with the more conservative management of breast cancer and especially with conservation of the breast, it was decided that a method of treatment consisting of local excision of the tumor plus axillary dissection should be added as a third option to this clinical trial." The WHO proposal for this international trial remained, however, at the stage of a project and never became operational. Many centers that had accepted in principle to participate performed their trials separately (Milan, Paris, Moscow, Bucharest). But the importance of the acceptance of the proposal by the WHO experts was fundamental in starting the trial at the Milan Institute, as the opposition of the more senior surgeons who considered the trial risky and unethical was rather strong.

Milan I Trial

The QUART technique was tested for its feasibility in pilot studies from 1970 to 1972, and in 1973 we started the randomization of patients who were subsequently steadily accrued in the following years at an average of 100 cases per year. At the beginning of 1980, the trial was concluded with 701 patients; 349 underwent the Halsted operation and 352 underwent QUART. The early results were published in 1981[1] with clear evidence of similar survival curves with the two procedures.

The impact on breast cancer treatment was considerable but slow, since, in the opinion of many surgeons, the results needed longer follow-up. It was suggested that patients might have unfavorable events many years after the operation, that the number of women who, after conservative treatment, would need salvage mastectomy for a local recurrence should be evaluated, and that to evaluate any oncogenic risk of breast irradiation, a very long follow-up is required. In 1990, a final evaluation was presented[2] confirming the original trend.

The 13-year survival data of small breast cancer showed that QUART gave identical results to those of Halsted mastectomy. Subdivision of the patients by size of tumor, site, and age did not reveal any difference between the treatments.

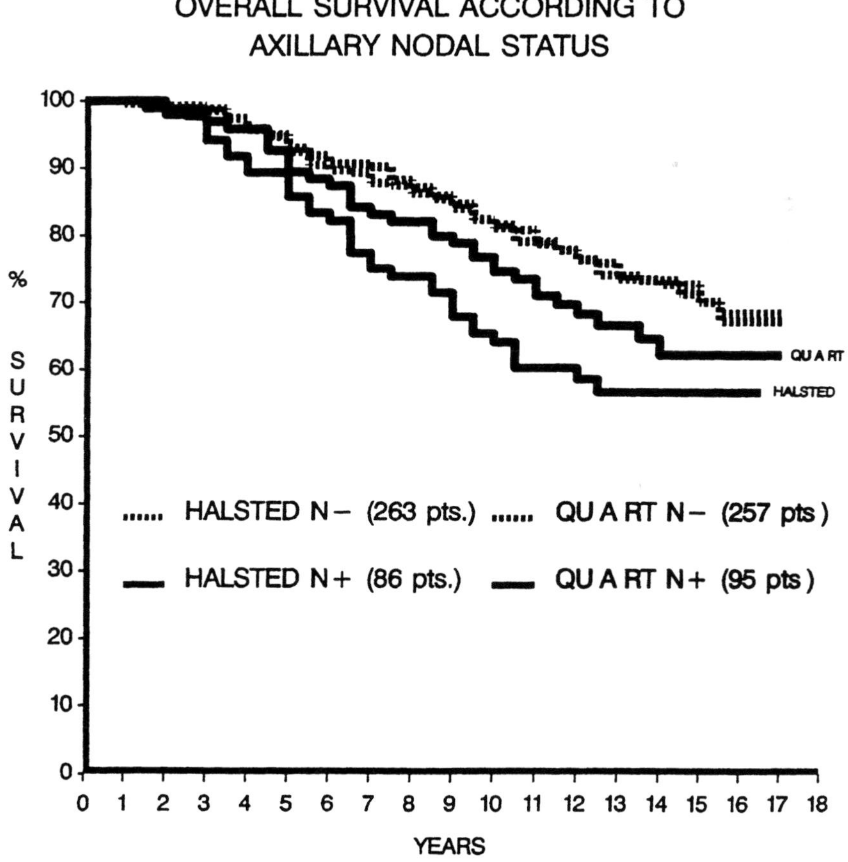

Figure 1: *Milan Trial I: overall survival rates according to type of treatment.*

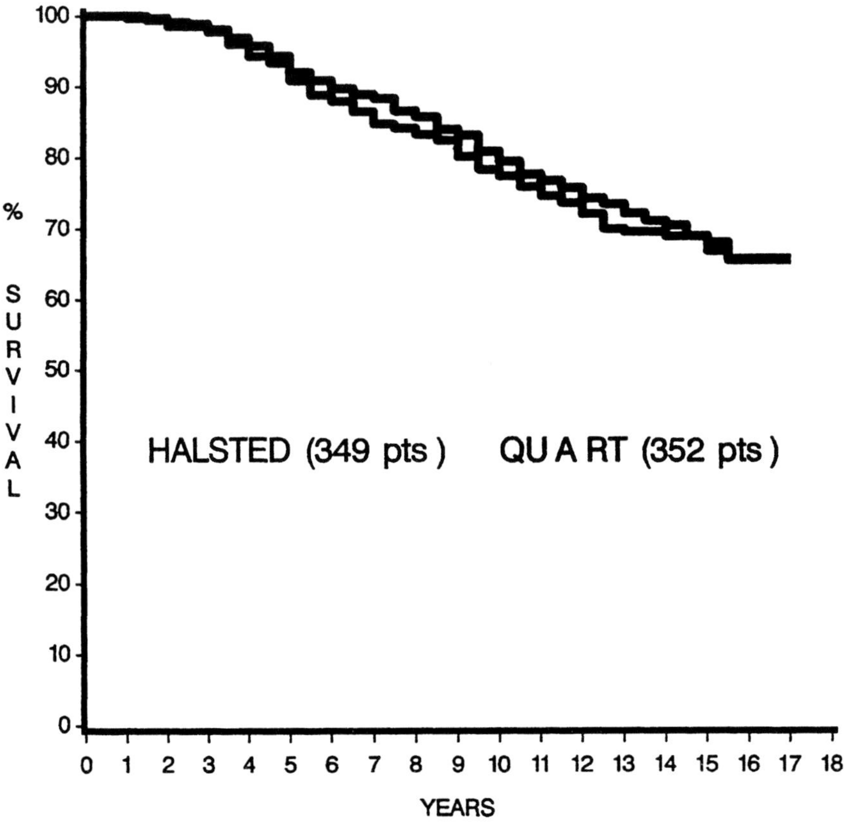

Figure 2: *Milan Trial I: overall survival rates according to axillary nodal status.*

On the contrary, QUART was superior to Halsted mastectomy in patients with positive axillary nodes, without being statistically better (Figs. 1 and 2).

The risk of late oncogenic action of radiotherapy appeared nonexistent. There were nine new ipsilateral cases in patients with heavily irradiated breasts, while in the contralateral breasts there were 19 cases. It appeared, therefore, that breast irradiation, at the doses we used, might perhaps protect the breast either by destroying occult foci of in-situ carcinomas or by inactivating any proliferative precancerous lesions. During the heavy irradiation on the operated breast in the QUART group, the contralateral breasts received a low dose of scattered irradiation. The dosage was calculated to be from 0.5 Gy in the lateral part to 5–15 Gy in the medial part. Nineteen carcinomas appeared in the contralateral breasts of the QUART patients, which is the same as the number of new carcinomas that appeared in the contralateral nonirradiated breasts of the Halsted patients. This indicates that low-dose irradiation is not oncogenic, at least in a population of adult women.

We therefore concluded that QUART is safe and that traditional mastectomy in small breast carcinomas should have no role.

Milan II Trial

The results of the Milan I trial were confirmed by subsequent publications of other trials,[3-6] and the new problem was the identification of the most appropriate type of treatment that could maximize both the local control of the disease and the cosmetic outcome. A number of second-generation trials were then implemented in various centers.[7-9]

A randomized trial was done at the Milan Cancer Institute in 1985–1987 to compare classic quadrantectomy, axillary dissection, and radiotherapy (QUART) with a more limited treatment, consisting of a tumorectomy followed by external radiotherapy and a boost with ^{192}Ir implantation (TART).[10]

TART consisted of excision of the primary tumor with a margin of normal breast tissue of 1 cm. The overlying skin was not removed, except for a very thin portion for histologic examination. Axillary dissection was done with a separate incision and was total. Radiotherapy was both external and interstitial. External irradiation was started 4 weeks after surgery, and the technique was the same as that given after quadrantectomy in equipment, field arrangements and volume irradiated. The difference was the total dose (45 Gy) given over 5 weeks with a daily dose of 0.9 plus 0.9 Gy. After 2–3 weeks, wires of ^{192}Ir were implanted interstitially to give a boost of 15 Gy directly to the tumor bed. A total dose of 60 Gy was thus given to both groups of patients. Nodal sites were never irradiated.

Seven hundred and five patients were evaluable; 360 were treated with QUART while 345 received TART. The two groups had similar characteristics. Different adjuvant treatments were equally distributed.

Local failures sited in the area of previous surgery (i.e., cutaneous, subcutaneous, or parenchymal lesions) that appeared within 3–5 cm from the line of quadrantectomy and lumpectomy scars, respectively, were considered as true local recurrences. At the time of the last review, there were 15 local recurrences in the QUART group and 34 in the TART group (Table 1). The survival is identical in the two groups.

Is a higher rate of local recurrences an acceptable price for better cosmetic results? Local recurrence is a psychological trauma to patients. Their hope for cure is undermined by the new event and intense anxiety may reappear. Because of our improved surgical technique, quadrantectomy may offer cosmetic results

Table 1
Trial II: First Unfavorable Event According to Treatment

	QUART	TART
Local recurrence	15	34
Second ipsilateral carcinoma	2	7
Contralateral carcinoma	14	17
Distant metastases	57	45

that, although inferior to those usually obtained with lumpectomy, are generally well accepted by patients. Since local recurrences are in many cases treated with mastectomy, an excessive number of salvage operations would frustrate the original objective of conservation. Thus, we feel that any radiosurgical procedure that results in an elevated rate of local recurrences should be discouraged.

Milan III Trial

The objective of this randomized trial conducted in the years 1987 and 1988 on 579 patients was to evaluate the efficacy of the quadrantectomy with or without postoperative radiotherapy. Out of the 579 women affected by a breast carcinoma of less than 2.5 cm, 294 were treated with quadrantectomy plus axillary dissection and radiotherapy while 273 were treated with quadrantectomy, axillary dissection, and no radiotherapy. Although it is too early to give significant results, it appears from the first available data that withdrawing the radiotherapy exposes the patients to an increased risk for local recurrences. The results will soon be available for publication.

Milan IV Trial

This trial has the limited objective to compare the efficacy of the traditional boost with an external beam of photons with the irradiation given from implantation of radioactive iridium in patients treated with wide excision, axillary dissection, plus external radiotherapy through two opposing fields with high-energy radiations. The study is in progress, and the accrual of patients is not yet completed.

Preoperative Chemotherapy

The finding that chemotherapy may induce regression of the primary breast carcinoma in a high number of patients with locally advanced disease[11,12] has led to its introduction in patients with a mass of intermediate size, large enough, however, to be treated with mastectomy. A series of 165 cases of patients with primary tumors larger than 3 cm treated with various regimens of preoperative chemotherapy has been reported recently at the Milan Institute.[13] The results showed that in 90% of the cases, the originally planned mastectomy could be substituted with a conservative procedure (QUART).

More recently, encouraged by these results, we have started treating patients with smaller tumors from 1 to 2.5 cm with preoperative chemotherapy with various combinations of drugs. In two subgroups of patients, primary radiotherapy (20 Gy as a boost) was also associated with chemotherapy while the remaining radiotherapy dosage was usually performed after the resection. The objective of this preoperative radio-chemotherapeutic approach is the reduction of both the surgical resection and the risk of local recurrences.

References

1. Veronesi U, Saccozzi R, Del Vecchio M, et al: Comparing radical mastectomy with quadrantectomy, axillary dissection, and radiotherapy in patients with small cancers of the breast. N Engl J Med 1981; 305:6–11.
2. Veronesi U, Banfi A, Salvadori B, et al: Breast conservation is the treatment of choice in small breast cancer: long-term results of a randomized trial. Eur J Cancer 1990; 26:668–670.
3. Sarrazin D, Le M, Fontaine MF, Arriagada R: Conservative treatment versus mastectomy in T1 or small T2 breast cancer: a randomized clinical trial. In: Harris JR, Hellman S, Silen W (eds): Conservative Management of Breast Cancer. JB Lippincott, Philadelphia, pp 101–111, 1983.
4. Fisher B, Bauer M, Margolese R, et al: Five-year results of a randomized clinical trial comparing total mastectomy and segmental mastectomy with or without radiation in the treatment of breast cancer. N Engl J Med 1985; 312:665–673.
5. Van Dongen J: Randomized clinical trial to assess the value of breast conserving therapy in stage I and II breast cancer: EORTC trial 10801. Proc NIH Consensus Development Conf (abstr) pp 25-27, 1990.
6. Lichter AS, Lippman M, Danforth DN, et al: Mastectomy versus breast-conserving therapy in the treatment of stage I and II carcinoma of the breast: a randomized trial at the National Cancer Institute. J Clin Oncol 1992; 10:976–983.
7. Stewart HJ, Prescott RJ, Forrest PA: Conservation therapy of breast. Lancet 1989; 2:168–169.
8. Ribeiro GG, Dunn G, Swindell R, Harris M, et al: Conservation of the breast using two different radiotherapy techniques: interim report of a clinical trial. Clin Oncol 1990; 2:27–34.
9. The Uppsala-Orebro Breast Cancer Study Group: Sector resection with or without postoperative radiotherapy for stage I breast cancer: a randomized trial. J Natl Cancer Inst 1990; 31:277-280.
10. Veronesi U, Volterrani F, Luini A, Saccozzi R, et al: Quadrantectomy versus lumpectomy for small size breast cancer. Eur J Cancer 1990; 6:671–673.
11. De Lena M, Zucali R, Viganotti G, et al: Combined chemotherapy-radiotherapy approach in locally advanced (T3b-T4) breast cancer. Cancer Chemother Pharmacol 1978; 1:53–59.
12. Rubens RD, Sexton S, Tong D, et al: Combined chemotherapy and radiotherapy for locally advanced breast cancer. Eur J Cancer 1980; 16:351–356.
13. Bonadonna G, Veronesi U, Brambilla C, et al: Primary chemotherapy to avoid mastectomy in tumors with diameters of three centimeters or more. J Natl Cancer Inst 1990; 82(19):1539-1545.

13

Radiation Therapy and Limited Surgery Are Not Necessarily as Good as Modified Radical Mastectomy for the Treatment of Breast Cancer

Murid A. Chaudary, John L. Hayward

Introduction

During the first half of this century, the Halsted radical mastectomy was essentially the only operation carried out for breast cancer.[1] When first introduced, the aim behind the technical design of the operation was to eliminate totally all local disease and, as a result, to improve the cure rate. It was largely successful in the first of these aims, but it became evident that a cure was not achieved in many cases because occult metastases were already present. Thus, in the large number of patients who presented with apparently operable tumors, the extent of the primary operation had little or no material effect on survival.

To cut down the extent of mutilation, the operation itself was amended. For instance, the modified radical mastectomy was introduced; this operation did not involve removal of pectoralis major, and treatment by total mastectomy with radiation to the axillary nodes was also used. Nevertheless, the breast still had to be removed, with all the psychological trauma that was involved, and without any real evidence that this affected the cure rate.

The impetus to find an acceptable operation, in which the breast was conserved, began during the second half of this century. By the late 1950s, it was becoming obvious that procedures in which the tumor could be treated by a

From: Wise L, Johnson H Jr (eds): *Breast Cancer: Controversies in Management.* Futura Publishing Company, Inc., Armonk, NY, © 1994.

combination of limited surgery and radical radiotherapy were becoming a real possibility. This was due partly to improvements in radiotherapeutic techniques and partly to the fact that patients were being seen with tumors at a much earlier stage than had been evident when the radical mastectomy was first designed. Early advocates were Mustakallio[2] in Finland, Crile[3] in the United States, Baclesse[4] in France, and Keynes[5] in Great Britain.

Recent years have seen the publication of results from a number of prospective studies that have compared conservative surgery and radiotherapy with mastectomy in patients with early breast cancer.[6–11] The findings from these controlled studies indicate that breast preservation treatment is a viable alternative to mastectomy in a proportion of patients. The questions remaining to be answered are (1) how many can be treated in this way, (2) how should they be selected, and (3) is there still a place for mastectomy? This chapter will try to answer these questions and detail some of the potential disadvantages and possible long-term adverse effects of breast preservation treatment compared to modified radical mastectomy.

Local Recurrence

There is little doubt that local-regional recurrence is higher after conservative treatment than after modified radical mastectomy. As experience with conservative surgery is maturing, the natural history and prognosis of those patients experiencing a local recurrence in the treated breast are beginning to unfold.[12–15] It appears that local recurrence in the conservatively treated breast has a different natural history and the patient has a different prognosis than is the case with chest wall recurrences following mastectomy. There have been divergent reports in the literature addressing the clinical and pathological features of local recurrence in the treated breast and how these features might impact on prognosis.[15–18] Some investigators have concluded that survival is independent of local treatment failure and that a local recurrence is simply a marker of tumor behavior with no impact on survival. Other studies have suggested that inadequate primary treatment, in patients undergoing radiation therapy and conservative surgery, has resulted in an unacceptably high incidence of local recurrence, which is associated with an increased incidence of systemic disease and shorter survival.

Crile et al.[19] published a study of partial mastectomy performed in 173 patients with primary breast cancer, 83% of whom were considered to be clinical stage I. A local recurrence rate of 23% was reported in these patients at 5 years, either at the local excision site, the axilla, or elsewhere in the breast. This failure of local control was associated with a poor 10-year survival rate of 44% in this selected group of patients with favorable disease. Tagart[20] attempted to repeat this study but observed an unacceptably high local recurrence rate and abandoned it. Another nonrandomized study of clinical stage I patients was carried out in Finland by Mustakallio,[21] a study that is often cited as demonstrating that radiation therapy and breast conservative surgery is as effective as radical surgery in controlling breast cancer. But there appears to have been an initial bias in the selection of patients for this study: 46% of those treated conservatively had T1 lesions (less than 2 cm in diameter) compared with 15% of the mastectomy group. Five-year survival rates were 82% for radical mastectomy and 79% for the conservative group. At 10 years, however, a significant difference in survival rate emerged between the two groups in those patients with T2 lesions: 65% survived after radical mastectomy compared with 49% on conservative treatment. With a follow-up of 15 years, a survival rate difference also became apparent in favor of the radical mastectomy patients with T1 lesions. These results stress the need for prolonged follow-up of patients to assess the efficacy of treatments in breast cancer, particularly where early stage I breast cancers are concerned.

The first indication from a clinical trial that radiation therapy and conservative surgery may not be the right approach in all patients with early breast cancer came from a study at Guy's Hospital, London, comparing wide excision with radical mastectomy, which was first reported in 1972.[22] Both groups of patients received postoperative radiotherapy. This prospective randomized study showed that in patients with clinically involved axillae, radical mastectomy gave significantly better results in terms of local and distant recurrence and survival, compared with wide excision with radiation therapy to the breast and axilla. On the other hand, in patients with clinically uninvolved axillae, although there was a higher incidence of local recurrence in patients who had a wide excision, this did not affect the development of distant metastases nor was survival impaired.

The design of this trial was widely criticized because the dose of radiation therapy given to the axilla of those women who were treated by wide excision was suboptimal by today's standards. Nevertheless, the fact that conservative treatment was effective in patients with clinically negative axillae seemed definite and persuaded the authors of the study to start a second series in which only patients with clinically negative axillae (T1, T2, or T3: N0 or N1A) were entered. This second series was completed by 1975, and reports of the results were published in 1976[23] and in more detail in 1983.[6] Results of this second trial did not, as had been expected, confirm those of the first. In the second series, patients who had a wide excision, and the same dose of radiation therapy to the breast and axilla as was used in the first series, did significantly worse than those who had radical mastectomy—not only in the incidence of local recurrence but also in the incidence of metastatic disease and in survival.

These results posed two fundamental questions: (1) was the survival rate in patients who had wide excision low because the treatment failed to achieve local control of disease (almost all the local recurrence in these patients was in the axillary lymph nodes)? This would indicate that local control of disease is important and contrary to a current suggestion that breast cancer is a systemic disease at first presentation. (2) If the outcome is predetermined, why did patients with clinically uninvolved axillae who had wide excision do so well in the first series but so badly in the second, although the treatment appeared to be identical? Hayward and Caleffi[24] recently reported the updated results of this trial and attempted to explain these paradoxical findings. The new analysis showed that the difference in survival between the two groups was confined to patients with T1 tumors. There was no significant difference in the survival of patients with T2 tumors in the two series. There were significantly more patients with T1 tumors in the second study than in the first, and this accounted for the difference in survival. These findings emphasize some points that are fundamental to the effective treatment of patients with early breast cancer, and provide strong evidence of the importance of achieving local control in the primary treatment of the disease, particularly in patients with small tumors where failure of local control will significantly affect survival.

Recently, further evidence has come from the preliminary results of the National Surgical Adjuvant Breast Project (NSABP) B-06 trial reported by Fisher and colleagues in 1985.[25] In this study, total mastectomy was compared with segmental mastectomy with or without radiation therapy. The initial 5-year report of this trial suggested that when the groups treated with partial mastectomy with or without radiation were compared, the disease-free survival of node-negative patients was higher among those women treated with radiation than in those treated with partial mastectomy alone, in whom a significantly higher incidence of local recurrence was observed. In the more recent results of this study,[6] the significant difference in distant disease-free survival rates between the two groups has disappeared. It has been suggested that the difference observed in the earlier report may have been related to a lead-time bias in the identification of distant disease in the lumpectomy alone group. As these patients had a significantly greater number of breast recurrences, they were subjected to more thorough screening for metastatic disease at that time which resulted in earlier detection of distant metastases. It has been suggested that the additional follow-up time presumably has removed this bias. This conclusion may be premature, as the follow-up on these patients is still short.

Stotter et al.[26] have recently argued that in the absence of a very large randomized controlled trial, a survival deficit due to local-regional recurrence following breast conservation therapy could not be discounted. They postulated that local-regional recurrence after breast conservation treatment might be associated with an additional survival hazard, similar to that of a second primary tumor with the same extent of local and regional disease. Using this hypothesis, they examined the probable effect of local-regional recurrence on the clinical course of disease in patients who were treated with conservative surgery and radiation therapy at their institution. Their calculations indicated that no statistically significant survival deficit due to local-regional recurrence following breast conservation therapy would be detectable until a randomized controlled trial comparing breast conservation with mastectomy had monitored more than 10,000 patients for more than 10 years. These authors argue that so far, no randomized prospective study comparing breast conservation therapy with mastectomy has the statistical power to demonstrate a survival deficit due to local-regional failure if it was of the magnitude of that associated with a comparable primary, and hence no reproducible survival difference has been demonstrated. The most cogent arguments that support the concept that local-regional treatment influences survival come from the results of the population-based breast cancer screening programs conducted both in Europe and the United States. The results of these studies unequivocally show that early detection reduces mortality rates. If screening reduces mortality, this effect must result from treatment at an earlier stage, achieving local control in a greater number of patients. As a direct consequence of this, the likelihood of metastatic disease becomes reduced and mortality is decreased. The Guy's Hospital trials[24] suggest that local control is most important in patients with small tumors. This underlines the potential hazards of treatment that conserves the breast. Conservation treatment is used most frequently in the very patients in whom there is a vital need to control local disease, and the methods used must be as effective as in mastectomy. In a large proportion of these patients, total cure is possible and it must not be compromised by the use of ineffective surgical and radiotherapeutic treatments. This is not to say that it is not important to achieve local control in patients with large tumors, but rather that an effect on survival in these patients may be small and has not been demonstrated with certainty so far. The prevailing concept that preventing recurrence in the local-regional area is unimportant is fraught with danger and encourages the use of trivial and ineffective treatment.

Long-Term Complications Resulting from Radiation Therapy

Breast-conserving therapy differs from primary radical surgery not only in the preservation of the diseased breast but in the need for breast irradiation. Since radiation is an established breast carcinogen,[27] it might be argued that patients who are treated with breast conservation are subjected to serious potential risks not necessarily shared by their surgically treated counterparts. Discounting the local side effects of radiotherapy, which are seldom of functional consequence, these risks fall into four categories: (1) the possible induction of contralateral breast cancer due to scatter radiation to the opposite breast[28,29]; (2) the induction of sarcomas in the high-dose region of the breast and chest wall,[30,31] (3) a potential increase in the rate of second malignancies at other anatomical regions,[32] and (4) excess mortality from nonmalignant causes. Cuzick et al.[33] carried out an overview of 10 randomized trials of postoperative adjuvant radiotherapy in breast cancer, in which the difference between the two groups was solely whether or not the patients had been irradiated postoperatively. This overview showed no significant effect on survival after 10 years, but beyond 10 years the mortality in the irradiated patients was significantly increased. The largest trial in Cuzick et al.'s overview was the Cancer Research Campaign Study (Kings/Cambridge Trial), which compared simple mastectomy and postoperative radiotherapy with simple mastectomy followed by a watch policy. Subsequent to the report by Cuzick et al., Haybittle et al.[34] carried out a detailed analysis of the data from this particular trial on causes of death in the two groups. Their findings confirmed that adjuvant radiotherapy after simple mastectomy for early breast cancer produced a small excess late mortality from other cancers and cardiac disease. Analysis of the causes of death after 5 years showed a relative risk of 2.11 (1.25–3.59) for new malignancies and of 1.65 (1.05–2.58) for cardiac disease, the risk in cardiac mortality being most pronounced in patients who had tumors of the left chest and whose treatment had included orthovoltage radiation. The fact that excess malignancies in this study were not predominantly in or close to the parts of the body that would have received the highest dose of radiation lends some support to the suggestion that radiotherapy may adversely affect the immune system and that its effect may be mediated by irradiation of the circulating lymphocytes. These findings have implications for the use of radiation therapy following conservative surgery in patients with small breast cancers, perhaps detected by mammography. Such patients have an excellent chance of surviving beyond 10 years and would then be at greatest risk of developing the long-term unwanted effects of radical radiotherapy. These patients may do far better in the long term with more radical primary surgical treatment and subsequent reconstruction.

Breast Conservation Treatment and Psychological Morbidity

At present, there is a lack of convincing evidence of a more favorable psychological adjustment after breast conserving treatment, although breast conservation does reduce the body image disturbances associated with mastectomy.[35–37] Apart from this benefit, studies using standardized psychological measures have shown no difference in the postoperative incidence of anxiety states and depressive illness among women undergoing either mastectomy or conservative surgery and radiation therapy.[35–39] The loss of sexual interest also appears to occur at the same rate in patients undergoing breast conservation and mastectomy. Fallowfield et al.,[39] in a retrospective study, reported that over 30% of patients in both the mastectomy and breast conservation group described loss of libido. While patients undergoing breast conservation treatment do not face the prospect of a markedly different body image, they may have additional worries. They may worry about whether the radiation therapy will have long-term ill effects, in addition to whether it will be really effective in eradicating local disease. Following radiation therapy, the texture of the breast changes and, as a result of this, a number of women worry about whether they should examine the treated breast and what they could tell if they did: Is any lumpiness or hardness a direct result of therapy? Is anything that feels unusual there to be considered a warning signal of recurrent disease? The results of present studies suggest that there is a need to consider both the potential psychological value and the medical efficacy of breast conservation therapy. Continued psychological assessment of these women is necessary to evaluate their quality of life.

The Influence of Delay from Tumorectomy to Radiation Therapy

There is a paucity of data about the effect of the interval between surgery and the start of radiotherapy on the risk of local recurrence in patients undergoing breast conservation treatment. A number of studies have suggested that the likelihood of local recurrence is high in those patients in whom radiation therapy is delayed for several weeks. In a series from the Institute Gustave Roussy,[40] patients treated within 7 weeks of conservative surgery had a local-regional failure rate of 5% compared with 14% for patients who did not start radiotherapy until 7 weeks or more after surgery (P = 0.01). Recht et al.[41] reported on 295 patients who underwent breast conservation treatment at the Joint Center for Radiation Therapy and affiliated institutions. The authors assessed breast failure rates in relation to the sequencing of radiotherapy and chemotherapy. The actuarial 5-year local failure rate was 5% for 252 patients irradiated within 16 weeks of surgery compared with 35% for 34 patients irradiated more than 16 weeks after surgery. Although the numbers in this study are small, and the sequencing of surgery, radiotherapy, and adjuvant systemic therapy was not done on a random basis, the results suggest that a delay in initiation of radiotherapy may result in increased risk of breast recurrence. Hayward et al.[42] have attempted to overcome this problem by giving a boost dose of radiation to the tumor site within 48 hours of excision, by immediate implantation with iridium-192. The sequencing of the various treatment modalities in breast preservation treatment remains controversial, and controlled randomized trials are necessary to assess survival and quality of life issues among patients treated by different sequences of conservative surgery, radiotherapy and chemotherapy.

Tumor Size

All prospective randomized trials of conservative surgery and radiation therapy have, for various reasons, considered patients with tumor sizes of 4 cm or less as being eligible for this form of treatment. Tumor size can affect both prognosis and cosmesis and the latter is discussed later in this chapter. A number of studies have examined the influence of tumor size on local recurrence of the disease. Eberlein et al.[43] reported the results from the Joint Center for Radiation Therapy regarding local recurrence in the breast following excision and radiation therapy. There was a 13% recurrence among patients with T1 lesions compared with 12% among patients with T2 tumors. They concluded that tumor size was not predictive of a local recurrence, and tumor size therefore should not be a dominant factor in determining suitability for such treatment. One interesting finding from this study, however, was that the highest rate of local recurrence (21%) was observed in patients with tumors less than 1 cm. Zafrani et al.[44] updated an uncontrolled series of 434 patients from Institute

Curie and also found that tumor size did not predict local recurrence, but incomplete surgical excision, as ascertained microscopically, was highly predictive. Ryoo et al.[45] reported an uncontrolled series of 393 patients. Size of tumor did not predict local failure but a small size of the excised specimen correlated with local recurrence. In the uncontrolled series reported by Kantrowitz et al.,[46] size of tumor again did not correlate with local recurrence, but it was noticed much less frequently in patients undergoing the widest surgical excisions (quadrantectomy). In the study by Veronesi et al.,[8] the patients had small tumors and were treated with quadrantectomy. The rate of local failure remains the lowest ever reported following conservative surgery and radiotherapy. The strong inference from these studies is that although size per se may not be a critical variable for local recurrence, the adequacy of excision, which relates indirectly to size, certainly is. The size of primary tumor is critically important to the outcome of patients with breast cancer. Detection of cancer of small size by mammography is associated with improved survival; the size of primary tumors within the symptomatically encountered range strongly correlates with outcome; size correlates with prognosis even within subsets of patients with or without nodal metastases. Tumor size, indeed, is one of the most important variables related to whether the woman can be cured of her disease. Much work still needs to be done to assess the significance of tumor size in relation to local recurrence and its adverse effect on outcome.

Age

A number of studies have examined the relation between the age at treatment and first recurrence following breast conservation treatment.[47–51] Results of these studies clearly show that young women have a high risk of local recurrence although breast preserving therapy is more desirable aesthetically in this age group. Overall, the group under age 30 has a 30% breast relapse rate. The study with the shortest follow-up[50] has shown the least effect, but all show a consistently increased breast relapse rate in the younger group treated by radiotherapy. Fourquet et al.[52] confirmed the dominant influence of age on breast recurrence risk. Their data show that local control of the disease increased linearly with age; patients over 55 years had a 97% 10-year probability of local control, whereas younger patients (less than 32 years) had only a 75% 10-year probability of being free of disease in the breast. When adjusted for other clinical and pathological variables in multivariate analysis, and particularly to adequacy of surgical excision, age remained the most important factor contributing to breast recurrence. The physical and psychological morbidity associated with relapse of disease in the breast in this group and its effect on mortality still needs to be evaluated properly.

Tumor Histology

Tumors of certain histologic subtypes are more prone than others to recur locally after tumorectomy and radiation therapy. Available data suggest that extensive ductal carcinoma in situ (DCIS) may be an important marker of residual disease after tumorectomy for invasive cancer. In a study of reexcisions after initial gross excision of 71 infiltrating ductal carcinomas, Schnitt et al[53] found that the presence of extensive DCIS in the initial specimen correlated strongly with a likelihood of reexcision. Furthermore, for patients with positive reexcisions, primary tumors with extensive DCIS were associated with a significantly greater quantity of residual cancer, predominantly intraductal, than were tumors without this feature. These conclusions were strengthened by Holland et al.,[54] who studied 214 serial mastectomy specimens after simulated tumorectomy. Prominent residual DCIS, mostly in the vicinity of the primary lesion, was found in 44% of cases with extensive DCIS in the reference tumor, compared to 3% of cases without extensive DCIS. These authors emphasized that extensive residual DCIS was the major contributor to local failure after conservative excision and radiotherapy, either because of a greater tumor burden per se or possibly due to a lesser radiosensitivity of DCIS.[55] They have defined as high risk those tumors exhibiting both 25% or more DCIS within the primary tumor mass as well as DCIS in the surrounding breast tissue. Patients with pure infiltrating ductal carcinoma and those with intraductal carcinoma making up less than 25% of their primary tumor have local failure rates of 4% to 10% after excision and radiation therapy. In contrast, patients with extensive intraductal carcinoma have local recurrence rates of 22% to 71% after gross excision and radiation therapy. The data indicate that a limited breast resection is acceptable for a tumor with a low in-situ component, but that a more extensive resection is required in the presence of extensive DCIS. These findings have implications for cosmetic outcome as well as local control because cosmetic outcome after conservative surgery and radiotherapy is most adversely affected by the extent of resection.[56,57]

Infiltrating lobular carcinoma has been considered a contraindication to breast conserving treatment by some.[58,59] Schnitt et al.[58] reported on 49 cases of infiltrating lobular carcinoma among 561 patients treated with breast conservation therapy. The 5-year actuarial risk of local recurrence was 12% in patients with infiltrating lobular carcinoma, 23% for patients with infiltrating ductal carcinomas with an extensive intraductal component, and 5% in those without an extensive intraductal component. Mate et al.[60] reported on a small series of 12 patients with lobular carcinoma and also found an increase in local recurrence rates for lobular histology. It has been suggested that the increased recurrence rate in patients with lobular carcinoma may be due to a large residual tumor burden in the breast following first tumor excision. Studies also indicated that breast recurrences following conservative surgery for lobular carcinoma are often subtle, tend to be multifocal, involving multiple quadrants of the breast, and often difficult to detect.[58,61] The present data for invasive lobular carcinoma indicate that wide microscopically clear margins should be obtained in these patients.

Cosmesis

The only advantage of conservative surgery and radiation therapy over mastectomy is that the former attempts to preserve a cosmetically acceptable breast. However, while it is important, cosmesis is one of the most difficult areas to evaluate. The cosmetic results reported so far have generally ranged from being good to excellent,[62–64] while recognizing that patients tend to judge cosmetic outcome more favorably than medical observers. Recognition of factors that can modify cosmesis is important so that the physical and psychological sequelae of treatment can be minimized. Factors influencing cosmesis are related to surgical techniques, radiation techniques, and patient characteristics. One patient characteristic that has been identified to influence cosmesis is the size of the breast. Patients with large breasts achieve poorer cosmesis than patients with smaller breasts following radiation therapy, while the cosmetic result of local surgery is worse in patients with small breasts.[65] This poor cosmetic outcome from radiation in patients with large breasts may be due to increased fat content in these breasts, making them particularly sensitive to high doses of fractionated irradiation. Thus, careful attention to radiotherapy technique is especially important in these patients to achieve a good cosmetic result. Tumor size is also a factor that affects the cosmetic result.[65,66] Clarke et al.[65] reported that when tumor size was 4 cm or greater, excellent cosmetic results were achieved in only 7 of 15 (47%) of the patients. In breasts with tumors less than 4 cm, excellent results were noted in 86%.

The poor cosmetic results that are reported in patients with large tumors would not support the use of primary radiotherapy for lesions greater than 4 cm. Even in patients with tumors of 4 cm or less, the size of the tumor in relation to the size of the breast is of paramount importance in affecting the cosmetic outcome. To obtain the best local control and cosmetic result, full attention must be given not only to the excision biopsy and radiation therapy techniques but also to the individual patient characteristics.

Multiple Cancers

Although the multicentricity of breast cancer has traditionally been used as an argument against limited surgery,[67,68] long-term results of breast-conserving treatment with radiotherapy suggest that the clinical relevance of multiple cancer foci documented only on pathological examination is probably limited.[8,69–72] However, the presence of more than one macroscopically apparent tumor mass has been considered to represent a contraindication for breast preservation, even by those strongly advocating this form of treatment.[73] Such patients are commonly excluded from breast-conserving treatment programs because of the assumption that patients with macroscopically multiple tumors have a high risk of local recurrence. Data from two recently reported studies support this assumption. Kurtz et al.[74] reported on 586 unilateral stage I and stage II breast cancers treated with conservative surgery and radiotherapy of whom 61 presented with two or more macroscopic tumor nodules, diagnosed either clinically or mammographically or on gross pathologic examination. After a median follow-up of 71 months, 15 of 61 (25%) of the patients with multiple tumors developed recurrence in the treated breast compared to 56 of 525 (11%) of patients with a single cancer (P<0.005). Local failure occurred in 6 of 37 (16%)

bifocal tumors and in 9 of 24 (35%) patients with three or more tumor foci. Recurrence was more frequent for multiplicity diagnosed clinically or mammographically (36%) than when it was apparent only to the pathologist (18%). The other important findings in this study were that, in contrast to the recurrences of unifocal breast cancer, local failures in these patients tended to be located at a distance from the original foci, to be multifocal, or to be diffuse including skin involvement. Only four recurrences presented as a single focus in the vicinity of the original primary tumor. Leopold et al.[75] reported on the effectiveness of conservative surgery and radiation therapy in 10 patients with multiple lesions and 707 patients with single lesions treated at the Joint Center for Radiation Therapy. Four of the 10 patients with multiple lesions recurred in the treated breast (40%) compared to 77 of the 707 patients (11%) with single lesions. (P = 0.019). The results of these studies show that the presence of two or more separate primary tumors in the breast is associated with a high likelihood of local recurrence after treatment with conservative surgery and radiation therapy, even when all identified tumors are grossly resected. The optimal management of patients who present with clinically multiple primaries appears to be a modified radical mastectomy. The use of conservative surgery and radiation therapy in these patients is often complicated by the practical considerations of resecting two separate primaries. In many women this alone would result in considerable breast distortion so that mastectomy is a most reasonable option. In addition, the use of a boost to two separate areas in the breast may also result in an unacceptable cosmetic result. The use of conservative surgery and radiation therapy for patients with multiple lesions may be more feasible in those where the two lesions are in very close proximity and where the combined size of the lesions does not exceed 4 cm.

The Elderly

Age per se is not a contraindication to breast preservation treatment and, indeed, many older patients are as conscious of their body image as their younger counterparts. Breast conservation therapy, however, is no less intense in its radicality and can be much more demanding in elderly patients than mastectomy. Established techniques of breast conservation treatment all include surgical components (tumorectomy, axillary clearance) and external radiation therapy. The latter consists of treating the breast to a dose of 46–50 Gy with a boost to the tumor bed of between 15–20 Gy. This treatment is fractionated and is given on a daily basis and usually lasts for 6 weeks.The safe delivery of radiotherapy requires immobilization of the patient, generally in a supine position, and a high degree of collaboration between patient and staff. This can pose a problem in elderly patients with chronic arthritic conditions, respiratory insufficiency, and other debilitating conditions. Thus, protracted radiation treatment may impose a heavy burden on an elderly patient. A prolonged admission to hospital for this treatment again may not be acceptable to the patient and will also make the procedure less cost-effective. Attempts to use wide local excision together with systemic tamoxifen in the elderly have not proved universally acceptable. Certainly, the local recurrence rate is higher and there is a suggestion that survival may be compromised.[76] Modified radical mastectomy offers a quick and effective means of local-regional control of disease provided the patient is fit to withstand this procedure.

Pregnancy

Pregnancy contraindicates radiation therapy and hence breast conservative treatment. Using the standard technique of whole breast irradiation, followed by a boost dose to the tumor site, the dose scattered to the fetus is unacceptably high. Leakage from the radiotherapy unit and internal scatter from within the body account for most of the fetal irradiation. Leakage radiation is independant of field size or beam energy but can be modified by external blocking. However, the radiation reaching the fetus from internal scatter by the mother's tissues cannot be reduced by external shielding. The internal scatter is dependent on field size, photon energy, and proximity to the field edge. The internal scatter dose may range from 10 to 20 rads for a total course of treatment in early pregnancy to a dose of 100 rads or more for a total treatment course given in the last pregnancy trimester. Internal scatter dose carries risk, both in terms of teratogenicity and congenital fetal abnormalities. For these reasons, mastectomy is the preferred treatment for pregnant patients with operable breast cancer. Such a procedure carries minimal risk to the mother or the fetus and the pregnancy can be allowed to continue.

Conservative Surgery and Radiation Therapy for Ductal Carcinoma In Situ

Until recently, management of ductal carcinoma in situ was not much of an issue. First, such tumors were considered to be uncommon, accounting for less than 5% of all breast cancers, and second, mastectomy was the standard treatment for almost every breast cancer including in-situ disease. Two recent developments, however, have transformed management of ductal carcinoma in situ into an issue of increasing clinical importance. These are the widespread use of mammography where in-situ disease is most commonly diagnosed, and the realization that breast conservation therapy is a viable alternative to mastectomy in patients with early invasive breast cancer. Ductal carcinoma in situ is a lesion with a high potential to become invasive and therefore requires definitive therapy. The invasive potential appears to vary from tumor to tumor, and the factors that affect the prognosis in ductal carcinoma in situ are not clearly defined. The results of studies of estrogen receptor proteins, oncogene products, cellular DNA content, and measurement of tumor proliferative rate are emerging,[77–79] but at present, the prognostic value of the findings is unclear. The prognostic significance of the histologic subtypes of ductal carcinoma in situ also needs to be established. Of symptomatic patients who are found to have DCIS, without evidence of invasion, up to 40% will go on to develop infiltration in the ipsilateral breast after biopsy alone.[80,81] Among screen-detected cases with lesions measuring less than 2.5 cm treated by wide excision, the progression rate to invasion has been reported to be as low as 5%. A number of institutions have published results on the use of conservative surgery and radiation therapy for ductal carcinoma in situ and have reported local recurrence rates of 5.5% to 10% with follow-up ranging from 39 to 55 months.[82-84] Although recurrence in the breast following conservative surgery and radiation therapy is not common, the patient must be willing to accept regular mammographic and clinical follow-up examination and a risk of developing subsequent invasive disease, which remains constant for the rest of her life. Suitability for breast-conserving treatment depends on the extent of ductal carcinoma in situ. If complete excision is a prerequisite, then only 40% to 50% of all cases of ductal carcinoma in situ can be treated by breast conservation.[85] Prospective randomized trials are necessary to establish the efficacy of conservative surgery alone or in combination with radiation therapy in the treatment of ductal carcinoma in situ. A number of such trials are now in progress in the United States and Europe. Outside of clinical trials, however, there are as yet no established criteria identifying patients who may benefit most from breast conservation treatment. Mastectomy remains the only treatment which virtually guarantees cure and obviates the need for close follow-up. The availability of reconstruction assumes an important role in these circumstances.

Discussion

In 1982, a meeting was held at Leeds Castle in England, of approximately 25 breast cancer specialists drawn from many disciplines and many different countries. The aim of this meeting was to identify the state of the art at that time. Regarding conservative treatment, the rapporteurs in their report[86] remarked as follows: "Less mutilating local treatments allowing breast preservation are being explored. Early results suggest that this may be appropriate treatment for some patients; however, these results are preliminary and need further follow-up and confirmation." Four years later, in 1986, a second such meeting was held to try to determine whether attitudes had changed over the intervening period. In their report,[87] the rapporteurs remarked as follows: "One major change since the previous meeting is the general acceptance that a procedure in which the breast is conserved can now replace mastectomy in many patients."

Now, some 7 years later, many regard a mastectomy as outmoded and outdated and suggest that conservation treatment can be used in most, if not all, patients with operable breast cancer. The time scale of this immense change is only 10 years. Indeed, this change has occurred so rapidly that it is reasonable to question whether sufficient thought has been given to the disadvantages as well as the advantages of conservation treatment. In this chapter, an attempt has been made to identify areas where conservation treatment carries a material risk.

In general, this risk is of an excess of local-regional recurrence over that which would be expected by the standard modified radical mastectomy. The suggestion is that this excess of local recurrence may, in its own right, ultimately compromise survival. Not only does local recurrence carry with it this potential threat, but some features of conservative treatment itself, for instance, the long-term results of radiation therapy on mortality from other diseases, and the unsuitability of radiation therapy in the case of pregnancy or in the elderly, must also be taken into account. It may well be that the difficulties encountered in many of the groups mentioned in this chapter may be considered to be too minor to determine a change of treatment from conservation therapy. That may or may not be so, but it is important to realize that these disadvantages exist and not simply to ignore them. This is not only relevant to those working in the field, but also to the patients themselves, who should be given some idea of the potential risks and hazards of a treatment that has been tested for a period of only 10 or so years—a very short time span in terms of survival following treatment for primary breast cancer. An immense amount of work needs to be done to determine precisely the relative benefits and contraindications. This information must come from clinical trials that have been properly and specifically designed. Until these answers are available, it should be remembered that, as with any major change in the treatment of disease, the pendulum often swings violently from one extreme to another. We do not yet know where the pendulum will stop in relation to our approach to the local treatment of cancer of the breast.

References

1. Halsted WS: The results of operations for the cure of cancer of the breast performed at the Johns Hopkins Hospital, June 1889-January 1894. Johns Hopkins Hosp Bull 1894–95; 4:297.
2. Mustakallio S: Conservative treatment of breast carcinoma: review of 25 years of follow-up. Clin Radiol 1972; 23:110–116.
3. Crile G: Treatment of breast cancer by local excision. Am J Surg 1965; 109:400–403.
4. Baclesse F: Roentgentherapy as the sole method of treatment of cancer of the breast. Am J Roentgenol Rad Ther 1949; 62:311–318.
5. Keynes G: Conservative treatment of cancer of the breast. Br Med J 1937; 643–647.
6. Hayward JL: Prospective studies: the Guy's Hospital trial on breast conservation. In: Harris JR, Hellman S, Silen WJB (eds). Conservative Management of Breast Cancer. Lippincott, Philadelphia, pp 77–90, 1983.
7. Sarrazin D, Le MG, Arriagada R, et al: Ten-year results of a randomised trial comparing conservative treatment to mastectomy in early breast cancer. Radiother Oncol 1989; 14:177–184.
8. Veronesi U, Banfi A, Del Veccio N, et al: Comparison of Halsted mastectomy with quadrantectomy, axillary dissection and radiotherapy in early breast cancer: long-term results. Eur J Cancer Clin Oncol 1986; 22:1085–1089.
9. Fisher B, Redmond C, Poisson R, et al: Eight-year results of randomized clinical trial comparing total mastectomy and lumpectomy with or without irradiation in the treatment of breast cancer. N Engl J Med 1989; 320:822–828.
10. Van Dongen JA, Bartelinik H, Fentiman IS, et al: Factors influencing local relapse and survival and results of salvage treatment after breast conserving therapy in operable

breast cancer: EORTC 10801 Trial, comparing breast conservation with mastectomy in TNM stage I and II breast cancer. Eur J Cancer 1992; 28A:801–805.

11. Findlay PA, Lippman ME, Danforth D, et al: Mastectomy versus radiotherapy as treatment for stage I and II breast cancer: a prospective randomised trial at the National Cancer Institute. World J Surg 1985; 9:671–675.

12. Delouche G, Bachelot F, Premont M, et al: Conservation treatment of early breast cancer: long-term results and complications. Int J Radiat Oncol Biol Phys 1987; 13:29–34.

13. Harris J R, Recht A, Almaric R, Calle E, et al: Time course and prognosis of local recurrence following primary radiation therapy for early breast cancer. J Clin Oncol 1984; 2:37–41.

14. Kurtz JM, Almaric R, Delouche GL: Second ten years following long-term results of breast conservation. Int J Radiat Oncol Biol Phys 1987; 30:1327–1332.

15. Recht A, Silen W, Schnitt SJ, et al: Time course of local recurrence following conservative surgery and radiotherapy for early stage breast cancer. Int J Radiat Oncol Biol Phys 1988; 15:255–261.

16. Kurtz JM, Spitalier J, Almaric R, et al: Mammary recurrences in women younger than 40. Int J Radiat Oncol Biol Phys 1988; 15:271–276.

17. Kurtz JM, Spitalier JM, Almaric R, et al: Late breast recurrence after lumpectomy and irradiation. Int J Radiat Oncol Biol Phys 1983; 9:1191–1194.

18. Recht A, Rose MA, Silver B, et al: Prognosis following breast recurrence after conservative surgery and radiotherapy for early stage breast cancer (abstr). Int J Radiat Oncol Biol Phys 1987; 13(S1):162–163.

19. Crile G, Cooperman A, Essenstein CB, et al: Results of partial mastectomy in 173 patients followed from 5–10 years. Surg Gynecol Obstet 1980; 150:563–566.

20. Tagart REB: Partial mastectomy for breast cancer. Br Med J 1978; 2:1268.

21. Rissanen P, Holsti P: Long-term results of conservative and radical surgery, combined with radiotherapy in stage I carcinoma of the breast: 15-year follow-up and assessment of quality of life of 646 patients. Presented at the International Congress of Radiology, Madrid, October 1973.

22. Atkins H, Hayward JL, Klugman DJ, et al: Treatment of early breast cancer: a report after 10 years of a clinical trial. Br Med J 1972; 2:423–429.

23. Hayward JL: The Guy's trial of treatments of early breast cancer. World J Surg 1977; 1:314–316.

24. Hayward JL, Caleffi M: The significance of local control in the primary treatment of breast cancer. Arch Surg 1987; 122:1244-1247.

25. Fisher B, Bauer M, Margoles ER, et al: Five-year results of randomized clinical trial comparing total mastectomy and segmental mastectomy with or without radiation in the treatment of breast cancer. N Engl J Med 1985; 312:665–673.

26. Stotter A, Atkinson EN, Fairston BA, et al: Survival following locoregional recurrence after breast conservation therapy for cancer. Ann Surg 1990: 212: 166–172.

27. Land CE: Lower dose irradiation: a cause of breast cancer? Cancer 1980; 46:868–873.

28. Basco VE, Coldman AJ, Elwood JM, et al: Radiation dose and second breast cancer. Br J Cancer 1985; 52:319–325.

29. Hankey BF, Curtis RE, Naughton MD, et al: A retrospective cohort analysis of second breast cancer risk for primary breast cancer patients with an assessment of the effect of radiation therapy. J Nat Cancer Inst 1983; 70:797–804.

30. Fergusson DJ, Sutton HG Jr, Dawson PJ: Late effects of adjuvant radiotherapy for breast cancer. Cancer 1984; 54:2319-2323.

31. Soubaw W, McKenna RJ Jr, Benjamin R, et al: Radiation induced sarcomas of the chest wall. Cancer 1986; 57:610–615.

32. Harvey EB, Brinton LA: Second cancer following cancer of the breast in Connecticut 1935–1982. J Nat Cancer Inst 1985; 68:9-112.

33. Cuzick J, Stuart H, Peter P, et al: Overview of randomised trials of post-operative adjuvant radiotherapy in breast cancer. Cancer Treatment Rep 1987; 71:15–29.

34. Haybittle JL, Brinkley D, Houghton J, et al: Post-operative radiotherapy and late mortality: evidence from the Cancer Research Campaign Trial for early breast cancer. Br Med J 1989; 298:1611–1614.
35. Sanger CK, Reznikoff M: A comparison of psychological effects of breast saving procedures with modified radical mastectomy. Cancer 1981; 48:2341–2346.
36. Steinberg MD, Juliano NA, Wise L: Psychological outcome after lumpectomy versus mastectomy in the treatment of breast cancer. Am J Psychiatry 1985; 143:34–39.
37. DeHaes JCJM, Van Oostrom MA, Welvaart K: The effect of radical and conserving surgery on the quality of life for early breast cancer patients. Eur J Surg Oncol 1986; 12:337–342.
38. Schain W, Edwards BK, Gorrell CR, et al: Psychosocial and physical outcomes of stage I breast cancer therapy: mastectomy versus excisional biopsy and irradiation. Breast Cancer Res Treatment 1983; 3:377–382.
39. Fallowfield LJ, Baum M, MaGuire GP: Effects of breast conservation on psychological morbidity associated with the diagnosis and treatment of early breast cancer. Br Med J 1986; 293:1331–1334.
40. Clarke DH, Le MG, Sarrazin D, et al: Analysis of locoregional relapses in patients with early breast cancers treated by excision and radiotherapy: experience of the Institute Gustave Roussey. Int J Radiat Oncol Biol Phys 1985; 11:137–145.
41. Recht A, Come SE, Gelman RS, et al: Integration of conservative surgery, radiotherapy and chemotherapy for the treatment of early stage node positive breast cancer: sequence in timing and outcome. J Clin Oncol 1991; 9:1662–1667.
42. Hayward JL, Winter PJ, Tong D, et al: A new combined approach to the conservative treatment of early breast cancer. Surgery 1984; 95:270–274.
43. Eberlein TJ, Connolly JL, Schnitt SJ, et al: Predictors of local recurrence following conservative breast surgery and radiation therapy. Arch Surg 1990; 125:771–777.
44. Zafrani B, Vielh P, Fourquet A, et al. Conservative treatment of early breast cancer: prognostic value of the ductal in-situ component and other pathological variables on local control and survival. Eur J Cancer Clin Oncol 1989; 25:1645–1650.
45. Ryoo MC, Kagan AR, Wellin M, et al: Prognostic factors for recurrence and cosmesis in 393 patients after radiation therapy for early mammary carcinoma. Radiology 1989; 172:555–559.
46. Kantrowitz DA, Poulter CA, Rubin P, et al: Treatment of breast cancer with segmental mastectomy alone or segmental mastectomy plus radiation. Radiother Oncol 1989; 15:141–150.
47. Vilcoq JR, Cale R, Stacey P, et al: The outcome of patients with operable breast cancer. Int J Radiat Oncol Biol Phys 1981; 7:1327–1337.
48. Matthews RH, McNeese MB, Montague ED, et al: Prognostic implications of age in breast cancer patients treated with tumorectomy and irradiation or with mastectomy. Int J Radiat Oncol Biol Phys 1988; 14:659–663.
49. Recht A, Connolly JL, Schnitt SJ, et al: The effect of young age on tumour recurrence in the treated breast after conservative surgery and radiotherapy. Int J Radiat Oncol Biol Phys 1988; 14:3–10.
50. Kurtz JM, Spitalier JM, Amalric R, et al: Mammary recurrences in women younger than 40. Int J Radiat Oncol Biol Phys 1988; 15:271–276.
51. Kurtz JM, Jacquemier J, Spitalier JM, et al: Why are local recurrences after breast conserving therapy more frequent in young women? Proceed Am Soc Clin Oncol 1989; 8:19.
52. Fourquet A, Campana F, Zafrani E, et al: Prognostic factors of breast recurrence in the conservative management of early breast cancer: a 25-year follow-up. Int J Radiat Oncol Biol Phys 1988; 17:719–725.
53. Schnitt SJ, Connolly JL, Khettry U, et al: pathologic findings on re-excision of the

primary site in breast cancer patients considered for treatment by primary radiation therapy. Cancer 1987; 58:675–681.

54. Holland R, Connolly JL, Gelman R, et al: The presence of an extensive intraductal component following a limited excision correlates with prominent residual disease in the remainder of the breast. J Clin Oncol 1990; 8:113–118.

55. Osteen RT, Connolly JL, Recht A, et al: Identification of patients at high risk for local recurrence after conservative surgery and radiation therapy for stage 1 and 2 breast cancer. Arch Surg 1987; 122:1248–1252.

56. Olivotto IA, Rose MA, Austin RT, et al: Late cosmetic outcome after conservative surgery and radiotherapy: analysis of causes of cosmetic failure. Int J Radiat Oncol Biol Phys 1989; 17:747–753.

57. Materywe JR, Wertheimer M, Fitzgerald TJ, et al: Aesthetic result following partial mastectomy and radiation therapy. Plastic Reconstr Surg 1990; 85:739–746.

58. Schnitt SJ, Connolly JL, Silver B, et al: Infiltrating lobular carcinoma of the breast in patients treated with conservative surgery and radiotherapy. Int J Radiat Oncol Biol Phys 1988; 15(Suppl 1):194.

59. Kurtz JM, Jacquemier J, Torhost J, et al: Conservative surgery for brest cancers other than infiltrating ductal carcinoma. Int J Radiat Onol Biol Phys 1988; 15(Suppl 1):194.

60. Mate TP, Carter D, Fischer D, et al: The clinical and histopathologic analysis of the result of conservation surgery and radiation therapy in stage I and II breast carcinoma. Cancer 1986; 58:1995–2002.

61. Kurtz JM, Almaric R, Brandone H, et al: Results of wide excision for mammary recurrence after breast conserving therapy. Cancer 1988; 61:1969–1972.

62. Harris JR, Levene MB, Sevensson G, et al: Analysis of cosmetic results following primary radiation therapy for stages 1 and 2 carcinoma of the breast. Int J Radiat Oncol Biol Phys 1979; 5:257–261.

63. Beadle G, Silver B, Botnik L, et al: Cosmetic results following primary radiation therapy for early breast carcinoma. Carcinoma 1984; 54:2911–2918.

64. Beadle G, Come S, Henderson IC, et al: The effect of adjuvant chemotherapy on the cosmetic result after primary radiation treatment for early breast cancer. Int J Radiat Oncol Biol Phys 1984; 10:2131–2137.

65. Clarke D, Martinez K, Cox RS: Analysis of cosmetic results and complications in patients with stage 1 and 2 breast cancer treated by biopsy and radiation. Int J Radiat Oncol Biol Phys 1983; 9:1807–1813.

66. Bedwinek J: Treatment of stage I and II adenocarcinoma of the breast by tumour excision and irradiation. Int J Radiat Oncol Biol Phys 1981; 7:1553–1559.

67. Morgenstern L, Kaufman PA, Friedman NB: The case against tylectomy for carcinoma of the breast: a factor for multicentricity. Am J Surg 1975; 130:251–255.

68. Shah JA, Rosen BP, Robbins GF: Pitfalls of local excision in the treatment of carcinoma of the breast. Surg Gynecol Obstet 1973; 136:721–725.

69. Spitalier JM, Gambarelli J, Brandone H, et al: Breast conserving surgery with radiation therapy for operable mammary carcinoma: 25-year experience. World J Surg 1986; 10:1014-1020.

70. Clark R, Wilkinson RH, Miceli MT, et al: Breast cancer: experiences with conservation therapy. Am J Clin Oncol 1987; 10:461–468.

71. Fisher ER, Sass R, Fisher B, et al: Pathologic findings from the National Surgical Adjuvant Breast Project (Protocol 6) II: relation of local breast recurrence to multicentricity. Cancer 1986; 57:1717–1724.

72. Recht A, Silen W, Schnitt SJ, et al: Time course of local recurrence following conservative surgery and radiotherapy for early stage breast cancer. Int J Radiat Oncol Biol Phys 1988; 15:255–261.

73. Danoff BF, Haller DG, Glick JH, et al: Conservative surgery and irradiation in the treatment of early breast cancer. Ann Int Med 1985; 102:634–642.

74. Kurtz JM, Jacqueimer J, Amalric R, et al: Breast conserving therapy for macroscopically multiple cancer. Ann Surg 1990; 212:38–44.
75. Leopold KA, Recht A, Schnitt J, et al: Results of conservative surgery and radiation therapy for multiple synchronous cancers of one breast. Int J Radiat Oncol Biol Phys 1991; 16:11–16.
76. Fentiman IS: Breast cancer in the elderly. In: Fentiman IS (ed). Detection and Treatment of Early Breast Cancer. Martin Dunitz, pp 193–206, 1990.
77. Meyer JS: Cell kinetics of histologic variants of in-situ breast cancer. Breast Cancer Res Treatment 1986; 7:171–180.
78. Carpenter R, Gibbs M, Matthews J, et al: Importance of cellular DNA content in pre-malignant breast disease and pre-invasive carcinoma of the female breast. Br J Surg 1987; 74:905-906.
79. Van de Vivjver MJ, Peterse JL, Mooi WJ, et al: Neu-protein over expression in breast cancer: association with comedo type ductal carcinoma-in-situ and limited prognostic value in stage II breast cancer. N Engl J Med 1988; 319:1239–1245.
80. Betsill WL, Rosen PP, Lieberman PH: Intraductal carcinoma: long-term follow-up after treatment by biopsy alone. JAMA 1978; 293:1863–1867.
81. Page DL, DuPont WD, Rogers LW, et al: Intraductal carcinoma of the breast: follow-up after biopsy alone. Cancer 1982; 49:751-758.
82. Fisher ER, Sass R, Fisher B, et al: Pathologic findings from the National Surgical Adjuvant Breast Project (Protocol 6) 1: intraductal carcinoma (DCIS). Cancer 1986; 57:197–208.
83. Recht A, Danoff BS, Solin LJ, et al: Intraductal carcinoma of the breast: results of treatment with excisional biopsy and irradiation. J Clin Oncol 1985; 3:1339–1343.
84. Zafrani B, Fourquet A, Vilcoq JR, et al: Conservative management of intraductal breast carcinoma with tumourectomy and radiation therapy. Cancer 1986; 57:1299–1301.
85. Fentiman IS, Julien JP, Van Dongen JA, et al: Reason for non-entry of patients with DCIS of the breast into a randomised trial (EORTC 10853). Eur J Cancer 1991; 27:450–452.
86. Canellos GP, Hellman S, Veronesi U: The management of early breast cancer. N Engl J Med 1982; 306:1430–1432.
87. Hayward JL, Rubens RD: UICC multidisciplinary project on breast cancer management of early and advanced breast cancer. Int J Cancer 1987; 39:1–5.

The Examination of Resection Margins with Conservative Surgery:

What Is the Value?

*Umberto Veronesi, Salvatore Andreola,
Roberto Agresti, Viviana Galimberti,
Stefano Zurrida*

Introduction

The progressive introduction of conservative procedures in breast cancer treatment have opened an era of more acceptable and less traumatic management of patients affected by this dreadful disease. The avoidance of the mutilation and the preservation of the symmetrical image of the body certainly represents progress toward a better quality of life. However, new procedures have raised new problems and new dilemmas for the surgeon and the pathologist.

One of the most important problems is the risk of local recurrence after the surgical and radiological conservative management. Although there is enough evidence that a local recurrence by itself is not an instigator of new metastases because it does not influence the survival rate, as shown in many randomized trials, any measure to reduce its occurrence should be considered and applied. In fact, a local recurrence not only frustrates the objectives of breast conservation itself as it often leads to a mastectomy, but it represents a dramatic event in the history of the patient because of the painful conditions of anxiety and anguish that it creates.

One of the main problems in breast conservation treatment is, therefore, the definition of the quantity of normal breast tissue to be removed around the tumor to keep the risk of local recurrence very low. To give a quantitative answer

From: Wise L, Johnson H Jr (eds): *Breast Cancer: Controversies in Management.* Futura Publishing Company, Inc., Armonk, NY, © 1994.

to the question, a series of studies conducted by Holland[1] have clearly shown that the presence of cancer cells at the periphery of breast carcinoma decreases progressively with the distance from the tumor edge, whereas at 1 cm there are cancer foci in 59% of the cases (of which nearly half are in situ), at 3 cm the percentage drops to 17%.

Obviously, if after a breast resection one could select the cases that are likely to have no more cancer cells left in the breast, these cases could be considered practically safe from the risk of recurrence, perhaps not even needing postsurgical radiotherapy.

The pathologists have therefore developed a technique to evaluate the margins of the excised breast tissue. One of the major clinical randomized studies where margin assessment was considered a fundamental part of the treatment protocol was the National Surgical Adjuvant Breast Project (NSABP) trial B-06.[2] In that trial, the cases that were found to have positive margins after lumpectomy were immediately treated with mastectomy, while cases with negative margins were treated, in one subgroup, with lumpectomy alone without postoperative radiotherapy.

The technique utilized by pathologists is very uniform. The surface of the margins of the specimen must be marked so that they can be identified by microscope. This is easily done with India ink or tattoo dyes that remain adherent to the tissue and are microscopically recognizable. This procedure is not an impediment to performing frozen section, nor does it delay obtaining tissue for biological or receptor analysis. To orientate the specimen, the guidance of the surgeon is essential, this being easily accomplished with a few well-placed stitches.

Generally, a total of 10 sections are taken from different parts of the specimen. Regarding the reporting of the results, there is no standardization. While it is easy to define a "positive" case when the tumor cells actually involve the free margins, it is difficult to define the borderline cases which are sometimes vaguely indicated as "close to the margins."

The clinical significance of the assessment of the margins has not been defined, but at least for the "negative cases" the results accumulated until now are disappointing. In the NSABP trial, cases with negative margins treated with lumpectomy without radiotherapy showed a local recurrence rate of more than 40%, indicating that in two cases out of five the margin negativity was false. Similar results have been observed by other investigators, although the postoperative radiotherapy usually administered after breast resection has reduced the rate of local recurrences in negative-margin patients.[3] The experience of the Milan Cancer Institute, in our trial II comparing quadrantectomy plus radiotherapy with lumpectomy plus radiotherapy, has shown that positive margins were rare in the quadrantectomy patients (4%), but frequent in the lumpectomy patients (16%). Regarding false-negative cases, out of 169 sampled patients with negative margins treated with quadrantectomy, six developed a local recurrence (4.5%), and out of 243 patients with negative margins treated with lumpectomy, 21 developed a local recurrence (8.6%) (Table 1). It appears, therefore, that the pathological finding of clear margins is not a reassuring factor that will predict a

Table 1
Rate of Local Recurrences According to Positive and Negative Margins in the MILAN II Trial

| Margins | Quadrantectomy + RT | | | Lumpectomy + RT | | |
| | | Local | | | Local | |
	N.	Recurrences	%	N.	Recurrences	%
Cases with margin assessment	178	7	3.9	289	29	10.0
Positive	8	1	12.5	46	8	17.4
Negative	170	6	3.5	243	21	8.6
Margins not assessed	182	8	4.4	56	5	8.9
Total	360	15	4.1	345	34	9.8

low risk of recurrence. We can conclude that rather often cancer cells remain in the breast beyond the "negative" margins of resection and such cases are not identified by the pathologist.

There are several reasons for the failure of the procedure. The first is that breast specimens are often soft and irregular and it is difficult to evaluate the margins accurately. The second is that the biopsies are taken at the surface of the specimen at random and, although numerous, they cover only a small portion of all the surface area. Therefore, it may be that an invaded margin may escape observation. The third is that the cancer process around the primary carcinoma is not "continuous" and that areas of discontinuity are not infrequent. To at least partially avoid these shortcomings, we have devised a procedure that employs monoclonal antibodies to detect the presence of cancer cells on the surface of the specimen.[4]

What about the reliability of positive margins? In this case, at least theoretically, the predictability should be excellent. If the margins are positive, it is fairly certain that cancer cells could be left in the breast, and local recurrence seems almost unavoidable if no other treatments are performed. Obviously there is no experience where the margins were found positive and nothing was done, so we have no experimental evidence of the above-mentioned assumption. In most instances, a mastectomy or a breast re-resection is performed whenever positive resection margins are found. However, in our Milan II trial, the protocol implied that after lumpectomy with positive margins, radiotherapy would be done without any additional surgical correction. This decision was in line with the concept that lumpectomy by definition cannot be called a radical operation but simply a "debulking" type of surgery. The treatment with radiotherapy of cases with positive margins and therefore likely to have residual breast cancer has provided important information on the rate of radiosensitive and radioresistant cases. In our study, the fact that 8 out of 46 cases with positive margins have locally relapsed would lead to the assumption that in the other 38 cases radiotherapy was able to destroy the residual cancer tissue. These data would lead to the conclusion that the percentage of radiosensitive breast cancer cases is more than 80%. Although this figure may change with a longer follow-up, it will certainly give an indication on the radioresistance issue.

If we now consider that in the remaining 243 patients with negative margins, 21 recurred locally, and that this number represents only one-fifth of the cases that actually would have recurred without radiotherapy, one could conclude that some 100 cases out of 243 had in fact remaining cancer cells in the breast, in spite of the resection margin negativity, a percentage (41%) that is similar to the NSABP B-06 experience.

Summary

The finding of clear margins is not a reliable sign of reassurance from local recurrence and therefore should not abolish additional treatments such as radiotherapy, while on the other hand, the finding of positive margins is a likely expression of residual disease left in the breast, so that appropriate measures must be considered.

References

1. Holland R, Veling SHJ, Mravunac M, et al: Histologic multifocality of Tis, T1–2 breat carcinomas: Implications for clinical trials of breast-conserving surgery. Cancer 1985; 56:979–990.
2. Fisher B, Bauer M, Margolese R, et al: Five-year results of a randomized clinical trial comparing total mastectomy and segmental mastectomy with or without radiation in the treatment of breast cancer. N Engl J Med 1985; 312:665–673.
3. Veronesi U, Volterrani F, Luini A, et al: Quadrantectomy versus lumpectomy for small size breast cancer. Eur J Cancer 1990; 26(6):671–673.
4. Veronesi U, Farante G, Galimberti V, Greco M, et al: Evaluation of resection margins after breast conservative surgery with monoclonal antibodies. Eur J Surg Oncol 1991; 17:338–341.

15

The Role of Axillary Dissection in Managing Patients with Breast Cancer:

The Case for Complete Axillary Clearance

Hiram S. Cody III, Jerome A. Urban

Introduction

Throughout this century, most patients treated for operable breast cancer had radical mastectomy, and hence a complete axillary dissection. In recent decades, encouraged by the results of randomized trials,[1-3] the treatment options for breast cancer have proliferated rapidly, to the confusion and dismay of patients and practitioners alike. Local therapies have included radical mastectomy, modified radical mastectomy, simple mastectomy, quadrant excision, wide local excision, and narrow local excision, with varying degrees of axillary dissection (none, partial, full), and with or without postoperative radiotherapy, a total of 36 options for local therapy alone. Including the options for systemic adjuvant treatment (none, hormonal, "standard" cytotoxic, and "aggressive" cytotoxic) yields a total of 144 possible combinations! The traditional "Halstedian" concept of breast cancer has emphasized the importance of aggressive local treatment in preventing subsequent regional recurrence and distant spread; the more recent "Fisher hypothesis"[4] has emphasized the importance of occult systemic disease in determining outcome, independent of variations in local treatment. These two views are not mutually exclusive. It is our contention that further improvement in breast cancer survival will be achieved only by (1) continued efforts at earlier diagnosis and (2) a combination of meticulous and thorough local therapy with the systemic treatment of those patients most likely to have occult metastases. Only through complete axillary dissection can these objectives best be realized for most patients with operable breast cancer.

From: Wise L, Johnson H Jr (eds): *Breast Cancer: Controversies in Management.* Futura Publishing Company, Inc., Armonk, NY, © 1994.

Patient Selection

For a small minority of breast cancer patients, 1% to 2%, complete axillary dissection is not indicated.

1. For very elderly or medically poor-risk patients, the risks of general anesthesia and the underlying illness far outweigh those of the breast cancer; this group is best treated by simple tumor excision under local anesthesia, followed (optionally) by a systemic agent such as tamoxifen.

2. Lobular carcinoma in situ is a condition associated with a high risk (about 35% over 25 years, nine times normal) for the development of an invasive cancer in either breast, as demonstrated in a careful long-term study by Rosen et al.[5] Many such patients are simply followed closely with frequent examination and mammography. For the minority who elect mastectomy (for a variety of reasons), our current practice is to perform either a low (level I) axillary dissection or no axillary dissection at all. Past experience indicates that about 1% will have axillary metastases (presumably from an unrecognized area of invasive carcinoma elsewhere in the breast).

For patients with noninvasive intraductal carcinoma, the role of axillary dissection is increasingly controversial. Historically, intraductal carcinoma comprised about 5% of all breast cancers, with a 1% to 5% incidence of axillary metastases and 10-year NED (no evidence of disease) survival of about 95% after mastectomy. The few deaths presumably occurred in patients with undiscovered foci of invasive cancer, most of whom indeed had axillary metastases. In the current era of mammographic screening, about 15% of all breast cancers are intraductal, and fewer patients have axillary metastases, perhaps 1% to 2%. If patients with tumor microinvasion can be excluded by careful pathological review, the frequency of axillary metastasis may be even less. In a recent report from Kinne et al.[6] (Memorial Hospital), only one patient in 128 treated by mastectomy and axillary dissection for in-situ breast cancer had positive nodes. Our current practice for these patients is to perform a total mastectomy with low (level I) axillary dissection.

The remaining 85% of breast cancer patients with invasive carcinomas are best treated by full axillary dissection, for the following reasons:

1. The number of axillary node metastases remains overwhelmingly the most important prognostic factor in all patients with operable breast cancer. The choice among all treatment options, both local and systemic, is based directly on the presence and extent of axillary nodal involvement. The surgical removal and pathological evaluation of the axillary contents should thus be as complete and precise as possible.

2. Clinical evaluation of the axilla is notoriously inaccurate. The frequency of false-negative axillary exam has been as high as 50% in historical series. Tables 1–3 report our experience with 795 patients treated between 1971 and 1978, all by mastectomy (radical, extended, or modified) and full axillary dissection, correlating clinical and pathological findings in the axilla. Full axillary dissection is defined as complete removal in continuity of all tissue medial to (level III),

Table 1
Axillary Node Status, Clinical vs. Pathological
1971–1978 (795 Patients)

Clinical	Neg	Highest Level + (Pathological) I	II	III	Total
		Number (Percent)			
Neg	459 (69)	132 (20)	39 (6)	33 (5)	663 (100)
Pos	18 (14)	55 (42)	27 (20)	32 (24)	132 (100)
Total	477 (60)	187 (24)	66 (8)	65 (8)	795 (100)

Table 2
Axillary Node Status, Clinical vs. Pathological
1971–1978 (795 Patients)

Clinical	0	# Nodes + (Pathological) 1–3	4–6	7–10	>10	Total
			Percent			
Neg% (n=665)	69.5	22.0	4.4	1.8	2.3	100
Pos% (n=130)	14.2	45.7	13.4	11.0	15.7	100
Total% (n=795)	60.5	25.8	5.9	3.3	4.5	100

Table 3
Axillary Node Status by Tumor Size
1971–1978 (747 Patients)*

Tumor Size (M)	Neg	Highest Level + (Pathological) I	II	III	Total
0–1.0 (n = 111)	78.7	14.9	2.8	3.5	100
1.1–2.0 (n = 189)	65.2	22.4	6.2	6.2	100
2.1–3.0 (n = 98)	53.6	26.2	9.8	10.4	100
3.1–4.0 (n = 24)	32.0	34.7	21.3	12.0	100
4.1–5.0 (n = 13)	39.4	33.3	6.1	21.2	100
>5.0 (n = 8)	32.0	36.0	16.0	16.0	100

*Tumor size pathologically indeterminate in 48 patients.

posterior to (level II) and lateral to (level I), the pectoralis minor. Each level was tagged for orientation intraoperatively, and each specimen dissected without special "clearing" techniques; a mean of 23 nodes was obtained per specimen. False-negative clinical exam occurred in 26%, and false-positive exam in 2.3% of all patients: i.e., in expert hands, clinical evaluation was incorrect 28.3% of tbe time.

3. Precise pathological staging is essential for the comparison of results from different therapeutic protocols, and from different centers. The critical comparison of treatment results in breast cancer remains frustrated by inconsistent local therapy and inadequate use of precise clinical and pathological TNM staging for all treated patients. Single-surgeon[7-9] and single-institution[10] results for breast cancer are consistently superior to those reported from multi-institutional randomized trials, yet it remains unclear whether these survival differences (some quite large) are better explained by variations in treatment or stage of disease.

4. Complete dissection removes all axillary nodal metastases, thereby preventing either distant metastasis from residual axillary disease or subsequent reoperation for local recurrence. In our patients, an axillary dissection limited to level I would have left level II and III metastases behind in 10.9% of clinically node-negative and 44.7% of clinically node-positive patients. For breast cancers in the average size range (2.1–3.0 cm), a limited axillary dissection would miss axillary metastases in 20.2% of patients. Even if a limited dissection were performed only for 0–1.0 cm tumors, 6.3% would have disease left behind.

Auchincloss[11] has argued fatalistically that because only 4 of 38 patients (10.5%) with level III axillary node involvement followed 8–10 years were still disease-free, the value of full axillary dissection was "minimal if not zero." This influential 1963 study led to the widespread adoption of modified radical mastectomy with less-than-complete axillary dissection as the "standard of care" in the 1970s and 1980s, yet its conclusions were based on a group of only 107 node-positive patients treated by radical mastectomy from 1951 to 1953. In fact, our most recent analysis of 1,288 primary operable breast cancers (1965–1978) treated by mastectomy and full axillary dissection demonstrated 10-year overall and disease-free survivals of 43% and 34% for level III positive patients.[12] Clearly, many patients with level III positive node involvement are quite salvageable with adequate local therapy alone.

Fisher[4] has hypothesized that (1) axillary nodes are not instigators of metastases but rather indicative of the host-tumor relationship, (2) survival is dependent more on the presence at diagnosis of occult systemic spread than on variations in local treatment, and (3) subsequent relapses in either the axilla or the breast should thus have no adverse survival impact. Four separate prospective randomized trials—the National Surgical Adjuvant Breast Project (NSABP) B-04, NSABP B-06, and the first and second Guy's Hospital trials—directly address this issue.

In the NSABP B-04 trial[13] (accrued 1971–1974), Fisher's hypothesis was tested, for clinically node-negative patients, by randomization to radical mastectomy (RM), total mastectomy with postoperative nodal and chest wall radiotherapy (TMR), and total mastectomy alone (TM). In the 1985 follow-up report of this trial,[2] there was "no significant difference" at 10 years in overall, disease-free, or distant disease-free survival among the three groups, seeming to suggest that axillary dissection was of no value to the patients in whom it was done.

A close reading of this and other NSABP reports suggests quite the opposite:

1. Among the 365 patients randomized to TM alone, 129 (35%) had removal of "some" axillary nodes:[14] fewer than 6 in 23%, 6–10 in 6%, and more than 10 in 7% of all patients. This violation of the randomization procedure significantly confounds any analysis of the results. One might expect as a result an underestimation of the rate of subsequent axillary recurrence (in patients randomized to TM), and narrowing of any survival advantage occurring as a result of axillary dissection.

2. Patients in whom six or more axillary nodes were removed had no axillary recurrences at 8 years.[14] All axillary relapses occurred in patients with minimal or no removal of axillary nodes.

3. Among the 236 patients having TM without removal of axillary nodes, 21.2% had axillary relapse at 8 years.[14] Fisher et al. chose not to define these axillary recurrences as treatment failures, despite the necessity for reoperation in all of these patients. A reoperation rate this high for benign disease (for example, hernia) would be universally condemned; should not the same be true for patients with early stage, potentially curable malignancy?

4. Ten-year disease-free survivals for RM, TMR, and TM were 47%, 48%, and 42% (P = 0.2),[2] despite the neutralizing bias introduced by the removal of lymph nodes in 35% of the TM group. A clinical trial requires about 600 patients in each treatment arm to demonstrate a 10% survival advantage at the P<0.05 level of significance; the B-04 trial, with 384–389 patients per arm, simply does not have the statistical power to find significant a survival advantage on the order of 5% to 6%. This may represent a classic example of "type II error," i.e., finding "no statistically significant difference" when in fact one actually exists.

Does local relapse in the breast have the same adverse survival impact as failure in the axilla? The NSABP's B-06 protocol[15] was specifically designed to answer this question: patients (accrued 1976–1984) were randomized to TM, lumpectomy plus RT, and lumpectomy alone. Notably, all patients had level I and II axillary dissection, reflecting the adverse experience of the B-04 trial; 590–636 patients were enrolled in each arm. If, in fact, the type of local therapy and adequacy of regional control were unrelated to survival, then one would expect no differences among these three treatment arms. In 1989, at 81 months' mean follow-up, lumpectomy with or without RT was "not significantly different" from TM in rates of disease-free survival (58% vs. 54%, P = 0.3), distant disease-free survival (65% vs. 62%, P = 0.4), and overall survival (71% vs. 71%, P = 0.8).[16] However:

1. Ten percent of patients in each of the lumpectomy arms actually had mastectomy. Patients randomized to have lumpectomy but found at operation to have positive excision margins, a group most likely to fail locally, were treated by TM. In the survival analyses, these patients were included with the patients who actually had lumpectomy.

2. For lumpectomy patients, 8-year local relapse in the breast was 10% with RT and 39% without RT (P<0.001). These figures are particularly striking because the patients at greatest risk of local failure had already been allocated to mastectomy. Breast relapse was not considered to be a treatment failure despite the necessity for mastectomy in all patients with local recurrence! The incidence of local recurrence after lumpectomy with RT was 12% (axillary node-negative) and 6% (axillary node-positive); without RT, local recurrence was 37% (node-negative) and 43% (node-positive).

3. Eight-year disease-free survival was significantly better for TM and lumpectomy-RT than for lumpectomy alone: 65.5% and 65.6% vs. 60.7% (P = 0.05). Distant disease-free survival was better for TM than lumpectomy alone by a comparable margin: 73.8% vs. 69.6% (P = 0.03).

Both the B-04 and B-06 trials demonstrate a clear relation between local control and long-term disease-free survival, contradicting Fisher's hypothesis. Patients having more thorough local therapy (B-04: RM and TMR, B-06: TM and lumpectomy-RT) had significantly better local control than patients having TM alone (B-04) or lumpectomy alone (B-06). This is reflected in a long-term NED survival advantage of 5% to 6% (B-04: P = 0.2) and 5% (B-06: P = 0.05). In other words, whether patients relapsed in the axilla (17.8% of the TM-alone group in B-04), or in the breast (39% of the lumpectomy-only group in B-06), survival was worse by about 5% than for patients treated more thoroughly at the outset.

How significant is a survival advantage of 5%? In the United States, 150,000 women are projected to develop breast cancer during 1990 (and 44,000 are predicted to die of disease). Had all been treated by mastectomy without axillary dissection (as in the B-04 trial), by 10 years 26,700 would have required reoperation for axillary node relapse, and an additional 7,500 would have died of disease. Had all been treated with level I axillary dissection (assuming from Table 1, 16.6% residual nodal disease at levels II and III, and from the B-04 results, that about half of these would later become clinically evident), 12,200 would require reexploration of the axilla, with an excess mortality of perhaps 2,500.

The results of the Guy's Hospital trials, as recently summarized by Hayward,[17] also demonstrate the dependence of survival on local control of disease. Patients were randomized to radical mastectomy (RM) or to tumor excision and RT to the breast and axillary nodes (with doses of 3,500–3,800 R, low by contemporary standards). In the first trial (1961–1971), stage I patients had significantly more local recurrences with local excision than RM, 32% vs. 16%, two-thirds in the undissected axilla, but comparable survivals; for stage II patients, the respective local recurrence rates were 57% vs. 21%, and survival was significantly better for RM. Axillary node recurrence after local excision alone (and despite RT) was 19% for N0 and 21% for N1 patients, strikingly similar to that noted in the NSABP B-04 trial. The second trial (1971–1975) was limited to stage I patients, all treated by experienced surgeons in a dedicated breast cancer unit, and demonstrated significantly less frequent local recurrence and better survival for RM. When stratified by tumor size, this advantage was limited to patients with T1 tumors, precisely those chosen most often for breast conservation.

Breast conservation has become well-established over the past decade for patients with early disease, largely as a result of the Milan trial[1] (accrued 1973–1980): patients with T1N0 disease (tumors less than 2 cm and clinically negative axillae) were randomized either to RM or to quadrantectomy, complete axillary dissection, and full-dose radiotherapy (6,000 R). Follow-up now exceeding 10 years has shown no survival differences between radical mastectomy and breast conservation, and no local recurrences in the axilla. Historically, breast relapse has occurred in 1% to 2% of patients per year treated by primary radiation therapy, or about 22% at 15 years of follow-up.[18] In the most recent report of the Milan experience with 1,232 patients (1970–1983, 352 randomized and 880 off-trial), tumor relapse in the conserved breast was 4.3%.[19] Most importantly, these excellent results have been achieved by selecting for breast conservation patients with the most biologically favorable disease (T1N0), and by the use of aggressive local treatment: quadrant-wide tumor excision with an ellipse of overlying skin, full axillary dissection with pectoralis minor excision, and full-dose RT. Breast conservation as currently done in the United States is much less selective and considerably less radical than in Veronesi's trial, and long-term survival and local recurrence data are quite unlikely to be as good (results from the above NSABP trials would suggest that this is already the case).

Further progress in the management of operable breast cancer will depend on progressively earlier detection through widespread mammographic screening, the development of more effective hormonal and chemotherapeutic agents with further refinement of the prognostic criteria governing their use, and finally an ongoing and meticulous pursuit of maximal local control of disease. Complete axillary dissection remains an essential element in this effort.

References

1. Veronesi U, Banfi A, Del Vecchio M, et al: Comparison of Halsted mastectomy with quadrantectomy, axillary dissection, and radiotherapy in early breast cancer: long-term results. Eur J Cancer Clin Oncol 1986; 22:1085–1089.
2. Fisher B, Redmond C, Fisher E, et al: Ten-year results of a randomized clinical trial comparing radical mastectomy and total mastectomy with or without radiation. N Engl J Med 1985; 312:674-681.
3. Fisher B, Redmond C, Poisson R, et al: Eight-year results of a randomized clinical trial comparing total mastectomy and lumpectomy with or without irradiation in the treatment of breast cancer. N Engl J Med 1989; 320:822–828.
4. Fisher B: Laboratory and clinical research in breast cancer: a personal adventure: The David A. Karnofsky memorial lecture. Cancer Res 1980; 40:3863–3874.
5. Rosen P, Lieberman P, Braun D, et al: Lobular carcinoma in situ of the breast: detailed analysis of 99 patients with an average follow-up of 24 years. Am J Surg Path 1978; 2:225–251.
6. Kinne D, Petrek J, Osborne M, et al: Breast carcinoma in situ. Arch Surg 1989; 124:33–36.
7. Urban JA, Castro EB: Selecting variations in extent of surgical procedure for breast cancer. Cancer 1971; 28:1615-1623.

8. Cody HS, Bretsky SS, Urban JA: The continuing importance of adequate surgery for operable breast cancer: significant salvage of node-positive patients without adjuvant chemotherapy. CA 1982; 32:4–18.
9. Haagensen CD: The choice of treatment for operable carcinoma of the breast. Surgery 1976; 76:685–714.
10. Tapley ND, Spanos WJ, Fletcher GH, et al: Results in patients with breast cancer treated by radical mastectomy and postoperative irradiation with no adjuvant chemotherapy. Cancer 1982; 49:1316–1319.
11. Auchincloss H: Significance of location and number of axillary metastases in carcinoma of the breast: a justification for a conservative operation. Ann Surg 1963; 158:37.
12. Cody HS, Laughlin EH, Trillo C, Urban JA: Have changing treatment patterns affected outcome for operable breast cancer? Ten-year follow-up in 1288 patients, 1965–1978. Ann Surg 1991; 213:297–307.
13. Fisher B, Montague M, Redmond C, et al: Comparison of radical mastectomy with alternative treatments for primary breast cancer: a first report of results from a prospective randomized clinical trial. Cancer 1977; 39:2827–2839.
14. Fisher B, Wolmark N, Bauer M, et al: The accuracy of clinical nodal staging and of limited axillary dissection as a determinant of histologic nodal status in carcinoma of the breast. Surg Gynecol Obstet 1981; 152:765–772.
15. Fisher B, Bauer M, Margolese R, et al: Five-year results of a randomized clinical trial comparing total mastectomy and segmental mastectomy with or without radiation in the treatment af breast cancer. New Engl J Med 1985; 312:665–673.
16. Fisher B, Redmond C, Poisson R, et al: Eight-year results of a randomized clinical trial comparing total mastectomy and lumpectomy with or without irradiation in the treatment of breast cancer. New Engl J Med 1989; 320:822–828.
17. Hayward J: The significance of local control in the primary treatment of breast cancer: Lucy Wortham James Clinical Research Award. Arch Surg 1987; 122:1244–1247.
18. Harris JR, Recht A, Amalric R, et al: Time course and prognosis of local recurrence following primary radiation therapy for early breast cancer. J Clin Oncol 1984; 2:37–41.
19. Veronesi U, Salvadori B, Luini A, et al: Conservative treatment of early breast cancer: long-term results of 1232 cases treated with quadrantectomy, axillary dissection, and radiotherapy. Ann Surg 1990; 211:250–259.

16

How Important Is a Full Axillary Dissection:

The Case for Surgery Without Full Dissection

Henry R. Shibata

Introduction

In the past, the main objective of cancer surgery was, "a big operation for a small tumor, a small operation for a big tumor," signifying that locoregional control was paramount for the so-called early cancers. Those were the days when life was simple and there was little knowledge of the recent exciting developments in breast carcinogenesis (oncogenes, suppressor genes) or the burgeoning insight into biological prognosticators (ploidy, s-phase fraction, thymidine labeling index); there wasn't a precise understanding of hormonal influences (growth factors) or the mechanisms of tumor cell dissemination (clonal theory of metastases, fibronectin, integrin receptors, etc.); and we were not privy to the important results of prospectively randomized clinical trials aimed at answering important biological questions, such as whether regional nodes need to be removed at all.

However, despite this tremendous improvement in our knowledge of cancer biology, why is there still this controversy today regarding such a simple surgical technique as axillary dissection?

Lymphatic Drainage of the Breast

In order to understand what is meant by a "full axillary dissection," it is necessary to be familiar with the lymphatic drainage pattern of the breast.

From: Wise L, Johnson H Jr (eds): *Breast Cancer: Controversies in Management.* Futura Publishing Company, Inc., Armonk, NY, © 1994.

Although the normal lymphatic drainage of the breast is to the axillary nodes, the internal mammary lymph nodes, and the intrapleural lymph nodes, surgical staging is confined to the axillary lymph nodes since the most comprehensive lymphatic stream from all portions of the breast flows towards the axilla. The axillary nodes vary from 15 to 30 in number and are arranged into a lateral group, an anterior or pectoral group, a posterior or subscapular group, a central or intermediate group, and a medial or subclavicular group. The efferent vessels of the subclavicular lymph nodes can pass to the inferior deep cervical lymph nodes or join to become the subclavian trunk, which opens either directly into the junction of the internal jugular and subclavian veins or into the jugular lymphatic trunk; on the left, it may end in the thoracic duct, constituting the very important lymphaticovenous connection.

For the purposes of axillary lymph node dissection, the axilla is classically divided into three levels: *level I* containing the lateral nodes, *level II* containing the intermediate and deeper nodes, and *level III* containing the most medial or subclavicular group. Inclusion of the apical or most medial lymph nodes, i.e., level III nodes, is required to assure a full axillary dissection.

What Is the Role of the Axillary Lymph Nodes?

The interrelationship between the host and the malignant tumor it harbors is complex and poorly understood. Broadly, it can be categorized into a local interaction, a regional interaction and a systemic interaction, all of which are intimately interconnected.

The axillary lymph nodes play an important role at the regional level, probably interacting with the breast cancer cells ever since their inception, but much more intimately once the aggressive migratory clones of cells have invaded through the walls of the lymphatic vessels and are carried by the lymphatic stream as tumor emboli to the nodes. Why these tumor emboli involve some nodes and not others cannot be explained on the basis of mechanical flow alone since the more proximal nodes are usually involved, but rarely the more distant ones may be the only ones with skip metastases. It is also still unclear as to how the tumor cells may completely bypass the lymph nodes and gain access to the blood vascular system either through the larger lymphaticovenous pathways or those contained within the lymph nodes.

It has been assumed for a long time that lymph nodes are not only a barrier to bacterial dissemination, but similarly to tumor cell metastasis as well. Bernard Fisher and Edwin Fisher[1-6] have shown that lymph nodes are not very effective in containing tumor cells regionally and that the majority of these cells fail to establish and maintain permanent foci of metastases within these nodes. They also showed very clearly that lymphogenous spread of the tumor cells can reach the blood vascular system and disseminate widely, but that some of these cells find their way back into the lymphatic vessels, the nodes, and then back into the general blood circulation. Their concept is that the lymphatic and vascular systems are so interrelated that it is not realistic to think of them as independent routes of cancer dissemination.

As part of the host-tumor interaction, the regional lymph nodes contain immune cells that interact with the invading tumor cells and cause their destruction. These cells can be NK cells, cytotoxic T cells, and B cells capable of provoking an antigen-antibody reaction.[7] Such cells may play an active role at the beginning when the tumor burden is small, but with ever-increasing number of cells, the immune cell population undergoes a change that enables the metastatic cells to take firm root. Thus, nodes with no metastatic foci may be immunologically competent while those with metastases have incompetent cells. Therefore, the presence of negative or positive axillary nodes is not an indication of whether tumor cell spread has taken place or not. It can be postulated that patients with negative nodes (stage I) are regionally immuno-competent and capable of destroying all cancer cells traversing their axillary nodes, denoting a more favorable prognosis. Those patients with positive nodes (stage II) are immunologically incompetent, and the metastatic lymph nodes are indicative of a systemic weakness allowing metastases to occur in distant sites, and this results in a poorer prognosis.[8]

Breast Cancer Therapy in the Past: Advocates of Complete Axillary Dissection

The principle of cancer surgery for carcinomas of any site has been and in some cases still is wide local excision of normal tissue surrounding the cancer with "full" lymph node dissection, the so-called en bloc dissection. For breast cancer, this type of "curative" surgery is attempted in an anatomical and mechanistic way to remove all the axillary lymph nodes. In order to accomplish this, Halsted[9,10] and Meyer[11] simultaneously reported in 1894 that it was necessary to completely remove the pectoralis major and minor muscles. This operation is now known as the Halsted type or standard radical mastectomy. This operation was further made more radical by extending the operation to a forequarter amputation of the arm to remove the clavicle and facilitate excision of the deeper subclavian nodes, as well as the supraclavicular lymph nodes, which were often involved.

Another form of extended radical or supraradical mastectomy that became popular in the 1950s through the efforts of Urban[12] was removal of the internal mammary lymph nodes for cancers arising in the medial quadrants.

After such radical operations, failure to achieve a cure was regarded as being due to extension of the cancer beyond the confines of the dissection or inade-quacy of the operation. Locoregional recurrences were not considered to be a sign of systemic disease, but the result of not adequately removing the last nest of cells in the tissues or the last remaining lymph node in the axilla. Therefore, to supplement this inadequate surgery, locoregional irradiation was adminis-tered postoperatively to the chest wall and the regional lymph node-bearing areas in an attempt to improve survival by reducing locoregional recurrences.

In 1948, McWhirter of Scotland[13] challenged the necessity for surgical removal of the regional lymph nodes and advocated irradiation of the intact lymph nodes after simple (total) mastectomy alone. He showed results that implied a better 5-year survival rate after simple mastectomy and irradiation (62.5%) compared to radical mastectomy and postoperative radiotherapy (50.1%). McWhirter was concerned that the radical operation was still inadequate and that the trauma from the procedure resulted in an increase of metastases to other sites, and that if the axillary lymph nodes were intact, the metastasizing cells would be trapped by these nodes. His rationale was in keeping with the prevailing mechanistic approach towards breast cancer spread. The term "modified radical mastectomy" is associated with Patey,[14] who in 1948, advocated that a full axillary dissection could be accomplished without removal of the pectoralis major muscle but with excision of the pectoralis minor muscle to better reach the level III nodes. Modifications followed in the form of division only of the attachment of the pectoralis minor muscle to the coracoid process of the scapula and later of retraction only of the pectoralis muscles made easier by a free arm drape. This latter form of modified radical mastectomy is the most widely performed mastectomy operation in North America at present and became widely accepted without benefit of a prospective randomized trial comparing it with the standard Halsted radical mastectomy, even though the surgeons advocating this method insisted that a full axillary dissection was necessary.

Beginning in 1961, Crile of Cleveland[15] strongly advocated that simple mastectomy alone was adequate treatment for stage I breast cancer. Simple mastectomy without prophylactic irradiation appeared to be at least as effective as radical mastectomy with or without irradiation. In those patients treated by simple mastectomy without irradiation, the axillary nodes were removed when they became positive, and it was noted that the chances of survival were similar to those treated by radical mastectomy.

The Case for Surgery Without Full Dissection

With mounting evidence that the axillary lymph nodes are not a barrier to invading breast cancer cells and that hematogenous spread of such cells to distant sites dictates the eventual outcome of the patient, and with so many diverse opinions as to the best way to manage breast cancer on a locoregional basis, the time was ripe in 1971 for the National Surgical Adjuvant Breast Project (NSABP) under the leadership of Bernard Fisher to plan, initiate, and carry to fruition the landmark surgical trial, protocol B-04. This trial (Fig. 1) randomized women with clinically negative axillary lymph nodes into three therapy groups: (1) radical mastectomy (surgical removal of the lymph nodes); (2) total mastectomy with regional irradiation (irradiation of the chest wall, axillary, internal

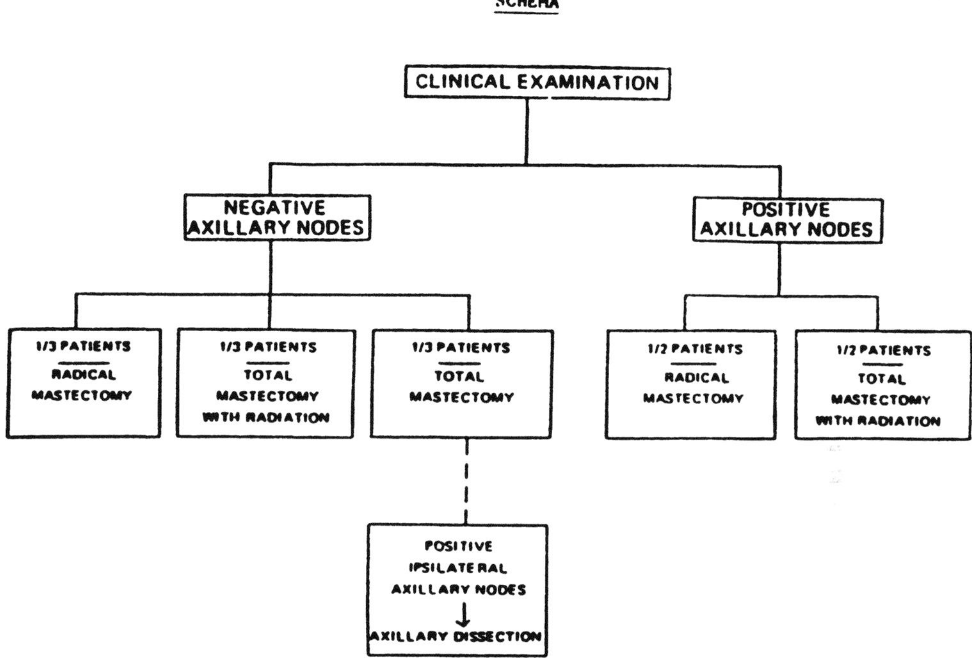

Figure 1: *The National Surgical Adjuvant Breast Project (NSABP) trial, protocol B-04. Women with clinically negative axillary lymph nodes were randomized into three therapy groups: (1) radical mastectomy (surgical removal of the lymph nodes); (2) total mastectomy with regional irradiation (irradiation of the chest wall, axillary, internal mammary, and supraclavicular lymph nodes); and (3) total mastectomy alone (observation of the lymph nodes) with removal of the nodes when they became positive.*

mammary, and supraclavicular lymph nodes); and (3) total mastectomy alone (observation of the lymph nodes) with removal of the nodes when they became positive. The women with positive nodes were randomized similarly to the first two arms. The total mastectomy alone was deemed unethical in this group of women since the clinically palpable nodes were considered to contain metastases and could not be left alone.

The results of this protocol at 5 years,[16] 10 years,[17] and now at an average follow-up of over 18 years, show no difference in disease-free survival, distant disease-free survival, and overall survival between the three clinically node-negative groups and the two clinically node positive groups. What does this mean in the clinically negative women? It means that complete surgical excision of the axillary nodes does not lead to improved survival. It means that irradiation of nodes with intent to ablate any microscopic foci of metastases does not improve survival over those patients treated with mastectomy alone, even though 20% of such patients later on underwent axillary dissection for metastatic lymph nodes.

One other interesting result of B-04 was that pathological analysis of the lymph nodes removed as part of the radical mastectomy showed 40% to contain metastases even though they were considered to be clinically negative. Therefore, in those randomized patients treated by mastectomy alone, the remaining axillary nodes should have 40% positive nodes. However, so far, even at 18 years, only 20% of such patients have undergone axillary dissection. The postulate is that 20% of patients still living either have lymph nodes with occult metastases or such metastases have been destroyed by the host defense mechanism. One other important pathological finding resulting from protocol B-04 was that even though occult micrometastases were detected in 24% of 78 patients considered to be negative after "routine" pathological examination, there was no correlation between any of the discriminants in these patients who have either died of their disease or are living with recurrence regardless of the presence of these occult metastases.[18] Fisher concludes that attempts to detect occult metastases by extending histopathological methods may be more academic than practical or therapeutically significant. These findings have shown that leaving positive nodes intact in the mastectomy-alone group has not led to increased incidence of distant metastases or overall failure, and provide further proof that involved axillary nodes are not the predecessors of generalized metastases, but are indicators of stage IV disease.[19]

Another interesting finding was that when the nodes were considered to be clinically positive, 30% of these patients had no metastatic foci in the dissected nodes. The most important finding concerning the resected lymph nodes is that the number of nodes involved with metastases is the most reliable indicator of prognosis. Patients with 1 to 3 nodes involved have a much better prognosis than those with 4 or more positive nodes. It appears that the number of nodes involved is much more important than the level of nodes involved, indicating that the level of axillary involvement for node-positive breast cancer is not of independent prognostic significance.[20]

The lessons that have been learned from NSABP protocol B-04 are as follows:

1. removal or irradiation of the axillary lymph nodes does not lead to improved survival;

2. removal of the axillary lymph nodes when they become clinically enlarged and positive is just the same as removing them when they are occult;

3. therefore, a full or not so full axillary dissection does not influence survival;

4. clinical assessment of the lymph nodes is very inaccurate, as noted above, so staging of the patient requires pathological examination;

5. pathological analysis of the number of nodes involved with cancer is one of the best indicators of prognosis;

6. thus, axillary dissection is necessary for staging and prognosis, not for increasing survival, as was fervently and blindly believed in the past.

What Is an Adequate Axillary Dissection for Staging?

Having established that axillary lymph node dissection is necessary for staging and prognosis, what are the guidelines as to what constitutes a good or adequate axillary dissection for this purpose?

The guidelines established by the NSABP for an adequate axillary dissection call for removal of level I and II lymph nodes, the highest or most medial landmark of dissection being up to the medial border of the pectoralis minor muscle.[21] With these criteria, the number of nodes removed has been fairly consistent whether the operation was a radical mastectomy, a modified radical mastectomy, or segmental mastectomy with axillary dissection (Fig. 2).

How extensive a dissection is required to determine whether ≥4 positive nodes exist in an axilla? The findings indicate that the more nodes removed, the probability increases that ≥4 positive nodes will be detected.[22] Therefore, to quantify accurately the number of positive nodes, a more extensive dissection (10 or more nodes) is required to determine negativity and positivity. There are some differences of opinion regarding the efficiency of lower axillary sampling.[23] This technique, which removes a few of the level I nodes, is considered inadequate for an accurate staging of the axillary nodes[24] and does not lend itself well to subsequent adjuvant therapy trials based on staging.[25]

The lymphedema of the upper extremity following this type of dissection

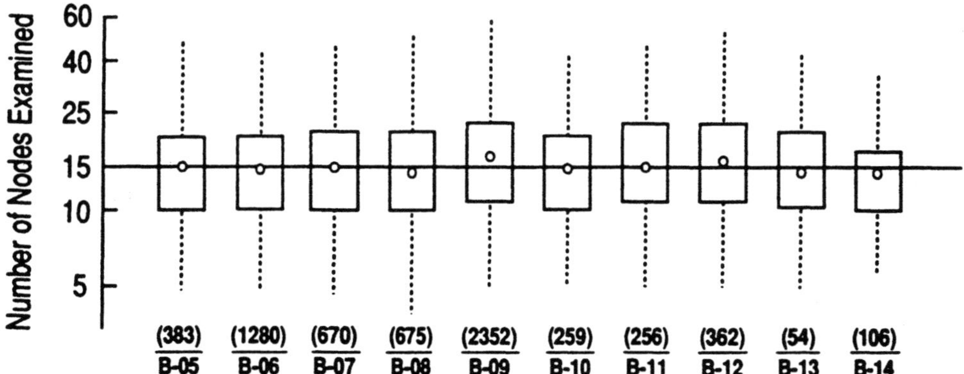

Figure 2: *Comparison of numbers of nodes reported pathologically in various NSABP protocols. In protocols B-05 and B-07 through B-12, operations included radical and modified radical mastectomy. Protocol B-06 included modified radical mastectomy, or segmental mastectomy with dissection in continuity or with use of two incisions. The circles indicate the median number of nodes removed. The ends of the "box" are the 75th and 25th percentiles.*

has been minimal and much less than that following removal of the level III lymph nodes with postoperative irradiation.

The Future: Can the Axillary Lymph Nodes Be Staged Without a Dissection?

Recently, there is increasing interest in imaging cancers, regional lymph nodes as well as distant metastases, utilizing monoclonal antibodies tagged with radioisotopes against tumor-specific antigens.[25] This interest has been further developed in detecting breast cancer metastases in axillary lymph nodes.[26] Tjandra et al.[27] used a 131-iodine labeled antibreast antibody (^{131}I RCC-1), which can be injected subcutaneously to image the axillary lymph nodes. By giving cold iodine-labeled antibody which does not react with breast cancer, they were able to successfully localize lymph node metastases in 88% of the cases. This compared favorably to preoperative clinical assessment, which was 58%. However, the results of immunolymphoscintography are still not as good as full axillary dissection and histological examination. Its accuracy in relation to lesser surgical procedures as axillary sampling is unknown. With further refinements such as a better defined breast cancer-specific antigen, this technique should lend itself well to nonsurgical determination of staging (positive or negative nodes) and prognosis (number of nodes involved) in patients with breast cancer.

Summary

The scientific acumen and diligence of surgical oncologists such as Bernard Fisher and contributors to NSABP protocol B-04 have provided unequivocal data that axillary lymph node dissection is not a curative procedure as once believed, but a technique for determining staging and prognosis of the patient with breast cancer.

The surgical technique to provide this vital information should be done properly to ensure a more accurate assessment of staging and prognosis and should at least include the levels I and II lymph nodes. This information is vital for assigning such patients into the proper biologically sound postoperative adjuvant therapy trials that are being conducted by several cooperative groups for the purpose of improving survival.

There is need for further elucidation of the role of the axillary lymph nodes in the complex host versus tumor interrelationship. The population of immune cells within the nodes and their alteration with changes in this interrelationship should be important factors in understanding the response of the host to the invading cancer cells. Utilizing specific radiolabeled antibodies against breast cancer-specific antigen may some day make axillary dissection obsolete.

References

1. Fisher B, Fisher E: Role of the lymphatic system in dissemination of tumor. In: Mayerson HS (ed). Lymph and the Lymphatic System. Charles C. Thomas, New York, pp 324–347, 1986.
2. Fisher B, Fisher ER: Transmigration of lymph nodes by tumor cells. Science 1966; 152:1397–1398.
3. Fisher B, Fisher ER: The barrier function of the lymph node to tumor cells and erythrocytes. I. Normal nodes. Cancer 1967; 20:1907–1914.
4. Fisher B, Fisher ER: The barrier function of the lymph node to tumor cells and erythrocytes. II. Effect of x-ray, inflammation, sensitization and tumor growth. Cancer 1967; 20:1914–1919.
5. Fisher B, Fisher ER: Interrelationship of hematogenous and lymphatic tumor cell dissemination. Surg Gynecol Obstet 1966; 122:791–798.
6. Fisher B, Saffer EA, Fisher ER: Studies concerning the regional lymph node in cancer. III. Response of regional lymph node cells from breast and colon cancer patients to PHA stimulation. Cancer 1972; 30:1202–1215.
7. Khuri N, Jothy SP, Shibata HR: Identification and importance of lymphocyte subpopulations in the regional nodes of breast cancer patients. Can J Surg 1989; 32:23–26.
8. Fisher B, Slack NH: Number of lymph nodes examined and the prognosis of breast cancer. Surg Gynecol Obstet 1970; 131:79-88.
9. Halsted WS: A clinical and histological study of adenocarcinoma of the breast. Ann Surg 1898; 28:557.
10. Halsted WS: The results of radical operations for the cure of carcinoma of the breast. Ann Surg 1907; 46:1–19.
11. Meyer W: An improved method of the radical mastectomy for carcinoma of the breast. Med Rec 1978; 46:351–359.
12. Urban JA: Clinical experience and results of excision of the internal mammary lymph node chain in primary operable breast cancer. Cancer 1959; 12:14–22.
13. McWhirter R: The value of simple mastectomy and radiotherapy in the treatment of cancer of the breast. Br J Radiol 1948; 21:599–610.
14. Patey DH, Dyson WH: The prognosis of carcinoma of the breast in relation to the type of operation performed. Br J Cancer 1948; 2:7–13.
15. Crile G Jr: Results of simple mastectomy without irradiation in the treatment of operative stage I cancer of the breast. Ann Surg 1968; 168:330–336.
16. Fisher B, Montague E, Redmond C, et al: Comparison of radical mastectomy with alternative treatments for primary breast cancer: a first report of results from a prospective randomized clinical trial. Cancer 1977; 39:2827–2839.
17. Fisher B, Redmond C, Fisher E, et al: Ten-year results of a randomized clinical trial comparing radical mastectomy and total mastectomy with or without radiation. N Engl J Med 1985; 312:674-681.
18. Fisher E, Swamidoss S, Lee CH, et al: Detection and significance of occult axillary node metastases in patients with invasive breast cancer. Cancer 1978; 42:2025–2031.
19. Fisher B, Wolmark N, Baver M, et al: The accuracy of clinical nodal staging and of limited axillary dissection as a determinant of histological nodal status in carcinoma of the breast. Surg Gynecol Obstet 1981; 152:765–772.
20. Barth RJ, Danforth DN Jr, Venzon DJ, et al: Level of axillary involvement by lymph node metastases from breast cancer is not an independent predictor of survival. Arch Surg 1991; 126:574-577.
21. Margolese R, Poisson R, Shibata H, et al: The technique of segmental mastectomy (lumpectomy) and axillary dissection: a syllabus from the National Surgical Adjuvant Breast Project workshop. Surgery 1987; 102:828–834.

22. Steele RJC, Forrest APM, Gibson T, et al: The efficiency of lower axillary sampling in obtaining lymph node status in breast cancer: a controlled randomized trial. Br J Surg 1985; 92:368-369.
23. Davies GC, Millis RR, Hayward JL: Assessment of axillary lymph node status. Ann Surg 1980; 192:148–151.
24. Kissin MW, Thompson EM, Price AB, et al: The inadequacy of axillary sampling in breast cancer. Lancet 1982; 1:1210–1212.
25. Fentiman, IS, Mansel RE: The axilla: not a no-go area. Lancet 1991; 337:221–223.
26. Epenetos AA, Britton KE, Mather S, et al: Targeting of Iodine -123-labelled tumour-associated monoclonal antibodies to ovarian, breast and gastrointestinal tumours. Lancet 1982; 2:999–1004.
27. Tjandra JJ, Sacks NP, Thompson CH, et al: The detection of axillary lymph node metastases from breast cancer by radio-labelled monoclonal antibodies: a prospective study. Br J Cancer 1989; 59:296–302.

17

The Role of Axillary Dissection in Operable Breast Cancer:

An Overview

*Nigel P.M. Sacks, Lester C. Barr,
Simon M. Allan, Michael Baum*

Introduction

The best treatment for axillary nodes in patients with operable breast cancer is currently a matter of intense debate in the United Kingdom.[1,2] There is controversy about the extent of axillary dissection required, and indeed whether any axillary surgery is necessary at all.[3,4]

The histologic status of the axillary nodes is still the best marker of disease behavior and ultimate outcome.[5] Even more importantly, it has been clearly shown that systemic adjuvant therapy given to patients with involved axillary nodes decreases the odds of dying from breast cancer by up to 30%.[6]

The aim of this chapter is to summarize the arguments for and against axillary dissection in patients with breast cancer and to recommend an appropriate management plan.

The Case in Favor of Axillary Dissection

Surgical clearance of the axilla in patients with operable breast cancer is undertaken to provide accurate staging and prognostic information upon which decisions about adjuvant treatment can be made and to provide local tumor control. Not only is it important to establish the histologic status of the axillary nodes (node-positive versus node-negative), but the prognosis of individual

From: Wise L, Johnson H Jr (eds): *Breast Cancer: Controversies in Management*. Futura Publishing Company, Inc., Armonk, NY, © 1994.

patients is directly related to the total number of nodes involved as well as the anatomical level of involvement.[7,8]

Staging

Clinical detection of axillary node involvement is notoriously unreliable with both high false-positive and high false-negative rates of approximately 25% and 30%, respectively (Table 1).[9–13] Attempts to study the axillary nodes using lymphoscintigraphy and mammography have been largely unsuccessful. Black et al.[14] have claimed that isotope-colloid preparations injected intradermally can accurately predict axillary node metastases but several others have not been able to reproduce these results.[15,16] The first successful report of specific detection of nodal metastases from breast cancer using antibody-targeted isotopes came from DeLand et al.,[17] using a polyclonal rabbit anti-CEA antibody administered subcutaneously. They were able to demonstrate axillary node metastases in two patients with histologic confirmation of positive nodes in both cases. This technique was based on the successful experimental mouse model of Weinstein et al.[18] and Goodwin et al.,[19] which first demonstrated the improved imaging obtained with intralymphatic delivery of isotope-antibody conjugate when compared with intravenous administration of the same conjugate. With the advent of monoclonal antibody technology, the potential to generate large volumes of tumor-specific antibodies was realized. Thompson et al.[20] reported the first study to accurately detect axillary node metastases in nine patients with breast cancer given radiolabeled antibreast monoclonal antibody subcutaneously. This work has recently been confirmed in one other small study,[21] and it is currently an area of active research interest. Attempts to use ultrasound to image axillary nodes and detect metastatic disease have not been successful,[22] and the place of magnetic resonance imaging is also under investigation.

The axillary lymph nodes are the principal site of regional metastases from carcinoma of the breast, and currently between 40% and 50% of patients with operable breast cancer have nodal metastases at presentation.[23] The likelihood of axillary node involvement is related directly to the size of the primary tumor,[24]

Table 1
Accuracy of Physical Examination in Predicting Histologic Involvement of Axillary Nodes in Patients with Operable Breast Cancer

	Clinical Assessment	
Series Reference no.	False-Positive (%)	False-Negative (%)
Butcher et al.[9]	25	32
Haagensen et al.[10]	24	32
Bucalosi et al.[11]	29	29
Schottenfeld et al.[12]	26	27
Danforth et al.[13]	11	38

both of which are directly related to the overall recurrence and mortality rates. There is also evidence that the incidence of axillary node metastases is somewhat higher with tumors involving the lateral quadrants of the breast than with those placed centrally or medially (Tables 2, 3, 4). One can conclude from the studies summarized in these tables[25–29] that axillary node involvements are nearly as common with medially positioned tumors as with lateral tumor sites. Although internal mammary node involvement is nearly always associated with positive axillary nodes, it occurs in isolation in 5% to 10% of cases and is largely independent of primary tumor site. These facts underline the lack of clinical importance associated with the presence of internal mammary node metastases.

The total number of histologically involved axillary nodes is related to the extent and technique of pathological analysis of the specimen as well as the completeness of axillary dissection. Clearance of the specimen with fat dissolution and more thorough sectioning of any nodes then found was first shown by Pickren to increase the yield of histologically positive nodes.[30] He was able to demonstrate that of 57 specimens routinely analyzed and reported as negative, 25% showed nodal metastases when fat was cleared from the specimen and more careful sectioning was performed. It was not until recently that the prognostic significance of these so-called micrometastases was demonstrated by

Table 2

Percentage of Cases with Histologically Positive Axillary Lymph Nodes in Relation to the Site of the Primary Breast Tumor

Quadrant Site	Series		
	Fisher et al.[25]	Handley[26]	Lacour et al.[27]
Upper Outer	52	55	
			58
Lower Outer	48	57	
Upper Inner	34	42	
			52
Lower Inner	46	41	

Table 3

Percentage of Cases with Histologically Positive Internal Mammary Lymph Nodes in Relation to the Site of the Primary Breast Tumor

Quadrant Site	Series			
	Handley[26]	Lacour et al.[27]	Margottini et al.[28]	Lacour et al.[29]
Upper Outer	14			
		22	18	16
Lower Outer	13			
Upper Inner	27			
		37	26	24
Lower Inner	33			

Table 4
Relationship Between Axillary and Internal Mammary Lymph Node Status in Patients with Primary Breast Cancer

	Handley[26]	Lacour et al.[29]	Lacour et al.[27]
Axillary Node-Positive and Internal Mammary Node-Negative	35%	—	33% (Inner Quadrants) 45% (Outer Quadrants)
Axillary Node-Negative and Internal Mammary Node-Positive	5%	10%	11% (Inner Quadrants) 8% (Outer Quadrants)

the International (Ludwig) Breast Cancer Study Group.[31] The axillary nodes from 921 breast cancer patients, treated by mastectomy and axillary clearance, who were originally reported as tumor-free were reexamined by serial sections at six levels with six 3-micron sections being cut at each level; two of these sections were examined using hematoxylin and eosin staining. The median number of nodes examined per patient was 14 and the mean number of node blocks examined per patient was 12.

Occult micrometastases were found in 83 (9%) of the 921 patients studied, and interestingly, these patients had a significantly worse disease-free and overall survival rate than did the patients whose nodes remained negative on serial sectioning (median follow-up of 5 years). While their presence was significantly correlated with vascular invasion and tumor size, occult micrometastases remained a statistically significant independent variable. This finding is in agreement with that reported by Friedman et al.[32] but is at variance with that reached by most other investigators.[30, 33–35] This technique is extremely time-consuming and its value over and above more established and new tumor markers awaits confirmation. Immunohistochemical staining of routine sections has recently been shown to increase sensitivity and provide similar prognostic information with a simpler technique.[36,37]

Local Tumor Control

Surgical clearance of the axilla in patients with operable breast cancer provides excellent tumor control with an axillary recurrence rate of 1% or less.[38,39] The value of treating axillary nodes was examined in the National Surgical Adjuvant Breast Project (NSABP) B-04 trial,[40] which randomized patients with clinically negative axillae to either radical mastectomy, total mastectomy and irradiation of the axillary nodes, or simple mastectomy with delayed axillary dissection if nodes became clinically involved. The analysis of results at 10 years showed no significant difference among the three groups of patients in terms of disease-free or overall survival rates (57%). Forty percent of patients with clinically negative nodes were found to have histologic involvement and yet only 18% of those treated by simple mastectomy alone required subsequent axillary dissection for the development of clinically positive nodes. In this trial, the axillary recurrence rate after surgical clearance was only 1%, whereas in those treated by axillary irradiation alone, it was 3%. These findings suggest that untreated nodes do not serve as a reservoir for further tumor dissemination and that not all histologically positive nodes will become biologically active. Similar results were found in the CRC Kings/Cambridge trial,[41] which demonstrated an increased local relapse rate without axillary dissection but again no effect on overall patient survival. Baum and Coyle[42] reported a personal series of 73 patients with early breast cancer treated by simple mastectomy alone with no treatment to the axilla. Spontaneous regression of palpably enlarged axillary nodes was a good prognostic indicator, whereas progression of axillary nodal disease (which was noted in 48% of the patients) was associated with the appearance of distant metastases within 8 months. The policy of not treating the axilla, adopting a watch policy, and treating the nodes on recurrence produces a risk that locoregional recurrence will be uncontrollable and cause significant patient morbidity.

Harris and Osteen[43] have pointed out several flaws in extrapolating the B-04 results to all patients. Thirty-five percent of patients assigned to treatment by simple mastectomy alone actually underwent a limited axillary dissection and this subgroup of patients had a significantly lower axillary recurrence rate. Many patients developed axillary metastases at the time of or subsequent to the appearance of distant metastases and some patients had uncontrolled axillary recurrences. The impact of axillary treatment on survival is also not known, as 60% did not have axillary involvement and many of the 40% who did also had occult distant metastases. Finally, they made the point that it is possible that the B-04 trial was too small to detect a clinically significant survival benefit from treating the axilla.

It has been claimed by some authors that axillary dissection, when performed as part of mastectomy, led to eradication of the disease in some longterm survivors even without any systemic treatment. Haagensen reviewed his 50-year personal experience with 1,036 patients treated with Halsted mastectomy alone.[44] Patients with one to three axillary nodes involved had a 10-year survival rate of 44% to 70%, four to seven involved nodes 36% to 43%, and eight or more involved nodes 16% to 19%; there was only one case of axillary recurrence. Similarly, the Milan group reported a series of 753 patients with a 10-year survival rate of 70% and 32%, respectively, for patients with one or more than four positive axillary nodes treated by radical mastectomy alone.[45]

Adjuvant Systemic Therapy

It is now well proven that premenopausal node-positive patients benefit from adjuvant cytotoxic chemotherapy with a reduction in the annual odds of dying of approximately 30%.[6] While there is also evidence that adjuvant cytotoxic chemotherapy can be of benefit in some node-negative patients, the absolute benefit is less and in this group the problem is to identify the 25% of patients who are destined to relapse who may potentially benefit. Several tumor-related factors have recently been shown to be associated with a worse prognosis independent of nodal status, size, tumor grade, presence of vascular invasion, absence of estrogen receptor, high proliferative index, tumor aneuploidy, and the presence of c-*erb* B-2 or cathepsin D.[46–54] There is as yet no direct evidence, however, to show that node-negative patients with these tumor factors are the only ones who will respond to potentially toxic combination chemotherapy regimes, underlining the importance of careful axillary staging. Interestingly, it has recently been suggested that patients whose tumors express a high level of c-*erb* B-2 are relatively resistant to cytotoxic chemotherapy.[55]

In postmenopausal patients, adjuvant tamoxifen improves survival of both node-positive and node-negative patients.[6,56,57] As this is a nontoxic drug, the importance of axillary staging in the postmenopausal patient is diminished, although axillary surgery may be needed to control clinically obvious disease and to avoid the need for radiotherapy.

The Case Against Axillary Dissection

The rationale for axillary clearance in the management of early breast cancer outlined above is that it provides an effective means of controlling axillary disease and that, in addition, it gives staging information upon which treatment decisions concerning adjuvant systemic therapy can be based. While these statements are true, control of axillary disease is not the exclusive property of surgery. Furthermore, decisions regarding adjuvant hormone therapy or cytotoxic chemotherapy can be made without a knowledge of axillary nodal status. The arguments surrounding axillary surgery in the management of breast cancer are thus not an "open and shut" case in favor, but rather the subject of a spectrum of opinion.

Staging

The information gained from studies that have included axillary lymph node dissection in the clinical protocol has been immensely important in enhancing our knowledge of the natural history of breast cancer and in formulating rational treatment policies over the last two decades. Despite these important epidemiologic and historical perspectives, the "staging" argument assumes importance to an individual patient with breast cancer only if a knowledge of the individual lymph node status will alter that patient's management. The undertaking of a surgical procedure for staging purposes if that surgery cannot influence the progress of the disease directly, or indirectly through its role in selecting therapy for high-risk patients, is difficult to justify.

Local Tumor Control

It is generally agreed that control of local disease within the axilla is essential regardless of any possible effect on survival. Uncontrolled axillary recurrence can be an unpleasant symptom that can markedly impair the quality of life.

It has been suggested that ineffective axillary treatment may also result in some survival disadvantage.[1,43,58] This argument appears to be supported by the Guy's Hospital trial (1961–1971) in which 370 women with T1–2, N0–1 breast cancer were randomized to either radical mastectomy or wide local excision; both groups received postoperative radiotherapy.[59] Patients in the latter group had a very high rate of locoregional recurrence compared with the mastectomy patients, probably reflecting the inadequate doses of radiotherapy—only 25–27 Gy tumor dose to the axilla and supraclavicular fossa. A second study from which a similar conclusion could be drawn is the Southeast Scotland trial, in which 275 stage I breast cancer patients were randomized to either radical mastectomy or total mastectomy with axillary irradiation. This latter group had a high rate of axillary recurrence (14%) and reduced survival compared with the radical mastectomy group.[60] Interpreting the results of these relatively small trials is of course difficult; Yarnold has argued that the survival disadvantage seen in the Guy's trial is nonsignificant and is unlikely to be related to failure of radiotherapy to control the axilla.[61] The effect of locoregional recurrence on overall survival should be clarified when the updated results of the next world overview are published.

A large number of studies have now demonstrated that radical axillary irradiation is an effective means of preventing axillary nodal recurrence, with control rates equivalent to that of axillary clearance.[43,62,63] Radiotherapy doses of at least 45–50 Gy in 2-Gy fractions to the axilla, with an additional local boost of 10–20 Gy in 2-Gy fractions in patients with clinically positive axillary nodes, result in an axillary recurrence rate of approximately 2% overall and less than 10% for patients with clinically obvious positive nodes.[61,64,65] For example, as already discussed above, the NSABP B-04 axillary irradiation arm had an axillary recurrence rate of 3%. Axillary irradiation is thus an acceptable alternative to axillary clearance, although of course the staging information is lost.

The concept of avoiding treatment of the axilla during the primary treatment of early breast cancer and treating only those patients who subsequently develop clinical axillary recurrence has had some supporters. The effect of delayed treatment of axillary disease on survival remains an open question, although the lack of significantly different survival rates in prospective trials suggests that any effect must be relatively small. It could thus be argued that a simple watch policy for patients with clinically uninvolved axilla is justified. However, the definitive management of axilla is probably better undertaken as part of the primary treatment, as the morbidity associated with both axillary surgery and axillary irradiation is small and this obviates the need for delayed treatment as well as the problem of uncontrolled local disease.

A number of authors have attempted to compare the complication rates following axillary clearance with axillary irradiation. It would appear that, when used as single modalities, similar rates of lymphedema of the arm are obtained, in the order of 2% to 8%, depending on definition.[63,66] The risk of limitation of shoulder movement is probably similar,[63] although Aitken et al.[67] have shown that radiotherapy significantly reduced shoulder mobility when compared with surgery to the axilla. The incidence of both complications increases dramatically up to nearly 40% if a combination of axillary surgery and axillary irradiation is used.[66]

Two long-term complications of axillary irradiation that have caused concern are radiation-induced brachial plexus neuropathy and radiation-induced secondary tumors, both of which are uncommon. The risk of neuropathy has been reported to be as high as 1% and is undoubtedly related to the radiotherapy technique, but the risk can be minimized by careful attention to fields and dosimetry.[68] The risk of radiation-induced sarcoma has been calculated to be 21 cases per 100,000 patient years in patients surviving beyond 5 years.[69] Whether or not a risk of this small magnitude should represent a deterrent to axillary irradiation is debatable, particularly as most patients treated by conservative surgery will be receiving irradiation to the breast with its own attendant increased risks of ischemic heart disease, pulmonary fibrosis, and radiation-induced sarcoma.

Axillary irradiation can thus be regarded as equivalent to axillary clearance both in terms of efficacy and incidence of complications. This of course is dependent on detailed attention to radiotherapy technique; a dose sufficiently tumorocidal must be carefully planned and executed in order to avoid overlap and damage to normal tissues.

Adjuvant Systemic Therapy

Probably the most important argument in favor of axillary surgery in breast cancer is that failure to clear the axilla leads to failure to diagnose nodal metastases, which in turn leads to failure to give adjuvant systemic treatment to patients who would benefit from it. However, rational decisions about systemic therapy can frequently be made without reference to nodal status.

The most obvious example is the large subgroup of breast cancer patients who are postmenopausal at diagnosis, since adjuvant therapy with tamoxifen is of benefit to both node-positive and node-negative women.[56,57] In these circumstances, the need to determine nodal status from a therapeutic point of view is lost.

The situation with premenopausal patients is more complex, since variations in opinions about the place of adjuvant cytotoxic chemotherapy have existed between the United States and the United Kingdom in recent years, and the general consensus of opinion has been shifting on both sides of the Atlantic. Many centers in the United Kingdom have until recently felt that the toxicity of chemotherapy regimens was not justified by the relatively small benefits obtained when used in an adjuvant setting, particularly when it was considered that this toxicity is suffered at a time when a woman with breast cancer might otherwise expect to feel physically well.[70] If a patient can expect 6 months of treatment-related toxicity, will she consider a 6-month improvement in disease-free survival a satisfactory result? Henderson et al.[23] have recently shown that the longer the potential prolongation of life, the more willing the woman will be to undergo the adjuvant therapy to gain this. Investigations from the International (Ludwig) Breast Study Group have recently proposed a more objective method to assess the quality of the disease-free survival with cytotoxic chemotherapy by studying the time spent without symptoms or toxicity.[71]

There has also been scepticism about the early published results of adjuvant chemotherapy trials in which impressive relapse-free survival differences between the treated and the nontreated groups were not translated into equally impressive differences in overall survival.[72] Furthermore, it has been suggested that a major mechanism of action of cytotoxic chemotherapy was that of drug-induced ovarian ablation and that the benefits of cytotoxic chemotherapy could be given with far less toxicity by offering other forms of hormonal manipulation such as ovarian ablation, lutenizing hormone-releasing hormone (LHRH) agonists, and/or tamoxifen.[73,74]

The opinion in the United Kingdom has now changed in the light of long-term follow-up of adjuvant chemotherapy trials and their meta-analysis to accept that polychemotherapy can be administered with minimum toxicity and result in significant survival benefit for node-positive premenopausal women. In the United States, the threshold for prescribing adjuvant cytotoxic chemotherapy has now been lowered to the extent that the majority of node-negative women are also being offered chemotherapy.[75] While the absolute improvements in survival for node-negative patients are not as great, it is likely that the relative risk reduction is equivalent to that achieved in node-positive patients. Thus, only those node-negative patients with a very low risk of disseminated disease (such as those with carcinoma in situ, "special type" histology, or invasive tumors less than 1 cm in diameter) would avoid chemotherapy.[76,77]

There is an obvious analogy here with the arguments for and against staging laparotomy in Hodgkin's disease, debated over a decade ago. The principle is similar in that the lower the threshold for giving chemotherapy, the lower the indication for accurate staging. Staging laparotomy was of benefit only to the small subgroup with low volume disease who could avoid chemotherapy if this laparotomy was normal. With the realization that chemotherapy was indicated for the majority of patients with Hodgkin's disease and that chemotherapy at first relapse for patients initially treated by radiotherapy alone gave equivalent results, the need for staging laparotomy was lost. If both node-positive and most node-negative breast cancer patients are to receive chemotherapy, which is the current position in the USA and likely to be the position adopted in the UK, then the only patients who will benefit from axillary surgical staging are those who by having a negative dissection could avoid the hazards of such cytotoxic chemotherapy.

Extent of Axillary Surgery

In an attempt to minimize the magnitude of the operation while still providing sufficient staging information and local tumor control, lesser procedures than full axillary clearance have been advocated. The underlying assumption, as yet unproven, is that lesser surgery does in fact further reduce the complication rate of approximately 5% associated with axillary clearance. Single axillary node biopsy has been shown to be inaccurate by Davies et al.,[78] who found that the procedure failed to detect metastases in 42% of cases who subsequently had immediate full axillary dissection. It must be pointed out, however, that sampling a single axillary node as part of a triple node (axillary, apical, and internal mammary) biopsy as practiced by DuToit et al.[79] has been shown by them to provide sufficient prognostic information to accurately predict patient outcome and select those suitable for adjuvant therapy,[80] but with an axillary recurrence rate of 21%.[81]

The technique of axillary sampling involves dissection of the axillary tail and tissue adjacent to it containing the central node group. This procedure can be inadequate, with 18% of specimens in Forrest's multicenter series containing no nodes.[82] The anatomical imprecision of this sampling technique was also demonstrated by Cant et al.,[83] who found that in 72% of cases no nodal tissue could be detected in the specimen, and by Kjaergaard et al.,[84] who did not achieve a satisfactory sample in 40% of patients. Kissin et al.[85] have prospectively studied the problem of adequate axillary sampling and found an overall error rate of 24% (12/50 patients) from whom an average of four nodes were yielded by sampling, whereas clearance provided an average of 14 nodes. In Edinburgh, however, the technique of axillary sampling is a well-defined, modified, level I dissection, reliably yielding at least four lymph nodes.[86] They have been able to show identical node positivity rates in over 400 patients randomized to sampling or clearance. Furthermore, in another 100 patients studied, who were randomized to receive either no further axillary surgery or full clearance, the node positivity rates were 45% and 38%, respectively.

Another alternative to axillary clearance is a limited axillary dissection. Fisher et al.[87] have claimed that a limited dissection alone is sufficient for accurate axillary staging (if at least 10 nodes are obtained) and for providing adequate local control. Veronesi et al.[38] concluded from their analysis of nearly 1,500 complete axillary dissections that the order of spread in the 839 cases with axillary metastases follows a regular advancing pattern with the lowest level involved first in 828 cases; in only 11 cases (1.3%) were the metastases in the second or third level in the absence of first-level involvement—so-called "skip metastases." The incidence of skip metastases varies, depending on the study cited and the criteria established for definitions of the axillary levels. Rosen et al.[88] noted a 1.6% incidence of discontinuous metastases in their series of 1,228 axillary dissections, whereas Smith et al.[89] and Boova et al.[90] noted 28% and 6% incidences of skip metastases. Thus, it can be claimed that a combined level I and level II dissection or even a level I dissection alone may adequately stage patients and control disease in the axilla. While a level I dissection would be adequate for staging purposes, nearly 50% of those with positive first-level nodes have residual nodal disease in the axilla.

The problem with these lesser axillary procedures is the management of the remaining nodes. Veronesi reported that 44% of those patients with positive level I nodes will have involvement of higher levels in the axilla as well.[38] In an earlier study by Danforth et al.,[13] it was shown that tumor-involved nodes would be left behind in 51% to 82% after a level I dissection and in 21% to 45% after level I and II dissection. Recurrence beyond the pectoralis minor muscle or at the apex of the axilla is difficult to detect, especially when a partial axillary dissection has previously been performed. Thus, there is a risk that axillary recurrence will invade the brachial plexus and subclavian vessels, causing distressing symptoms to the patient and perhaps posing the difficult management problem of uncontrolled axillary recurrence. To avoid these problems, patients with involved first-level nodes could receive axillary irradiation or undergo a second operation to complete the axillary dissection. However, the addition of axillary irradiation to surgery increases the risk of lymphedema to nearly 50%, and a second operation increases the risk of inadvertent damage to the neurovascular bundle.

Conclusion

What recommendations can now be made as to the indications for axillary clearance in patients with operable breast cancer? In premenopausal patients, the case for adjuvant cytotoxic chemotherapy is proven in node-positive patients but not for all those with node-negative disease. Hence, in the absence of a better predictor of response to chemotherapy, axillary clearance should be routine for all premenopausal women with a palpable primary tumor. The place of axillary clearance is questionable in the impalpable cancer or in the case of ductal in-situ disease, where less than 5% of patients will have histologic involvement of the axillary nodes. In patients with ductal carcinoma in situ (DCIS), where the optimal treatment is still uncertain, we would advocate entering eligible patients into the UK CCCR DCIS trial, which precludes axillary surgery.

As adjuvant tamoxifen improves survival in postmenopausal patients regardless of nodal status, axillary clearance is necessary only for local control. For those treated by mastectomy for whatever reason the axilla should be cleared as part of this operation. However, in those postmenopausal patients suitable for treatment by breast-conserving surgery, there is a genuine choice. The patient can undergo axillary clearance performed at the same time as excision of the primary tumor, and thus avoid axillary irradiation. Alternatively, the axilla can be left untouched and the patient can have axillary irradiation at the same time as the postoperative breast irradiation. From this review, it can be seen that there already exists sufficient information to enable rational treatment decisions to be made for individual patients, determined by the tumor type, resource availability, patient preference, and the treating surgeon or oncologist's skills.

References

1. Fentiman IS, Mansel RE: The axilla: not a no-go zone. Lancet 1991; 337:221–223.
2. O'Dwyer PJ: Axillary dissection in primary breast cancer. Br Med J 1991; 302:360–361.
3. Hellman S, Harris JR, Leverne MB: Radiation therapy of early carcinoma of the breast without mastectomy. Cancer 1980; 46:988–994.
4. Boote DJ, Stockdale AD, Phillips RH: Axillary dissection in breast cancer. Lancet 1991; 337:486.
5. Fisher ER: Prognostic and therapeutic significance of pathological features of breast cancer. NCI Mongr 1986; 1:29–34.
6. Early Breast Cancer Trialists Collaborative Group: Treatment of Early Breast Cancer, Volume I: Worldwide evidence, 1985–1990. Oxford Medical Publications, Oxford, 1990.
7. Fisher B, Bauer M, Wickerham DL, Redmonds CK, et al: Relation of the number of positive axillary nodes to the prognosis of patients with primary breast cancer. Cancer 1983; 52:1551–1557.
8. Veronesi V, Rilke F, Luimi A, et al: Distribution of axillary node metastases by level of invasion: an analysis of 539 cases. Cancer 1987; 59:682–687.
9. Butcher H: Radical mastectomy for mammary carcinoma. Ann Surg 1969; 170:883–884.
10. Haagensen CD: Diseases of the Breast, 2nd ed. WB Saunders, Philadelphia, pp 384–390, 1971.
11. Bucalosi P, Veronesi V. Zingo L, et al: Enlarged mastectomy for breast cancer: review of 1213 cases. Am J Roentgen Rad Ther Nuc Med 1971; 111:119–122.
12. Schottenfeld D, Nash AG, Robbins GF, et al: Ten year results of the treatment of primary operable breast carcinoma; a summary of 304 patients evaluated by the TMN system. Cancer 1976; 38:1001–1007.
13. Danforth DN, Findlay PA, McDonald HD, et al: Complete axillary lymph node dissection for stage I–II carcinoma of the breast. J Clin Oncol 1986; 4:655–662.
14. Black RB, Merrick MV, Taylor TV, et al: Prediction of axillary metastases in breast cancer by axillary lymphoscintigraphy. Lancet 1980; 11:15–17.
15. McLean RG, Ege GN: Prognostic value of axillary lymphoscintigraphy in breast carcinoma patients. J Nucl Med 1986; 27:1116–1124.
16. Black RB, Merrick MV, Taylor TV, et al: Lymphoscintigraphy cannot diagnose breast cancer. BR J Cancer 1980; 67:667–668.
17. DeLand FH, Kim EE, Corgan RL, et al: Axillary lymphoscintigraphy by radioimmunodetection of carcinoembryonic antigen in breast cancer. J Nucl Med 1979; 20(12):1243–1249.
18. Weinstein JN, Stellar MA, Keenan AM, et al: Monoclonal antibodies in the lymphatics: selective delivery to lymph node metastases of a solid tumor. Science 1983; 222:423–426.
19. Goodwin DA, Meares CF, McCall MJ, et al: Chelate conjugates of monoclonal antibodies for imaging lymphoid structures in the mouse. J Nuc Med 1985; 26:493–502.
20. Thompson CH, Stacker SA, Salehi N, et al: Immunoscintigraphy for the detection of lymph node metastases from breast cancer. Lancet 1984; 11:1245–1247.
21. Tjandra JJ, Russell IS, Collins JP, et al: Immunolymphoscintigraphy for the detection of lymph node metastases from breast cancer. Cancer Res 1989; 49:1600–1608.
22. Bruneton JN, Caramella E, Hery M, et al: Axillary lymph node metastases in breast

cancer: preoperative detection with ultrasound. Radiology 1986; 158:325–326.
23. Henderson IC: The treatment of metastatic breast cancer with adjuvant systemic therapy. Ann Oncol 1990; 1:9–11.
24. Fisher B, Slack NH, Bross IDJ, et al: Cancer and the breast: size of neoplasm and prognosis. Cancer 1964; 24:1071–1080.
25. Fisher B, Slack NH, Ausman RK, Bross IDJ: Location of breast carcinoma and prognosis. Surg Gynecol Obstr 1969; 129:705–716.
26. Handley RS: Carcinoma of the breast. Ann R Coll Surg 1975; 57:59–66.
27. Lacour J. Bucalossi P, Cacers E, et al: Radical mastectomy versus radical mastectomy plus internal node dissection. Cancer 1976; 37:206–214.
28. Margotinni WS, Jacobelli G, Cau M: The end result of enlarged radical mastectomy. Acta Unio Int Contra Cancrum 1963; 19:1555–1559.
29. Lacour J, Le M, Cacers E, et al: Radical mastectomy versus radical mastectomy plus internal mammary dissection. Cancer 1983; 51:1941–1943.
30. Pickren JW: Significance of occult metastases. Cancer 1961; 14:1266–1271.
31. International (Ludwig) Breast Cancer Study Group: Prognostic importance of occult axillary lymph node micrometastases from breast cancers. Lancet 1990; 335:1565–1568.
32. Friedman S, Bertin H, Mouriesse H, et al: Importance of tumour cells in axillary node sinus margins discovered by serial sectioning in operable breast carcinoma. Acta Oncol 1988; 27:483–487.
33. Fisher ER, Swamidoss S, Lee CH, et al: Detection and significance of occult axillary node metastases in patients with invasive breast cancer. Cancer 1978; 45:2025–2031.
34. Apostolikas N, Petraki C, Agnantis NJ: The reliability of histologically negative axillary lymph nodes in breast cancer. Pathol Res Pract 1989; 184:35–38.
35. Wilkinson EJ, Hause LL, Hoffman RG, et al: Occult axillary lymph node metastases in invasive breast carcinoma: characteristics of the primary tumour and significance of the metastases. Pathol Ann 1982; 17:67–91.
36. Wells CA, Heryet A, Brochner J, Gatter KC, et al: the immunocytochemical detection of axillary micrometastases in breast cancer. Br J Cancer 1984; 50:193–197.
37. Bussolati G. Gugliotta P, Morra I, Pietribiari F, et al: The immunocytochemical detection of lymph node metastases from infiltrating lobular carcinoma of the breast. Br J Cancer 1986; 54:631–641.
38. Veronesi U, Luini A, Galimberti V, et al: Extent of metastatic axillary involvement in 1446 cases of breast cancer. Eur J Surg Oncol 1990; 16:127–133.
39. Graverson HP, Blichert Toff M, Anderson JA, et al. Breast cancer, risk of axillary recurrence in node negative patients following partial dissection of the axilla. Eur J Surg Oncol 1988; 14:407–412.
40. Fisher B, Redmond C, Fisher ER: Ten-year results of a randomized clinical trial comparing radical mastectomy and total mastectomy with or without radiation. N Engl J Med 1985; 312:674–681.
41. Cancer Research Campaign Working Party: CRC (Kings/Cambridge) trial for early breast cancer: a detailed update at the tenth year. Lancet 1980; 11:55–60.
42. Baum M, Coyle PJ: Simple mastectomy for early breast cancer and the behavior of untreated axillary nodes. Bull Cancer (Paris) 1977; 64:603–610.
43. Harris JR, Osteen RT: Patients with early breast cancer benefit from axillary treatment. Breast Cancer Res Treat 1985; 5:17–21.
44. Haagensen CD, Bodian C: A personal experience with Halsted's radical mastectomy. Ann Surg 1984; 199:443–450.
45. Cascinelli N, Greco M, Bufalino R, et al: Prognosis of breast cancer with axillary node metastases after surgical treatment only. Eur J Cancer Clin Oncol 1987; 23:795–799.
46. Clark GM, Dressler LG, Owens MA, et al: Prediction of relapse or survival in patients with node-negative breast cancer by DNA flow cytometry. N Engl J Med 1989; 320:627–633.
47. Sigurdsson H, Baldetorp B, Borg A, et al: Indicators of prognosis in node-negative breast cancer. N Engl J Med 1990; 322:1045–1053.

48. Hery M, Gioanni J, Lalanne CM, et al: The DNA labelling index: a prognostic factor in node-negative breast cancer. Breast Cancer Res Treat 1987; 9:207–211.
49. Salmon DJ, Clark GM, Wong SG, et al: Human breast cancer: correlation of relapse and survival with amplification of the HER-2/*neu* oncogene. Science 1987; 235:177–182.
50. Van De Vijver MJ, Peterse JL, Mooi WJ, et al: Neu-protein overexpression in breast cancer: association with comedo-type ductal carcinoma in situ and limited prognostic value in stage II breast cancer. N Engl J Med 1988; 319:1239–1245.
51. Wright C, Angus B, Nicholson S, et al: Expression of *c-erb* B-2 oncoprotein: a prognostic indicator in human breast cancer. Cancer Res 1989; 49:2087–2090.
52. Paik S. Hazan R, Fisher ER, et al: Pathologic findings from the National Surgical Adjuvant Breast and Bowel Project: prognostic significance of *erb* B-2 protein overexpression in primary breast cancer. J Clin Oncol 1990; 8:103–112.
53. Sainsbury JRC, Farndon JR, Needham GK, et al: Epidermal-growth-factor receptor status as predictor of early recurrence of death from breast cancer. Lancet 1987; 1:1398–1402.
54. Tandon AK, Clark GM, Chamnes GC, et al: Cathepsin D and prognosis in breast cancer. N Engl J Med 1990; 322:297–302.
55. Gusterson G: Unpublished data.
56. Nolvadex Adjuvant Trial Organisation: Controlled trial of tamoxifen as single adjuvant agent in management of early breast cancer. Br J Cancer 1988; 57:608–611.
57. Breast Cancer Trials Committee: Adjuvant tamoxifen in the management of operable breast cancer: the Scottish Trial. Lancet 1987; 2:171–175.
58. Stotter A, Atkinson EN, Fairston BA: Survival following locoregional recurrence after breast conservation therapy for cancer. Ann Surg 1990; 212(2):166–172.
59. Hayward JL: The Guy's trial of treatments of "early" breast cancer. World J Surg 1977; 1:314–316.
60. Langlands AO, Prescott RJ, Hamilton T: A clinical trial in the management of operable breast cancer. Lancet 1980; 2:55–60.
61. Yarnold JR: Selective avoidance of lymphatic irradiation in the conservative management of breast cancer. Radiother Oncol 1984; 2 (2):79–92.
62. Amalric R, Santamaria F, Robert F, et al: Radiation therapy with or without primary limited surgery for operable breast cancer. Cancer 1982; 49:30–34.
63. Mazeron JJ, Otmezguine Y, Huart J, Pierquin B: Conservative treatment of breast cancer: results of management of axillary lymph node area in 3353 patients (letter). Lancet 1985; 1:1387.
64. Bataini JP, Picco C, Martin M, Calle R: Relation between time-dose and local control of operable breast cancer treated by tumorectomy and radiotherapy or by radical radiotherapy alone. Cancer 1978; 42:2059–2065.
65. Fletcher GH: Local results of irradiation in the primary management of localized breast cancer. Cancer 1972; 29:545–551.
66. Kissin MW, Querci della Rovere G, Easton D, Westbury G: Risk of lymphoedema following the treatment of breast cancer. Br J Surg 1986; 73:580–584.
67. Aitkin RJ, Gaze MN, Rodger A, Chetty U, et al: Arm morbidity within a trial of mastectomy and either nodal sample with selective radiotherapy or axillary clearance. Br J Surg 1989; 76:568–571.
68. Yarnold JR: Early stage breast cancer: treatment options and results. Br Med Bull 1991; 47:372–387.
69. Kurtz JM, Amalric R, Brandone H, Ayme Y, et al: Contralateral breast cancer and other second malignancies in patients treated by breast-conserving therapy with radiation. Int J Radiat Oncol Biol Phys 1988; 15(2):277–284.
70. Gough MH, Durrant KR, Giraud-Saunders AM, et al: A randomized controlled trial of prophylactic cytotoxic chemotherapy in potentially curable breast cancer. Br J Surg 1985; 72(3):182–185.
71. Goldhirsch A, Gelber R, Simes R: Costs and benefits of adjuvant therapy in breast cancer: a quality-adjusted survival analysis. J Clin Oncol 1989; 7:36–44.

72. Himel HN, Liberati A, Gelber RD, Chalmers TC: Adjuvant chemotherapy for breast cancer: a pooled estimate based on published randomized control trials. J Am Med Assoc 1986; 256(9):1148–1159.
73. Padmanabhan N, Howell A, Rubens RD: Mechanism of action of adjuvant chemotherapy in early breast cancer. Lancet 1986; 2:411–414.
74. Donaldson M, Bain J, Carter D: Consensus Development Conference: treatment of primary breast cancer. Br Med J 1986; 293:946–947.
75. DeVita VT: Breast cancer therapy: exercising all our options. N Engl J Med 1989; 320(8):527–529.
76. Rosner D, Lane WW: Node-negative minimal invasive breast cancer patients are not candidates for routine systemic adjuvant therapy. Cancer 1990; 66(2):199–205.
77. Rosen PP, Groshen S: Factors influencing survival and prognosis in early breast carcinoma (T1N0M0-T1N1M0): assessment of 644 patients with median follow-up of 18 years. Surg Clin North Am 1990; 70(4):937–962.
78. Davies GC, Millis RR, Hayward JL: Assessment of axillary node status. Ann Surg 1980; 192:148–151.
79. Du Toit RS, Locker AP, Ellis IO, Elston CW, et al: Evaluation of the prognostic value of triple node biopsy in early breast cancer. Br J Surg 1990; 77:163–167.
80. Todd JH, Dowle C, Williams MR, et al: Confirmation of a prognostic index in primary breast cancer. Br J Cancer 1987; 56:489–492.
81. Locker AP, Ellis IO, Morgan DAL, et al: Factors influencing local recurrence after excision and radiotherapy for primary breast cancer. Br J Surg 1989; 76:890–894.
82. Forrest APM, Stewart HJ, Roberts MM, Steele RJC: Simple mastectomy and axillary node sampling in the management of primary breast cancer. Am J Surg 1982; 196:371–378.
83. Cant ELM, Shivas AA, Forrest APM: Lymph node biopsy during simple mastectomy. Lancet 1975; 1:995–997.
84. Kjaergaard J, Blichert-Toft M, Anderson JA, et al: Probability of false negative nodal staging in conjunction with partial axillary dissection in breast cancer. Br J Surg 1985; 72:365–367.
85. Kissin MW, Thompson EM, Price AB, et al: The inadequacy of axillary sampling in breast cancer. Lancet 1982; 1:1210–1212.
86. Steele RJC, Forrest APM, Gibson T, et al: The efficacy of lower axillary sampling in obtaining lymph node status in breast cancer; a controlled randomised trial. Br J Surg 1985; 72:368–369.
87. Fisher B, Wolmark N, Bauer M, et al: The accuracy of clinical node staging and of limited axillary dissection as a determinant of histological nodal status in carcinoma of the breast. Surg Gynecol Obst 1981; 152:765–772.
88. Rosen PR, Lesser ML, Kinne DW, Beattie EJ: Discontinuous or skip metastases in breast cancer. Ann Surg 1983; 197(3):276–283.
89. Smith JA, Gamez Aranjo JJ, Gallager HS, White EC, et al: Carcinoma of the breast: analysis of total lymph node involvement versus level of metastases. Cancer 1977; 39:527–532.
90. Boova RS, Bonanni R, Rosato FE: Patterns of axillary nodal involvement in breast cancer. Ann Surg 1982; 196:642–644.

18

The Clinical Significance of Atypical Hyperplasia, Multicentricity, and Bilaterality

David L. Page

Introduction

Hyperplasia presages the development of epithelial malignant neoplasms in many body sites. In the breast, the borderline between a benign tumor and a malignancy has engendered many forms of inquiry and terminology. We are of the opinion that current knowledge supports risk assessment as an acceptable approach to stratification and definition in this area. Thus, specifically defined risk indicators are tested and, for simplification, may be found to fall within one or another of these groups: (1) unassociated with an increased cancer risk; (2) associated with increased risk of invasive cancer approaching double (1.5 to 2 times) that of a comparable group (slight); (3) associated with a risk of 4 to 5 times (moderate).

Thus, histopathologically defined lesions are assigned to categories with differing magnitudes of cancer risk (Table 1). Since the 1985 Consensus Conference,[1] few changes have been made in this general approach except for the placement of well-developed examples of sclerosing adenosis[2] within the slightly increased risk category.

Somewhat fewer than 5% of women in a large group undergoing surgical biopsy prior to mammography[3,4] had specific histopathological patterns of atypical hyperplasia (AH) that approached the patterns of carcinoma in situ (CIS). These women with AH had a risk of cancer four to five times that of the general population, or about one-half the risk associated with microscopic carcinoma in situ. When generally utilized criteria from original diagnoses of many pathologists were used in a similarly designed cohort study, AH still

---

Table 1
Relative Risk for Invasive Breast Carcinoma Based on Pathological Examination of Benign
Breast Tissues

Slightly Increased Risk (1.5 to 2 times)
Women with any lesion specified below in a biopsy specimen are at slightly increased risk for
invasive breast carcinoma relative to comparable women who have had no breast biopsy:
- Hyperplasia, moderate or florid, solid or papillary
- Papilloma with fibrovascular core
- Sclerosing adenosis, well-developed*

Moderately Increased Risk (4 to 5 times)
Women with a lesion specified below in a biopsy specimen are at moderately increased risk for
invasive breast carcinoma relative to comparable women who have had no breast biopsy:
- Atypical hyperplasia (borderline lesion)
     Specific patterns of atypical ductal hyperplasia
     Specific patterns of atypical lobular hyperplasia

---

*All forms of adenosis were accepted in 1985 as having no indication of increased cancer risk. Since
that time, well-developed examples of sclerosing adenosis, apart from other associations, indicate a
slightly increased risk.[2]

elevated the risk,[5] but only to about three times, supporting the use of more
stringently defined histologic criteria. Several recent studies support the utility
and predictiveness of specifically defined AH.[6,7] Follow-up studies of comparable type involving women with mammographically detected lesions are not
available. However, it is likely that the incidence of AH is higher in mammographically directed biopsies.[8]

Further studies have indicated an appreciable interaction between atypical
hyperplasia and other nonanatomical risk factors, particularly a family history of
breast cancer.[3,9] Also, lower dosage estrogen replacement (specifically conjugated preparation) after menopause does not appear to further affect risk in any
histologically defined group.[10]

Clinical Implications of Increased Cancer Risk

Breast cancer risk assessment is only of unquestioned clinical importance
when its magnitude approaches five times the general population. Note that
comments on magnitude of relative risks (RR) are inherently confusing without
an immediate reference group. This reference or comparison group is usually to
the general population of women without the risk factor. The age of a patient as
well as the number of years at risk are of great importance in the evaluation of the
impact these risk statements should have in the clinical setting. Thus, in the
clinical setting relating to a single patient, absolute risk (AR) statements are more
relevant. However, these statements rendered as a single fraction or percentage
must be known to have relevance to comparable women over a similar period of
time. It is important not to extrapolate such risks to time intervals that are longer
than those documented by follow-up studies in the literature. In particular, the

discussion above indicates that projecting risk over the entire lifetime of an individual patient is misleading and usually overstates the magnitude of the patient's absolute risk.[11,12]

For most, women in their late forties may be taken to represent the average experience of the follow-up studies that have assessed cancer risk. Thus, the absolute risk figures may be taken to apply to them and should be altered for younger and older women accordingly. Thus, the experience of comparable women is taken to relay the information in a more direct way as in AR, e.g., 10% likelihood of developing invasive carcinoma in 10–15 years. A specific period of time is necessary in the statement. In general terms, we do not feel that prediction of breast cancer risk should be extended beyond 10 to 15 years[12] because the stability of risk with time is unproven. It is our experience, particularly with older women, that these elevated risks will fall, at least in relative terms, 10 to 15 years after detection.[12] Thus, AR should be used preferentially in the clinical setting with an individual patient, but should be carefully sculpted to the setting. AR may be derived from RR.[11] However, overestimates of AR will occur even if the relative risk is assumed to be constant for a full 20 years, when in fact, RR falls with greater time since biopsy. This is precisely what happens for proliferative disease.[12] Thus, it is the AR that is most useful in the clinical setting,[13] but it must be derived with care for each individual patient, assessing the relevance of published figures to the specific patient being advised. For example, few women under age 30 and over age 60 were present in our studies, and risk figures for atypical lesions must be understood to be less certain for women in these young and older age groups.[13,14]

Moderately Increased Risk

This term was originally chosen by the 1985 Consensus Conference[1] in order to place the atypical hyperplasia lesions in perspective between mild or slight and microscopic examples of in-situ carcinoma. The relative risk for subsequent invasive carcinoma of the atypical hyperplasias within this group is four to five times that of the general population. This is approximately half the risk experienced by women with microscopic in-situ carcinoma, specifically LCIS[15] and microscopic DCIS of the noncomedo variety.[16]

There is such a strong interaction with family history and AH that it is relevant to consider women with atypical hyperplasia who have a positive family history of breast cancer separately from those who do not. The definition of a positive family history in these studies was at least a first-degree relative (mother, daughter, sister) with proven breast cancer. The absolute risk of breast cancer development in women with atypical hyperplasia without a family history was 8% in 10 years, whereas those with a positive family history experienced a risk of about 20% to 25% at 15 years. This strong interaction with family history has been supported in a recent study.[5] This magnitude of risk for women with AH and family history is closely analogous to that accorded lobular carcinoma in situ.[15,17–19]

Confirmatory studies linking more complex and "atypical" lesions to future risk of breast cancer are several.[5,20] Most recently, London et al.[21] have used the original histologic criteria[4,22] and found the same risks for atypical hyperplasia in a very large cohort from the 1970s and 1980s primarily. This extends the relevance of AH because the initial studies[3,4] involved a cohort biopsied in the 1950s and 1960s. Also, Tavassoli and Norris have documented the experience of a reference center with atypical hyperplasia.[6] Using criteria similar to those of Page et al.,[4] but including a criterion of size up to 2–3 mm in greatest dimension, they found similar risks for later carcinoma development as previously recorded for AH based on specific histologic criteria.

Mammographic surveillance is widely accepted as a clinical alternative over extirpative surgery for most women with increased risk. The logic of this decision rests largely in the knowledge that: (1) mastectomy would remove many more breasts than ever would develop cancer, (2) the patient's breast cancer risk will more closely approximate that of slightly elevated risk if she remains free of cancer for 10 years after biopsy indicating moderate risk,[12] and (3) the current era of mammography should only improve the good prognosis after treatment of later developing breast cancer in women with moderate and high risk followed closely by palpation.[23]

Multicentricity

The occurrence of two or more physically separate lesional foci of breast carcinoma constitute multifocality. The term does not necessarily indicate tumors of independent origin, and is usually confined to tumors within the same breast. Bilaterality, the occurrence of carcinoma in the contralateral breast, is usually excluded by definition and is discussed separately.

The terms *multicentricity* and *multifocality* have been used for decades to indicate seeming or real multiplicity of cancer throughout an individual breast. The terms have no intrinsically different meanings, but have in recent decades been interpreted as follows: multicentricity has been used to indicate multicentric origin, usually in sites remote or relatively so from the initially identified neoplasm, and multifocality has been used in recent years to indicate foci of the same tumor, relatively close to each other, usually in the same quadrant. Earlier studies that are reviewed by Fisher et al.[24] were concerned primarily with establishing the concept of multicentric origin and were not focused on the specific anatomical features of whether tumor foci were adjacent to, connected by in-situ disease, or remote from the dominant mass. One of the first studies distinguishing between cancerous foci in the vicinity of the primary mass and those that may be regarded as distant was that of Qualheim and Gall.[25] They found that 54% of mastectomy specimens contained multiple foci of carcinoma, but their study was limited to one or two large sections of the breast without three-dimensional examination, excluding the possibility that apparently separate foci were connected. This approach obviously maximizes the apparent incidence of multicentricity. One study that analyzed grossly inapparent disease within radical mastectomy specimens found 7% of cases to have "precancerous or early intraductal carcinomatous lesions."[26] Thus, many of these studies are hampered by failing to indicate the precise location as well as leaving unclear the distinction between cancers and atypical hyperplasia. Some studies, for example, indicate only that the distant carcinomas were "microscopic."

Recent studies have been concerned with practical questions that are precisely defined in space and time, such as the occurrence of cancer in remote quadrants, whereas the concept of multicentric origin was the focus of earlier studies.[24] Other recent studies have added both the elements of time and biology (natural history) by observing the evolution (or nonevolution) of clinical disease in the living breast after partial mastectomy. These have given a clear focus and better understanding to our clinical decisions as these empirical observations relative to various therapeutic strategies are recorded.

Anatomy

A perfect definition of multicentricity referable to all settings is either unobtainable or of practical impossibility because of the inherent difficulties in understanding and studying the three-dimensional microanatomy of the breast. Distinguishing between separate breast carcinomas and intramammary spread of breast carcinoma, particularly along ducts, is difficult and requires three-dimensional reconstruction. Therefore, any definition of multicentricity is necessarily arbitrary and will be situationally confined, i.e., bound by the method utilized for detection.

The breast is a branching (racemose) gland with 15–20 collecting (lactiferous) ducts exiting at the nipple. Each of these ductal systems or lobes subserves hundreds of lobular units, which are collections of acinar elements. The lobes are not defined anatomical units separated by septa, and adjacent radiating lobar units may overlap. Thus, if apparent multicentricity is due to spread along ducts of the originating lobe, they will be preferentially arranged in a radial fashion from nipple to periphery in whatever quadrant they appear. Thus, the irregular branching system of breast ducts in three dimensions easily explains why those numerous breast cancers that spread along the ducts appear as separate foci in the two-dimensional slides routinely utilized.

Prevalence

Partly because of difficulties with definitions of multicentricity, the exact prevalence of multicentricity is uncertain but is more frequent with some forms of carcinoma. The reported prevalences of multicentricity have ranged from 9% to 75%.[27] In a complete review of these diverse studies, McDivitt[28] concluded that the prevalence of multicentricity probably lay between 25% and 50%, with approximately 5% to 10% of secondary lesions being invasive. This tremendous disparity in prevalence rates is attributable to many variables, including (1) which definition of multicentricity is used, (2) the method of examining mastectomy specimens employed, (3) the number of quadrants sampled and number of sections from each quadrant examined, (4) which subsets of patients are included in or excluded from the study, (5) whether the lesions were detected clinically or mammographically, and (6) the age of patients in the group, among others.

One should be aware of the method used to study breasts in a series looking for multicentricity. The most thorough method involves combined examination of breast tissue using radiographs, a dissecting microscope, and microscopic examination of whole tissue sections from breasts that have been frozen and serially sectioned at 2.5-mm intervals.[27,29] This method is thorough and best captures the three-dimensional anatomy of the breast, but uses technology that may not be available at all centers, and may force investigators to elect between examining large numbers of slides on a small number of specimens, and examining a smaller number of less extensive sections of a much larger sample.[30]

In-Situ Lesions

The prevalence of multicentricity can vary depending on whether the primary lesion is an in-situ or invasive lesion, and depending on the histologic type of the primary lesion. The risk of multicentricity associated with lobular carcinoma in situ is great, and is well accepted.[17,31]

Ductal carcinoma in situ is sometimes multicentric, but much less frequently than is lobular carcinoma in situ.[25] Lagios[27] noted that ductal carcinoma in situ had been reported to have varying rates of multicentricity and found in his own concurrent series that 29% of in-situ ductal lesions were multicentric. Of his cases of ductal carcinoma in situ, 19.5% were associated with occult foci of invasion. Size dependency of multicentricity was striking in all cases where the lesion was larger than 25 mm in its greatest extent. Gump[30] found an extremely high rate (81%) of multicentricity associated with ductal carcinoma in situ, but most of these studies were hampered by sample limitations in concurrent studies. Conservation surgical procedures have taught us the most about these matters, as recurrences after local resections are adjacent to the initial disease over 95% of the time.[32-34]

Patchefsky[35] examined the incidence of multicentricity associated with various subsets of ductal carcinoma in situ, finding that multicentricity was greatly increased with the micropapillary type of ductal carcinoma in situ and was much less common with the cribriform and solid types of ductal carcinoma in situ, leaving the comedo type in an intermediate position.

Invasive Lesions

Invasive mammary carcinoma of no specific type (invasive ductal carcinoma) is by far the most common type of invasive mammary carcinoma, and it is associated with one of the lowest rates of multicentricity. Gump[30] found that it was least likely to have multicentric disease, accounting for a 19% rate of multicentricity compared to a rate of 27% for all types. The rate of multicentricity increases when other factors are present. For example, the rate of multicentricity associated with minimally invasive (dominant in-situ disease) ductal carcinoma is apparently greater than that associated with the usual invasive ductal carcinoma.[36] This may not be related to the small size of the invasive component per se, but rather to the regular presence in such cases of extensive DCIS. The rate of multicentricity is also increased approximately twofold when infiltrating ductal carcinoma is associated with in-situ lobular carcinoma.[37]

Infiltrating lobular carcinoma is associated with elevated rates of multicentricity.[37] Fisher[24] showed that invasive lobular carcinoma was more frequently associated with invasive secondary lesions but that noninvasive secondary lesions were not more likely. Some authors have pointed out that most of the secondary lesions lie near the primary lesion and probably represent recurrence or spread of the original invasive lobular carcinoma rather than true multicentricity.[38]

Recent Studies

The most important recent addition to our knowledge of possible multicentricity has related to the recognition of the extensiveness of a ductal carcinoma in-situ component in association with invasive carcinomas. The definition of an extensive intraductal component (EIC) was first proposed by Connolly and Schnitt[39] and consisted of two criteria: (1) DCIS was present prominently within the infiltrating tumor, and (2) DCIS was present clearly extending beyond the infiltrating margin of the tumor. Note that tumors that were predominantly intraductal with little invasion were included. The studies of Holland et al.[40,41] have supported the studies of the Joint Center for Radiation Therapy.[39,42] One of these supportive studies described the histologic elements in reexcision specimens from 71 patients with infiltrating ductal carcinoma who initially underwent a limited excision of tumor.[43] Residual carcinoma on reexcision was present in 88% of patients with EIC, with one-half of these having a considerable quantity of residual DCIS. Only 2% of patients without EIC on initial biopsy had subsequent biopsies with extensive DCIS. These histological findings mirror very closely the predictability of EIC with regard to local recurrence after local excision and radiotherapy as definitive therapy for breast cancer. In these latter studies, most of the local recurrences within 5 years of follow-up were predicted by EIC. These clinical follow-up studies of the predictive utility of EIC have been confirmed from Amsterdam[44] and London.[45]

Two studies have not agreed with the predictive utility of EIC with regard to local treatment failure. This disparity may be explained by the fact that one of these studies employed a large resection[46] and the other required tumor-free margins.[47] These wider initial resections are accompanied by a lower rate of local failure and may well largely negate the importance of EIC and its predictive value because little or no DCIS is left behind in the breast. All of these observations are compatible with the contention that residual foci of DCIS left within the breast at the time of radiation after local resection of primary breast cancer are largely responsible for local recurrence.

It is evident, in summation, that most apparent multifocality is due to the tendency of DCIS to spread through the duct system. This spread may be extensive but seems usually to be within a segment (quadrant) or into adjacent quadrants rather than being truly separate foci. It takes three-dimensional reconstruction to prove that apparently distant deposits of disease are actually continuous.[41]

Second Primary or Bilateral Primary Breast Cancer

Although discussion of a second primary breast cancer has usually assumed that it would take place in the contralateral breast, that is no longer true because of the advent of therapy conserving major portions of the ipsilateral breast. However, the second primary breast cancer occurring within the same breast as the first is considered to be multicentricity and is covered in the preceding discussion.

Considerations of bilateral primary breast cancer are plagued by concerns of unpredictability. This eventuality is unavoidable because the event is uncommon and case definition is inconsistent between publications on the subject. This presentation will emphasize invasive mammary carcinoma. Certainly there is a special place for lobular histology in increased bilaterality.[48,49]

The first major paper on the subject of bilateral primary mammary carcinoma was written only in 1921.[50] Many reports in the literature have subsequently documented this condition and have only recently advanced us in a major way beyond the conclusions of Foote and Stewart in 1945[51] that the risk to the second breast after a woman had a cancer in one breast represented the most frequent antecedent of breast cancer. Although this increase in risk is well understood, it is still apparent that bilateral disease occurs only rarely, but it is an important consideration because its spectre dictates that it be considered in the management of the contralateral breast after a breast carcinoma. Several subsequent studies reported in the 1970s and 1980s form the basis of our current understanding. These various studies have differed, particularly with regard to prognosis, but there is a striking similarity with regard to the yearly incidence of carcinoma that may be expected in the contralateral breast.

Some of the difficulty with understanding this situation clearly is the unavoidable trade-off between precise case definition in a small series of patients likely to recruitment bias and larger series that may be population-based but often have poor case definition. Studies that are done with good case definition based on material from one institution may be biased because of selection of the patient material, while population-based studies such as from regional tumor registries, for various reasons lack careful case definition. This weakness is compensated in the latter case by the unbiased nature of the study and the large numbers involved. Separate consideration should be given to the bilateral breast cancers that occur simultaneously in time as opposed to metachronous tumors.[52] There is certainly no widely accepted definition to separate the considerations of synchrony and metachrony; the former have been defined as occurring within one month or within the same hospitalization or before the first cancer is treated. Certainly this definition will be of extreme importance because the major clinical concern in this area is how to deal with the spectre of contralateral breast cancer following treatment. When the second breast carcinoma has occurred within the time frame that the first has been clinically managed, then its therapeutic decision-making will be more straightforward. Mammography has made a huge difference in all of these considerations, greatly raising the incidence of synchronous breast cancers to the range of 2% to 3%. Prior to the advent of mammography, the risk of synchronous bilateral primary cancers in different studies averaged about 1%.

The case definition should guarantee that the second lesion is primary and not a metastasis. This has been a consideration for 100 years since the time that Billroth established criteria for multiple primary neoplasms. His considerations with some modification have recently been recorded by Chaudary et al.[53] and are as follows:

1. The demonstration of the in-situ change in the contralateral tumor was considered absolute proof that the contralateral lesion was a primary tumor.

2. The tumor in the second breast was considered to be a new primary lesion if it was histologically different in type from the cancer in the first breast.

3. In the absence of definite histologic difference, a carcinoma in the breast was considered to be compatible with an independent lesion provided there was no evidence of local, regional, or distant metastases from the cancer in the ipsilateral breast.

The study by Chaudary et al.[53] may be taken to be a model. Case accrual was performed during the mammographic era and consequently bilateral breast cancers occurring simultaneously (in the same hospital admission) in 3% of women was much higher than in earlier series. The problem of breast case selection is well-demonstrated in this study because it is stated that there was a greater awareness of the opposite breast. Every lump in the contralateral breast was biopsied in order to determine whether it was a second primary tumor, leading to a greater number of nonsimultaneous primary breast carcinomas diagnosed during this study than in previous years. In the presence of wide-spread metastases, lumps in the contralateral breast were also biopsied, whereas they might have been ignored previously. Some of the cases in the study were from such lesions, but the number is not stated.

The annual rate of occurrence of the second primary cancer was constant for 20 years at a rate of 7.6 second cancers occurring per 1,000 patients at risk per year.[53] The relative risk of a second nonsimultaneous primary carcinoma was 5.9 times that of a risk of occurrence of cancer in the first breast in the general female population. There was a very important age consideration demonstrated in this study in that a woman less than 40 years old presenting with a first breast cancer had a three times greater chance of developing a second cancer than a woman over the age of 40. Actually, in each decade, the incidence of second cancer per 1,000 women per year fell, being 12 in the age group 40 to 49, 6 in 50 to 59, 8 in 60 to 69, and 4 in women over 70. The nonsimultaneous bilateral breast cancers arose in the 2,454 survivors of 4,656 patients with a unilateral breast cancer seen and treated from 1950 onwards and who were studied for the occurrence of a nonsimultaneous bilateral breast carcinoma from January 1980 to March 1982. Fifty-four bilateral primary breast cancers were seen, with 40 of these being nonsimultaneous.

The indication that young women have a greater risk of a second tumor was also presented in the large study of Robbins and Berg in which those developing cancer by the age of 50 years had almost twice the risk of a second tumor per year of exposure as women entering the series after the age of 60 years.[54]

Most models that study relative hazards assume that prognostic variables maintain the same hazard irrespective of the length of time after diagnosis. This is really not the case in this situation. It is quite clear that poor prognosis attends women with bilateral carcinomas presenting synchronously or within a close time frame. The overall prognosis is better as the metachronous carcinomas occur farther apart. It seems clear from life table analysis and comparisons with unilateral cancer cases that the second cancer adds an independent risk. If prognosis is determined from the onset of the initial carcinoma, then the occurrence of the metachronous carcinoma many years later will be happening in women who have already identified themselves as having a quite good prognosis from the first tumor. Metachronous bilateral disease has a similar prognosis to unilateral cancer when survival is calculated from the date of the second diagnosis.

The National Surgical Adjuvant Breast Project added confirmatory information to most of these elements in a carefully done ten-year follow-up study of over a thousand patients with breast cancer. The largest incidence of carcinoma diagnosis in a contralateral breast was in the first year after treatment.[55] However, the subsequent incidence per year following that remained approximately the same, at just under 1% for those surviving in each year. With only 10 years of follow-up, there was no difference in survival between patients who did and those who did not develop contralateral carcinoma. However, studies reporting 20-and 30-year follow-up after the first carcinoma have indicated that the prognosis is slightly less favorable overall for women developing a second breast carcinoma, and that this survival difference is totally dependent upon the second carcinoma. These observations are, of course, strongly biased by the fact that women have to survive a long period in order to develop a second carcinoma.

The study by Fisher et al. at 10 years[55] did indicate that many factors were associated with a somewhat increased risk of developing contralateral carcinoma within the group of women having a first cancer. These included original lesions greater than 2 cm in diameter, histology of lobular carcinoma in situ or lobular invasive type, as well as invasive tubular carcinoma. None of these features, however, indicated a relative risk greater than two or occasionally three times that of the other women. Considering that the absolute risk for all patients is less than 1% per year, the absolute magnitude in the group with a higher risk is not greatly increased. The elevation of risk for women with a family history of breast carcinoma as well as carcinoma of their own was approximately double that of women without a positive family history, but is not statistically reliably greater than 1.5% per year.

Two of the more interesting recent developments relate to the possibility that contralateral biopsy may be used to reduce risk of cancer in the second breast,[56] and to reduce contralateral cancers in women being treated by tamoxifen.[57,58] The latter seems quite certain and is probably at the level of a 50% reduction. The former is not confirmed by other studies.

References

1. Hutter RVP: Consensus meeting: is "fibrocystic disease" of the breast precancerous? Arch Path Lab Med 1986; 110:171–173.
2. Jensen RA, Page DL, Dupont WD, Rogers LW: Invasive breast cancer risk in women with sclerosing adenosis. Cancer 1989; 64:1977–1983.
3. Dupont WD, Page DL: Risk factors for breast cancer in women with proliferative breast disease. N Engl J Med 1985; 312:146-151.
4. Page DL, Dupont WD, Rogers LW, Rados MS: Atypical hyperplastic lesions of the female breast: a long-term follow-up study. Cancer 1985; 55:2698–2708.
5. Carter CL, Corle DK, Micozzi MS, Schatzkin A, et al: A prospective study of the development of breast cancer in 16,692 women with benign breast disease. Am J Epidemiol 1988; 128:467-477.
6. Tavassoli FA, Norris HJ: A comparison of the results of long-term follow-up for atypical intraductal hyperplasia and intraductal hyperplasia of the breast. Cancer 1990; 65:518-529.
7. Connolly JL, Schnitt SJ, London SJ, Colditz G: Benign breast disease and risk of subsequent breast cancer: the experience in the nurses' health study (abstr). Lab Invest 1991; 64:10.
8. Rubin E, Alexander RW, Visscher DW, Urist MM, et al: Proliferative disease and atypia in biopsies performed for mammographically detected nonpalpable lesions. Cancer 1988; 61:2077–2082.
9. Dupont WD, Page DL: Breast cancer risk associated with proliferative disease, age at first birth, and a family history of breast cancer. Am J Epidemiol 1987; 125:769–779.
10. Dupont WD, Page DL, Rogers LW, Parl FF: Influence of exogenous estrogens, proliferative breast disease, and other variables on breast cancer risk. Cancer 1989; 63:948–957.
11. Dupont WD: Converting relative risks to absolute risks: a graphical approach. Stat Med 1989; 8:641–651.
12. Dupont WD, Page DL: Relative risk of breast cancer varies with time since diagnosis of atypical hyperplasia. Hum Pathol 1989; 20:723–725.
13. Page DL, Dupont WD: Histopathologic risk factors for breast cancer in women with benign breast disease. Semin Surg Oncol 1988; 4:213–217.
14. Dupont WD, Page DL: Risks factors for breast carcinoma in women with proliferative breast disease. In: Bland KI, Copeland EM (eds). The Breast. W.B. Saunders, Philadelphia, pp 292–298, 1991.
15. Gump FE: Lobular carcinoma in situ: pathology and treatment. Surg Clin NA 1990; 70:873–883.
16. Page DL, Dupont WD, Rogers LW, Landenberger M: Intraductal carcinoma of the breast: follow-up after biopsy only. Cancer 1982; 49:751–758.
17. Frykberg ER, Santiago F, Betsill WL, O'Brien PH: Lobular carcinoma in situ of the breast. Surg Gynecol Obstet 1987; 164:285–301.
18. Wapnir IL, Rabinowitz B, Greco RS: A reappraisal of prophylactic mastectomy. Surg Gynecol Obstet 1990; 171:171-184.

19. Hutter RVP: The management of patients with lobular carcinoma in situ of the breast. Cancer 1984; 53:798–802.
20. Palli D, Rosselli del Turco M, Simoncini R, Bianchi S: Benign breast disease and breast cancer: a case-control study in a cohort in Italy. Int J Cancer 1991; 47:703–706.
21. London SJ, Connolly JL, Schnitt SJ, Colditz GA: A prospective study of benign breast disease and risk of breast cancer. JAMA, in press.
22. Page DL, Anderson TJ, Rogers LW: Epithelial hyperplasia. In: Page DL, Anderson TJ (eds). Diagnostic Histopathology of the Breast. Churchill Livingstone, Edinburgh, pp 120–156, 1988.
23. Haagensen CD, Lane N, Lattes R, Bodian C: Lobular neoplasia (so-called lobular carcinoma in situ) of the breast. Cancer 1978; 42:737–769.
24. Fisher ER, Gregorio R, Redmond C, Velljos F, et al: Pathologic findings from the national surgical adjuvant breast project (Protocol No. 4). I. Observations concerning the multicentricity of mammary cancer. Cancer 1975; 35:247–254.
25. Qualheim RE, Gall EA: Breast carcinoma with multiple sites of origin. Cancer 1957; 10:460–468.
26. Kern WH, Brooks RN: Atypical epithelial hyperplasia associated with breast cancer and fibrocystic disease. Cancer 1969; 24:668–675.
27. Lagios MD, Westdahl PR, Rose MR: The concept and implications of multicentricity in breast carcinoma. Pathol Annu 1981; 16(Pt 2):83–102.
28. McDivitt RW: Breast cancer multicentricity. In: McDivitt RW, Oberman HA, et al. (eds). The Breast, 25th ed., Williams and Wilkins, Baltimore, pp 139–148, 1984.
29. Lagios MD: Multicentricity of breast carcinoma demonstrated by routine correlated serial subgross and radiographic examination. Cancer 1977; 40:1726–1734.
30. Gump FE, Habfi DV, Logergo P, Shikora S, et al: The extent and distribution of cancer in breasts with palpable primary tumors. Ann Surg 1986; 204:384–388.
31. Page DL, Kidd TE, Dupont WD, Simpson JF, et al: Lobular neoplasia of the breast: higher risk for subsequent invasive cancer predicted by more extensive disease. Hum Pathol 1991; 22:1232–1239.
32. McCormick B, Rosen PP, Kinne D, Cox L, et al: Duct carcinoma in situ of the breast: an analysis of local control after conservation surgery and radiotherapy. Int J Radiat Oncol Biol Phys 1991; 21:289–292.
33. Solin LJ, Recht A, Fourquet A, Kurtz J, et al: Ten-year results of breast-conserving surgery and definitive irradiation for intraductal carcinoma (ductal carcinoma in situ) of the breast. Cancer 1991; 68:2337–2344.
34. Lagios MD, Margolin FR, Westdahl PR, Rose MR: Mammographically detected duct carcinoma in situ. Cancer 1989; 63:618–624.
35. Patchefsky AS, Schwartz GF, Finkelstein SD, Prestipino A, et al: Heterogeneity of intraductal carcinoma of the breast. Cancer 1989; 64:731–741.
36. Schwartz GF, Patchefsky AS, Feig SA, Shaber GS, et al: Multicentricity of non-palpable breast cancer. Cancer 1980; 45:2913–2916.
37. Lesser ML, Rosen PP, Kinne DW: Multicentricity and bilaterality in invasive breast carcinoma. Surgery 1982; 91:234-240.
38. Schnitt SJ, Connolly JL, Recht A, Silver B, et al: Influence of infiltrating lobular histology on local tumor control in breast cancer patients treated with conservative surgery and radiotherapy. Cancer 1989; 64:448–454.
39. Schnitt SJ, Connolly JL, Harris JR, Hellman S, et al: Pathologic predictors of early local recurrence in stage I and II breast cancer treated by primary radiation therapy. Cancer 1984; 53:1049–1057.
40. Holland R, Connolly JL, Gelman R, Mravunac M, et al: The presence of an extensive intraductal component (EIC) following a limited excision correlates with prominent residual disease in the remainder of the breast. J Clin Oncol 1990; 8:113.
41. Holland R, Hendriks JHCL, Verbeek ALM, Mravunac M, et al: Extent, distribution, and mammographic/histological correlations of breast ductal carcinoma in situ. Lancet 1990; 335:519–522.

42. Harris JR, Connolly JL, Schnitt SJ, Cohen RB, et al: Clinical-pathologic study of early breast cancer treated by primary radiation therapy. J Clin Oncol 1983; 1:184–189.
43. Schnitt SJ, Connolly JL, Khettry V: Pathologic findings on re-excision of the primary site in breast cancer patients considered for treatment by primary radiation therapy. Cancer 1987; 59:675–681.
44. Bartelink JH, Borger JH, van Dongen JA, Peterse JL: The impact of tumor size and histology on local control after breast-conserving therapy. Radiother Oncol 1988; 11:297–303.
45. Lindley R, Bulman A, Parsons P: Histologic features predictive of an increased risk of early local recurrence after treatment of breast cancer by local tumor excision and radical radiotherapy. Surgery 1989; 105:13–20.
46. Van Limbergen E, Van der Schueren E, Van den Bogaert W, Van Wing J: Local control of operable breast cancer after radiotherapy alone. Eur J Cancer 1990; 26:674–679.
47. Fisher B, Redmond C, Poisson R, Margolese R, et al: Eight-year results of a randomized clinical trial comparing total mastectomy and lumpectomy with or without irradiation in the treatment of breast cancer. N Engl J Med 1989; 320:822–828.
48. Dixon JM, Anderson TJ, Page DL, Lee D, et al: Infiltrating lobular carcinoma of the breast: an evaluation of the incidence and consequence of bilateral disease. Br J Surg 1983; 70:513-516.
49. Baker RR, Kuhajda FP: The clinical management of a normal contralateral breast in patients with lobular breast cancer. Ann Surg 1989; 210:444–448.
50. Kilgore AR: The incidence of cancer in the second breast. JAMA 1921; 77:454–457.
51. Foote FW, Stewart FW: Comparative studies of cancerous versus noncancerous breasts. Ann Surg 1945; 121:6–53;197–222.
52. Fracchia AA, Robinson D, Legaspi A, Greenall MJ, et al: Survival in bilateral breast cancer. Cancer 1985; 55:1414-1421.
51. Chaudary MA, Millis RR, Hoskins EOL, Halder M, et al: Bilateral primary breast cancer: a prospective study of disease incidence. Br J Surg 1984; 71:711–714.
54. Robbins GF, Berg JW: Bilateral primary breast cancers. Cancer 1964; 17:1501–1527.
55. Fisher ER, Fisher B, Sass R, Wickerham L, et al: Pathologic findings from the national surgical adjuvant breast project (Protocol No. 4). XI. Bilateral breast cancer. Cancer 1984; 54:3002–3011.
56. Wanebo HJ, Senofsky GM, Fechner RE: Bilateral breast cancer: risk reduction by contralateral biopsy. Ann Surg 1985; 201:667-677.
57. Fornander T, Cedermark B, Mattsson A, Skoog L, et al: Adjuvant tamoxifen in early breast cancer: occurrence of new primary cancers. Lancet 1989; 21:117–120.
58. Andersson M, Storm HH, Mouridsen HT: Incidence of new primary cancers after adjuvant tamoxifen therapy and radiotherapy for early breast cancer. JNCI 1991; 83:1013–1017.

The Management of Lobular Carcinoma In Situ of the Breast

Paul H. O'Brien

Introduction

The lesion that is now commonly called lobular carcinoma in situ (LCIS) of the breast was first described in 1898.[1] A description that would be acceptable today was "a morbid proliferation of the acinous epithelium which represents the earliest change usually observable by the microscope in carcinoma of the mamma." Other investigators agreed, without naming this particular condition, that it is the very early stage of "acinar carcinoma." In Ewing's classic text, *Neoplastic Disease*, published in 1919, the entity was described and considered to be an atypical proliferation of acinar cells "which was felt to represent" precancerous changes.[2] Again, no name was offered. It was simply felt to be a documentation of a very early stage of breast cancer.

The first extensive histologic description, which also included a specific title, was published in 1941, by Drs. Foote and Stewart. This lesion was described as *lobular carcinoma in situ* and was considered a rare form of mammary cancer.[3] The lesion was felt to be an initial stage of breast cancer, and was, from 1941 to 1969, reported in only 235 patients. However, with further education and attention directed towards this lesion, it was found to be much more frequent than originally suspected.[4] Furthermore, the initial premise that this cancer was inevitably the prologue to invasive breast cancer has not been the destiny of the great majority of patients with LCIS. Indeed, LCIS has taken on an identity of its own, separate and distinct from invasive adenocarcinoma of the breast. Because of its growing incidence and the conflicting therapeutic strategies recommended for the treatment of this entity, we feel the review and discussion of LCIS is warranted.

From: Wise L, Johnson H Jr (eds): *Breast Cancer: Controversies in Management.* Futura Publishing Company, Inc., Armonk, NY, © 1994.

Clinical Patterns and Incidence of Lobular Carcinoma In Situ

Lobular carcinoma in situ of the breast is routinely diagnosed in women between 44 and 48 years of age. This represents a population that is significantly younger by a decade than the population that presents with invasive carcinoma of the breast.[5] Approximately 90% of the women with LCIS are premenopausal. There are no physical findings or symptoms associated with the patient that has LCIS. When the diagnosis is made, it is from a breast biopsy that was indicated by other pathology, which represented either a density, mass, or suspicious shadow on mammography. The incidence of LCIS being found from breast biopsy varies from 1% to 7% of breast biopsy specimens.[6] As with patients with invasive carcinoma of the breast, in patients with LCIS, a familial history of breast cancer is found in 15% to 20%. LCIS has never been found in men because the male breast does not have the lobular elements in which this lesion originates.

The major problem is determining the most appropriate therapeutic strategy once LCIS has been diagnosed.[7] The original premise that this lesion inevitably progressed to invasive cancer mandated mastectomy. The awareness of multicentric foci alerted early investigators to suspect a high incidence of bilaterality of LCIS.[8] This has been reported to be present in 25% to 70% in the opposite grossly normal breast. With this information, it was strongly urged that a blind biopsy of the opposite breast be performed in a mirror-image location of where the first LCIS was identified. Indeed, if LCIS was found, the patient would then be urged to undergo a second mastectomy. Such a strategy clearly protected the patient from the high risk of developing a lethal invasive breast cancer.

However, the exact risk of developing a life-threatening invasive cancer in women with LCIS has been difficult to quantitate. There is a significant variation in the percentage of patients with LCIS who subsequently develop breast cancer, from 6% to 67%. The respective studies generally concur in an incidence rise in the range of 25% to 35%.[9] Furthermore, in those patients with LCIS who subsequently develop invasive cancer, the temporal relationships vary enormously, with more than 50% of the cancers occurring 15 years post LCIS diagnosis and another 38% developing 20 years post LCIS diagnosis.

Pathology of LCIS

As we stated in the beginning, while there were many early investigators aware of this lesion, it was the definitive study by Foote and Stewart that provided the most widely accepted name and a microscopic description that is still considered the "gold standard." The normal lobular anatomy, with an outer layer of myo-epithelial cells and an inner layer of cuboidal cells, undergoes a "sudden and abrupt alteration in lobular cytology." There is disorderly proliferation within the lobular and terminal ducts of a distinctive epithelial cell that is larger than the cells normally lining these structures. This cell contains pale acidophilic cytoplasm, ill-defined borders, and enlarged, rounded uniform nuclei with rare mitoses. While the normal nuclear cytoplasmic ratio is maintained, the epithelial arrangement becomes disorganized. There is progressive displacement of the proliferating cells toward the lumen. This process is confined to the investing borders of the lobular and terminal ducts. The overall glandular picture is maintained. There is a homogenous pattern with an absence of necrosis. The definitive diagnosis of LCIS requires an experienced pathologist.[6] Being able to distinguish LCIS from other benign diseases of the breast is not easy. Borderline proliferative lesions such as atypical lobular hyperplasia (ALH) can easily be confused with LCIS. Indeed, a premise that ALH should be treated very similarly to LCIS in being simply a precursor questions the older concept of rigid distinction being defined between ALH and LCIS.[9]

Controversy over the proper title for this lesion named by Foote and Stewart is of many years' duration. If LCIS represents a true malignant disease that has not reached an invasive stage, the use of *carcinoma* seems justified. If, however, what we call lobular carcinoma in situ is simply a benign lesion that becomes malignant once invasion occurs, then possibly Haagensen's term, *lobular neoplasia* would be justified. The reason for selecting the more benign-appearing lobular neoplasia was to counter what was felt to be inappropriate aggressive therapy as we have outlined earlier.[10] The invasive cancers that do develop in patients with LCIS differ from those seen in patients without LCIS. There is a much higher incidence of invasive lobular carcinoma, approximately 35% to 50% of cancers found in patients with LCIS, in contrast to an incidence of no more than 5% to 10% incidence in patients who have not been diagnosed with LCIS.[8] Also, we have the frequent presence of intraductal carcinoma or ductal carcinoma in situ in the breast that has LCIS. This has been estimated to be found in 60% to 70% of the patients carrying a diagnosis of LCIS.[11,12]

The Role of Mammography

Mammography has certainly shown its ability to detect occult malignant disease from 1 to 3 years before such an occult malignant disease becomes palpable. The ability of mammography to specifically identify LCIS is very limited, however, because there are no clinical signs or symptoms associated with LCIS, and there are no diagnostic links and patterns for LCIS. There are studies in which patients with documented LCIS had obtained mammograms prior to biopsy. On review of the mammograms, 50% of the mammograms showed no roetgenographic findings whatsoever.[13] Mammography does, however, provide us with a very important tool for detecting early cancer in this high-risk group of females. Indeed, as Lewison observed in 1965, "mammography may very well hold the key to the dilemma of the treatment of LCIS."[14] In order to have a coherent treatment strategy for LCIS, one must understand its high degree of multicentricity within the diagnosed breast, the high incidence of bilaterality, and the previously mentioned risk factors of developing a future invasive carcinoma. This author believes the multicentricity of LCIS precludes the success of a subcutaneous mastectomy as definitive treatment of this condition. The obvious advantages would be the retention of the nipple and its sensation. However, the residue of breast tissue left behind, particularly under the nipple, makes this procedure questionable. The most commonly recommended approaches for the management of LCIS are:

1. Mastectomy with contralateral biopsy. This is often a mirror-image biopsy on the opposite breast.

2. Bilateral mastectomy, wherein the patient has been completely protected from subsequent development of breast cancer.

3. No further surgical treatment beyond a diagnostic biopsy, but with very careful, lifelong follow-up study of both breasts.

The more aggressive surgical approach enjoyed great popularity in the 50s and 60s. However, during the 70s, many studies encouraged a more conservative approach. The bilaterality of the disease became more widely understood and documented. The patient's preference post education becomes a deciding factor. The paradox of recommending more extensive surgery for LCIS than was now known to be statistically justified for more aggressive, invasive lesions supported a conservative strategy.[9,10,15]

Always, the pivotal decision about therapy for LCIS has to include, if possible, patient participation. It may well be that a subset of the population with LCIS is not interested in having mammograms every 9 months, seeing a physician for an examination every 6 months, and undergoing self-examination every month. They simply would rather undergo bilateral mastectomy with or without reconstruction. I consider this to be an acceptable therapeutic strategy, assuming the patient's educated approval.

References

1. Shield AM: A Clinical Treatise on Disease of the Breast. Macmillan and Co., Ltd., London, p 3, 1898.
2. Ewing J: Neoplastic Disease. First ed. W.B. Saunders, Philadelphia, 1919.
3. Foote FW, Stewart FW: Lobular carcinoma in situ: a rare form of mammary cancer. Am J Pathol 1941; 17:491–495.
4. Warner NE: Lobular carcinoma of the breast. Cancer 1969; 23:840–846.
5. Newman W: Lobular carcinoma of the female breast: report of 73 cases. Am Surg 1966; 164(2):305–315.
6. Schwartz GF, Feig SA, Rosenberg AL, et al: Staging and treatment of clinically occult breast cancer. Cancer 1984; 53:1379–1384.
7. Farrow JH: Current concepts in the detection and treatment of the earliest of early breast cancers. Cancer 1970; 25:468–477.
8. McDivitt RW, Hutter RVP, Foote FW: In situ lobular carcinoma: a prospective follow-up study indicating cumulative patient risks. JAMA 1967; 201:96–100.
9. Hutter RVP: The management of patients with lobular carcinoma in situ of the breast. Cancer 1984; 53:798–802.
10. Gump FE: Premalignant diseases of the breast. Surg Clin North Am 1984; 64:1051–1059.

11. Fisher ER, Fisher B: Lobular carcinoma of the breast: an overview. Ann Surg 1977; 195:377–385.
12. Rosen PP: Lobular carcinoma in situ and intraductal carcinoma of the breast. Monogr Pathol 1984; 25:59–105.
13. Hutter RVP, Snyder RE, Lucas JC, et al: Clinical and pathologic correlation with mammographic findings in lobular carcinoma in situ. Cancer 1969; 23:826–839.
14. Lewison EF: Lobular carcinoma in situ of the breast. Ann Surg 1965; 31:787–789.
15. Powers RW, O'Brien PH, Kreutner A: Lobular carcinoma in situ. J Surg Oncol 1980; 13:269–273.

20

Wide Local Excision is Adequate Treatment for Microscopic Ductal Carcinoma In Situ

Frank E. Gump

Introduction

Widespread application of screening mammography has resulted in a dramatic increase in in-situ breast cancers. Physicians are under tremendous pressure to reward patients for such an early diagnosis, and for most women the reward would be keeping their breasts. Can this be done without compromising the more important reward: survival? Recent evidence suggests that this is possible, but the issue is complex and a careful definition of terms is necessary.

Intraductal Carcinoma in Situ

Intraductal carcinoma in situ (DCIS) has been reevaluated since it became associated with microcalcifications seen on mammography. It is necessary to carefully define this lesion as a first step in any defense of wide excision. Intraductal carcinoma existed long before mammography because the presenting symptom was a mass in the breast.[1] It was categorized as intraductal because the cancer was to a large extent contained within the ducts on histologic examination. The other intraductal presentation was purely microscopic disease that constituted an incidental finding in association with excision of a benign tumor, examination of "normal" breast tissue removed in conjunction with reduction mammoplasty or on retrospective slide reviews.[2-4] Mammographic detection of DCIS came later and constitutes yet another category of intraductal disease.

Patients that present with a mass, nipple discharge, or Paget's disease are

From: Wise L, Johnson H Jr (eds): *Breast Cancer: Controversies in Management.* Futura Publishing Company, Inc., Armonk, NY, © 1994.

not at issue in this discussion even if the pathologist sees no evidence of invasion. I have called this *gross*, as opposed to microscopic, DCIS, and such patients behave very much like patients with invasive cancer.[5]

Microscopic DCIS, on the other hand, can be defined simply as tissue that looks like normal breast tissue to the surgeon doing the biopsy, but when the slides come out, the pathologist reports DCIS. This category includes both DCIS as an *incidental finding* and DCIS diagnosed following needle localization biopsy for *mammographic microcalcifications*. A further distinction is also worth noting. Microscopic DCIS can be subdivided according to its histologic appearance. When DCIS appears as an incidental finding it presents a cribriform or papillary pattern. When the diagnosis is made following biopsy of mammographic microcalcifications, the appearance of the ducts is altered and central necrosis is usually a prominent feature. This has also been described as the comedo form of DCIS but I would prefer central necrosis since "comedo" is a term derived from the toothpaste-like material that oozes from the cut surface of the intraductal cancer that forms a mass. In other words, comedo suggests an abnormality that can be seen without the aid of a microscope (gross disease) as opposed to central necrosis which is a microscopic finding.

To summarize, this discussion of wide excision for DCIS will be restricted to microscopic in-situ disease. The histologic pattern, papillary, cribriform or ducts with central necrosis, is also important in any discussion of wide excision and will be considered in the next section.

Multifocal Disease or Multicentricity

Efforts to preserve breast tissue have focused attention on the extent and distribution of cancer in the breast. The concept of multicentricity was the rationale for treatment of the entire breast whenever cancer was diagnosed in any quadrant. However, recent studies suggest that multicentricity in the sense of random distribution of cancer cells throughout the breast does not exist.[6,7] Instead, there is a geographic relationship of secondary cancer foci to the index lesion with the result that the term "multicentric" has been replaced by "multifocal." This is not simply a matter of semantics since a geographic relationship implies that a proper match between the lesion and the size of the circle selected to remove it will rid the patient of the cancer without resort to mastectomy or radiation.

Previous studies on multicentricity have focused on invasive cancers but much of this information is relevant for in-situ lesions as well. The first problem is the disparity in the reported incidence of multifocal deposits with figures that vary from 9% to 75%.[8] A number of factors are responsible but the technique used to examine the breast is most important. At one end of the spectrum are whole mount studies where sections of the entire breast are made into large slides. This is a laborious procedure and it is not surprising that only a limited number of specimens have been studied in this fashion.[9] Random sampling of four quadrants represents the opposite extreme and studies utilizing this approach will show the lowest rates of multifocal disease.[10] Occupying an intermediate position are studies that utilize mammography of breast slices (Egan's method) to identify suspicious areas for microscopic study.[11] The incidence of multifocal disease will reflect the method of examination but it also depends on how the pathologist chooses to characterize proliferative lesions. The criteria for differentiating between ductal hyperplasia and atypia on the one hand and carcinoma in situ on the other are not always clear cut. The 75% figure recorded by Gallagher and Martin included proliferative lesions that fell short of DCIS so their high figure for multifocality becomes understandable.[12] One of the most important distinctions made by the pathologist relates to lobular carcinoma in situ (LCIS). This lesion continues to provoke controversy but most oncologists now feel that it should be regarded as a marker of increased risk rather than a precancerous lesion.[13] The distinction is important since inclusion of LCIS as cancer will not only increase the incidence of multifocal disease but will affect reports regarding the geographic distribution of cancer cells in the breast. LCIS is widely distributed in both breasts and does indeed constitute random distribution. Any thought that wide excision has a role in the treatment of LCIS would be unrealistic given this pattern of distribution.

DCIS, on the other hand, is not a bilateral process, nor is its distribution in the breast random. The best evidence to support this statement comes from two recent studies, one of which was limited to invasive cancers[7] while the other included both invasive and in-situ lesions.[6] The latter study was reported by Holland who broke new ground in that he documented geographic spread from the primary tumor. Egan's method was utilized as the starting point but was combined with detailed measurements so that a topographic diagram would be created. Thirty-two of Holland's patients were intraductal. It is important to note that 11 of the patients had palpable tumors, but 21 were diagnosed as the result of mammographic microcalcifications. These 21 patients are relevant to the present discussion since they represent microscopic DCIS and they show the lesion to be geographically localized in the breast. While Holland's work makes it clear that local excision has a rational basis, the large area of involvement reported in his paper can present a technical problem for the surgeon. Holland went on to divide his DCIS patients into papillary-cribriform and "comedo," stating that there was reasonably good correlation between mammographic lesion and size on his pathological topographic representation for the latter but not for the former. This distinction plays a role in the debate about wide excision in two ways. First of all, it helps in patient selection for excision and secondly it relates to the other issue in the debate: will DCIS inevitably progress to invasive cancer? If it routinely does, the pressure on the surgeon to achieve complete excision is obviously greater.

Natural History of DCIS

Much of the information regarding the progression of DCIS comes from two retrospective studies. It is of more than passing interest that neither study was designed to look at DCIS. Dr. Rosen was interested in lobular carcinoma in situ

(LCIS) and for that reason reviewed all the benign breast biopsies in the Memorial Hospital file between 1940 and 1950.[2] He found approximately 100 patients with LCIS but was alert enough to pick up 25 patients with DCIS that had been overlooked at the time of the original biopsy. Since the original tissue was read as benign, no treatment had been instituted. Dr. Page also carried out an extensive review of benign biopsies, but his interest was in features of benign disease that might increase the risk of breast cancer in the future.[3] He found 28 patients with DCIS that had been initially overlooked. Long-term follow-up information was available for most of the patients and it was clear that the majority did not develop invasive cancers during this time period. Interpretation of these results requires a closer look at the histology of the DCIS lesions that had been previously overlooked. All of the 25 patients in Dr. Rosen's series had papillary DCIS, while 25 of the 28 lesions reported by Dr. Page also had this histologic pattern. This is an important point since the boundary between benign proliferative lesions with or without atypia and papillary DCIS is not always clear cut. Once the ductal cells have progressed to filling the ducts—especially if they are dividing rapidly enough to create a central zone of necrosis, they are out of the gray area and into the cancer side of the boundary.[14] That is why central necrosis is an important finding, and it is worth noting that no lesions of this sort were overlooked by the original pathologists. When microcalcifications are associated with DCIS, they are usually in the area of central necrosis. When we reviewed the pathology on 60 consecutive DCIS patients biopsied for microcalcifications, we found that 55 had central necrosis while there were only four patients with papillary lesions. This preponderance of patients with central necrosis has not always been confirmed.[15,16] For example, Holland's report of 85 DCIS patients reported 50 with central necrosis and 32 that were classified as micropapillary.[16] However, 14 of the 32 actually also had central necrosis; of the 18 pure micropapillary lesions, 15 had no calcifications. The obvious question would be: how were they detected on mammography if there was no calcium? The answer is provided in the article since 30 of the 85 were picked up on physical exam because of the presence of a mass.

If we restrict the discussion to microscopic DCIS detected mammographically as stated previously, it is clear that we are dealing with DCIS that has central necrosis. For that reason, the uncertain natural history of DCIS as an overlooked incidental finding is not the issue. Since the vast majority of DCIS patients seen at the present time are diagnosed because of an abnormal mammogram (microcalcifications), this is the group that we would like to treat by wide excision.

Wide Excision as an Option for DCIS

The foregoing discussion is essential in order to provide a rational basis for wide excision. First of all, the malignant potential of DCIS lesions picked up mammographically must be stressed. These lesions will show central necrosis, possibly not in every section, but as a rule this is the histologic pattern in sections showing the calcifications. The two often quoted retrospective studies[2,3] deal with DCIS as an initially overlooked incidental finding. The uncertain natural history of papillary DCIS will always be a problem, but is not relevant when patients present with central necrosis. Such patients require excision of the lesion. Holland's studies and the topography information provided make it clear that there is a geographic relationship between the cancer and the area of microcalcifications that led to detection. His studies also illustrate the problem facing oncologists and patients interested in breast preservation. While these intraductal lesions are not multicentric (randomly distributed throughout the breast), they may occupy such an extensive area that total mastectomy is necessary.

There are two general approaches to breast preservation for DCIS. The traditional approach is designed to ensure complete removal of the lesion, which implies patient selection and attention to margins.[17] This approach was applied to both arms of the National Surgical Adjuvant Breast Project (NSABP) B-17 protocol but one arm also received postoperative radiation treatment. Provided the initial surgery was properly carried out, as judged by clear margins and no remaining calcification on postoperative mammography, it is not clear if there was any residual cancer to be radiated. Although no results are available at this time, I would not expect to see a difference between the two groups. Numerous patients were considered ineligible for B-17 because there was uncertainty regarding residual disease. This led to a new protocol, B-24, designed to evaluate wide excision in this group of patients. This protocol incorporates a different concept. It accepts residual disease and asks whether it will progress to invasive cancer when subjected to radiation and tamoxifen. This formulation is based on the old concept of multicentricity as discussed previously but to my mind it is not relevant for DCIS associated with microcalcifications. The data from this new protocol, when available, will certainly provide important information, but at the present time I would favor wide excision based on the results of recent studies that suggest a geographically localized lesion.

Technical Considerations

The foregoing makes it clear that wide excision constitutes definitive treatment for some but not all patients with DCIS. Since the discussion is limited to DCIS picked up by mammographic microcalcifications, the mammogram is the starting point in patient selection. A single cluster or area of suspicious microcalcification would be necessary since widespread calcifications are not well suited to wide excision. Secondly, the area of microcalcifications has to be small. Lagios places a limit of 25 mm and I would agree that this would be the upper limit.[15] The first step is needle localization and biopsy since approximately 70% to 80% of microcalcifications judged to need biopsy are benign.[18,19] Once the diagnosis of cancer is made, wide excision is the next step. If the specimen X-ray documents complete removal of the suspicious area of calcifications, it does not insure that there is no more DCIS in the breast. While the lesion has a geographic relationship to the area of calcification, it is inevitably more extensive than the calcifications that led to the diagnosis. The extent of the resection needed to encompass the lesion is obviously the critical issue. Since the "lesion" is microscopic, the surgeon is guided by the previous biopsy cavity which should be excised with a 1–2 cm margin. At times sections through this specimen will show no further DCIS, suggesting that the initial needle-guided biopsy done for diagnosis removed the disease. If DCIS is found in the wide excision, a more complicated situation exists. Clear margins sound nice but there are many artifacts that cloud the issue. I have found the quantity of DCIS judged by the number of involved ducts to be a valuable criterion and this has also been noted by others.[20] The techniques used to document complete excision will vary from surgeon to surgeon and some patients will become ineligible along the way, necessitating mastectomy or radiation. There is no question that we need better techniques for assessing the extent and location of DCIS lesions in the breast. Until these become available, we must rely on microscopic examination of resected tissue and postoperative mammography to search for residual calcifications. Even then there is no absolute certainty regarding the remaining breast tissue. The surgeon's goal is to utilize patient selection and surgical excision so that the likelihood of cancer in the remaining breast is on a par with the contralateral breast.

Summary

Evidence has been presented that DCIS diagnosed following needle-guided biopsy for microcalcifications will show central necrosis, and progression to invasive cancer would be expected. Under these circumstances, complete excision of the lesion is mandatory. Recent studies of the extent and distribution of cancer in the breast show DCIS to be a localized process amenable to wide excision. Selection of patients and documentation of the completeness of the excision are critical in the successful application of this form of treatment.

References

1. Haagensen CD: Diseases of the Breast. WB Saunders, Philadelphia, pp 782–789, 1986.
2. Betsil WL, Rosen PP, Lieberman PH: Intraductal carcinoma: long-term follow-up after treatment by biopsy alone. JAMA 1978; 239:1863–1867.
3. Page DL, Dupont WD, Rogers LW: Intraductal carcinoma of the breast: follow-up after biopsy only. Cancer 1982; 49:751–758.
4. Ringberg A, Palmer B, Linell F: The contralateral breast at reconstructive surgery after breast cancer operation: a histological study. Breast Cancer Res Treat 1982; 2:151–161.
5. Gump FE: In situ cancers. In: Harris JR, Hellman S, Henderson IC (eds). Breast Diseases. JB Lippincott, Philadelphia, pp 359–368, 1987.
6. Holland R, Solke HJ, Veling M: Histologic multifocality of Tis, T1–2 breast carcinomas. Cancer 1985; 56;979–990.
7. Gump FE, Shikora S, Habif DV: The extent and distribution of cancer in breasts with palpable primary tumors. Ann Surg 1986; 204:384–390.

8. Lagios MD, Westdahl PR, Rose MR: The concept and implications of multicentricity in breast carcinoma. In: Sommers SG, Rosen PP (eds). Pathology Annual. Appleton Century Crofts, New York, pp 83–102, 1981.

9. Nielson M, Jensen J, Anderson J: Precancerous and cancerous breast lesions during lifetime and at autopsy. Cancer 1984; 54:612–615.

10. Fisher ER, Gregario R, Redmond C: Pathologic findings from the National Surgical Adjuvant Breast Project. Cancer 1975; 35:247–254.

11. Egan RL, McSweeney MB: Multricentric breast carcinoma. In: Brunner S (ed). Recent Results in Breast Cancer Research. Springer Verlag, Berlin, pp 28–35, 1984.

12. Gallagher IS, Martin JE: The study of mammary carcinoma by mammography and whole organ sectioning. Cancer 1969; 23:855–873.

13. Gump FE: Lobular carcinoma in situ. Surg Clin NA 1990; 70:873–884.

14. Gump FE, Jicha D, Ozzello L: Ductal carcinoma in situ (DCIS): a revised concept. Surgery 1987; 102:790–795.

15. Lagios MD: Duct carcinoma in situ: pathology and treatment. Surg Clin NA 1990; 70:853–871.

16. Holland R, Hendriks JHCL, Verbeek ALM: Extent, distribution and mammographic histological correlations of breast ductal carcinoma in situ. Lancet 1990; 335:519–522.

17. Schnitt SJ, Silen W, Sadowsky NL: Ductal carcinoma in situ (intraductal carcinoma of the breast). N Engl J Med 1988; 318:898–903.

18. Lanyi M: Microcalcifications in the breast: a blessing or a curse. Diagn Imag Clin Med 1985; 54:126–145.

19. Citoler P: Microcalcifications of the breast. In: Grundmann E, Beck L. Early Diagnosis of Breast Cancer. Gustav Fischer, Stuttgart, 1978.

20. Patchefsky AS, Schwartz GF, Finklestein SD: Heterogeneity of intraductal carcinoma of the breast. Cancer 1989; 63:731-741.

21

Is Wide Local Excision Adequate Treatment for Ductal Carcinoma In Situ?

Gordon Francis Schwartz

Introduction

How easy it would make the practice of medicine if we could easily type a few observations into a computer and await precise instructions for care, based upon an audit and analysis of these observations, however complicated we make the algorithm. (Perhaps fortunately for those of us who still take pride in our clinical skills, that millennium has not yet arrived.) Certainly the entity that we designate by a hodgepodge of names, including DCIS, intraductal, noninvasive, noninfiltrating ductal carcinoma, and in-situ ductal carcinoma, might benefit from such an inflexible system, since there is almost no more currently controversial diagnosis in the breast cancer spectrum. Admittedly, the options of therapy are few—the treatment of the breast and attention to the axilla—but the differences between these treatments is formidable to the patients who must make these decisions and live with them.

The diagnosis of DCIS (ductal carcinoma in situ) (our choice of term, only because it is more easily spoken and written) has become commonplace within the past few years, as the ubiquitous use of mammography for screening asymptomatic women has been embraced as a major advance in the discovery of earlier malignancies, and as notable improvements in mammographic technique have allowed the detection of smaller and smaller areas of subtle change within the breast.

As implied by the name, DCIS seems to arise within the ducts of the breast that become greatly dilated as the process evolves. In the usual scenario, when necrosis occurs within the lumina of the ducts, the precipitation of radiographi-

From: Wise L, Johnson H Jr (eds): *Breast Cancer: Controversies in Management.* Futura Publishing Company, Inc., Armonk, NY, © 1994.

231

cally opaque inorganic material, usually containing calcium, leads to the mammographic discovery of these areas of intraductal disease as areas of clustered calcifications. According to tradition, if the process continues without detection and interference, the involved ducts coalesce into a mass, growing in volume until finally discovered by the patient or physician as a palpable mass. At some time in this process, the formerly intraductal, cytologically malignant but biologically noninvasive cells penetrate through the basement membrane of the ducts, and the disease becomes invasive, with all of the implications of any invasive carcinoma.

Within the past generation, the inevitable progression of DCIS to invasive carcinoma has been challenged. Whether there are circumstances such that the identification of DCIS at some early stage in its natural history will obviate the obligatory treatment of the entire breast and/or axilla with a minimum risk to the patient of developing a subsequent life-threatening cancer has become a topic of great debate. If, indeed, DCIS is not always accompanied by invasion and/or does not necessarily progress to this stage, to prescribe lesser treatment for DCIS than for invasive carcinoma implies an obligation to recognize the time at which the identification and excision of DCIS might be treatment enough. This maneuver, however, also implies that the detection and eradication of DCIS at one location satisfies the possibility that the site detected was no greater in significance than another location within the same breast that might harbor the same or even more aggressive disease, as yet undetected.

Controversy about the treatment of DCIS probably has its most significant origins in terms of the definitions of the disease itself. Initially, Haagensen and others were careful to separate the term *intraductal* from the term *noninfiltrating*.[1] The terms were not then considered synonyms! Those cases of intraductal carcinoma described by Haagensen were also palpable lesions, and many (29%) were accompanied by metastasis to axillary lymph nodes.[2] Although many similar tumors may fail to exhibit areas of invasion when examined under light microscopy, it is probably preferable to comment that invasion may not have been seen "in the sections studied." As the mammographic detection of smaller masses, then areas of nonpalpable calcifications, became more common as radiographic techniques improved, these distinctions became blurred and, over time, the terms *noninvasive, intraductal, noninfiltrating,* and *DCIS* have become interchangeable; as currently used, they imply the absence of invasive carcinoma. The separation of *clinical* from *subclinical* DCIS to permit a more careful comparison of equivalent diseases was first suggested by Gump et al., and their distinction also has great implications for treatment.[3] DCIS presenting as a palpable mass, as nipple erosion (Paget's carcinoma), and as nipple discharge, is not the same as DCIS presenting as an area of calcification on a screening mammogram or discovered as an incidental finding in a specimen of breast tissue removed for another reason.

In any discussion about treatment, therefore, it is first appropriate to define the disease. Inasmuch as staging systems for breast cancer have not yet addressed this issue, DCIS is considered stage 0, Tis, so that the subdivision of DCIS into categories for consideration is somewhat arbitrary.[4] It is easier to discuss *clinical* DCIS, that producing palpable mass, nipple erosion, or nipple discharge, from the treatment viewpoint than *subclinical* DCIS detected by mammography or as an incidental finding. If, as questioned previously, there are patients in whom DCIS is not an obligate precursor of invasive cancer, we have not considered those with clinical DCIS among that group. Currently, we believe that, almost without exception, until data are available that refute this recommendation, patients with clinical DCIS should continue to undergo treatment that includes the entire breast and usually the axilla.

The term, *palpable DCIS* is virtually an oxymoron. As a palpable mass, a carcinoma may be largely intraductal, but it should not be considered noninvasive. As already noted, the appropriate designation should probably be "not invasive in the sections studied." These allegedly intraductal but palpable lesions are often accompanied by invasion, even when not seen, and the appropriate treatment addresses both the breast and the axilla. Whether irradiation is an alternative to mastectomy is another contentious point in the contemporary literature, but, except for the likelihood of recurrence in the same breast that may occur after irradiation, with careful follow-up, the long-term survival for carefully selected patients should be similar.[5] The importance of an extensive intraductal component (EIC) would be mitigated, if it is at all significant, by careful attention to wound margins at the time of local excision. Carefully excising the wound margins and base separately and affixing small metallic clips to these sites for subsequent radiographic localization of this area aids the radiotherapist and makes subsequent mammography easier to interpret.

Some of these (predominantly intraductal) lesions can achieve considerable size, i.e., more than a 5-cm diameter, and can be accompanied by clinically involved axillary nodes. They are characterized by their firmness, their fairly well-delimited margins, and an abundance of malignant-appearing calcifications on mammography. These large lesions are often not candidates for treatment by irradiation because of the difficulty of excising all of the calcifications that permeate the ducts contiguous to and even at great distance from the mass itself. The palpable masses of DCIS that radiotherapists currently covet remain small ones, amenable to wide local excision with clear surgical margins.

Paget's carcinoma, presenting as a nipple erosion, is a form of breast carcinoma that grows initially within the milk sinuses of the nipple and extends within the ducts beneath the nipple in an apparently intraductal but not necessarily in-situ manner. The development of the disease may be multicentric within the breast, and patients with Paget's disease may have axillary node metastasis, although uncommonly. Tempting as it may be to perform less aggressive surgical procedures, mastectomy with axillary dissection remains the treatment of choice except in unusual situations.

The mammograms in Paget's disease may be helpful in defining the retroareolar spread of disease. Not well described in the literature, it has been our observation that calcifications in a branching distribution in the retroareolar area may help outline the intraductal spread of Paget's disease, proving its widespread character and the need for mastectomy. Although it is not necessarily true that the absence of retroareolar calcifications proves a more limited distribution of disease, when the calcifications are seen to be distributed in this pattern, the failure of any procedure that does not treat the entire breast can be appreciated. Nevertheless, we have treated several women with Paget's carcinoma by irradiation only, not even excising the nipple and areolar complex, but this choice is tenable only when the biopsy of the nipple indicates what we believe is a relatively confined distribution of disease. These several patients have also been quite vocal and unequivocal in their desire to retain their breasts. Despite this limited success with what should be considered less-than-adequate treatment, Paget's carcinoma should be considered as *clinical* DCIS, at the very least. Untreated, Paget's carcinoma is inevitably progressive and fatal.

Patients presenting with spontaneous nipple discharge that proves to be due to intraductal carcinoma are tempting candidates for treatment by something less than mastectomy. The argument is often made that, since the mammograms in these patients rarely show evidence of mass or calcifications, and the usual microscopic appearance of the malignant cells is less rather than more aggressive, why not consider that these patients within the group be followed by local excision and surveillance alone? Indeed, that had been our initial suggestion as we began to search for patients with DCIS who might be candidates for local excision alone.

After the first two patients so treated had recurrences relatively promptly, and we reviewed the mastectomy specimens in other patients with this same presentation, we became more convinced that nipple discharge as the first sign of DCIS implies an uncertain intraductal and usually multicentric distribution peripherally, and, at least in the traditional sense, it is impossible to perform a "lumpectomy" in these patients that conclusively circumscribes the macroscopic disease. Irradiation as an alternative to mastectomy is not usually suitable; there is no specific site to target, and if one believes that the macroscopic extent of the disease must be excised prior to irradiation, the nipple and areola must be part of the tissue sacrificed.

Treatment of the axilla in patients with clinical DCIS detected as nipple discharge is more controversial than the same consideration in patients with intraductal carcinoma detected as Paget's disease or as a palpable mass. If frank invasion is present, treatment includes the same attention to the axilla as for any other invasive cancer. When invasion is questioned, even if termed *focal* or *microinvasion*, at least a level I dissection is a reasonable recommendation.

It is more difficult to justify treatment of the entire axilla when the microscopic sections fail to detect any question of invasion whatsoever. However, most of these patients are currently treated by mastectomy, and a *total* mastectomy includes the removal of the axillary prolongation (tail of Spence) of the breast. Thus, the lowermost axillary lymph nodes, those in what would be called by anatomists the external mammary group, and some of those in the central or scapular group of the level I nodes, which are impossible to separate from the axillary tail tissue, are included within the specimen.

It adds little morbidity or time to the operative procedure to dissect the axillary contents at level I completely and anatomically, from the point at which the axillary vein crosses the white tendon of the latissimus dorsi muscle, along the axillary vein medially to the lateral border of the pectoralis minor muscle, the medial border of level I. When addressing frankly invasive breast cancer, the likelihood of overlooking involved nodes at levels II or III is about 10% if only level I is dissected.[6] Because the likelihood of axillary metastasis in these carefully selected patients is itself very small, the additional probability of missing a "skip" metastasis to levels II or III if level I is negative is remote.

The current controversy, therefore, with respect to DCIS, concerns the patients who have *subclinical* disease, that which is detected by mammography within areas of clustered calcifications or as an incidental finding when biopsy is performed for another reason, whether palpable or not. In the latter cases, the detection of DCIS is truly serendipitous.

Although it is accepted that many patients with DCIS, if untreated, do not subsequently develop invasive carcinoma of the same breast, the ability to distinguish which women will be spared has eluded us.[7] The few reports that discuss the implied natural history of this disease in patients untreated because the diagnosis was initially overlooked fail to demonstrate that even a simple majority of these patients progressed to invasive carcinoma. Nevertheless, until recently, mastectomy had been the overwhelming choice of treatment for this disease and, currently, the generally accepted choice is either mastectomy or irradiation, depending upon the availability and influence of radiation therapists on local traditions.

In our own practice, needle-guided biopsy for mammographically detected lesions was initiated in 1973 and, until 1978, mastectomy was the customary "reward" for those patients who were diligent enough to have their "cancers" (DCIS) detected in such an "early" stage. As the exponential increase in patients with subclinical DCIS was noted in response to technical improvements in mammograms and a greater acceptance of screening mammography by the medical profession as well as the public, questions relating to the extent of disease within the breast, the possibility of occult invasion, and the likelihood of axillary metastasis began to be addressed. In 1975, Lagios et al. began to offer selected patients with DCIS the possibility of local excision only—neither mastectomy nor irradiation.[8] Their studies of these women have been the most elegant, and their follow-up has been the longest. Thus far, 12.6% of their patients have developed local recurrence, either further DCIS or invasive duct carcinoma, after a median follow-up of 68 months.[9]

Independently influenced by similar observations and in response to patients' greater participation in their own health care, in 1978 we began to offer highly selected patients the same option—local excision alone—with the caveat that perhaps as many as 30% to 40% (our initial estimates, subsequently revised downward) of patients so treated would develop a subsequent invasive carcinoma of the same breast. Having championed the surveillance option for patients with lobular carcinoma in situ (LCIS or lobular neoplasia) from the inception, extrapolation from LCIS to DCIS was understandable if not accurate. The observations of Haagensen about LCIS afforded a more firm commitment to the surveillance option for LCIS,[10] but at the time this study was initiated, there was only a smattering of information available about patients with DCIS treated by local excision alone. Since that time, other reports have been published, but they have almost invariably addressed DCIS generically, without separating those we consider subclinical from the others. Thus, it is almost impossible to glean meaningful information about the treatment of subclinical DCIS from the extant literature. In addition to the 79 patients reported by Lagios, however, there have been both British and Swedish reports of patients with *subclinical* DCIS, detected by mammographic screening, treated by excision and surveillance alone.[11,12] The group of patients reported by Carpenter et al. from Charing Cross Hospital in London includes 28 women treated by excision alone, four women (14%) having subsequent local recurrence with a mean follow-up of about 3 years. The group of women reported by Arnesson from the University Hospital of Linköping, Sweden, includes 38 treated by local excision alone. After a mean follow-up of 60 months, five patients (13%) had recurrence.

We have previously reported our own limited experience with subclinical DCIS treated by local excision and surveillance in 75 breasts (73 women), followed for a mean of 39 months.[13] In this group of 75 breasts, recurrence occurred in nine, or 12%, between 8 and 85 months after the initial diagnosis. Of the initial group, however, two patients developed subsequent invasive cancer of the same breast; the others developed only further DCIS at the same site. Overall recurrence was comparable in frequency to that reported by Lagios, and we differ only in the likelihood of an invasive recurrence. Half of the recurrences in his series were invasive. Arnesson observed 40% (2/5) invasive recurrence, and Carpenter noted DCIS only in the four patients who developed recurrence after local excision alone. None of these studies, our own, those of Lagios, or the two European series, includes enough patients to speak authoritatively about the subsequent danger of developing "worse," i.e., invasive, cancer after initial treatment for DCIS. Certainly this will be an important observation, since, if careful surveillance will detect recurrence while it is yet noninvasive, patients may be more enthusiastic about this alternative to mastectomy or irradiation, since this implies that recurrence (as DCIS only) does not endanger the patient. However, if a sizeable segment of the group treated by surveillance alone develops invasive carcinoma as the first sign of recurrence, there will be a small fraction of this group who will undoubtedly succumb to this disease, and for those women, however few, the price of surveillance was too high.

Therefore, the challenge to those of us who would advocate local excision and surveillance as an option for those women whose subclinical DCIS is detected by screening mammography is to define with precision the ultimate risk of developing invasive cancer, not only the likelihood that this unfortunate event might occur, but also within what period of time. Additionally, we must try to determine whether specific subsets of patients with DCIS of various histologies are more likely than others to develop recurrence.

Most investigators divide DCIS into several separate subsets; these usually include comedo, cribriform, solid, papillary, and micropapillary types, and each has distinctive morphological features. Attempts to correlate cytometric and histologic characteristics of these several varieties of DCIS have been undertaken, and the comedo type is considered the most biologically aggressive.[14]

Our own comparisons of the findings within biopsies and those within subsequent mastectomy specimens (when we used to treat all patients with DCIS this way) have helped to define the risks of multicentricity and microinvasion associated with these various subsets of subclinical DCIS.[15,16] For example, the incidental finding of DCIS in a specimen of tissue removed for another reason has not been associated with either microinvasion or multicentricity, and no patient with incidental DCIS treated by excision and surveillance has yet developed recurrence. When we reviewed our mastectomy specimens, we also noted the tendency for the comedo type of DCIS to be more likely accompanied by microinvasion and/or multicentricity. Similarly, although there was no maximum or minimum number of involved ducts that guaranteed the presence or absence of multicentricity or microinvasion, there was a trend, as might be expected, that the greater the volume of DCIS, the more likely there was to be accompanying microinvasion and/or multicentricity.

This analysis of microinvasion and multicentricity in mastectomy specimens has not yet been related to clinical observations of recurrence in similar patients treated by excision and surveillance. One would expect a greater incidence of recurrence in the patients with the comedo type of DCIS than the other histologic categories if recurrence were related directly to these cytologic and cytodynamic traits. Although this premise has not been completely validated, in our own series of patients treated by excision alone, eight of the nine patients who have had recurrences had comedo type DCIS as the initial finding.

The morphology and nuclear grade of the malignant cells and the degree of intraductal necrosis have also been considered features that may predict local recurrence, but these associations have not been fully substantiated. Perhaps the current division of DCIS into the five subsets named is not precise enough. Because the vast majority of DCIS is detected within clustered calcifications, and intraductal cellular necrosis leading to calcification is the hallmark of detection of these lesions, it is not surprising that the diagnosis of comedo carcinoma is the most common. Pathologists may differ in the appreciation of intraductal necrosis that provokes the term *comedo* as a modifier. Perhaps the implication of intraductal necrosis needs to be reconsidered. All of these lesions that were formerly defined as the comedo type of DCIS may need tc be reclassified, based upon other attributes, possibly biological (cytometric) as well as morphological.

For the time being, a pragmatic approach should be adopted to allow the accrual of patients into clinical trials that employ local excision only with careful, lifetime surveillance, as an alternative to mastectomy or irradiation, for highly selected patients with subclinical DCIS. Our own approach is quite similar to that advocated by Lagios.[7] At the time of needle-guided biopsy, since no treatment plans depend upon them, frozen sections of excised tissue are not performed. All of the fresh tissue is examined by the surgical pathologist. We do differ with Lagios in our perception of the importance of inking surgical margins. The careful excision of a small area of calcifications is more difficult than a breast biopsy performed for a palpable lesion, especially if the surgeon wishes to spare a small breast from a significant cosmetic deformity. Not infrequently, it may require a second specimen to insure that the mammographic abnormality has been removed.

Since the majority of needle-guided biopsies still prove to be for benign disease (about 70% within our own experience of about 3,000 such biopsies since 1973), the pathologist's enthusiasm for the appropriately defined specimen must be tempered by the surgeon's and the patient's concern about the overall outcome. Moreover, these specimens are not like smooth marbles that lend themselves to being coated by India ink in a uniform way. The excised tissue contains "nooks and crannies" related to varying proportions of fat, stromal elements, and glandular breast tissue that may be encountered.

Rather than sacrifice a large volume of normal tissue to insure that margins are clear, since margins are irrelevant in benign disease, reexcision of the primary site with separate dissection of the margins and the base of the wound and the application of metallic clips to these sites is our preferred alternative. This is especially appropriate for the many patients with DCIS who have been referred for treatment recommendations following initial biopsy and diagnosis elsewhere.

Reexcision of the primary site and dissection of wound margins and base are more precise than inking the margins of the specimen, since the specimen is almost never uniform in its consistency or shape. Additionally, the application of metallic clips to wound margins and base offers precise localization of this site on subsequent mammograms. Since recurrence, when it ensues, is most commonly detected as new calcifications at the same site as the primary lesion, "boxing in" this area on subsequent mammograms by these clips facilitates the radiologist's detection of a new problem. We have used this technique of clipping wound margins and base for almost 10 years to prepare patients for irradiation following local excision (and axillary dissection) for invasive carcinomas; both radiation therapists and radiologists have found it most helpful to determine the site of the previous lesion accurately in this way.

When the specimen is sent to the pathologist, grossly apparent areas of abnormality may be examined by frozen section, and if malignancy is confirmed, a portion of the specimen may be saved for receptor and cytometric studies. It is more important, however, to determine invasion, if present, than these other studies, since treatment decisions in these particular cases are currently more likely related to the presence of invasion than to the quantification of receptors, etc. Moreover, these studies may be performed subsequently on fixed tissue from the paraffin blocks if desired.

The earlier detection of mammographic abnormalities has even led to greater technical difficulties for the surgeon and surgical pathologists. More often than not, there are no grossly apparent abnormalities in the breast tissue even though the calcifications are known to be within the specimen. We rely upon the radiologist to confirm the presence of the calcifications within the excised tissue by specimen radiography, and often a clip is placed at the exact site; both the specimen and the specimen radiograph are sent to the pathologists so they can be alerted to the exact site of the area of greatest concern, even within a small specimen.

With respect to other clinical decisions about the choice of patients with DCIS for treatment by local excision and surveillance, we agree that the lesion must be subclinical, found on the basis of mammographic calcifications or as an incidental finding. The diameter of the area of calcifications should usually be 2.0 cm or less as measured on the mammogram, with minor exceptions, such as a patient with a marginally larger area of calcifications but a large enough breast to allow the removal of a greater volume of tissue without creating a major deformity. The specimen radiograph should confirm the excision of the area in question, or a postoperative mammogram is indicated to substantiate this important criterion.

That the patient must recognize the limits of our current knowledge about this disease is implicit in the mutual agreement between patient and physician to choose surveillance as an option. A clear understanding of the biology and natural history of the disease that we call subclinical DCIS still eludes us. As clinicians, we have been involved in the care of too many women with often lethal breast cancers, so that reluctance to abandon traditional treatment in favor of lesser options is understandable. Our respect for breast cancer is too great! When dealing with malignancy, "overkill" has always been assumed to be a more sound philosophy than "underkill." If we could be convinced that certain diseases that we currently call malignant, such as DCIS, are not inevitably followed by invasive, life-threatening cancers, and that, even if recurrence does occur, there is a second opportunity for successful interference, perhaps there would be greater enthusiasm for less rather than for more treatment. Unless we can, however, enroll our patients in programs that follow rather than always treat this disease, we will never know which, if any, women with DCIS will be not affected by the subsequent specter of invasive breast cancer.

References

1. Haagensen CD: Diseases of the Breast, Third Edition. W.B. Saunders Co., Philadelphia, p 782, 1986.
2. Haagensen CD: Diseases of the Breast, Third Edition. W.B. Saunders Co., Philadelphia, p 788, 1986.
3. Gump FE, Jicha DL, Ozello L: Ductal carcinoma in situ (DCIS): a revised concept. Surgery 1987; 102:790–795.
4. Manual for Staging of Cancer, Third Edition. American Joint Committee on Cancer, Chicago, pp 145–150, 1988.
5. Solin LJ, Recht A, Fourquet A, et al: Ten-year results of breast-conserving surgery and definitive irradiation for intraductal carcinoma of the breast. Cancer 1991; 68:2337–2344.
6. Schwartz GF, D'Ugo DM, Rosenberg AL: Extent of axillary dissection preceding irradiation for carcinoma of the breast. Arch Surg 1986; 121:1395–1398.
7. Betsill WL Jr, Rosen PP, Lieberman PH, et al: Intraductal carcinoma: long-term follow-up after treatment by biopsy alone. JAMA 1978; 239:1863–1867.
8. Lagios MD, Westdahl PR, Margolin FR, et al: Duct carcinoma in situ: relationship of extent of noninvasive disease to the frequency of occult invasion, multicentricity, lymph node metastasis and short-term treatment failures. Cancer 1982; 59:1309–1314.
9. Lagios MD: Duct carcinoma in situ: pathology and treatment. Surg Clin NA 1990; 70:853–871.
10. Haagensen CD, Lane N, Lattes R, Bodian C: Lobular neoplasia (so-called lobular carcinoma in situ) of the breast. Cancer 1978; 42:737–769.

11. Carpenter R, Boulter PS, Cooke T, Gibbs NM: Management of screen detected ductal carcinoma in situ of the breast. Br J Surg 1989; 76:564–567.
12. Arnesson LG, Smeds S, Fgerberg G, Gröntoft O: Follow-up of two treatment modalities for ductal cancer in situ of the breast. Br J Surg 1989; 76:672–675.
13. Schwartz GF: Treatment of in situ duct carcinoma of the breast. Presented at the 18th Annual Symposium of the New York Metropolitan Breast Cancer Group, Inc., January 19, 1991.
14. Locker AP, Horrocks C, Gilmour AS, et al: Flow cytometric and histological analysis of ductal carcinoma in situ of the breast. Br J Surg 1990; 77:564–567.
15. Schwartz GF, Patchefsky AS, Finkelstein SD, et al: Nonpalpable in situ ductal carcinoma of the breast. Arch Surg 1989; 124:29–32.
16. Patchefsky AS, Schwartz GF, Finkelstein SD, et al: Heterogeneity of intraductal carcinoma of the breast. Cancer 1989; 63:731–741.

The Contralateral Breast

Sir Patrick M. Forrest

Introduction

It is now accepted that breast cancer is initiated in the epithelium that lines the terminal ductules and acini that compose the lobular unit.[1-3] It is easy to understand that although the final genetic changes that lead to a cancer may be a focal phenomenon, there are widespread changes in the epithelium that increase its susceptibility to transformation to a malignant phenotype, setting the stage for the known multifocality of both invasive and noninvasive cancer.[4-6] Once malignant transformation has occurred, a second series of genetic changes are believed to be necessary for the property of invasiveness, leading to dissemination and a fatal outcome.[7,8] The changes that precede cancer of the breast are less well understood in genetic terms than those that predispose to colonic cancer. Nevertheless, there is no doubt that the development of breast cancer, particularly one that is invasive, denotes an increased risk of a further cancer in the remaining breast tissue which, in the days of mastectomy, was represented solely by the contralateral breast. As indicated by Foote and Stewart,[9] "the most frequent antecedent of cancer in one breast is a history of having had cancer in the opposite breast." The existence of this risk is not controversial, but the management of the opposite breast in women with proven unilateral breast cancer most certainly is (Table 1).

Incidence of Contralateral Cancer

Contralateral breast cancer, as a clinical entity, may present at the same time as the initial cancer (simultaneous or synchronous) or at a variable time following the treatment of the first cancer (nonsimultaneous or metachronous). Reported estimates of the risk of contralateral cancer vary greatly from 0.3% to 1.9% for

From: Wise L, Johnson H Jr (eds): *Breast Cancer: Controversies in Management.* Futura Publishing Company, Inc., Armonk, NY, © 1994.

Table 1
Incidence of Ductal Cancer In Situ in Normal Autopsy Breasts and Contralateral Breasts
from Women with Breast Cancer* (Reference 6)

Source	No. of Patients	DCIS Present (%)	Average No. of Lesions/Involved Breasts
Normal autopsy	185	11 (6.0%)	1.5
Contralateral breast	44	21 (47.7)	13.0

*No invasive cancers were identified. DCIS = ductal carcinoma in situ.

simultaneous and from 1.0% to 8.9% for nonsimultaneous cancer.[10] This variation depends upon a number of factors, such as the origin of the reported series of cases, the degree of selectivity of evaluated patients, and the completeness and duration of follow-up. Of critical importance are the criteria which were applied to determine whether the second mammary cancer was truly a second primary, which has developed ab initio in the remaining breast, or whether it was a metastasis from the original tumor. As originally defined by Robbins and Berg, this opinion is usually based on the site of the second tumor and its gross and histologic characteristics.[11] Thus:

1. Metastatic tumors were more likely to be situated in the fat that surrounds the breast proper, most often either in that part of the breast nearest to the midline or in the tail of the breast (this is due to retrograde lymphatic spread). Primary tumors arise within the breast parenchyma, and are more common in the upper outer quadrant of the breast.

2. Metastases are more commonly multiple, grow in an expansile fashion (rather than the crablike stellate growth of a primary tumor), and histologically resemble the most malignant parts of the first cancer.

3. Metastatic tumors are *not* associated with contiguous in-situ carcinoma, such foci of in-situ disease being the rule with a primary tumor.

Review of pathological material is thus an essential safeguard against overestimating risk.

In their report from the Breast Cancer Unit in Guy's Hospital, London, Chaudary and colleagues also stressed the importance of in-situ change which they regarded as providing absolute proof that a contralateral tumor represented a new primary tumor.[12] But in the absence of in-situ change, they also accepted as new primary tumors those which were histologically different in type, or which histologically demonstrated "distinctly greater differentiation" than the first one. They also introduced a criterion based on clinical findings, suggesting that in the absence of the above histologic differences, a carcinoma in the opposite breast *was compatible* with a second primary tumor, provided that there was no evidence of local-regional or distant metastatic spread from the cancer in the ipsilateral breast, but this definition is too "soft" for general use. In that used by the Scottish Cancer Trials Office, a contralateral tumor is regarded as being compatible with a new primary tumor only if there is no evidence of relapse at other sites within 12 months of the detection of the second tumor.[13]

The extent to which these various criteria have been used to determine the true incidence of contralateral disease is not always clear in published reports.

Impact of Mammography

The impact of mammography on increasing diagnostic efficiency is also a matter to take into account. There is no doubt that mammography increases detection rates of tumors in either breast, and therefore will uncover a larger number of both simultaneous and nonsimultaneous contralateral cancers. In a recent report from Edinburgh of 200 operable cancers of less than 4 cm in size, seven had suspicious microcalcifications (one with a mass) on the contralateral mammogram, of which five proved to be malignant.[14] The sharp increase in detection rate of simultaneous cancers coincidental with the introduction of mammography is well shown in the Guy's Hospital series[12] (Fig. 1). However, mammography only introduces "lead-time" into diagnosis by discovering a

OCCURRENCE OF SIMULTANEOUS CONTRALATERAL BREAST CANCER IN 3032 CASES OF PRIMARY BREAST CANCER

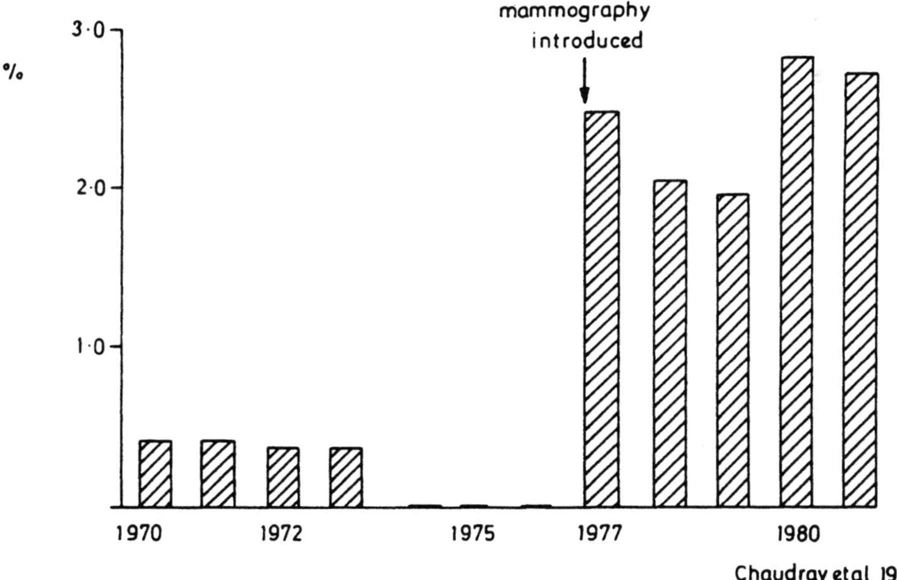

Figure 1: *Detection of simultaneous contralateral cancer before and after introduction of mammography. From Chaudary MA, et al.,[12] with permission.*

malignant lesion at an earlier date. It should not influence actual incidence rates, unless it leads to overdiagnosis of cancer. The cumulative incidence curves would but be "shifted to the left."

Mammography also has a role in differentiating the infiltrating spiculated primary cancer from a smooth "pushing" metastasis.

Assessment of Risk

To express the incidence of contralateral *primary* cancer as a percentage is misleading. It is preferable to express this as a rate, i.e., related to the number of women at risk. These are those who survive from their initial cancer. In the Memorial Hospital and Guy's Hospital series, incidence was expressed as the rate per 1,000 patient years. It is also relevant to know the relative risk that a woman with a first breast cancer has of developing a second contralateral cancer compared to that which is present for the development of the first cancer. This comparison requires knowledge of incidence rates in age-matched women in the general population. When such strict criteria for assessment of risk are applied, it is apparent from the Memorial and Guy's Hospital series that simultaneous clinically detectable cancer of the contralateral breast is a relatively rare event, occurring in less than 1% of all patients, and that nonsimultaneous second primary cancers can be expected to accumulate at a rate of less than 1% of those women at risk each year. The similarity of the data from these two series is striking (Table 2). Further, both studies indicate that the cumulative incidence of second cancers increments at a constant exponential rate, not showing any trend to increase or decrease with time (Fig. 2). In the study from Guy's Hospital, in

Table 2
Risk of Nonsimultaneous Contralateral Breast Cancer from Two Hospital Cohort Studies*

Hospital	Annual Rate Nonsimultaneous Cancers	Relative Risk Compared to Primary Cancer
Memorial Hospital (New York)		
Comparison with		
New York State	0.71	5.0
Connecticut		4.8
10 US cities		3.7
Guy's Hospital (London)		
Comparison with		
South-Thames	0.76	5.9

*From references 11 and 12.

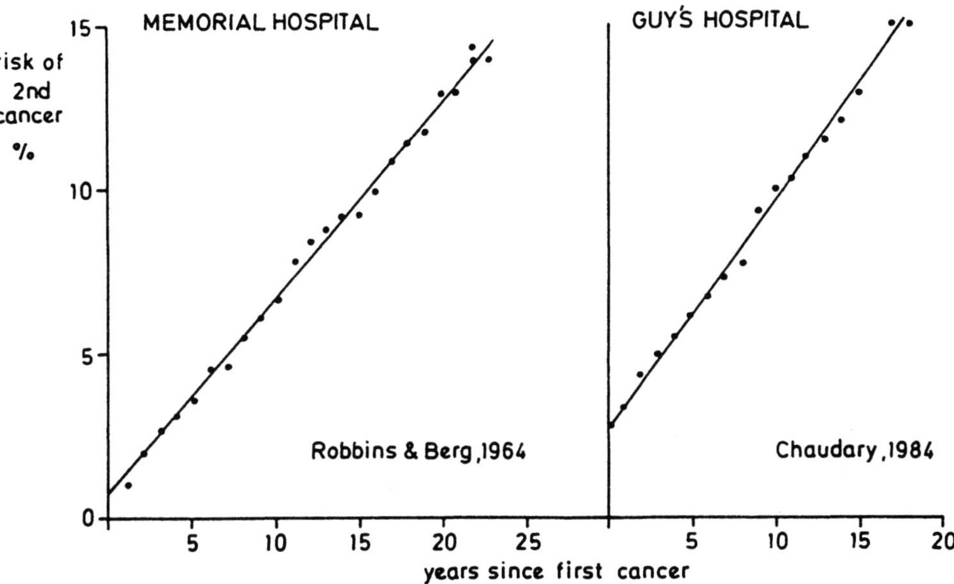

Figure 2: *Cumulative net risk of developing a second primary breast cancer in two hospital cohorts. From Robbins GF, et al.,[11] with permission.*

which the incidence rates of second contralateral cancers were compared with age-specific rates for first cancers in the general population, the relative risk was 5.9%, a figure rather in excess of those reported by Robbins and Berg (Table 2).

Evidence on the incidence of nonsimultaneous contralateral breast cancer is also available from multicentric trials, such as that of the National Surgical Adjuvant Breast Project (NSABP).[15] In their report on 1,578 women enrolled in Protocol 4 (in which those with bilateral disease were excluded from entry), the annual rate based on patients at risk was again constant at less than 1%.

Population studies of the risk of contralateral cancer have been reported from England, the United States, and Denmark. These suggest that the computation of risk from cohort studies may have overestimated risk (Table 3).[16–18] In a report from Birmingham, England, in which 21,967 cases of breast cancer were considered, the relative risk of developing a second contralateral tumor in women with cancer of one breast compared to the incidence of primary breast cancer in the general population was 3.0% (when both simultaneous and nonsimultaneous tumors were included) and 2.4% (when simultaneous tumors were excluded). These figures are in agreement with the other two studies. The Danish study, which included 56,237 women with breast cancer, followed up over 38 years, with a relative risk for nonsimultaneous contralateral cancer of 2.8%, gave the 95% confidence limits to be 2.7–3.0%.

Table 3
Population Studies of Computing Relative Risk of Invasive Second Breast Cancer*

		Relative Risk of Second Cancer	
	No. of Patients	Overall	Nonsimultaneous
Birmingham			
England (1978)	21,967	3.0	2.4
Connecticut			
USA (1983)	27,175	3.2	2.9
Denmark (1986)	56,237	—	2.8

*From references 16–18.

Risk Factors

Attention has been paid to the factors that may increase the risk for developing contralateral disease in a woman with breast cancer. Of these, age is by far the most significant. All reports have indicated that the younger a woman at the time of diagnosis of her first tumor, the more likely she is to develop a second one in the opposite breast. This is true of population as well as cohort studies (Table 4). This effect may be due to the longer period of follow-up that youth provides. But there is also the possibility that it is influenced by the greater likelihood of genetically inherited disease in the younger age group. Truly familial breast cancer, genetically determined, is more commonly expressed in young premenopausal women, in whom it is frequently shown to be bilateral.[19] And although not significant, the NSABP study showed a trend in favor of a higher incidence of bilaterality in those with a family history of breast cancer. A recent report from Sweden, however, casts doubt on the relationship between

Table 4
Effect of Age on Risk of Nonsimultaneous Contralateral Cancer*

	Relative Risk	
Age at Diagnosis	England	USA
<45	5.3	4.9
45–49	3.0	3.2
≥60	1.0	2.1
Total	2.4	2.9

*From references 16 and 17.

age, bilaterality, and family history.[20] The influence of other factors, such as exposure to ionizing radiation, the histologic type and stage of the first tumor, and the frequency of multicentricity and in-situ involvement, are more open to debate. Ionizing radiation has assumed particular importance on account of its increasing use in breast-conserving methods of management; but to date there is no evidence that a spill-over to the opposite breast puts it at increased risk (Table 5).[21] In the Danish population study,[18] women who were irradiated at the time of primary treatment had a significantly greater risk of contralateral cancer after 10 years than those who had not been irradiated. The relative risks were 2.6% and 2.0%, respectively (Table 6).

Some have reported that the more advanced the stage of the first cancer, the more common is contralateral disease.[17] In the NSABP study, first cancers larger than 2 cm were more likely to be associated with the subsequent development of a second contralateral tumor than were smaller first cancers.[15] Proliferative fibrocystic disease in the vicinity of the dominant mass, nipple involvement, multicentricity, and tubular and lobular invasive types were also factors of significant risk. Others have stressed the association between lobular invasive cancer and bilaterality.[22,23] Lobular carcinoma in situ (LCIS) in the vicinity of the dominant first tumor was also related to risk; and again, LCIS in one breast is known to be a precursor of cancer in either breast. LCIS is not cancer, but it is a marker of increased risk.

Table 5
Risk of Contralateral Breast Cancer in Irradiated and Nonirradiated Patients in Milan Trial*

Primary Treatment	No of Patients	No. of Contralateral Cancers (9–16 Year Follow-up)
Halsted mastectomy	349	20
Quadrantectomy + irradiation	352	19

*From reference 21.

Table 6
Effect of Irradiation on Relative Risk of Breast Cancer in Danish Population Study*

Primary Treatment	No. of Cancers	Relative Risk
Irradiated	327	2.6 (2.3–2.9)
Nonirradiated	118	2.0 (1.7–2.4)
Total	445	2.4 (2.2–2.6)

*From reference 18.

Prognosis

The effect that the development of either a simultaneous or a nonsimultaneous cancer of the contralateral breast bears on eventual outcome is controversial. This is not surprising, as the incidence of simultaneous contralateral tumors is low, while the potential difficulty of distinguishing between a second primary tumor and a metastatic tumor makes interpretation of survival times after the appearance of the second tumor difficult. The NSABP study indicated that apart from those contralateral tumors that appeared within 2 years, the outcome of patients overall was similar from the time of diagnosis for those with unilateral and bilateral disease[15] (Fig. 3). It is difficult to find evidence to support the statement that "the presence of bilateral invasive cancers places the patient in double jeopardy."[22]

Biopsy of the Contralateral Breast (Urban's Series)

It was knowledge of the risk of bilaterality in his own cases (9% within 10 years) and the difficulty of detecting these, particularly in women who defaulted from follow-up, that prompted Urban into performing a biopsy of the opposite breast at the time of primary treatment of the presenting tumor.[24] His series of 954 biopsies, performed between 1964 and 1975, has been frequently quoted as the "gold standard" for this procedure.[25]

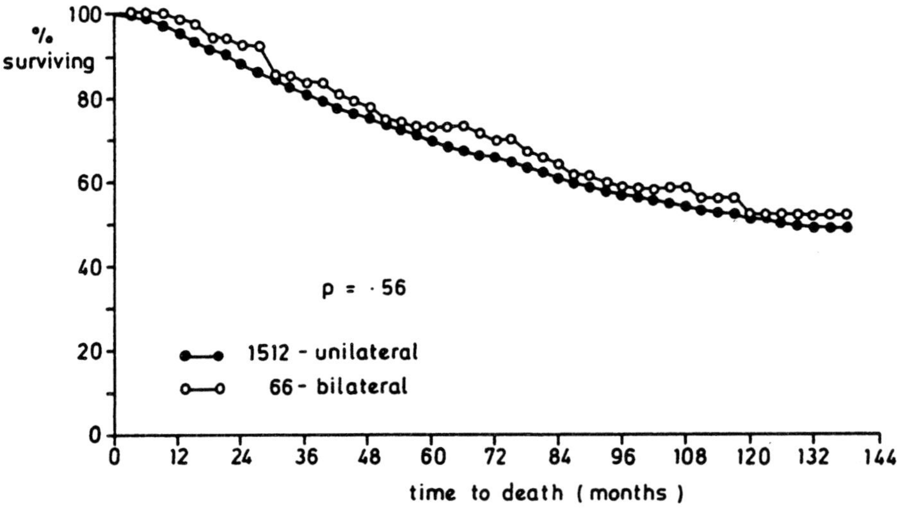

Figure 3: *Survival of patients with unilateral and bilateral breast cancer in NSABP Protocol 4. From Fisher ER, et al.,[15] with permission.*

In 653 of his 954 patients, there were positive (28) or suspicious (625) clinical or mammographic signs in the opposite breast, the latter being minimal indefinite thickening or mammographic density, even if thought to be benign. In both of these groups he advocated a generous biopsy of the suspicious area of the breast. In the remaining 301 patients, the other breast was apparently completely normal. The biopsy included a fusiform area of glandular tissue, comprising 20% to 25% of the breast parenchyma, from the tail of the breast plus a biopsy of the mirror-image site of the first tumor.

The results are given in Table 7. In biopsies of breasts without positive but suspicious signs of simultaneous contralateral cancer, 11.8% indicated malignancy; the corresponding figure for the truly random biopsies was 7.6%.

These data, originally reported in 1977, have formed the base on which the performance of contralateral biopsy has been advised. However, the high incidence of noninvasive cancer should be noted (only 2% of the 301 random biopsies were of invasive cancer); there is no indication whether the findings were subject to pathological review; and one cannot assess the extent to which the high incidence of patients with positive and suspicious signs in the opposite breast indicated bias from the referral pattern to a specialist hospital.

Other Series

Other series of contralateral biopsies at the time of primary surgery have been reported, but with variable results (Table 8).[22,23,25-31] The sites for biopsies have varied, as have the amounts of breast tissue removed. From those series that detail findings, the incidence of invasive cancer is 2.4%, and that of noninvasive cancer 5.9% (Table 9).

The criteria for a diagnosis of noninvasive cancer, and in particular the

Table 7
Urban's Data on Contralateral Breast Biopsy in Women with Primary Breast Cancer*

	Contralateral Cancers Detected		
Clinical and/or Mammographic Evaluation of the Contralateral Breast	Histology Invasive	Histology Noninvasive	Total
Positive clinical or mammographic signs 28	20	2	22
Suspicious clinical or mammographic signs 625	30	44	74
Other breast normal 301	5	18	23
Total: 954	55	64	119

*There were 838 primary invasive and 116 noninvasive primary cancers. From reference 25.

Table 8
Incidence of Contralateral Malignancy on Random Biopsies

		Cancers Detected		
Author/Year	No. of Patients	Invasive	Noninvasive	Total
Fenig (1975)	314	NA	NA	23
King (1976)	109	1	4	5
Urban (1977)	301	5	18	23
Leis (1978)	321	10	14	24
Anderson (1980)	170	7	3	10
Fracchia (1985)	150	NA	NA	20
Wanebo (1985)	62[1]	10[1]	3	13
Pressman (1986)	226	4	28[2]	32

[1]Mostly LCIS.
[2]Included patients with mass.
NA = not available.

Table 9
Contralateral Malignancy on Random Biopsies (Five Series with Clinically and
Mammographically Normal Opposite Breasts)

	Cancers Detected		
Total No. of Biopsies	Invasive	Noninvasive	Total
1,127	27 (2.4%)	67 (5.9%)	94 (8.3%)

differentiation of ductal and lobular types, are not generally apparent in these reports.

Contralateral Mastectomy

The "ultimate" biopsy is a mastectomy. Evidence of the incidence with which malignancy is diagnosed comes from a small series of patients having a "prophylactic" contralateral mastectomy at the time, or within a few months of their primary treatment. This approach has been promoted in "high-risk" women by Leis, these being defined as women who are less than 50 years of age, who have a family history of the disease, and who have small node-negative cancers associated with multicentric spread.[32] In 112 such cases, none of whom had clinical or mammographic anomalies in the breast, Leis reported histologic evidence of malignancy in 19 (16.9%), and atypical change in an additional 21 (18.7%). Seven invasive cancers were present. Supportive evidence for these findings is hard to find.

Opinion

From this survey it can be concluded that a woman who develops a cancer of one breast is more at risk for a second primary tumor of the opposite breast than is a normal woman at risk from breast cancer as a primary phenomenon. The relative risk lies somewhere between 2% and 5% and is inversely related to age at presentation of the first primary cancer. But in terms of a woman treated for breast cancer, the absolute risk approximates 0.5% per annum for at least the next 15 years. Evidence that delay in the diagnosis of this second cancer adversely affects prognosis is far from validated. The view expressed by Leis, that the second breast remains as a "useless, nonfunctioning, questionable sex symbol" is no longer tenable, particularly as in most patients the first breast need no longer be removed to treat cancer. Prophylactic mastectomy has a place only for the woman who expresses a wish to be free of the risk of contralateral cancer.

In the Sloan-Kettering Memorial Cancer Center, biopsy of the contralateral breast is still advised as a routine procedure, this being carried out through a circumareolar incision (Fig. 4). It is difficult to justify such "random sampling" of breast tissue, knowing that it can only investigate a small part of the total breast tissue. And despite the view of some that lobular invasive cancer is a positive indication for contralateral biopsy, the lack of congruity between histologic types (Table 10) suggests that chance may also enter this equation.[33]

TECHNIQUE FOR BLIND BIOPSY

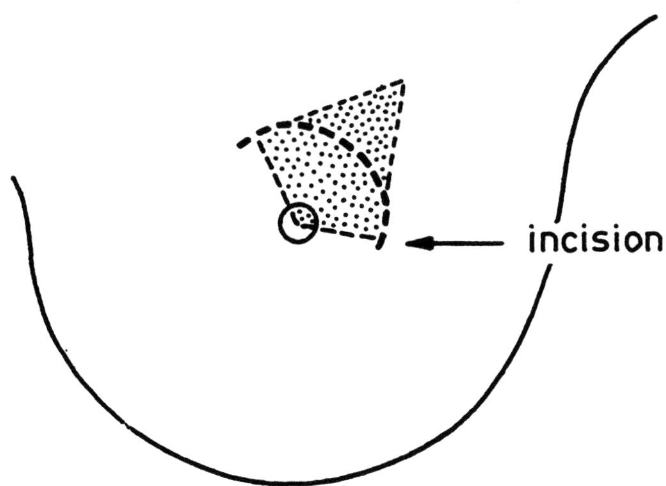

Figure 4: *Biopsy recommended, by Fracchia. From Fracchia AA, et al.,[22] with permission.*

Table 10
Relationship of Histological Types of Primary and Nonsimultaneous Contralateral Tumors*

First Tumor Histology	No. of Primary Tumors	Contralateral Tumor Histology		
		Lobular	Tubular	Other
Lobular	12	6	0	6
Tubular	1	1	0	0
Other	75	16	4	55

*From reference 33.

It is now firmly established that high-quality mammography can detect both invasive and noninvasive cancer with a lead-time of several months before they reach a clinically detectable stage. Mammography, unlike a biopsy, can examine the whole breast when both mediolateral oblique and craniocaudal projections are used, and effort is better expended to ensure that women treated for breast cancer have continuous surveillance of the remaining breast tissue by annual mammography, which a random biopsy, by causing distortion of breast tissue, may make less reliable.

References

1. Wellings SR, Jensen HM: On the origin and progression of ductal carcinoma in the human breast. J Natl Cancer Inst 1973; 50:1111.
2. Azzopardi JG: Problems in breast pathology. WB Saunders, London, 1979.
3. Page DL, Anderson TJ: Diagnostic histopathology of the breast. Churchill-Livingstone, Edinburgh, 1988.
4. Qualheim RE, Gall EA: Breast carcinoma with multiple sites of origin. Cancer 1957; 10:460–468.
5. Tinnemans JG, Wobbes T, Van der Sluis RF, Lubbers EJ, et al: Multicentricity in non-palpable breast carcinoma and its implications for treatment. Am J Surg 1986; 151:334–348.
6. Alpers CE, Wellings CR: The prevalence of in situ carcinoma in normal and cancer associated breasts. Human Pathol 1985; 16:796–807.
7. Editorial: Metastatic fundamentals. Lancet 1989; 1:1052–1054.
8. Liotta LA: Gene products which play a role in cancer invasion and metastases. Breast Cancer Res Treatment 1988; 11:113–124.
9. Foote FW, Stewart FW: Comparative study of cancerous versus non-cancerous breasts. Surgery 1946; 19:74–99.
10. Eremin A: Second primary breast cancer. Br Med J 1988; 296:1755–1756.
11. Robbins GF, Berg JW: Bilateral primary breast cancers: a prospective clinicopathological study. Cancer 1964; 17:1501–1527.
12. Chaudary MA, Millis RR, Hoskins EOL, Halder M, et al: Bilateral primary breast cancer: a prospective study of disease incidence. Br J Surg 1984; 71:711–714.
13. Stewart HJ: Personal communication. 1992.
14. Dixon JM, Chetty U: Mammography in the management of patients with small breast cancers. Br J Surg 1991; 78:218–219.
15. Fisher ER, Fisher B, Sass R, Wickerham L, et al: Cancer 1984; 54:3002–3011.

16. Prior P, Waterhouse JAH: Incidence of bilateral tumours in a population-based series of breast cancer patients: two approaches to an epidemiological analysis. Br J Cancer 1978; 37:620–634.
17. Hankey BF, Curtis RE, Naughton MD, Boice JD, et al: A retrospective cohort analysis of second breast cancer risk for primary breast cancer patients with an assessment of the effect of radiation therapy. J Nat Cancer Inst 1983; 70:797–804.
18. Storm HH, Jensen OM: Risk of contralateral breast cancer in Denmark 1943–80. Br J Cancer 1986; 54:483–492.
19. Anderson DE: Breast cancer in families. Cancer 1977; 40:1855.
20. Adami HO, Hansen J, Jung B, Rimsten A: Characteristics of familial breast cancer in Sweden: absence of relation to age and unilateral versus bilateral disease. Cancer 1981; 48:1688–1695.
21. Veronesi U, Banfi A, Salvadori B: Breast conservation is the treatment of choice for small breast cancer: long-term results of a randomised trial. Eur J Cancer 1990; 26:668–670.
22. Fracchia AA, Robinson D, Legaspi A, Greenall MJ, et al: Survival in bilateral breast cancer. Cancer 1985; 55:1414–1421.
23. Andersen LI, Mucharett O: Simulataneous bilateral cancer of the breast: evaluation of the use of a contralateral biopsy. Acta Chir Scand 1980; 146:407–409.
24. Urban JA: Bilaterality of breast cancer; biopsy of the opposite breast. Cancer 1967; 20:1867.
25. Urban JA, Papachriston D, Taylor J: Bilateral breast cancer: biopsy of the opposite breast. Cancer 1977; 40:1968–1973.
26. King RE, Terz JJ, Lawrence W: Experience with opposite breast biopsy in patients with operable breast cancer. Cancer 1976; 37:43–45.
27. Fenig J, Arlen M, Livingston SF, Levowitz BS: The potential for carcinoma existing synchronously on a microscopic level within the second breast. Surg Gynecol Obstet 1975; 141:394–396.
28. King RE, Terz JJ, Lawrence W: Experience with opposite breast biopsy in patients with operable breast cancer. Cancer 1976; 37:43–45.
29. Leis HP: Bilateral breast cancer. Surg Clin N Am 1978; 58:833–841.
30. Martin JK, van Heerden JA, Gaffey TA: Synchronous and metachronous carcinoma of the breast. Surgery 1982; 91:12–16.
31. Wanebo HJ, Senofsky GM, Fechner RE, Kaiser D, et al: Bilateral breast cancer: risk reduction by contralateral biopsy. Ann Surg 1985; 201:667–677.
32. Leis HP: Selective elective prophylactic contralateral mastectomy. Cancer 1971; 23:956–961.
33. Dawson PJ, Maloney T, Gimothy P, Junean P, et al: Bilateral breast cancer: one disease or two. Breast Cancer Res Treatment 1991; 19:233–244.

23

Clinical Issues Regarding Breast Cancer and Pregnancy

Charles L. Loprinzi

Introduction

It is hardly a surprise that the relatively rare combination of pregnancy and breast cancer is a challenging clinical problem that encompasses many moral and ethical issues. Breast cancer and pregnancy has been the subject of a recent comprehensive review article.[1] This present chapter will address a few selected clinical issues concerning breast cancer and pregnancy.

Does Pregnancy Change the Prognosis of Concurrently Diagnosed Breast Cancer?

In the distant past, it was generally felt that pregnancy had a negative impact on the prognosis of a young woman with breast cancer.[2-4] However, at the present time, an overwhelming body of evidence[5-11] supports the conclusion that pregnancy in and of itself does not portend a diminished prognosis. Rather, the relatively poor prognosis of breast cancer patients who have a concurrent pregnancy appears to be related to patient age, as young women with breast cancer have a poorer prognosis than do older women.[10,11]

What Are Appropriate Treatment Principles for Women With Breast Cancer and a Concurrent Pregnancy?

Treatment decisions are often quite difficult in pregnant breast cancer patients. They need to be individualized on a case-by-case basis, taking into

From: Wise L, Johnson H Jr (eds): *Breast Cancer: Controversies in Management.* Futura Publishing Company, Inc., Armonk, NY, © 1994.

255

account medical, ethical, and moral issues. Several involved physicians, including a medical oncologist, an obstetrician, a surgeon, and a radiation oncologist, are often simultaneously involved in the patient's care. One of these physicians should act as a primary spokesperson. The following paragraphs will discuss a few relevant guidelines regarding the use of surgery, radiation therapy, chemotherapy, and hormone therapy in pregnant women with breast cancer.

Surgery can usually be safely performed in pregnant women, and it is the recommended primary treatment for such women with newly diagnosed localized breast cancer. If a mastectomy is to be performed in the postpartum period, lactation suppression is recommended to decrease the breast size and vascularity, and thus allow for a safer surgical procedure.[12-14] Primary radiation therapy is appropriate in many newly diagnosed breast cancer patients.[15] Nonetheless, it should not be utilized in pregnant patients in view of the risk of radiation effects on the developing fetus.

Cytotoxic drugs result in a higher than otherwise expected incidence of fetal wastage and fetal malformations if they are administered in the first trimester of pregnancy.[16] The folate antagonists (e.g., methotrexate) appear to be particularly toxic, and it is recommended that they not be given to pregnant women. In the later stages of pregnancy, most cytotoxic drugs can be administered with less of an apparent effect on the fetus. Nonetheless, the potential beneficial effects of chemotherapy for the patient need to be weighed against the potential for toxicity to both the patient and the fetus prior to chemotherapy administration in each individual case. Finally, postpartum women receiving chemotherapy should not breast-feed their infants because chemotherapeutic drugs can be passed on to an infant through breast milk.[16]

Scant data are available regarding the use of hormone modulatory treatments in pregnant breast cancer patients. Similarly, little is known regarding the toxicity of hormonal agents such as tamoxifen or megestrol acetate on a developing fetus. The current opinion is that pregnancy termination does not alter the course of breast cancer in afflicted patients.[1]

The following is an interesting case presentation concerning a young woman who was diagnosed with breast cancer while she was pregnant. The management of this patient required several physicians with different areas of expertise. Despite a very poor prognosis at the time of primary disease diagnosis, this patient has fared well to date.

Case History

The patient was a 34-year-old woman in 1985 when she presented with a tender right breast during the middle trimester of her second pregnancy. On examination, she had a large, ill-defined right upper breast mass without clear-cut clinical evidence of inflammatory breast cancer. On 12/30/85, she underwent a right modified radical mastectomy. Histologic findings revealed an 11

× 11 × 5 cm grade 4 breast adenocarcinoma. There was pathological evidence of inflammatory breast cancer with extensive cancer
cells in the lymphatics of the skin, nipple, and breast. The cancer
involved the deep fascia. All 21 examined axillary lymph nodes
contained cancer. The patient had an uneventful postoperative
course. Following extensive discussion regarding the patient's
diagnosis, prognosis, and treatment options, she started chemotherapy with cyclophosphamide, doxorubicin, and 5-fluorouracil,
20 days postoperatively, at a time when she was in her sixth
month of pregnancy. Following two cycles of chemotherapy and
evidence of mature fetal lungs obtained by an amniocentesis
procedure, a Cesarean section resulted in a healthy-appearing
baby girl. Subsequently, chemotherapy was restarted and continued for a total of 10 months. Following chemotherapy, the patient
received local-regional irradiation therapy (50.4 cGy in 28 fractions). The patient finished all of her treatment in March 1987 and
has received no subsequent breast cancer treatment. Five years
following initial diagnosis, this patient is doing well without any
evidence of recurrent breast cancer. Her daughter appears to be
developing normally without any apparent sequelae resulting
from her in-utero chemotherapy exposure.

What Should Young Women With Breast Cancer Be Told Regarding Subsequent Pregnancy?

It is generally agreed that subsequent pregnancy following a diagnosis of
breast cancer does not appreciably alter a patient's prognosis.[9,17–20] Nonetheless,
it appears wise to recommend to young primary breast cancer patients that they
use effective, nonhormonal birth control methods to assure that they do not
become pregnant for at least 5 years following the diagnosis of breast cancer. The
primary basis for this recommendation is that it is usually within the 5 years
following diagnosis when most breast cancer relapses will become evident.
Thus, particularly difficult treatment decisions regarding the therapy of metastatic breast cancer in a pregnant woman involving many moral, ethical, and
psychosocial concerns can be avoided. It should be recognized that this recommendation may translate into "no subsequent pregnancy," as a 5-year period
may put the woman past the age of child-bearing potential, especially if adjuvant
chemotherapy has been administered.

There are rare patients who are 5 years status post diagnosis and wish to
become pregnant. In this situation, the patient should be carefully evaluated for
any evidence of metastatic disease. Subsequently, it should be explained to the
patient and her partner the risk of subsequent cancer recurrence. Also, precon-
ception consultation with an obstetrician is recommended. Women should not
attempt to become pregnant while concurrently receiving adjuvant tamoxifen or
other systemic antitumor treatment.

Summary

In conclusion, the simultaneous presentation of breast cancer and pregnancy occurs rarely in clinical practice. Appropriate treatment of such cases needs to be individualized based on multiple medical, moral, and ethical issues. Often, several physicians need to be intimately involved in the care of the pregnant breast cancer patient.

References

1. Gallenberg MM, Loprinzi CL: Breast cancer and pregnancy. Semin Oncol 1989; 16(5):369–376.
2. Kilgore AR: Tumors and tumor-like lesions of the breast in association with pregnancy and lactation. Arch Surg 1929; 18:2079–2098.
3. Harrington SW: Carcinoma of the breast: results of surgical treatment when the carcinoma occurred in the course of pregnancy or lactation and when pregnancy occurred subsequent to operation (1910–1933). Ann Surg 1937; 106:690–700.
4. Haagensen CD, Stout AP: Carcinoma of the breast. Ann Surg 1943; 118:859–870.
5. Haagensen CD: Cancer of the breast in pregnancy and during lactation. Am J Obstet Gynecol 1967; 98:141–149.
6. Treves N, Holleb AI: A report of 549 cases of breast cancer in women 35 years of age or younger. Surg Gynecol Obstet 1958; 107:271–283.
7. Horsley JS, Alrich EM, Creighton BW: Carcinoma of the breast in women 35 years of age or younger. Ann Surg 1969; 169:839–843.
8. Peters MV, Meakin JW: The influence of pregnancy in carcinoma of the breast. Prog Clin Cancer 1965; 1:471–493.
9. Nugent P, O'Connell TX: Breast cancer and pregnancy. Arch Surg 1985; 120:1221–1224.
10. Host H, Lund E: Age as a prognostic factor in breast cancer. Cancer 1986; 57:2217.
11. Adami HO, Malker B, Holmberg L, et al: The relation between survival and age at diagnosis in breast cancer. N Engl J Med 1986; 315(9):559–563.
12. Ribeiro GG, Palmer MK: Breast carcinoma associated with pregnancy: a clinician's dilemma. Br Med J 1977; 2:1524–1527.
13. Anderson JM: Mammary cancers and pregnancy. Br Med J 1979; 1:1124–1127.
14. Horstein E, Skornick Y, Rozin R: The management of breast carcinoma in pregnancy and lactation. J Surg Oncol 1982; 21:179–182.
15. Fisher B, Redmond C, Poisson R, et al: Eight-year results of a randomized clinical trial comparing total mastectomy and lumpectomy with or without irradiation in the treatment of breast cancer. N Engl J Med 1989; 320:822–828.
16. Doll DC, Ringenberg S, Yarbro JW: Antineoplastic agents and pregnancy. Sem in Oncol 1989; 16(5):337–346.
17. Bunker ML, Peters MV: Breast cancer associated with pregnancy or lactation. Am J Obstet Gynecol 1963; 85:312–321.
18. Peters MV: The effect of pregnancy in breast cancer. In: Forrest AP, Kunkler PB (eds). Prognostic Factors in Breast Cancer. William & Wilkins, Baltimore, pp 65–80, 1968.
19. Ribeiro GG, Jones DA, Jones M: Carcinoma of the breast associated with pregnancy. Br J Surg 1986; 73:607–609.
20. Mignot L, Morvan F, Sarrazin D, et al: Breast carcinoma and subsequent pregnancy. Proc Annu Meet Am Soc Clin Oncol 1986; 5:57.$

24

Breast Reconstruction After Mastectomy:

An Update

John Bostwick, III

Introduction

Women now expect the treatment of their breast cancer to include either breast preservation or a breast reconstruction. For a woman, losing a breast from the treatment of breast cancer often leads to significant emotional difficulties. This can lead to a deleterious impact on her emotional stability and body image. An external prosthesis is not effective in improving body image. Techniques have been developed to restore the breast form and to improve the body image of these patients. Breast reconstruction following mastectomy has now become a part of the treatment of the woman with breast cancer. Since breast cancer typically strikes a woman in the prime of her life, and the overall survival rate is not improving, breast reconstruction focuses on the quality of life.

Breast reconstruction is designed to satisfy the patient's expectations both psychologically and aesthetically. This must be done within the principles of sound oncologic management. The opposite breast serves as the guide for the reconstructed breast; however, the oncologic status of the opposite breast is also considered in planning the operation.

Breast Cancer Management Team

The complexity of the treatment of women with breast cancer has prompted the development of a team of medical specialists focusing on the best management of each patient. Included on this team are the general surgeon, the medical

From: Wise L, Johnson H Jr (eds): *Breast Cancer: Controversies in Management.* Futura Publishing Company, Inc., Armonk, NY, © 1994.

oncologist, and the radiation therapist. The reconstructive surgeon contributes to the rehabilitation of the breast cancer patient who does not want to experience permanent breast loss after a mastectomy. Other members of the breast management team include the family physician, pathologist, psychiatrist, social workers, and nurses.

Role of Breast Reconstruction in Treating the Breast Cancer Patient

Breast reconstruction contributes to the management and rehabilitation of the woman with breast cancer. The treatment focus remains on the oncologic aspects. The patient's sense of deformity and compromised body image is a constant reminder of her life-threatening disease. The external prostheses are never incorporated into their body image as a restored breast, and therefore it is necessary to restore the breast form to manage the patient's sense of deformity. In the past 15 years, breast reconstruction has developed from an unusual and rare request to an integral part of the treatment of the woman who has had a mastectomy. These newer techniques give more natural-appearing and aesthetically acceptable breasts. Breast reconstruction has been shown not to hide potential local recurrences. It does produce positive psychological benefits for women which leads to a renewed sense of wholeness and a return to normalcy.

Timing of Breast Reconstruction

During the development of breast reconstruction, it was usually delayed until after the primary local treatment and adjuvant therapy. During the past few years, there has been an increase in the number of requests for immediate breast reconstruction; it is not necessary for a woman to live with her mastectomy defect in order to appreciate her reconstructed breast. Some women may delay or refuse mastectomy because of the fear of losing their breast, and immediate reconstruction can give them encouragement and present an alternative to lumpectomy-radiation if a mastectomy is determined to be the best management of the breast cancer.

For immediate breast reconstruction, a breast implant or a breast tissue expander is positioned beneath the musculofascial layer after the mastectomy. While the reconstruction is initiated at the time of the mastectomy, a secondary procedure is often necessary to complete the reconstruction and the nipple-areola reconstruction. When reconstruction is delayed until after the mastectomy and any other adjunctive treatments, it is often initiated about 3 to 9 months after the mastectomy. This reconstruction is done in two operations. The breast and chest wall are reconstructed during the first operation as well as correction of the opposite breast. The nipple-areola is reconstructed at the time of the second operation. The tissue expansion technique usually adds an additional operation to place the permanent implant.

Techniques of Breast Reconstruction

The reconstructive surgeon selects the method of breast reconstruction to meet the patient's expectations and breast symmetry after careful patient evaluation. The reconstructive surgeon first evaluates the oncologic status and then the other breast to determine its appearance as well as its oncologic status. A woman with breast reconstruction who must still wear an external prosthesis will usually be very unhappy.

Breast reconstruction with the tissues remaining after mastectomy together with a breast implant beneath the musculofascial layer is usually the preferred method of breast reconstruction after total mastectomy and modified radical mastectomy. A decision should be made during the initial planning if the available tissues are suitable or whether distant tissue in the form of a flap will be necessary.

Breast implants have been the subject of an evaluation by the FDA, and currently, implants filled with saline solution are available for breast reconstruction. Implants made of silicone gel are currently not available for implantation. There is no scientific evidence that silicone implants increase the incidence of breast cancer, although they may cause some problems with mammographic interpretation, especially if there is a capsular contracture that develops after implantation. There has been some concern about the possibility of an association of the silicone breast implant and autoimmune conditions. While no direct association has been shown, larger controlled studies are necessary to evaluate this possible association. Tissue expansion can permit the breast reconstruction without the need of a flap.

Since there is usually a significant deficit of tissue after a mastectomy, additional skin and/or muscle may be necessary to supplement the available tissues for the breast reconstruction. The transverse rectus abdominis musculocutaneous (TRAM) flap can provide abundant tissue from the lower abdomen to permit a breast reconstruction without a breast implant. This TRAM flap can also be moved to the breast region and reattached with microsurgical technique. The latissimus dorsi flap from the back is also a versatile and reliable source of skin and muscle to use for breast reconstruction. Breast reconstruction with microsurgical transfer of tissue from the buttocks region using a gluteus maximus musculocutaneous flap is another technically demanding method of breast reconstruction. These microsurgical techniques are selected as a method by an experienced surgeon when the other methods are not suitable. The method also permits breast reconstruction with autogenous tissue and without the need for breast implants.

Breast Reconstruction With Available Tissue

This method requires less surgical intervention than the other more complex methods. It involves the placement of a breast implant beneath the musculofascial layer of the tissues remaining after the mastectomy. By using the technique of modified tissue expansion, a larger silicone breast implant is placed during the second operation at the time of the reconstruction of the nipple-areola. The reconstruction is usually performed through the mastectomy scar without a second incision and scar. Since the implant is retromuscular, any possible local recurrences of the breast cancer are not masked by the breast reconstruction and can be detected in front of the breast implant.

This is an excellent method when the tissues after the total mastectomy or modified radical mastectomy are of good quality and breast symmetry can be achieved with one or two procedures. Other methods, such as autogenous tissue, should be used when the skin is tight, irradiated, or if the opposite breast is large and pendulous. After a radical mastectomy, autogenous tissue is usually necessary to achieve the best result, especially in the anterior axillary fold area.

Complications after this method are less frequent than with the other techniques. There can be the development of a fibrous capsule about any silicone breast implant. This results in a reconstructed breast that seems firm and spherical. When an unacceptable capsular contracture develops, an open release of the scar tissue may be helpful. The introduction of textured surface expanders and implants seems to reduce the incidence of capsular contracture.

Reconstruction With Tissue Expansion

Tissue expansion involves the gradual stretching of the tissues of the chest wall so that they can accommodate a larger breast implant so the breast reconstruction can appear more natural with some ptosis. Tissue expansion permits more patients to have breast reconstruction with their available tissues and reduces the need for the more complex autogenous tissue flaps.

A tissue expander is a saline-inflatable implant made with an outer elastomer similar to the cover of the silicone breast implant. There is a separate implantable fill valve or, as in some devices, the fill valve is located on the device. For breast reconstruction, the tissue expander is positioned in the submusculofascial position and the attached fill valve is placed subcutaneously lateral to or below the reconstructed breast. Saline is placed into the device at the time of the initial breast reconstruction. During the postoperative period, it is gradually filled incrementally about every week with 50 to 200 cc of normal saline. The fill must be done very slowly in order to obtain the best possible result.

After some overexpansion of the tissue expander and after it has been in place for a few additional months, the tissue expander is removed and replaced by a permanent breast implant of the size to give symmetry with the opposite breast. Nipple-areola reconstruction is usually done at this time or a few months later.

Tissue expansion is a good choice when there is enough skin cover and the breast reconstruction needs to be larger than can be achieved with a silicone breast implant in one operation (>400 cc). Tissue expansion is often unsatisfactory when the skin cover is thin or there are marked radiation changes. The patient should be told that the method is slow and includes several stages.

Tissue expansion breast reconstruction can have a few more complications than breast reconstruction with breast implants alone. In addition to the capsular contracture, failures of the tissue expander device can occur, and infection can be introduced when the device is filled utilizing external punctures.

Breast Reconstruction with Autogenous Tissue

Breast Reconstruction with the TRAM Flap

The lower abdominal skin and fat can be an excellent source of tissue for the woman who requests a breast reconstruction without a silicone breast implant and who also would benefit from a reduction of her lower abdomen. The transverse rectus abdominis musculocutaneous (TRAM) flap is a ellipse of skin and fat taken from the lower abdomen. Using this tissue, the breast reconstruction can usually be done without a silicone breast implant. The TRAM flap is also indicated when the opposite breast is attractive and there are hopes of matching it with the replacement of tissue. The symmetry obtained with this operation when there is a significant tissue deficit can be excellent. This TRAM flap procedure is versatile, and the large amount of skin and fat provides tissue for achieving symmetry within a broad range of shapes and sizes of the opposite breast.

Careful patient selection is necessary for the TRAM flap in order to avoid serious potential complications. Heavy radiation to the base of the flap or to the mediastinum, or surgical division of the superior epigastric artery pedicle can lead to flap necrosis. Obese patients, patients older than 65 years, and those with problems with their microcirculation, such as diabetes mellitus, should usually be reconstructed with other methods. Long-term cigarette smoking over one pack per day for 20 years has an acute and chronic effect on the microcirculation and the reliability of the flap is reduced in these patients. The TRAM flap location is often the tissue usually discarded during the aesthetic abdominoplasty.

Complications of the TRAM flap such as flap necrosis and fat necrosis are primarily related to poor vascular perfusion. Abdominal wall complications develop when there is a protrusion of the intra-abdominal contents against the weakened abdominal wall. A secure abdominal closure, enhanced when necessary with Prolene mesh, usually avoids this problem. If protrusion occurs, the abdominal wall is plicated and this closure is supported with Prolene mesh.

The use of microsurgery can give the TRAM flap additional versatility. The deep inferior epigastric artery is dissected and is used to revascularize the flap to the vessels in the axilla. This technique requires excellent experience and technique, and is currently being done in a few centers.

Breast Reconstruction with the Latissimus Dorsi

When the implant and expander type of breast reconstructions are not sufficient to provide a satisfactory breast reconstruction, tissue needs to be brought to the breast region in the form of a flap. When the opposite breast is attractive and symmetry with this breast is the goal of breast reconstruction, a flap is often necessary. A donor scar either on the back or lower abdomen may be preferred to a scar on an attractive opposite breast.

The latissimus dorsi provides skin to supplement any missing skin, and its muscle can cover a silicone breast implant. This often leads to a softer and more natural breast reconstruction. This flap is a good choice when a flap is needed and the patient is interested in axillary fill or has had a radical mastectomy. It can provide additional fullness in the lower outer quadrant of a breast reconstruction and add ptosis to the final reconstruction.

The volume of the latissimus dorsi flap gives fullness in the lower portion of the breast reconstruction. After a modified radical mastectomy, the latissimus dorsi muscle is used to give coverage for the breast implant. Usually the skin island is positioned in the opened mastectomy scar or when it is low it is placed through a separate oblique incision in the lower outer quadrant of the reconstructed breast.

Complications after the latissimus dorsi flap include partial or total flap necrosis. The incidence of total flap necrosis has been less than 1%, and partial necrosis less than 5%. Seroma of the back donor site is the most common problem and is seen in 20% of the operations. This is one of the most predictable and reliable flaps for breast reconstruction.

Gluteus Maximus Musculocutaneous Flap and Microsurgical Transfer

When autogenous tissue is needed and other flap techniques are not suitable, the breast can be reconstructed with tissue from the buttocks. Many women have an excess of tissue in this area. The technique uses autogenous tissue, usually without the need for an implant, and provides an attractive result. The donor scar is either on the buttocks or in the lower buttocks crease.

The tissue needed for the breast reconstruction is designed and planned on the buttocks region. The flap is elevated on its vascular pedicle and transferred to the breast region. The vessels of the breast area are prepared in the axillary region and the inferior gluteal artery is anastomosed to the internal mammary artery. Breast reconstruction with this microvascular technique is highly refined and technically demanding. Success requires a successful anastomosis of the vessels and maintenance of patency in the postoperative period. Failure of nourishing blood flow can result in death of the tissues unless the flow is reinstated.

Reconstruction of the Nipple-Areola

Nipple-areola reconstruction is done after there is symmetry in the reconstructed breasts. The position, size, shape, and projection of the opposite nipple-areola is the model for the reconstruction. The patient can help determine the nipple-areola position.

Nipple reconstruction is done with donor material in the region of the nipple either on the flap skin or the mastectomy skin. The skate flap is elevated in the deep dermis and is based on the central blood flow into it through a central fat and subcutaneous pedicle. Often the areola can be tattooed later and a graft is not needed. When there is the need for a graft for the areola, the diameter of the areola graft should be identical to the recipient site so that it does not distort the new areola.

When the opposite nipple is larger than can be produced with the local flap techniques, it is a good choice both for color match, texture, and symmetry.

Selected Bibliography

1. Davis JH (ed): Clinical Surgery. CV Mosby, St. Louis, pp 1358–1390, 1987.
2. Holleb AI: The American Cancer Society Cancer Book. Doubleday and Co., New York, 1986.
3. Harris JR, Hellman S, Henderson IC, Kinne D: Breast Diseases. JB Lippincott Co., Philadelphia, 1987.
4. Fisher B, Redmond C, Poisson R, Margolese R, et al: Eight-year results of a randomized clinical trial comparing total mastectomy and lumpectomy with or without irradiation in the treatment of breast cancer. N Engl J Med 1989; 320:822–828.
5. Bostwick J: Plastic and Reconstructive Breast Surgery. Quality Medical Publishing Co., St. Louis, 1990.
6. Pearl RM, Wisnicki J: Breast reconstruction following lumpectomy and irradiation. Plast Reconstr Surg 1985; 76;83–86.
7. Berger K, Bostwick J: A Woman's Decision: Breast Care, Treatment and Reconstruction. CV Mosby, St. Louis, 1984.
8. Noone RB, et al: Patient acceptance of immediate reconstruction following mastectomy. Plast Reconstr Surg 1982; 69:632.
9. Little JW, Golembe EV, Fisher JB: The "living bra" in immediate and delayed reconstruction of the breast following mastectomy for malignant and non-malignant disease. Plast Reconstr Surg 1981; 68: 392.
10. Dick GO, Brown SA: Breast reconstruction using modified tissue expander. Plast Reconstr Surg 1986; 77:613–619.
11. Bostwick J: (ed)? (eds?) Breast reconstruction using modified tissue expansion for matching a small opposite breast. In: Perspectives in Plastic Surgery, Vol. 1:1. Quality Medical Publishing Co., St. Louis, pp 79–92, 1987.
12. Becker H: Breast reconstruction using an inflatable breast implant with detachable reservoir. Plast Reconstr Surg 1984; 70:678.
13. Dinner MI, Dowden RV, Scheflan M: Refinements in the use of the transverse abdominal island flap for postmastectomy reconstruction. Ann Plast Surg 1983; 11:362.
14. Biggs TM, Cronin ED: Technical aspects of the latissimus dorsi flap in breast reconstruction. Ann Plast Surg 1981; 6: 381.
15. Shaw WW: Breast reconstruction by superior gluteal microvascular free flaps without silicone implants. Plast Reconstr Surg 1983; 72:490–499.
16. Truppman ES, Ellenby JD: A 13-year evaluation of subpectoral augmentation mammaplasty. In: Owsley JQ Jr, RA Peterson (eds.) Symposium on Aesthetic Surgery of the Breast. Mosby, St. Louis, pp 341–343, 1978.

17. Anderson DE, Badzioch MD: Bilaterality in familial breast cancer patients. Cancer 1985; 56:2092.
18. Woods JE, Irons GB, Arnold PG: The case for submuscular implantation of prostheses in reconstructive breast surgery. Ann Plast Surg 1980; 5:115.
19. Little JW, Spear S: Nipple-areola reconstruction. In: Perspectives in Plastic Surgery, Vol. 2:1. Quality Medical Publishing Co., St. Louis, 1988.

25

Prophylactic Mastectomy: An Assessment of the Key Factors Involved in Decision-Making

Joel Lundy

Introduction

If one takes a "pro" position for prophylactic mastectomy, then an intellectually honest statement must precede any discussion. There are no absolute indications for this operation. Decision-making is based upon a clear understanding that there is no controlled study that has been done to show that survival, the true "punch line," is altered by prophylactic removal of the breast.

This being the case, then the relative indications are based on (1) a thorough assessment of risk factors, (2) a clear understanding by the patient of those findings that indicate a "high risk" of developing a breast cancer, (3) an assessment of the psychological makeup of the patient, and (4) a detailed discussion of all options available.

The purpose of this chapter will be to define what is known about risk factors, i.e., who is the high-risk patient, and to put into perspective options of dealing with some of these difficult problems.

Patients Who Have Had Breast Biopsies for Benign Disease

It has been stated in several studies that patients who have had breast biopsies for benign disease are at increased risk of developing a breast cancer.[1-3] This statement needs to be examined in a very critical manner. Does sclerosing adenosis carry the same risk as atypical duct hyperplasia?

From: Wise L, Johnson H Jr (eds): *Breast Cancer: Controversies in Management.* Futura Publishing Company, Inc., Armonk, NY, © 1994.

Perhaps the most comprehensive series of studies on patients with benign breast biopsies was done by Dupont and Page.[4-6] Almost 4,000 patients underwent follow-up for a median of 17 years. Patients with no proliferative changes (i.e., fibroadenoma, sclerosing adenosis, papillary apocrine change, cysts, and mild hyperplasia) had no greater absolute risk of developing cancer over this time period than age-matched controls (i.e., about 2%). This group represented almost 70% of all biopsies done for benign disease. The group with proliferative disease without atypia (an additional 25% of all biopsies) had only a small increase in absolute risk to 4%.

The group with atypical duct or atypical lobular hyperplasia represented only about 3.5% of all biopsies performed. This group had an absolute risk of cancer of 8% over the 15-year time period involved. It should be pointed out that cancers in patients with atypia have about an equal chance of appearing in the contralateral breast.[7] To put the high-risk group (i.e., atypia) into perspective, women with carcinoma in situ would have a 20% risk of developing invasive cancer over this same time period.

The conclusion to be drawn from the data available is that atypia alone is not a significant enough risk factor to warrant prophylactic mastectomy. Also, unless other factors are present, patients who have had a previous benign breast biopsy that does not show atypia require no intensive type of follow-up.

Carcinoma in One Breast

It is recognized that carcinoma in the ipsilateral breast puts one at increased risk for carcinoma in the contralateral breast. Reviews by Robbins and Berg, as well as other investigations, indicate that the incidence of second contralateral primary cancers is essentially constant and does not show any tendency to increase or decrease with the follow-up period.[8-10] This rate is a little less than 1% annually, or expressed as about seven cancers per 1,000 patients at risk per year. For a period of 10 years, 1,578 patients were followed who were enrolled in the National Surgical Adjuvant Breast Project (NSABP) B-04 protocol.[11] There was a 4.2% incidence of clinically metachronous second breast cancers; 3.7% were invasive and 0.5% were in situ. Importantly, estimated survival following the first cancer in patients with bilateral cancer was similar to patients with unilateral disease only. Specific histologic types of cancer (excluding lobular carcinoma in situ, LCIS) do not serve as a significant enough discriminant to warrant prophylactic mastectomy. This includes lobular invasive or tubular cancers that are claimed to be predictors of bilaterality. Familial occurrence of breast cancer (other than strictly defined genetic breast cancer) does not serve as such a discriminant. Although the risk has been stated to increase when the patient gets the first cancer before age 40, other data does not confirm this finding.[11,12]

Finally, since according to Fisher et al., 80% of second cancers are found within 5 years of the first cancer, there is a reasonable possibility that these are truly synchronous tumors.[11] Evidence to support this view also comes from the increased incidence of synchronous cancers being detected by modern technique mammography of the contralateral breast.[12]

In conclusion, as an isolated risk factor this can be looked at in the following way:

1. Improved mammography has resulted in an increase in the detection of synchronous cancers.

2. The risk of developing a second (or contralateral) breast cancer is not exceedingly high and warrants only close follow-up by physical examination and mammography.

3. Routine contralateral biopsy is not indicated in the absence of physical or mammographic findings. This will not aid in patient selection for prophylactic mastectomy.

4. There are no solid data to indicate that overall survival is affected by the development of contralateral cancer.

Lobular Carcinoma In Situ

This clinical entity was first described by Stewart and Foote in 1941.[13] Lobular carcinoma in situ (LCIS) represents only about 25% of all in-situ cancers. There are really two hypotheses that have been advocated to describe the biological behavior of this entity. The first states that if followed long enough, LCIS progresses to invasive lobular cancer. The second views LCIS not as a precursor lesion but as a marker, indicating that the patient is at high risk of development of a de novo breast cancer.

Natural history studies of this entity are not extensive, they are all retrospective, and the methodology is less than ideal. However, as a basis for decision-making, the following facts are suggested. LCIS is a multicentric lesion found in 60% to 85% of mastectomy specimens in which the operation was performed for this diagnosis.[14] Five percent will have invasive cancer if mastectomy is performed on the ipsilateral side. Bilaterality of LCIS is seen in 35% to 50% of cases. If patients are followed with this diagnosis (rather than an ipsilateral mastectomy done at the time of diagnosis), about 25% of patients will develop an invasive cancer over a 20-year period.[15–18] However, two factors are significant in this regard. Almost an equal number of cancers will be found in the contralateral breast. Also, most of these cancers will be infiltrating duct, *not* infiltrating lobular. Thus, the second hypothesis, i.e., that LCIS is a biological marker, is suggested from the above data. More importantly, the logic of unilateral "prophylactic" mastectomy is flawed in a disease with an equal propensity to occur in an ipsilateral or a contralateral breast. There is no histologic marker to indicate which breast will get the cancer. Preventive therapy here takes on a "radical" look and must be weighed in the light of overall risk, as will be explained later in the chapter.

Lumpectomy with axillary dissection is not a viable alternative in LCIS. You should not expect to get margins free in this multicentric entity and really cannot equate it with duct carcinoma in situ (DCIS). The incidence of positive axillary nodes is extremely rare.

Duct Carcinoma In Situ

Screening studies have taken a relatively uncommon lesion in the past (0.8–5.0% of all breast cancers) and pushed it into the limelight to account for 15% to 20% of breast cancers.[19,20] In contrast to older studies in which DCIS was frequently a larger gross (palpable) tumor, the most recent studies find these tumors often as small, nonpalpable mammographically detected lesions. There is very limited data on the latter in terms of natural history.

Older natural history studies are based upon patients followed who had biopsy alone. Two such studies have identified patients with DCIS found during a histologic review of biopsies originally called benign. In patients followed for a mean of 6.1 years, Page noted ipsilateral invasive breast cancer in 7 of 28 patients.[22] In patients followed for an average of 9.7 years, Rosen reported 8 of 30 (27%) who developed invasive cancers. In such studies, several aspects are important.[23] First, no attempt was made on the initial biopsies to obtain cancer-free margins. Secondly, the invasive cancers were found at or near the original biopsy site.

The gold standard for DCIS has traditionally been total mastectomy. Recurrence rates are less than 3% and survival rates approach 100%.[16,21,24] Nobody would argue that axillary dissection is an unnecessary component of the operation. If one is dealing with DCIS without microinvasion, retrospective data indicate in series such as Kinne's an incidence of axillary metastases of less than 1% (1/128).[25]

The argument thus centers on whether or not total mastectomy is required as "prophylaxis," i.e., to prevent invasive cancer from developing in the DCIS patient. What data are available to indicate which patients can have breast conservation with DCIS? No controlled studies are available to answer this question. NSABP protocol B-17 will hopefully give us the answer in a few years.

Until such information is available, retrospective data tell us the following. Lagios' studies indicate that the extent of DCIS should be a major consideration in selecting patients for breast conservation. Multicentric foci of DCIS were present in 54% of cases in which the primary lesion was *greater than* 25 mm, but only 14% of cases in which the lesions were *less than* 25 mm. Foci of invasive carcinoma were present in mastectomy specimens in 46% of cases in which DCIS was *greater than* 25 mm but in none of the cases in which DCIS was 25 mm or smaller.[26]

In the NSABP protocol B-06 (total mastectomy, excision plus radiation versus excision alone for the treatment of T1, T2 invasive breast cancer), 78 cases of DCIS were retrospectively evaluated.[27] Twenty-nine were treated by excision and radiation therapy and 22 by excision alone. The average size of tumors was

2.2 cm, and only one was picked up by mammography alone. With a mean follow-up of less than 4 years, 7% recurred in the excision/radiation therapy group and 23% in the excision alone group. Similar studies on palpable DCIS with short-term follow-up show recurrence rates of 5% to 10%.[28,29] In many studies, margins were not evaluated. In some studies, 50% of the recurrences were invasive.[30]

Where does this leave us with DCIS today? Clearly, total mastectomy should not be uniformly applied to DCIS. If patients have limited DCIS with clear margins of excision, and a postoperative mammogram that shows no residual calcification, the option of breast conservation should be offered, or the patient should be considered a candidate for the NSABP B-17 protocol. Total mastectomy does have a place in the armamentarium of treatment for DCIS. In such cases, total mastectomy is really "prophylactic," in that it prevents the development of invasive cancer. DCIS is a precursor lesion (although not obligate in 100% of cases) and the invasive cancers do occur in the ipsilateral breast. Bilaterality of DCIS is less than 5%.

Nonhistologic Risk Factors

The Family History

Terms need to be clarified when dealing with the genetics of breast cancer in order to more accurately quantify risk. There is familial breast cancer and hereditary breast cancer. They are not synonymous, but both are associated with an increased cancer risk.

Lynch defines hereditary breast cancer as a pattern of cancer distribution in a family compatible with segregation of an autosomal dominant disease susceptibility gene.[31] Hereditary breast cancer is characterized by (1) early age of onset (average age 40–45), (2) transmission through three generations, (3) an excess of bilaterality (approaching 50%), and (4) association with other cancer syndromes (i.e., breast and ovary, etc.). Familial breast cancer involves two or more first-degree relatives in a family with breast cancer, without the other described characteristics.[31] The genetics of familial breast cancer are not well understood. However, a first-degree relative of an affected individual has about three times the lifetime risk of getting breast cancer as a patient with no familial background.

In the studies of Dupont and Page, having a single first-degree relative with breast cancer resulted in only a modest twofold increase in "relative risk" over a 15-year period of observation.[4]

It behooves the physician to document (with a careful nuclear pedigree and pathological confirmation) the family cancer history. Patients with hereditary breast cancer should have prophylactic mastectomy as an available option, particularly if they have cancer in one breast and are young.

Interaction of Risk Factors

Can we say that risk factors are synergistic, additive, or multiplicative? It is difficult to quantitate risk in this fashion. However, in a retrospective study such as that of Page, an interaction was seen with atypia and family history.[4] The relative risk of atypia was 4.5, of family history 2, and if a patient had both, the relative risk was 9. This translated into an actual risk of almost 20% of getting an invasive breast cancer over a 15-year period (at least equivalent to the risk associated with DCIS). However, other epidemiologic factors such as age of first pregnancy or nulliparity had no such interaction to increase the risk of atypia. In fact, first pregnancy before age 20 reduced the risk of atypia.

The Operation

Does prophylactic subcutaneous or total mastectomy reduce the cancer incidence to zero? The answer is clearly no, and facts will be given to support this. In addition, if any breast tissue remains, isn't it subject to the same risk as the breast tissue removed? If you remove 95% of the breast tissue, is the corresponding risk of cancer reduced by 95%?

In C3H mice, spontaneous mammary tumors develop with increasing age. If you perform unilateral mammectomy or bilateral mammectomy, the tumor incidence is the same as controls.[32] It is probably not possible to remove all mammary tissues in these animals, and the residual breast tissue would actually appear to have a relative increased risk of tumorogenesis.

In the human, it has been shown that it is extremely difficult, even with "total" mastectomy, to remove all breast tissue.[33,34] The largest series of prophylactic mastectomy reported shows a less than 1% incidence of invasive cancer developing with a short follow-up (less than 10 years) in relatively young patients.[35] This suggests that the incidence will be higher with long-term follow-up.

Conclusions

There are select circumstances under which prophylactic mastectomy should be offered as an option to a patient. A young woman with a documented history of genetic breast cancer falls into this category. Even if the risk is not reduced to zero, you are starting with a risk of 50%. If a 35-year-old patient has lobular carcinoma in situ, and her mother died at age 50 of breast cancer and a sister had breast cancer at age 40, bilateral mastectomy should be offered as an option. It is difficult to quantitate interaction of risk factors in this setting, but common sense would indicate that this is a "high-risk" patient. She is also in an age group where mammography may not be helpful in finding an early cancer, and she has many years "at risk" for developing an invasive cancer.

There are patients with duct carcinoma in situ who cannot have breast conservation, and total mastectomy is the treatment of choice, not just to clear the DCIS, but also to prevent the future development of an invasive cancer.

The patient who has had multiple biopsies for fibrocystic disease and now has a cosmetically distorted breast and fear of cancer falls into a different category. In the absence of premalignant histology, she may warrant prophylactic mastectomy on a cosmetic and/or a psychological basis.

If prophylactic mastectomy is offered as an option, it must be clearly explained to the patient that (1) survival differences have never been shown in controlled studies, (2) it is not possible to reduce the cancer incidence to zero, and (3) if the patient is in a "high-risk" categorys long-term follow-up is still required after prophylactic mastectomy, as residual breast tissue may remain even after "total" mastectomy.

References

1. Ernster VL: The epidemiology of benign breast disease. Epidemiol Rev 1987; 3:184–202.
2. Love SM, Gelman RS, Silen W: Fibrocystic "disease" of the breast: a non-disease? N Engl J Med 1982; 307:1010–1014.
3. Davis HH, Simons M, Davis JB: Cystic disease of the breast: relationship to carcinoma. Cancer 1964; 17:957–978.
4. Dupont WD, Page DL: Risk factors for breast cancer in women with proliferative breast disease. N Engl J Med 1985; 312:146–151.
5. Page DL, Dupont WD, Rogers LW, Rados MD: Atypical hyperplastic lesions of the female breast: a long-term follow-up study. Cancer 1985; 55:2698–2708.
6. Dupont WD, Page DL: Breast cancer risk associated with proliferative disease, age at first birth and a family history of breast cancer. Am J Epidemiol 1987; 125:769–779.
7. Black MM, Barclay THC, Cutler SJ, Hankey BF, et al: Association of atypical characteristics of benign breast lesions with subsequent risk of breast cancer. Cancer 1972; 29:338–343.
8. Robbins GF, Berg JW: Bilateral primary breast cancers: a clinicopatholgic study. Cancer 1964; 17:1501–1527.
9. Bailey MJ, Royce C, Sloane JP, Ford HT, et al: Bilateral carcinoma of the breast. Br J Surg 1980; 67:514–516.
10. Leis HP: Bilateral breast cancer. Surg Clin N Am 1978; 58:833–841.
11. Fisher ER, Fisher B, Sass R, Wickerham L: Pathologic findings from the National Surgical Adjuvant Breast Project (protocol No. 4). XI Bilateral breast cancer. Cancer 1984; 54:3002–3011.
12. Chaudary MA, Millis RR, Hoskins EOL, Haldes M, et al: Bilateral primary breast cancer: a prospective study of disease incidence. Br J Surg 1984; 71:711–714.
13. Foote FW, Stewart FW: Lobular carcinoma in situ. Am J Pathol 1941; 17:491–495.
14. Schwartz GF, Feig SA, Patchefsky AS: Significance and staging of non-palpable carcinomas of the breast. Surg Gynecol Obstet 1988; 166:6–10.
15. Ringberg A, Palmer B, Linell LF: The contralateral breast at reconstructive surgery after breast cancer operation: a histopathologic study. Breast Cancer Res Treat 1982; 2:151–161.
16. Farrow JH: The James Ewing lecture: current concepts in the detection and treatment of the earliest of the early breast cancers. Cancer 1970; 25:468–477.
17. Rosen PP, Seine R, Schottenfeld D, Ashikari R: Noninvasive breast carcinoma: frequency of unsuspected invasion and implications for treatment. Ann Surg 1979; 189:377–382.

18. Carter D, Smith RRL: Carcinoma in situ of the breast. Cancer 1977; 40:1189–1193.
19. Rosner D, Bedwani RN, Vana J, Baker HW, et al: Noninvasive breast carcinoma: results of a national survey by the American College of Surgeons. Ann Surg 1980; 192:139–147.
20. Baker LH: Breast Cancer Detection Demonstration Project: five-year summary report. CA 1987; 32:194–225.
21. Ashikari R, Huvos AG, Snyder RE: Prospective study of non-infiltrating carcinoma of the breast. Cancer 1977; 39:435–439.
22. Page DL, Dupont WD, Rogers LW, Landenberger M: Intraductal carcinoma of the breast: follow-up after biopsy only. Cancer 1982; 49:751–758.
23. Betsill WL Jr, Rosen PP, Lieberman PH, et al: Intraductal carcinoma: long-term follow-up after treatment by biopsy alone. JAMA 1978; 239:1863–1867.
24. Sunshine JA, Moseley HS, Fletcher WS, et al: Breast carcinoma in situ: a retrospective review of 112 cases with a minimum 10-year follow-up. Am J Surg 1985; 150:44–51.
25. Kinne DW, Petrek J, Osborne MP, et al: Breast carcinoma in situ. Arch Surg 1989; 124:33–36.
26. Lagios MD, Westdahl PR, Margolin FR, et al: Duct carcinoma in situ: relationship of extent of occult invasion, multicentricity, lymph node metastases, and short-term treatment failures. Cancer 1982; 50:1309–1314.
27. Fisher ER, Sass R, Fisher B, et al: Pathologic findings from the National Surgical Adjuvant Breast Project (protocol No. 6). I. Intraductal carcinoma (ductal carcinoma in situ). Cancer 1986; 57:197–208.
28. Recht A, Danoff BS, Salin LJ, et al: Intraductal carcinoma of the breast: results of treatment with excisional biopsy and irradiation. J Clin Oncol 1985; 3:1339–1343.
29. Montague ED: Conservation surgery and radiation therapy in the treatment of operable breast cancer. Cancer 1984; 53(Suppl 3):700–704.
30. Gallagher WJ, Koaner FC, Wood WC: Treatment of intraductal carcinoma with limited surgery: long-term follow-up. J Clin Oncol 1989; 7:376–380.
31. Lynch HT: The family history and cancer control: hereditary breast cancer. Arch Surg 1990; 125:151–152.
32. Nelson H, Miller SH, Buck D, et al: Effectiveness of prophylactic mastectomy in the prevention of breast tumors in C3H mice. Plast Reconst Surg 1989; 83:662–669.
33. Goldman LD, Goldwyn RM: Some anatomic considerations of subcutaneous mastectomy. Plast Reconst Surg 1973; 51:502–508.
34. Holleb A, Montomery R, Farrow JH: The hazard of incomplete simple mastectomy. Surg Gynecol Obstet 1965; 121:819–820.
35. Pennisi VR, Capozzi A: Subcutaneous mastectomy data: a final statistical analysis of 1500 patients. Anesth Plast Surg 1989; 13:15–21.

26

Does Prophylactic Mastectomy Have a Significant Role in the Management of Breast Cancer?

Mary Jane Houlihan, William Silen

Introduction

The use of prophylactic mastectomy for the prevention of invasive breast cancer depends upon the physician's concepts of the disease and the patient's perspective of the chances for her to develop breast cancer. While the place of prophylactic mastectomy may change in the future, in our opinion it has a small role in the management of the patient with breast cancer and should be employed only after serious consideration.

Historical Perspective

Prior to the 1890s, most women with breast cancer inevitably developed large ulcerated, infected tumors prior to their death. In the 1890s, a presumably logical concept about the spread of breast cancer emerged, i.e., that the malignancy was initially confined to the breast with a subsequent orderly spread to the axillary nodes and, finally, it spread systemically. Halsted, Meyer, and others reasoned that if an operation could encompass the tumor, its surrounding apparently normal tissues, and the axillary nodes, breast cancer could be cured. In 1894, Halsted[1] reported that radical mastectomy had resulted in a local recurrence rate of only 6%, a remarkable improvement over previous treatments. Because of this achievement as well as the seeming logic of this treatment, radical mastectomy became the treatment of choice for the next 50 to 60 years. Once the possibility of "cure" with radical mastectomy became apparent, the concept of possibly prevent-

From: Wise L, Johnson H Jr (eds): *Breast Cancer: Controversies in Management.* Futura Publishing Company, Inc., Armonk, NY, © 1994.

ing breast cancer by prophylactic removal of the breast began to evolve. While radical mastectomy for the treatment of breast cancer left a large cosmetic defect and frequent functional loss due to the development of a "frozen" shoulder or chronic lymphedema, a prophylactic mastectomy required removal of the breast alone, sparing arm function, and providing a better cosmetic result. It was reasoned that if women at high risk of developing breast cancer could be identified, these patients could be offered an operation that would be both lifesaving and less debilitating. Prophylactic mastectomy thus became an integral part of the management of breast cancer, at least as practiced by some, for the next 60 years.

Since the 1970s and 1980s, much has changed in the understanding and the management of breast cancer. As breast-conserving operations have been shown to be comparable to radical mastectomy for the local regional control and survival of most patients with invasive breast cancers, patients and physicians have questioned the need for a more radical procedure such as mastectomy to effect prophylaxis. At a time when women are choosing breast-conserving procedures for clinically documented cancers, the argument for prophylactic mastectomy becomes difficult. There probably remains a small place for mastectomy to protect against potential future cancer, and this chapter will define the circumstances under which it remains an option for the high-risk patient.

Risk Factors for Development of Breast Cancer

A high risk for the future development of breast cancer is the only logical reason to consider prophylactic mastectomy. The estimation of this risk is influenced by a variety of clinical factors including the family history, a prior history of breast cancer, the presence of carcinoma in situ or benign proliferative lesions, the ease with which the breasts can be evaluated by physical examination and mammography, and the individual woman's perceptions about her own breast or breasts.

Family History

A family history of breast cancer has for many years been recognized as a risk factor for the development of breast cancer. Observations prior to the 20th century that certain families had a higher incidence of breast cancer among female members than the general population led to studies in this century that have better defined the influence of a family history of breast cancer. While many authors have proposed that a family history of breast cancer increases the chances of developing cancer by two-to fourfold over those in the general population,[2-7] these data do not take into consideration the many factors that influence risk in an individual patient. Recent studies have reported a difference in risk assessment based on a number of variables, including the relation of affected family members, the number of affected family members, whether the disease is premenopausal or postmenopausal, and whether it is unilateral or bilateral. Table 1 lists the frequency and relative risk of breast cancer when one

Table 1
Frequency of Breast Cancer When a Single Family Member is Affected

	Relative at Risk	Total Familial Incidence (%)	* Control Incidence (%)	Relative Risks (Total: Control)
Anderson	mother	3.7%	4.6%	0.8 ± 1.8
	sister	6.2%	2.3%	2.8 ± 1.5
	daughter	3.7%	0.8%	5.1 ± 3.0
	Total first-degree relatives	4.9%	2.7%	1.8 ± 1.4
Adami et al.	mother	3.8%	2.7%	1.4
	sister	3.8%	1.9%	2.1
	daughter	0.5%	0.2%	2.4
	Total first-degree relatives	2.9%	1.6%	1.7

*Control = no family member with breast cancer.
Adapted from Anderson[6] and Adami et al.[7]

family member is affected. Relative risk ranges from one to five depending upon whether the relative is a mother, sister, or daughter. In the Anderson[6] and Adami et al.[7] studies, the respective control values of 2.7% and 1.6% were less than the usual frequency of 6% to 7% cited for the general population, but may be accounted for by the fact that the controls had not lived their theoretical full 83-year life span. If a second-degree relative (grandmother, aunt, first cousin) was affected, Adami et al.[7] reported a relative risk of only 1.5. However, when two or more first-or second-degree relatives have breast cancer, risk may be increased fivefold or greater.[6,8,9] These figures are difficult to validate because neither study has a large number of families with multiple affected members.

A number of reports have suggested that premenopausal breast cancer and bilateral disease are both associated with an increased incidence of breast cancer in first-degree relatives in comparison with a control population. The frequency of breast cancer in premenopausal women with bilateral disease in the Anderson study of familial breast cancer was 32-fold in excess of older controls.[8] Adami et al.,[7] however, were unable to confirm in their studies that young age or bilateral disease were associated with an increased risk of familial breast cancer.

The frequency of a family history of breast cancer in women with established breast cancer may also shed some light on the influence of a family history of the disease. In a study by Lynch et al.,[9] only 18% of the women had a close relative with breast cancer. Thus, for the majority of women, the absence of a family history of breast cancer suggests that genetic factors may be of relatively little importance. For women who have a family history of breast cancer, risk is influenced by a number of factors.[10,11] The risk for a woman with a single postmenopausal relative with unilateral breast cancer is near that of the general population, whereas a history of two or more relatives with premenopausal bilateral breast cancer increases the risk to almost 50%. Clearly, the considerations for prophylactic mastectomy in these two subsets of patients would be very different.

A strong genetic effect has been recognized in some rare syndromes. Cowden's disease (multiple hamartomas syndrome) is transmitted as an autosomal dominant trait.[12] Hyperkeratotic cutaneous and gingival lesions are markers of the disease. There is a high frequency of breast cancer at an early age in the affected women. In one family kindred reported by Walton et al.,[13] 10 of 21 women had developed breast cancer at the median age of 36 years.

Muir's syndrome[14,15] is characterized by polyps and adenocarcinomas of the gastrointestinal tract, skin tumors, and breast cancers in female family members. It has been suggested that these breast cancers usually occur at a postmenopausal age, but the relative lifetime risk is still not known. Muir's syndrome is inherited as an autosomal dominant trait.

Li-Fraumeni syndrome[16] is transmitted as an autosomal dominant trait and is characterized by a predisposition to a number of malignancies including sarcoma, brain tumor, leukemia, lung cancer, and breast cancer. In some pedigrees, breast cancer is the predominant phenotype.

For the woman with a high-risk family history or the woman who is a member of a cancer syndrome family, prophylactic mastectomy is an option. If prophylactic mastectomies are to be considered or performed on the basis of a strong family history of breast cancer, that history must be confirmed. In the past, mastectomies were occasionally performed for an erroneous frozen section diagnosis of breast cancer and at other times for lobular carcinoma in situ, not now considered an invasive lesion, or even for benign disease. Patients and families often erroneously assumed that if a mastectomy had been performed, cancer must have been present. In addition, women with a factitious family history have sometimes requested prophylactic mastectomy (Munchausen's syndrome).[17] Frequently these women are cancerophobic and have underlying psychological problems. By documenting the family history, error may be avoided.

It is important to emphasize that the vast majority of women who develop breast cancer do not have a family history of breast cancer. For those women who do have a single first-degree family member with breast cancer, the risk of developing breast cancer over a lifetime appears to be 8% to 9%, a number that in our opinion does not warrant prophylactic mastectomy. For the small percentage of women who are at an increased risk of developing breast cancer because there are multiple family members with premenopausal and/or bilateral breast cancer, or for those with a strong family history who are desirous of avoiding the constant emotional turmoil of doubt, prophylactic mastectomy should be included in management options.

Prior History of Contralateral Breast Cancer

A number of studies have demonstrated that a woman who has had one breast cancer is at increased risk of developing a second breast cancer in her contralateral breast, not surprising since the breasts are paired organs presumably under similar genetic, hormonal, and environmental influences. Despite many studies, no clear consensus has been reached as to the risk for the contralateral breast. Even the definition of contralateral breast cancer has varied, making comparison among studies difficult.

In the first detailed study of contralateral breast cancer, Kilgore[18] recognized the importance of distinguishing between a new primary cancer and metastatic disease. He defined a new primary cancer as arising in the absence of metastases in other parts of the body and running a clinical course similar to that of the first primary cancer. Robbins and Berg[19] distinguished primary from metastatic disease on the basis of a number of pathological factors: (1) metastases usually occur in the fat surrounding the breast parenchyma, whereas primary cancers arise in the glandular breast parenchyma; (2) metastases tend to be multiple, whereas primaries are usually single; (3) histologically, metastases grow in an expansile fashion, while a stellate pattern is characteristic of new primaries; and (4) metastases are not usually associated with adjacent in-situ carcinomas, whereas new primaries might have an in-situ component. Others[20] have suggested that a new primary is more likely if the interval between the first and second tumor is 5 years or longer. Mider et al.[21] proposed that the location in the breast might be of value in making this distinction, and that medial lesions were to be considered metastatic unless of a different histologic type than the original lesion. Fisher et al.[22] have pointed out that the gross, pathological, and mammographic features of primary versus metastatic disease are overlapping and, in the past, criteria to determine second primary cancers have frequently been too restrictive.

The reported incidence of contralateral breast cancer may underestimate the true incidence because of an overestimation of the incidence of metastases. The reported incidence of contralateral breast cancer ranges from 3% to 6%[18,19,21–25] (Table 2). Viewed in another way, this frequency is about three to six times greater than that of expected cases in the general population (Table 3).

A number of different factors affect the risk of developing contralateral breast cancer. In their detailed clinicopathological study of 1,458 women with breast cancer, Robbins and Berg[19] found that women 28 to 52 years old comprised 59% of their series and were responsible for 77% of the contralateral cancers. Multicentric breast cancer in the first breast was also associated with an increased risk of contralateral breast cancer. Patients with earlier-stage cancers were also more likely to live longer and be at greater risk of developing a contralateral cancer.[18,19] Fisher et al.[22] examined the potential predictive value of 32 pathological and clinical features for the development of contralateral breast cancer. Factors found to increase the risk of a contralateral breast cancer were tumors greater than 3 cm in size, proliferative benign breast lesions in association with the primary tumor or in other parts of the breast, multicentric breast cancer, the absence of histiocytosis, the presence of tubular and lobular invasive histologic types, and the presence of lobular carcinoma in situ in the vicinity of the dominant mass. While Anderson[8] demonstrated an increased incidence of bilateral breast cancer in the family members of women with breast cancer, Fisher et al.[22] and Adami et al.[7] failed to demonstrate a similar risk.

Table 2
Incidence of Cancer in the Second Breast

Author/Reference	No. of Patients	No. of Patients with Contralateral Breast Cancer	Incidence in %	Follow-up (Years)
Kilgore[18]	1,100	37	7.3%	15
Ryan et al.[23] (1935–1953)	8,396	272	3.2%	
Mider et al.[21] (1932–1939)	941	59	6.2%	
Hubbard[24] (1932–1939)	272	17	6.2%	10
Robbins, Berg et al.[19] (1940–1943)	1,458	91	6.2%	20
Fisher et al.[22] (1971–1974)	1,578	66	4.2%	9.6
Egan[25] (1967–1973)	1,112	67	6.2%	

Table 3
Incidence of Contralateral Breast Cancer

Author/Reference	Incidence Rates %	Controls
Kilgore[18]	4.0	
Hubbard[24]	5.8	Connecticut Tumor Registry general population
Mider et al.[21]	3.5	New York State Department health data
Robbins and Berg et al.[19]	4.8	Connecticut Tumor Registry general population
Ryan et al.[23]	5.3	Connecticut Tumor Registry general population

Although a consensus cannot be developed from the various studies regarding the definition of bilateral breast cancer or the subgroups at highest risk of developing contralateral breast cancer, the data suggest that the contralateral breast of a woman with breast cancer is at greater risk of developing breast cancer compared to breasts of women in the general population. The NSABP study[22] found that the overall survival of women with breast cancer is not influenced by the development of contralateral breast cancer. In that study, the second primary was at a comparable or earlier stage to the initial breast cancer. This and other more recent studies imply that contralateral breast cancers can be detected at an earlier stage by placing women who have had a prior cancer under closer surveillance with more frequent physical examinations and regular mammograms. Studies by Egan,[25] Senofsky et al.,[26] and Mellinick et al.[27] have examined the role of mammography in the detection of contralateral breast cancer. Egan[25] found that a population of 1,112 patients with breast cancer who had had at least one mammographic study had a higher incidence of smaller simultaneous bilateral tumors but no difference in axillary node status when compared to historical controls reported by Robbins and Berg in the premammographic era. Senofsky et al.[26] compared 496 women from 1969 to 1975 in the premammographic era to 559 women from 1977 to 1984 followed with mammography. He found only an 11% incidence of stage III or IV breast cancer in the contralateral breast of the mammography group compared to a 36% incidence in the premammography group. In a study of 1,291 women, Mellinick et al.[27] showed improvement in the early detection of contralateral breast cancer when a routine of regular mammography and physical examination was compared to regular physical examination alone. Although the incidence of contralateral cancers was comparable in the two groups (3%), 75% were axillary node-negative in the mammography/physical examination group compared to 57% in the physical examination only group. These data suggest that a routine of regular mammography and careful physical examination would lead to the earlier detection of contralateral breast cancer with improved survival. However, all of these studies suffer from relatively small numbers of patients, the use of historical controls,[25,26] and a short follow-up time.[27] Therefore, firm conclusions cannot be reached with certainty.

The use of random biopsy of the contralateral breast at the time of operative treatment of the affected breast has been advocated as a technique to discover early contralateral breast cancer. Urban et al.[28] felt that the 6% incidence of contralateral breast cancer reported in the literature and his own 12.5% incidence of simultaneous breast cancers justified biopsy of the contralateral breast. Urban "removed" 20% to 25% of the upper outer portion of the contralateral breast and the mirror-image area at the time of mastectomy. Of 1,204 patients available for study, 954 biopsies were performed, of which 301 were truly random. The remaining 653 had clinical signs suggesting an abnormality. Cancer was demonstrated in 7.6% of the random biopsies but 6.0% of these were of the noninfiltrating type (Table 4). Twenty of 278 patients who had an initial negative contralateral breast biopsy subsequently developed a contralateral breast cancer. At the time of diagnosis 50%

Table 4

Biopsy of the Contralateral Breast at the Time of Mastectomy, 1,204 cases, 80% biopsy rate

Number of Biopsies	Cancer Infiltrating	Noninfiltrating
301 Random	5	18
	(1.6%)	(6.0%)
653 Clinical signs of abnormality	50	44
	(7.6%)	(6.7%)

Adapted from Urban JA et al.[28]

were axillary node-positive and only 10% had noninvasive breast cancer. The impact of random biopsy on subsequent survival was not reported. King et al.[29] found five contralateral cancers (4.6%) of which one was invasive and four were noninvasive among 109 patients who had contralateral biopsies. Although none of the lesions were palpable, the infiltrating cancer was suspected on the mammogram. Based upon this experience, biopsy of the contralateral breast in a random fashion was discontinued by King et al.[29]

In the absence of definitive data with regard to outcome, a number of approaches have been developed to manage potential contralateral breast cancers: (1) perform a contralateral prophylactic mastectomy at the time of mastectomy for primary breast cancer, (2) random biopsy of the contralateral breast with subsequent mastectomy if contralateral cancer is found at the time of biopsy, (3) prophylactic mastectomy 2 to 3 years after initial mastectomy if a patient has an ongoing favorable prognosis, and (4) close follow-up.[30-36]

We have favored close follow-up, but counsel patients about the option of prophylactic mastectomy and biopsy. In most cases, we recommend a semiannual physical examination and a yearly mammogram. Patients receiving systemic therapy as part of their initial treatment are examined more frequently. Biopsies are dictated by abnormal findings on either physical examination or mammogram. Rarely, we perform a prophylactic contralateral mastectomy on a woman who has several risk factors such as multicentric disease, lobular carcinoma in situ, multiple family members with breast cancer, especially if the patient is extremely concerned about her contralateral breast. Random biopsy of the contralateral breast is discouraged if the breast examination and mammogram are normal. Our policies are based upon the assumption that most contralateral breast cancers will be detected as either noninvasive lesions or in an early stage by close follow-up and will not impact upon survival.

Carcinoma In Situ

In the days of radical mastectomy, the use of the term *carcinoma*, whether invasive or in situ, meant that the patient would undergo a radical mastectomy. It was taught that invasion would always be found if the pathological examination was sufficiently compulsive. Twenty-five years ago, the diagnosis of noninvasive carcinoma was given to about 3% of patients with cancer, whereas today the incidence is as high as 20%. In our opinion, it is likely that many of the long-term cures attributable to radical mastectomy were in patients with what today would be regarded as noninvasive carcinomas. Total mastectomy has been shown to cure virtually 100% of patients with carcinoma in situ (Table 5). There are two types of carcinoma in situ that are reasonably distinct clinically and microscopically, lobular carcinoma in situ, and ductal carcinoma in situ.

Lobular carcinoma in situ (LCIS) is usually an incidental finding at biopsy performed for either a palpable mass or a mammographic abnormality. Without any further treatment, subsequent cancer will develop in 16.3% of women over a 15-year period (Table 6). The cancers do not arise adjacent to or in the prior

Table 5
Mastectomy for Carcinoma In Situ

Author/ Reference	No. of Patients	Type of Carcinoma In Situ	Follow-Up (Years)	Local Recurrence	Survival
Ashikari et al.[30]	74	ductal	11	0	100%
Sunshine et al.[31]	68	ductal	10	0	95%
Farrow[32]	181	ductal	5.2	2	98%
Kinne et al.[33]	31	lobular	11.5	0	100%

Table 6
Subsequent Invasive Cancers in Patients with Lobular Carcinoma In Situ

Author	No. of Patients	Cancers During Follow-Up			Total	Years of Follow-Up
		Ipsilateral	Contralateral	Bilateral		
Haagensen et al.[34]	210	16	17	3	36 (17.1%)	14
Wheeler et al.[35]	38	1	3	0	4 (10.5%)	15
Total	248	17 (6.8%)	20 (8.1%)	3 (1.2%)	40 (16.3%)	

Adapted from Houlihan and Goldwyn.[35]

biopsy site as would be expected with a precancerous lesion, but rather develop in either breast and are more likely to be infiltrating ductal carcinomas rather than infiltrating lobular carcinomas. Thus, in our opinion and in that of most authorities, LCIS should be considered a histologic marker of an increased risk to develop breast cancer rather than a precancerous lesion itself.

Management of LCIS has varied from bilateral mastectomies, to unilateral mastectomy with mirror-image biopsy of the contralateral breast (and subsequent mastectomy if positive), to close observation. The only logical alternatives in our opinion are either bilateral prophylactic mastectomies or close observation with semiannual breast examinations and annual mammograms. Haagensen[37] noted that the rate of observed to expected cases of breast cancer in patients with LCIS was 6.9% to 1.0%. The risk ratio is similar to that of women whose mothers had had bilateral breast cancer. Since mastectomy is not generally advocated for the latter group, Haagensen[37] advocated a policy of observation for women with LCIS as well. We concur with the policy of close surveillance for patients with LCIS. Prophylactic mastectomies for LCIS in our institution are reserved for women who strongly request this option.

Ductal carcinoma in situ (DCIS) is a heterogeneous lesion whose biological behavior is not completely understood. DCIS has a number of histologic patterns: comedo, solid, cribriform, papillary, and micropapillary. All of these forms of DCIS are thought to be premalignant, i.e., they have the potential to become infiltrating carcinomas if left untreated. DCIS is thought to arise in a duct, and some believe that it extends along that ductal system. Most DCIS lesions are discovered as a result of excision of a nonpalpable mammographic lesion, although occasionally a mass is the presenting sign. The mammographic abnormality is usually a discrete cluster of microcalcifications involving less than 1 cm of tissue but in some instances extensive involvement of a quadrant, half, or all of a breast may be encountered. The goal in management is to excise all DCIS with a margin of healthy surrounding breast tissue, achieving a postoperative magnification mammogram that demonstrates no residual microcalcifications.[38] Wide excision with or without radiotherapy may be done for relatively limited DCIS, but partial or total mastectomy may be required for more extensive lesions (Tables 5, 7).

In our practice, the management of ductal carcinoma in situ is guided by the principle that complete excision of the lesion is desirable if not mandatory. If complete excision requires the removal of the breast, or so much of it that there will be a marked deformity, mastectomy is recommended. Such a mastectomy is regarded as therapeutic rather than prophylactic. In patients with small lesions (1–2 cm) and in whom clear margins can be achieved without gross deformity of the breast, observation is usually recommended. Where there is a strong desire for conservation of the breast, radiotherapy should probably be added to excision, especially if tumor-free margins are difficult to achieve.

Ductal carcinoma in situ confers an increased risk to the contralateral breast similar to that of a patient with invasive carcinoma.[39–47] We follow the guidelines for management of the contralateral breast previously outlined in the section *Prior History of Contralateral Breast Cancer.*

Table 7
Results of Treatment for DCIS

Author	No. of Patients	Treatment	Recurrence	Follow-Up (Years)
Ashikari et al.[30]	112	TM	1 (0.9%)	
Fisher et al.[40]	27	TM	0 (0%)	
Rosner et al.[41]	182	TM	19 (10.4%)	
Recht et al.[42]	40	WLE + XRT	4 (10%)	3 8/12
Montague et al.[43]	56	WLE + XRT	2 (3.6%)	4
Zafrani et al.[44]	54	WLE + XRT	4 (7.4%)	5
Solin et al.[45]	261	WLE + XRT	28 (16%)	10
Lagios et al.[46]	79	WLE	8 (10%)	3 8/12
Carpenter et al.[47]	28	WLE	5 (18%)	5

DCIS = ductal carcinoma in situ; TM = total mastectomy; WLE = wide local excision; XRT = radiation therapy.

Benign Breast Lesions

The relationship between benign breast lesions and breast cancer has been muddled and misunderstood. Fibrocystic disease, cysts, fibrosis, papillomas, and other benign breast lesions have at one time or another been considered either precancerous or markers of increased risk of breast cancer. In either case, these lesions were frequently used to justify prophylactic mastectomies. Love and Silen[48] have questioned the value of the term *fibrocystic disease* since it added little if at all to the management of women with breast problems. They felt that the term *fibrocystic disease* was so nonspecific that it should be abandoned. In reality, until recently, little was known about the natural history of benign breast disease. Fibrocystic disease was a term used for widely different clinical presentations ranging from breast pain to gross cystic disease. Also included in the diagnosis were the pathological diagnoses of papillomatosis, apocrine metaplasia, ductal hyperplasia, sclerosing adenosis, fibroadenoma, and others. In 1986, the College of American Pathologists issued a consensus statement about benign diseases and the risk of subsequent breast cancer[49] after study of a large number of surgical biopsies.

Breast lesions were grouped into three categories: no increased risk, slightly increased risk of 1.5 to 2 times, and moderately increased risk of 4 to 5 times (Table 8). A moderately increased risk (atypical ductal or lobular hyperplasia) was one-half that of a woman with in-situ carcinoma. Pathologists continue to refine their criteria and to modify their classifications.

Some investigators feel that the risk after 15 years actually decreases, and thus the assumption that the risk remains constant after 15 years may overestimate an individual woman's risk.[50] Dupont and Page[51] reviewed more than

---

Table 8
Relative Risk of Subsequent Breast Cancer in Patients with Benign Breast Biopsies
(Compared to General Population)

No Increased Risk

adenosis	*fibroadenoma*
apocrine metaplasia	*fibrosis*
cysts: micro and/or macro	*mastitis*
hyperplasia: mild	*periductal mastitis*
duct ectasia	*squamous metaplasia*

Slightly Increased Risk *(1.5–2 times)*
hyperplasia: moderate or florid, solid or papillary
papilloma with fibrovascular core
well-developed sclerosing adenosis

Moderately Increased Risk *(4–5 times)*
atypical hyperplasia: ductal or lobular

From Page and Dupont.[50]

10,300 benign breast lesions and found that most women with benign breast lesions were not at increased risk for the development of subsequent breast cancer. Patients with an atypical proliferative lesion such as atypical ductal and lobular hyperplasia exhibited a risk 5.3 times that of those with nonproliferative lesions in the absence of a family history, and 11 times greater with a family history (Table 9).

Since nearly 70% of women with prior benign breast biopsies are not at any increased risk of subsequent breast cancer, a benign biopsy should reassure the patient rather than suggest any radical prophylactic surgical procedure (Table 10). For the small number of women with a family history of breast cancer and a biopsy that demonstrates an atypical proliferative lesion, close surveillance rather than prophylactic mastectomy is recommended.

Miscellaneous

Prophylactic mastectomy has been recommended in the past and even today for indications ranging from "lumpy breasts" too difficult to examine, to breasts

Table 9
Effect of Family History and Atypical Proliferative Lesions on
Subsequent Development of Breast Cancer

Numerator of Relative Risk	Denominator of Relative Risk	Relative Risk
PDWA/no FH	Non-PD/no FH	1.9
PDWA/(+) FH	Non-PD/(+) FH	2.0
PDWA/(+) FH	Non-PD/(−) FH	2.7
AH/no FH	Non-PD/no FH	4.3
AH/(+) FH	Non-PD/(+) FH	8.4
AH/(+) FH	Non-PH/(−) FH	11.0

From Dupont and Page.[51] PDWA = proliferative disease without atypia; Non-PD = nonproliferative disease; AH = atypical hyperplasia; FH = family history.

Table 10
Relative Risk of Breast Cancer

Diagnosis	No of Biopsies	% of Benign Lesions	Relative Risk	Absolute Risk—15 Yrs.
Nonproliferative Disease	7,221	69.7	0.89	2%
Proliferative Disease without Atypia	2,768	26.7	1.6	4%
Atypical Hyperplasia	377	3.6	4.0–6.5	
Total	10,366	100%		

Adapted from DuPont and Page.[51]

with marked tissue defects due to many biopsies for benign disease, to abnormal Wolfe mammographic patterns. In these patients, mastectomy is being recommended for what we consider dubious indications.

The 'Difficult Breast'

The degree of difficulty in clinical evaluation is related to the experience and expertise of the examiner. Many women have been deformed by repeated biopsies for clinically palpable benign irregularities, on occasion prompting the suggestion that a mastectomy be done because of the difficulty in assessing breasts with multiple defects and scars. Physicians who feel uncomfortable with the burden of following "difficult breasts" should refer such patients to clinicians willing to accept this responsibility. There are, however, some with especially firm breast tissue and an uninterpretable mammogram due to the excessive density of their breasts that make clinical surveillance difficult if not nearly impossible. The care of these women must be individualized. Prophylactic mastectomy is an option for such a patient who has already had breast cancer, has a strong family history of breast cancer, or a diagnosis of LCIS or atypical hyperplasia, but we recommend this only with the greatest reluctance.

Wolfe Patterns

With the advent of screening mammography, attempts have been made to correlate certain mammographic patterns with the risk of developing breast cancer. In 1976, Wolfe established a classification system that grouped women's breasts into four separate categories based upon mammographic appearance[52,53] (Table 11). Using a case control method study of mammograms taken within 8 weeks of surgery, Wolfe established the N1 pattern as normal and the DY pattern as most likely to be associated with an increased risk of developing breast cancer—37 times greater than the normal pattern.[53]

Depending upon a woman's body habitus, age, and menopausal status, the proportion of fat and mammary glandular tissue varies. Since breast cancers arise in mammary glandular tissue rather than fat, it is not surprising that the incidence of breast cancer might be increased in areas of mammographic nodular densities compared to fat. Wolfe's N1 pattern may be the norm in postmeno-

---

Table 11
Wolfe Pattern: Mammographic Density and Risk of Breast Cancer

N1	Breast with almost all fat – "normal."
P1	Fatty breast with nodular densities occupying less than 25% of the breast.
P2	Fatty breast with nodular densities more than 25% of the breast.
DY	Diffuse density of the breast.

Adapted from Saftlas.[53]

pausal, obese women, but the DY pattern is more likely to be found in the young, nulliparous woman. Since the incidence of breast cancer increases with age, it is difficult to ascribe a particular Wolfe pattern to increased risk for breast cancer. Furthermore, recent studies[52] show that while there is a somewhat increased incidence of cancer in patients with the DY pattern, differences in risk among the different Wolfe patterns are not so distinctive that patients should either be overly frightened or reassured by a particular mammographic pattern. Prophylactic mastectomies based upon Wolfe patterns are not warranted.

Cancerophobia

Cancerophobia is defined by psychiatrists as "the negative reaction to cancer in our society that often makes it the object of excessive fear..." Transient cancerophobia may be a response to a specific event, such as a cancer death in the family, or may develop when new staff begin work on a cancer ward, or when close friends develop malignancy. Fixed cancerophobia ranges from a neurotic symptom to a hypochondriacal fixation, an obsession or a somatic delusion. It is associated with a broad spectrum of diagnoses, and management depends upon making the appropriate diagnosis.[54] To the clinician, cancerophobia implies that a patient has such an excessive fear of developing cancer that this phobia impinges adversely on life, causing insomnia, eating disorders, and interpersonal strife. Whether cancerophobia should ever be an indication for prophylactic mastectomy is a difficult question that should be considered on a patient-by-patient basis. Psychiatric consultation in conjunction with medical review of risk factors is mandatory before prophylactic mastectomies are recommended. Such instances should be extremely rare.

Choice of Procedure

If a prophylactic mastectomy is indicated, it should, in our opinion, be a total mastectomy rather than a subcutaneous mastectomy. A total mastectomy removes the nipple-areolar complex, all breast tissue, and pectoralis major fascia. Skin flaps should be reasonably thin because breast tissue is commonly present in close approximation to the skin.[55] Subcutaneous mastectomy unfortunately preserves both the nipple-areolar complex and pectoralis fascia. Breast tissue is regularly left beneath the nipple[55,56] and with the pectoralis fascia[57] after subcutaneous mastectomy. Since breast cancer may arise in the residual breast tissue, complete prophylaxis is not achieved, and there are reports of patients who have developed breast cancer years after undergoing subcutaneous mastectomy.[36,58]

Animal studies have given additional support to total mastectomy rather than subcutaneous mastectomy for prophylaxis of breast cancer. Jackson et al.[59] and Wong et al.[60] found that the risk of breast cancer induced by dimethylbenzanthracene in rats was not reduced by removal of portions of the breast. Nelson et al.[61] confirmed this finding in a spontaneously occurring mouse mammary cancer. Total mastectomy, which aims to remove all of the breast tissue by the construction of thin skin flaps, the removal of the nipple-areolar complex, and pectoralis major fascia, is the only truly prophylactic operation if prophylaxis is deemed appropriate. Although subcutaneous mastectomy still has some advocates, the use of the procedure for prophylaxis has declined and probably should be eliminated completely.

In recent years, we have found that most women who have prophylactic mastectomy also desire reconstruction. The choice of the timing of the reconstruction (immediate or delayed) and the type of reconstruction is made by the patient in consultation with the reconstructive surgeon.

Conclusion

Specific guidelines and indications for prophylactic mastectomy cannot be defined with confidence at this time. Risk factors and emotional considerations must be weighed in each individual patient. When prophylactic mastectomy is deemed advisable or appropriate, total mastectomy is the only reasonable operation. Hopefully, tests will become available which better define high-risk women who might benefit from prophylactic mastectomy. In concert with these, it would be even more useful to have regimens that would reduce the risk of breast cancer in high-risk women, sparing them the possibility of prophylactic mastectomy. Studies testing the value of retinoids and tamoxifen for prophylaxis are now ongoing in Europe and the United States.

References

1. Halsted WS: The results of operations for the cure of cancer of the breast performed at Johns Hopkins Hospital from June 1889 to January 1894. Johns Hopkins Hosp Bull 1894–1895; 4:297.
2. Brinton LA, Williams RR, Hoover RN, et al: Breast cancer risk factors among screening program participants. J Natl Cancer Inst 1979; 62:37–43.
3. Hauge M, Marvald B, Fischer, et al: The Danish Twin Register. Acta Genet Med 1968; 17:315–331.
4. Henderson BE, Powell D, Rosario I, et al: An epidemiologic study of breast cancer. J Natl Cancer Inst 1974; 53:609–614.
5. Lilienfield AM: The epidemiology of breast cancer. Cancer Res 1963; 23:1503–1513.
6. Anderson DE: A genetic study of human breast cancer. J Nat Cancer Inst 1972; 48:1029–1034.
7. Adami HO, Hansen J, Jung B, Rimsten A: Characteristics of familial breast cancer in Sweden: absence of relation to age and unilateral versus bilateral disease. Cancer 1981; 48:1688–1695.
8. Anderson DE: Genetic study of breast cancer: identification of a high risk group. Cancer 1974; 34:1090–1097.
9. Lynch HT, Guirgis HA, Brodkey F, et al: Early onset of age in familial breast cancer. Arch Surg 1976; 111:126–131.
10. Harris RE, Lynch HT, Guirgis HA: Familial breast cancer: risk to the contralateral breast. J Natl Cancer Inst 1978; 60:955–960.

11. Lynch HT, Albano WA, Heieck JJ, et al: Genetics, biomarkers and control of breast cancer: a review. Cancer Genet Cytogenet 1984; 13:43–92.
12. Brownstein MH: Cowden's disease: a possible new symptom complex with multiple system involvement. Ann Int Med 1978; 48: 136–142.
13. Walton BJ, Morain WD, Baughman RD: Cowden's disease: a further indication for prophylactic mastectomy. Surgery 1986; 99: 82–86.
14. Muir EG, Yates-Bell AJ, Barlow KA: Multiple primary carcinomata of the colon, duodenum, larynx associated with keratatocanthomata of the face. Br J Surg 1966; 54:191–195.
15. Anderson DE: An inherited form of large bowel cancer, Muir's syndrome. Cancer 1980; 45:1103–1107.
16. Li FP, Fraumeni JF Jr: Soft-tissue sarcomas, breast cancer and other neoplasms: a familial syndrome? Ann Int Med 1969; 71: 747–751.
17. Grenga TE, Dowden RV: Munchausen's syndrome and prophylactic mastectomy. Plast Reconstruct Surg 1987; 80:119–120.
18. Kilgore AR: Incidence of cancer in second breast: after radical removal of one breast for cancer. JAMA 1921; 77:454–457.
19. Robbins GF, Berg JW: Bilateral primary breast cancers: a prospective clinicopathological study. Cancer 1964; 12:1501–1527.
20. Leis, HP Jr: Selective, elective prophylactic contralateral mastectomy. Cancer 1971; 28:956.
21. Mider GB, Schilling JA, Donovan JC, Rendall ES: Multiple cancer: a study of other cancers arising in patients with primary malignant neoplasms of the stomach, uterus, breast, large intestine, or hematopoietic system. Cancer 1959; 5:1104–1109.
22. Fisher ER, Fisher B, Sass R, et al: Pathologic findings from the National Surgical Adjuvant Breast Project (Protocol no. 4). XI. Bilateral breast cancer. Cancer 1984; 54:3002–3011.
23. Ryan RJ, Griswold MH, Allen EP, et al: Breast cancer in Connecticut, 1935–1953: study of 8,396 proved cases. JAMA 1958; 167: 298–307.
24. Hubbard TB: Non-simultaneous bilateral carcinoma of breast. Surgery 1953; 34:706–723.
25. Egan RL: Bilateral breast carcinomas: role of mammography. Cancer 1976; 38:931–938.
26. Senofsky GM, Wanebo HJ, Wilhelm MC, et al: Has monitoring of the contralateral breast improved the prognosis in patients treated for primary breast cancer? Cancer 1986; 57:597–602.
27. Mellinick WAM, Holland R, Hendriks JHCL, et al: The contribution of routine follow-up mammography to an early detection of synchronous contralateral breast cancer. Cancer 1991; 67:1844–1848.
28. Urban JA, Papachristou D, Taylor J: Bilateral breast cancer: biopsy of the opposite breast. Cancer 1977; 10:1968–1973.
29. King RE, Terz JJ, Lawrence W: Experience with opposite breast biopsy in patients with operable breast cancer. Cancer 1976; 37:43–45.
30. Ashikari R, Huvos AG, Snyder RE: Prospective study of non-infiltrating carcinoma of the breast. Cancer 1977; 39:435–439.
31. Sunshine JA, Moseley HS, Fletcher WS, Krippaehne WW: Breast carcinoma in situ: a retrospective review of 112 cases with a minimum 10-year follow-up. Am J Surg 1985; 150:44–51.
32. Farrow JH: Current concepts in detection and treatment of the earliest of the early breast cancers. Cancer 1970; 25:468–477.
33. Kinne DW, Petrek J, Osborne MP, et al: Breast carcinoma in situ. Arch Surg 1989; 124:33–36.
34. Haagensen CD, Lane N, Lattes, et al: Lobular neoplasia (so-called lobular carcinoma in situ) of the breast. Cancer 1978; 42:737–769.

35. Wheeler JE, Enterline HT, Roseman JM, et al: Lobular carcinoma in situ of the breasts: long-term follow-up. Cancer 1974; 34:554–569.
36. Houlihan MJ, Goldwyn RM: Role of prophylactic mastectomy. In: Stoll BA (ed). Approaches to Breast Cancer Prevention. Stoll BA (ed). Kluwer Academic Publishers, Dordrecht, p 139, 1991.
37. Haagensen CD: Diseases of the Breast, 3rd ed. W.B. Saunders, Philadelphia, p 269, 1986.
38. Schnitt SJ, Silen W, Sadowsky NL, et al: Ductal carcinoma in situ (intraductal carcinoma) of the breast. N Engl J Med 1988; 318: 898–903.
39. Ashikari R, Hajdu SI, Robbins GF: Intraductal carcinoma of the breast (1960–1969). Cancer 1971; 28:1182–1187.
40. Fisher ER, Sass R, Fisher B, et al: Pathologic findings from the National Surgical Adjuvant Breast Project (Protocol No. 6). I. Intraductal carcinoma (DCIS). Cancer 1986; 57:197–208, 1986.
41. Rosner D, Bedwani RN, Vana J, et al: Noninvasive breast carcinoma: results of a national survey by the American College of Surgeons. Ann Surg 1980; 192:139–147.
42. Recht A, Danoff BS, Solin LJ, et al: Intraductal carcinoma of the breast: results of treatment with breast biopsy and irradiation. J Clin Oncol 1985; 3:1339–1343.
43. Montague ED: Conservation surgery and radiation therapy in the treatment of operable breast cancer. Cancer (Suppl 3) 1984; 53:700–704.
44. Zafrani B, Fourquet A, Vilcog JR, et al: Conservative management of intraductal breast carcinoma with tumorectomy and radiation therapy. Cancer 1986; 57:1299–1301.
45. Solin LJ, Recht A, Fourquet A, et al: Ten-year results of breast-conserving surgery and definitive irradiation for intraductal carcinoma (ductal carcinoma in situ) of the breast. Cancer 1991; 68:2337–2344.
46. Lagios MD, Margolin FR, Westdahl PR, Rose MR: Mammographically detected duct carcinoma in situ: frequency of local recurrence following tylectomy and prognostic effect of nuclear grade on local recurrence. Cancer 1989; 63:618–624.
47. Carpenter R, Boulter PS, Cooke T, Gibbs NM: Management of screen detected ductal carcinoma in situ of the female breast. Br J Surg 1989; 76:564–567.
48. Love SM, Gelman RS, Silen W: Fibrocystic "disease" of the breast: a non-disease? N Engl J Med 1982; 307:1010–1014.
49. Winchester DP: Consensus statement: the relationship of fibrocystic disease to breast cancer. Bull Am Coll Surg 1986; 71: 29–31.
50. Page DL, Dupont WD: Histologic indicators of breast cancer risk. Bull Am Coll Surg 1991; 76:16–23.
51. Dupont WD, Page DL: Risk factors for breast cancer in women with proliferative breast disease. N Engl J Med 1985; 312:146–151.
52. Saftlas AF, Hoover RN, Brinton L, et al: Mammographic densities and risks of breast cancer. Cancer 1991; 67:2833–2838.
53. Wolfe JN: Risk for breast cancer development determined by mammographic parenchymal patterns. Cancer 1976; 37:2486–2492.
54. Kaplan HI, Sadock BJ (eds): Comprehensive Textbook of Psychiatry, V. Baltimore, pp 1253, 1989.
55. Goldwyn RM (ed): Plastic and Reconstruction Surgery of the Breast. Little, Brown, Boston, pp 441–454, 1976.
56. Menon RS, VanGeel AN: Cancer of the breast with nipple involvement. Br J Cancer 1989; 59:81–84.
57. Urbanski SJ, Temple WJ, Magi E: Is total mastectomy adequate for prophylactic procedure? Lab Invest 1986; 54:65A.
58. Eldar S, Mequid MM, Beatty JD: Cancer of the breast after prophylactic subcutaneous mastectomy. Am J Surg 1984; 148:692–693.

59. Jackson, CF, Palmquisr M, Swanson J, et al: The effectiveness of prophylactic subcutaneous mastectomy in Sprague Dawley rats with 7,12-dimethylbenzanthracene. Plast Reconstruct Surg 1984; 73:249–255, 256–260.
60. Wong JH, Jackson CF, Swanson JS, et al: Analysis of the risk reduction of prophylactic partial mastectomy in Sprague Dawley rats with 7,12-dimethylbenzanthracene induced breast cancer. Surgery 1986; 99:67–71.
61. Nelson H, Miller SH, Buck D: Effectiveness of prophylactic mastectomy in the prevention of breast tumors in C3H mice. Plast Reconstruct Surg 1989; 83:662–669.

The Role of Mammography

Editorial Commentary

Chapters 27–30

Professor Forrest describes the British system for screening and the significantly higher benign/malignant ratio in the biopsy rates in the United Kingdom versus the United States (0.61 vs. 3.9 in the HIP and 5.7 in the BCDDP trial). It is Professor Baum, however, who compares the cost benefit of screening for breast cancer in the UK and the US. Professor Baum, in his usual entertaining style, states that in his view the American Cancer Society's current recommendation for patients to have screening mammograms under age 50 is unwarranted, and even over age 50 not more than 1% of patients who undergo screening will benefit from it. The very small benefit resulting from cancer screening with mammography is further emphasized by Professor Wright from Canada; using the latest Canadian data (*Canada Med Assoc J* 1992; 147:1459) he also comes to the conclusion that mammography as a mass screening procedure should be abandoned. In contrast, although Dr. Feig agrees that the benefit with screening mammography in the 40–50 year age group is questionable, he feels that the value of mammographic screening is well justified in patients above the age of 50. I believe that the reading of these chapters should be mandatory for anybody who advocates the use of screening mammography.

27

The Mammographic Abnormality and Its Assessment

Sir Patrick M. Forrest

The United Kingdom Program

In February 1987, having considered a report from a Working Group (Forrest Report) set up by the Health Ministers of England and Wales, Scotland, and Northern Ireland, the United Kingdom government decided to introduce, as part of the National Health Service, a program for the early detection of breast cancer by mammographic screening.[1] This is now offered to women of 50 to 64 years of age who are invited by personal letter to attend for a single mediolateral oblique-view mammogram of each breast every 3 years at no personal cost. This service includes not only the basic screening mammogram, but provision for the assessment of those abnormalities detected by the screening mammogram, the performance of biopsies, their histopathological diagnosis, and the treatment of screen-detected cancers, with appropriate counseling and aftercare.[2] Although the target group is restricted to women of 50 to 64 years, older women can be screened on demand; but women under the age of 50 must be referred for mammography by their primary care physician, in UK terms, their general practitioner.

The program for mammographic screening is population-based. Screening centers equipped with dedicated mammographic equipment have been set up in cities, supported by mobile units that go out into the surrounding country towns. Films from mobile units are processed centrally in the urban screening center. As each mammographic X-ray unit can screen some 10,000 women each year, if there is 70% compliance, a single unit can serve 45,000 women in the target population. This is equivalent to a total population of one half of a million.

In the design of these centers care has been taken to ensure that surroundings are pleasant and attractive to the women so that acceptance of the invitation

From: Wise L, Johnson H Jr (eds): *Breast Cancer: Controversies in Management.* Futura Publishing Company, Inc., Armonk, NY, © 1994.

is encouraged. Training of all staff, including radiographers, has also been a priority. For this purpose, six training centers were set up. The attitude of the staff in the screening units also determines the acceptability of the procedure. Currently, 70% of over 1 million invited women in the UK have had their first screening and 65% have had a second screening.

The Basic Screen

It must be emphasized that a screening mammogram is not a diagnostic procedure. A radiologist, who under the national program is expected to read the mammograms of 5,000 to 6,000 women each year (to ensure quality), is asked only to record whether he or she believes a woman's mammogram to be normal, whether there is an abnormality, or whether the films are of insufficient quality to allow such an assessment to be made. Those women with an abnormal mammogram (or one of insufficient quality) must be recalled for further diagnostic tests, which include physical examination, additional X-rays, ultrasonography and, if indicated, fine-needle aspiration, which, if a lesion proves to be solid, is supported by aspiration cytology. In the UK screening service, these investigations are generally arranged in the main screening centers and their related National Health Service hospitals, by agreement with the women's general practitioners, who are happy to regard these further tests as an integral part of the screening service. But they are carried out not by an individual radiologist or surgeon but by a multidisciplinary team, equipped with the expertise and experience necessary to resolve the nature of a mammographic abnormality, preferably without the need for a surgical exploratory operation performed solely for diagnostic purposes.

Assessment of Abnormalities

Some abnormalities on a woman's single-view oblique mammogram, such as the composite shadow due to overlapping parenchymatous tissue, may cause a localized increase in density and this may require only an additional craniocaudal view to eliminate suspicion. But it has been accepted that a physical examination of the breasts should be performed on all recalled women. As in other European countries with national screening programs, a physical examination of the breasts is not part of the basic screening procedure, for provided the quality of mammography is high, this will detect less than 5% of additional cancers.[3] If both mediolateral oblique and craniocaudal views are used for the basic screen (as in the Netherlands), the additional detection rate of clinical examination is even less.

Should there be a discrete mammographic abnormality, it is critical to know whether this is physically palpable or not. For should that mammographic abnormality be associated with a palpable mass, its further investigation is no different from that of other women with a palpable abnormality in the breast.

Fine-needle aspiration is performed to determine whether the lesion is cystic or solid; if cystic, it is used to aspirate the fluid and, if solid, to obtain a specimen for cytology. A definitive diagnosis can be quickly established. A diagnostic operation is not required.

It is not necessary, nor a good use of surgical "time," that the physical examination of all recalled women be carried out by a surgeon; in most screening centers in the UK, the radiologist or a clinic doctor usually performs this task. But it is important that a surgeon should have the opportunity to examine all *solid* lesions before they are needle-aspirated, so that their size and clinical characteristics can be recorded. For this reason, most radiologists will perform an ultrasonic scan of a palpable mass, and only "needle" those that are demonstrably cystic.

The Nonpalpable Breast Abnormality

The ideal diagnostic objective for the nonpalpable mammographic abnormality is no different from that which is physically palpable. This is to reach a preoperative diagnosis, so that the number of *diagnostic* surgical operations can be reduced to a minimum. A diagnostic biopsy that reveals only benign change causes unnecessary physical stress and psychological anxiety for the patient and is wasteful of resources. Further, by distorting the breast tissues, a biopsy makes subsequent mammograms more difficult to interpret. In the United States, there may also be financial implications for the patient that are not evident in the UK scene. Reduction in the number of diagnostic surgical operations to a defined level of safety is an accepted objective of the UK national screening program.

In addition to diffuse asymmetry (usually due to overlapping parenchymatous tissues), nonpalpable mammographic abnormalities include three main groups of change. These are:

1. Opacities, i.e., discrete areas of increased density which are clearly delimited from surrounding breast tissue. Their border may be smooth and uniform (as in a benign cyst), spiculated and irregular (as in invasive cancer), or mixed.

2. Calcifications. Most are coarse, forming a round dense shadow within a lobule, an irregular "blob" within a fibroadenoma; crescent-shaped shadows in the wall of a cyst; or casts of ectatic ducts. These coarse calcifications are characteristic of benign disease and do not require further investigation. It is the fine, irregular, jagged, and sharp microcalcifications that are suspicious of malignancy. These may occur in clusters, may be diffusely scattered throughout a segment of the breast, or form fine linear branching shadows within ducts. Microcalcifications within an opacity are particularly suspicious of intraductal and invasive cancers.

3. An architectural abnormality distorting the parenchymal pattern of the breast. This may be associated with a small mass.

It is important that previous mammograms are available for review. The development of a new lesion or change in one already observed demands further investigation.

The investigation of these nonpalpable mammographic abnormalities is initially radiological. Ultrasonography is helpful in determining whether a small opacity is solid or cystic and, if cystic, to guide an aspirating needle into the lesion. It is not helpful in the differential diagnosis of calcifications, which, as they do not alter acoustic impedence, are not visualized. For further definition of the solid opacity, microcalcifications, and the architectural abnormality, magnification mammography is an essential investigation. Observation of the contour of a radiological opacity, the shape and pattern of microcalcifications, and the nature of an architectural abnormality allows the radiologist to determine the level of suspicion of malignancy. In a well-organized screening program, this is a matter for discussion with other members of the diagnostic team, including the surgeon, and should not be relegated to the generation of a formal written report upon which a surgeon unacquainted with the significance of these changes is expected to act. Yet this is accepted practice in countries without a formalized program of screening.

While the surgeon and radiologist together may decide whether or not a biopsy is indicated, their decision can be greatly simplified by collaboration with a cytologist, who will examine a specimen obtained by fine-needle aspiration. In many screening/assessment centers in the UK, a cytologist is a full member of the multidisciplinary assessment team. In order to obtain a fine-needle aspirate of a nonpalpable lesion, stereotactic radiology, with a computerized simulator, is used to localize the lesion and to guide the aspirating needle into it.[4] For success, this method of investigation requires dedication, skill, and regular experience. It should not be left in the hands of inexperienced and occasional practitioners. As the required equipment is expensive, it is justified only if regularly used.

The prime role of cytology is to confirm a diagnosis of cancer in a suspicious lesion. If it is confirmed that this contains malignant cells, the surgeon's task is greatly simplified, as the operation becomes one for the treatment of cancer, which will be performed only after further investigation of the patient and her counseling by skilled staff. The participation of the trained nurse counselor is now also regarded as an essential component of the UK screening program. Before stereotactic fine-needle aspiration cytology was available in our unit, it was routine that a woman in whom a *diagnostic* localization biopsy gave proof of cancer would require a second operation, either a wide local excision or a mastectomy. This approach was justified by our report of the finding of residual tumor in almost half (44%) of 144 patients in whom such second operations were performed.[5] Now that a preoperative diagnosis can be made in the majority of malignant nonpalpable lesions, a second operation is required only when histological examination of the excised cancer demonstrates its incomplete removal.

Stereotactic fine-needle aspiration cytology is of value not only in confirming malignancy. The demonstration of benign epithelial cells can support the radiologist in his/her view that a mammographic abnormality is benign. In a report from Stockholm, Sweden, 2,005 women with nonpalpable mammographic abnormalities, which neither radiologically or cytologically were regarded as suspicious of cancer, were observed over a period of 2 to 6 years. In only one patient had a cancer been falsely regarded as being benign.[6]

The Team Approach

It is apparent that, in the UK, the assessment of a nonpalpable mammographic lesion is not regarded as a procedure that can be left to the discretion of a radiologist or surgeon who is practicing as an individual. Rather, it is the responsibility of a multidisciplinary team, of which the surgeon, although important, is but one member. In our assessment center, it is a rule that the radiologist, the surgeon, and the cytologist together reach a decision, and if one of the team is convinced that the lesion is malignant and should be removed, they will follow through based on that decision.

The value of this team approach is obvious when one considers the biopsy rates and the ratio of benign to malignant histology in biopsies generated by mammographic screening. In both Holland and the UK, where the multidisciplinary assessment procedure is practiced, the biopsy rates are considerably lower than in the United States, where no such arrangements generally exist [7-10] (Table 1). Even before the availability of localization fine-needle aspiration cytology, the value of the stringent multidisciplinary approach was apparent to us. In a study of 434 localization biopsies for nonpalpable lesions, 304 generated from the screening clinic with its formal multidisciplinary procedure of assessment, and 130 from a symptomatic hospital clinic in which the decision to perform a biopsy was left to the attending surgeon who had the radiologist's report of the mammogram, the higher efficiency of the stringent assessment procedure was in no doubt (Table 2).

Table 1
Biopsy Rates on Prevalence Screen in USA, Holland, and UK

Screening Program	Age Group Years	Biopsy Rate per 1000 Screened	Benign:Malignant Ratio
USA			
HIP Trial	40–64	32.1	3.9
BCDDP	35–74	99.6	5.7
Holland			
Nijmegen	35–49	12.3	1.7
	50–64	16.2	0.8
UK			
NHS program	50–64	10.0	0.61

From references 7–10.

Table 2
Experience of 434 Localization Biopsies, Generated from Screening Clinics with Multidisciplinary Assessment and from Symptomatic Hospital Clinic (Surgical Decision)

	Screening Team	Symptomatic Breast Clinic
Number of biopsies	304	130
Malignant	108 (35.5%)	17 (13.1%)
Benign:malignant ratio	1.8 to 1	6.6 to 1

The addition of fine-needle aspiration cytology further reduces biopsy rates and the ratio of benign to malignant histology. In a recent Italian study,[11] it was reported that following the introduction of fine-needle aspiration cytology, the biopsy rate was reduced from 1.7:1 to 0.5:1.[12] But even more important is the ability to reach a preoperative diagnosis of malignancy and its implications for patient care.

Biopsy

As has been indicated, the number of diagnostic biopsies generated by a properly regulated screening program should be low. Biopsy of the nonpalpable lesion, like the assessment procedure, requires a multidisciplinary approach. In the UK program, the surgical member of the assessment team, together with the radiologist and pathologist, is responsible for performing biopsies on nonpalpable lesions requiring localization. Our preferred method of localization is the hooked wire designed by Frank.[13] This is inserted by the radiologist either freehand or using stereotactic guidance. Guidelines have been laid down for the technique of excision biopsy of nonpalpable lesions to ensure that the accuracy of placement of localization wires and care to excise minimal volumes of tissue are achieved.

Radiological Examination

Confirmation of excision of the lesion by specimen-mammography is an essential step, which is most conveniently performed on a dedicated apparatus (Faxitron) in the operating suite. Usually the lesion should be present in the first piece of tissue removed, but excision of a second or even third piece of tissue may be necessary (Table 3). Any palpable nodules within the breast tissue must also be removed. It was our experience that if the lesion was not seen on the specimen-mammogram after removal of a second piece of tissue, it was best to close the wound and perform a mammogram postoperatively, usually in 3 months' time, to determine if further exploration was necessary.[15]

Table 3

Outcome of 503 Localization Biopsies for Nonpalpable Mammographic Abnormalities:
Number of Attempts Required to Excise the Mammographic Abnormality

Abnormality Identified on Specimen Radiology	
In first piece of tissue	402 (79.9%)
In additional tissue	74 (14.7%)
TOTAL	476 (94.6%)
Abnormality Not Identified on Specimen Radiology	27 (5.4%)

From: Br J Surg 1990; 77:673–676, with permission.

Histopathological Examination

Strict guidelines have also been laid down for the histopathological examination of excised material.[14,16] The pathologist must obtain a fresh specimen so that it can be sliced, the slices X-rayed, and the area for examination defined. He/she may also wish to obtain an aspirate for immunocytochemical analysis of estrogen receptor.

Frozen-section examination has no place in the diagnosis of the small screen-detected lesion. Not only do these sections require careful preparation and evaluation, but review sessions, at which the pathologist discusses the findings with radiological and surgical members of the screening team, are critical to the maintenance of quality. In Edinburgh, these are held every 2 weeks and are attended by all members of the screening team.

Treatment

The objective of screening is to detect so-called "minimal" cancer, i.e., that which is noninvasive or, if invasive, is of nonpalpable size. In their initial report, Gallagher and Martin[17] described the threshold of minimal invasive cancer as being 0.5 cm in size or less (volume 0.125 mL), indicating that in such tumors the incidence of metastases in the axillary nodes was less than 10%. As a result of the findings in the Breast Cancer Detection Demonstration Project (BCDDP),[8] this threshold was increased to 1.0 cm. The survival for women with such "minimal" cancers is reported to be over 90% at 10 years.

Current reports of the two-counties trial in Sweden indicate the yield of "minimal" and node-negative cancers[18] in high-quality population screening (Table 4). It is generally considered that for the small noninvasive and invasive

Table 4
Cancers Detected Among Screened and Nonscreened Populations in the Two-Counties Trial in Sweden

| | Characteristics of Cancers in Swedish Trial | | | |
| | Size | | Node Status | |
Population	Number Detected	% Under 15 mm	Number Detected	% Node Negative
Controls	572	22.6	548	54.4
First screen	281	55.5	271	78.6
Later screens	373	53.3	380	84.2

From: NE Day, Br Med Bull 1991; 47:400–415, with permission.

cancers, mastectomy is not necessary. But the safety of local excision alone, i.e., without the administration of postoperative radiotherapy, is still a matter for debate. In the UK and Europe, as in the US, controlled randomized trials comparing local excision with and without radiotherapy are being carried out for ductal carcinoma in situ. In the trial currently in progress in the UK, women in each arm are being randomized into two groups, one of which will receive tamoxifen.[19]

For the small invasive cancer, controlled randomized trials of conservation therapy are also being mounted. One, in Sweden, in which cancers less than 2 cm in size are being treated by "sector resection" alone or resection with radiotherapy, has reported preliminary results (which are also now available from Milan)[20,21] (Table 5). Local relapse rates are greater in nonirradiated cases, but there is no evidence that they compromise survival. Further follow-up time is clearly required.

Not all "minimal" noninvasive and small invasive cancers can be treated safely by breast conservation regimes. Noninvasive cancers that extend widely within the breast and some biologically aggressive cancers may be better treated by mastectomy, but we need to know what is best; this requires further evidence from well-designed and carefully controlled clinical trials.

It is critical to avoid overtreatment of borderline lesions. The interpretation of noninvasive cancers and atypical hyperplastic lesions can be particularly difficult, and pathology review panels are a necessary part of screening programs. So also is the close monitoring of surgical procedures generated by screening programs. From a study of two in-patient operations in two regions in Sweden, it was apparent that although there is a "hump" of operations for cancer during the early years of a screening program, this is temporary and is not accompanied by any increase in benign biopsies.[22] Further, recent evidence from the screening program in the Netherlands does not indicate any degree of overtreatment.[23]

Table 5
Comparison of Treatment of Tumors Equal to or Less Than 2 cm in Size by Wide Local Excision (Sector Resection) Alone or the Same Procedure Followed by Radical Radiotherapy

Procedure	Number of Patients	Mean Follow-Up (months)	Local Relapse Rate
Sector resection alone	194	29.3 ± 2.4	7.6 (3.0–12.3)
Sector resection plus radical radiotherapy (54 Gy)	187	32.9 ± 2.2	2.9 (0.1–5.8)

From: J Natl Cancer Inst 1990; 82:277–282.

Conclusions

It is essential in a program of mammographic screening that risks do not outweigh benefits. Excessive numbers of unnecessary biopsies are a risk in poorly controlled screening programs. In the UK, biopsy rates and the ratio of benign to malignant biopsies are strictly monitored nationwide[10] (Table 6). The diagnosis and treatment of the nonpalpable mammographic lesion demand expertise and experience, which require the services of a multidisciplinary assessment team, whose members constantly keep their findings under critical review.

Table 6
Recent Results of the UK Screening Program

	First Screen	Second Screen
Number of patients invited	957,326	38,760
response to invitation (%)	71.4	65.5
recall rate (%)	7.1	4.9
biopsy rate (%)	1.0	0.5
Benign:malignant ratio	0.61	0.30
Cancer detection rate per 1,000 women screened	6.3	4.0
noninvasive ductal (%)	17.6	17.6
Invasive less than 1 cm (%)	20.9	20.6

From: National Screening Program News Release October 7, 1991.

References

1. Breast cancer screening: report to the Health Ministers of England, Wales, Scotland and Northern Ireland by a Working Group chaired by Sir Patrick Forrest. Her Majesty's Stationery Office, London, 1987.
2. Parliamentary Debates (Hansard), Vol 1, second series, Report of House of Commons, 25 February 1987.
3. Roberts MM, Alexander FE, Anderson TJ, Chetty U, et al: Edinburgh trials of screening for breast cancer. Lancet 1990; 335:241–246.
4. Bolmgrehn J, Jacobson B, Nordenstrom B: Stereotaxic instrument for needle biopsy of the mamma. Am J Radiol 1977; 129:121–125.
5. Aitken RJ, Macdonald HL, Kirkpatrick AE, Anderson TJ, et al: The outcome of surgery for nonpalpable lesions of the breast. Br J Surg 1990; 77:673–676.
6. Azavedo E, Svene G, Aner G: Stereotactic fine-needle biopsy in 2,594 mammographically detected nonpalpable lesions. Lancet 1989; 1:1033–1035.
7. Shapiro S, Venet W, Strax P, Venet L: Periodic screening for breast cancer. The Health Insurance Plan Project and its sequelae 1963–1986. John Hopkins University Press, Baltimore and London, 1988.
8. Seidman H, Gelb SK, Silverberg E, La Verola N, et al: Survival experience in the Breast Cancer Detection Demonstration Project. CA 1987; 37:258–290.

9. Peeters PHM, Verbeek ALM, Hendricks JHCL, van Bon MJH: Screening for breast cancer in Nijmegen: report of six screening rounds 1975–86. Int J Cancer 1989; 43:226–230.

10. National Breast Screening Program News Release. October 7, 1991.

11. Aitken RJ: Personal communication.

12. Ciatto S: Usefulness of needle aspiration in a screening program. In: Practical Modalities of an Efficient Screening for Breast Cancer in the European Community. International Congress Series 865. Excerpta Medica, Amsterdam, pp 83–94, 1989.

13. Frank HA, Hall FM, Steer ML: Preoperative localization of non-palpable breast lesions demonstrated by mammography. N Engl J Med 1976; 295:259–260.

14. Guidelines for Pathologists: Prepared by the Department of Health Royal College of Pathologists Working Party. NHS Breast Screening Programme, 1989.

15. Pathology Reporting in Breast Cancer Screening: Prepared by a Royal College of Pathologists Working Group. NHS Breast Screening Programme, 1989.

16. Anderson TJ: Breast cancer screening: principles and practicalities for histopathologists. Recent Adv Histopathol 1989; 14:43–61.

17. Gallagher HS, Martin JE: An orientation to the concept of minimal breast cancer. Cancer 1971; 28:1505–1507.

18. Day NE: Screening for breast cancer. Br Med Bull 1991; 47:400–415.

19. Protocol of the UK Randomised Trial for the Management of Screen-Detected Ductal Carcinoma in-situ (DCIS) of the Breast. NHS Breast Screening Programme, 1989.

20. The Uppsala-Orebro Breast Cancer Study Group: Sector resection with or without postoperative radiotherapy for stage I breast cancer. J Nat Cancer Inst 1990; 82:277–282.

21. Salvadori B, Saccozzi R: No radiotherapy following conservative surgery. Eur J Cancer 1991; Suppl 2:S18.

22. Holmberg L, Adami H-O, Persson I, Lundstrom T, et al: Demands on surgical inpatient services after mass mammographic screening. Br Med J 1988; 293:779–782.

23. Peeters PH, Verbeek AL, Straatman H, Holland R, et al: Evaluation of overdiagnosis of breast cancer in screening with mammography: results of the Nijmegen program. Int J Epidemiol 1989; 18:259.

28

Routine Mammographic Screening: Does It Reduce Mortality?

Stephen A. Feig

Introduction

Early detection affords a more favorable balance between tumor and host so that treatment will be more effective. Breast cancer survival depends on lesion size and lymph node status. Smaller lesions with no histologic evidence of axillary metastases have the best prognosis,[1-3] (Table 1). Screening mammography can frequently detect such early cancers, long before they are clinically palpable[4] (Table 2). Among the screening methods, mammography has a much lower detection size threshold and a better documented record of benefit than physical examination[5,6] or breast self-examination.[7]

Although there has been general agreement that such screening should be performed on women age 50 and older, some investigators have questioned the advisability of screening women between 40 and 50 years of age.[8,9] The reluctance to screen younger women may be partially attributed to concern about radiation risk. However, such risk is negligible or nonexistent at the low doses of current mammographic techniques.[10]

Skeptics also question whether early detection and increased survival necessarily result in mortality reduction.[11,12] This line of reasoning may be understood by means of the models seen in Figure 1 which show possible relationships of early detection to breast cancer mortality.

Model 1 depicts the classic description of the natural history of breast cancer. A tumor will grow over time and metastasis may occur after point A. In the absence of screening, the cancer will not be diagnosed until point C, usually as a chance discovery by the patient herself, less frequently by a physician after development of signs or symptoms.[13] At that time, more than 50% of patients have axillary node metastases on pathological examination. The true frequency

From: Wise L, Johnson H Jr (eds): *Breast Cancer: Controversies in Management.* Futura Publishing Company, Inc., Armonk, NY, © 1994.

Table 1
Relative Breast Cancer Survival (%) According to Pathological Stage of Disease and Method of Cancer Detection*

Pathological Stage of Disease	5-Year Survival	10-Year Survival	20-Year Survival
Minimal	98**	95**	93***
Negative nodes	85	74	62
Positive nodes	55	39	23
Distant metastases	10	2	0

*Data compiled from Wanebo et al.,[1] Frazier et al.,[2] NIH.[3]
**Five- and 10-year survival for minimal breast cancer as defined by Wanebo et al.[1]
***Twenty-year survival for minimal breast cancer as defined by Frazier et al.[2]

Table 2
Accuracy of Mammography and Physical Examination in Breast Cancer Screening According to Stage of Disease

	Percent Detection	
Stage of Disease	Mammography	Physical Examination
Minimal carcinoma	97	33
Negative nodes	92	51
Positive nodes	93	77

Source: Beahrs et al.[4]

of metastasis is even greater since over 70% of patients eventually die from the disease at point D.[13,14]

In model 2, the natural history of disease is altered by mammographic detection at point A prior to metastasis. Alternatively, for those who subscribe to the theory that breast cancer is a disseminated disease from time of inception, then point A could represent an early stage where the balance between tumor and host is still favorable to curative treatment. In both cases, a breast cancer death is averted or significantly postponed by early detection.

Model 3 postulates that metastases occur prior to detection by mammographic screening at point A. The patient will still die from her disease at time point D as in model 1. Actual survival is not prolonged, though it may seem to be since it is now measured as A to D rather than C to D. This model is known as the *lead time bias hypothesis* since it postulates that the lead time from screening (A to C) will not alter the predetermined time of the patient's demise.

Model 4 illustrates the *length bias hypothesis* which postulates the existence of slow-growing cancers that have little or no potential for metastatic spread. These nonaggressive lesions are presumed to have favorable survival rates even if they remain undetected in the absence of screening.

Finally, model 5 acknowledges that mammographic screening can detect cancers at an earlier stage (A) than is possible with clinical screening (B).

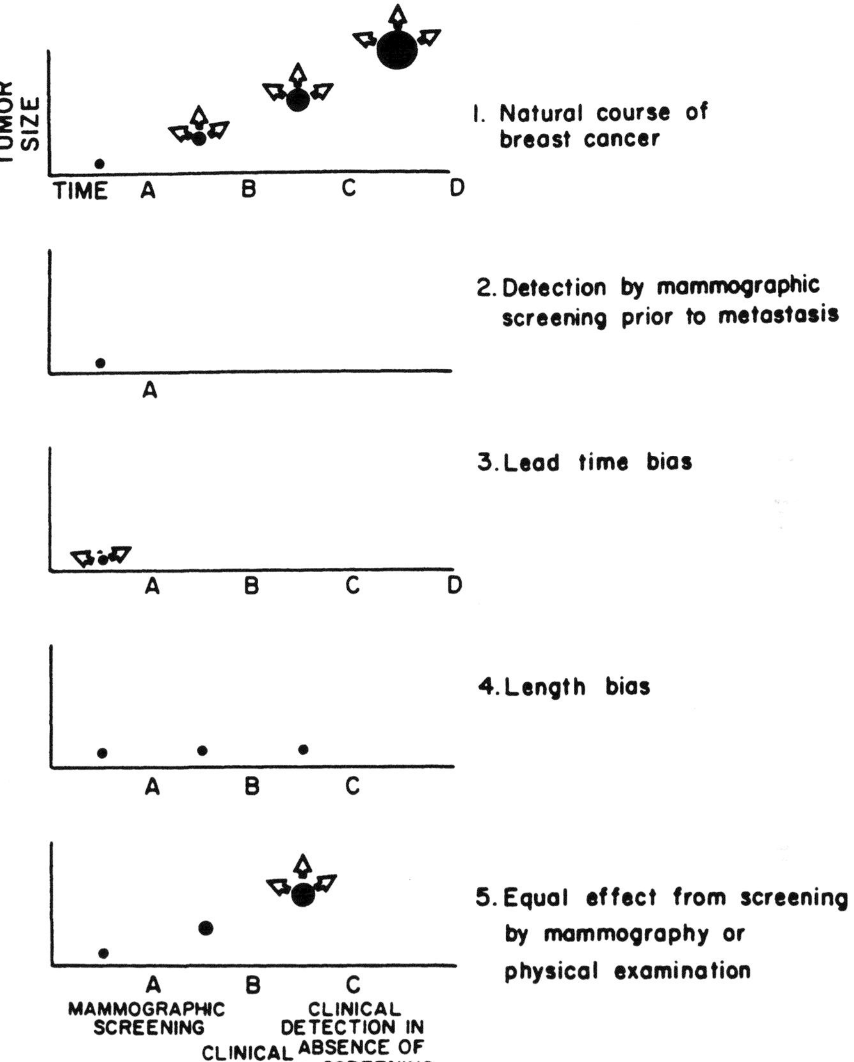

Figure 1: *Models for possible effect of early detection and treatment on breast cancer mortality.*

However, it speculates that either modality can achieve similar cure rates because significant metastatic spread does not occur between points A and B.

It can be appreciated that the theories of lead time bias and length bias are mutually exclusive when applied to a specific cancer. If a lesion has metastasized prior to detection (lead time bias), then it cannot be so biologically inert that it would never threaten patient life if undetected (length bias). However, if either of these two hypotheses were to apply to a given lesion, then its detection on screening would have no impact on mortality reduction. As postulated by the length bias hypothesis, some detected lesions such as lobular neoplasia in situ may not behave as true cancers[15] and, as predicted by the lead time bias theory, some very small minimally invasive ductal carcinomas may have already metastasized at that stage.[16] Thus, the effectiveness of screening would depend on the relative magnitude of these models in the population. Although a recent review of clinical-pathological correlation studies suggested that the lead time bias and length bias models apply to an insignificant minority of cancers detected on screening, such studies provide only indirect evidence of benefit.

The effectiveness of screening is best evaluated by means of a randomized clinical trial. In such a trial, breast cancer mortality (breast cancer deaths/population) rather than survival (percent of patients alive at given time after diagnosis) is measured simultaneously in control and study populations. Both populations are similar except that only women in the study group are offered screening. The results from such a study cannot be negated by the arguments of lead time bias and length bias, which apply only to length of survival but not to mortality rates in a randomized trial. Thus, results from such a trial can offer incontrovertible proof of benefit from screening.

HIP Study

In a randomized trial conducted by the Health Insurance Plan of New York (HIP) from 1963–1970, about 31,000 women between 40 and 64 years old on entry were offered an initial screening and three additional examinations at annual intervals by mammography and physical examination. A control population of about 31,000 women was not offered screening. After 5 years from entry, a 50% reduction in breast cancer mortality was demonstrated among study group women age 50 and older at the time of entry.[17] The numerical gains from screening are still evident on 18-year follow-up (Fig. 2). However, since screening was not continued beyond the three annual follow-up exams, the percent difference in breast cancer deaths between study and control group women age 50 and older at entry diminishes to 23% on 18-year follow-up due to the damping effect in both groups of breast cancer deaths still accumulating from cancers diagnosed within 5 years of entry (Fig. 2).

Mortality reduction was calculated on the basis of the entire study population (women offered screening) rather than women actually screened. However, only 65% of the study population appeared for the initial examination, 57% had two or more and 39% received all four examinations.[18,19] Thus, it is possible that an even greater mortality reduction could have been demonstrated if the entire study population had attended each of the four annual screenings.

Early follow-up studies (5 years from entry into the screening program) of women between 40 and 49 years old at entry, did not show any difference in reduction in breast cancer deaths among study and control groups. As follow-up continued, a reduction in breast cancer mortality did emerge (Fig. 3) and has been maintained on the most recent 18-year follow-up.[17] At present, the reduction in breast cancer deaths among study women 40–49 years old on entry

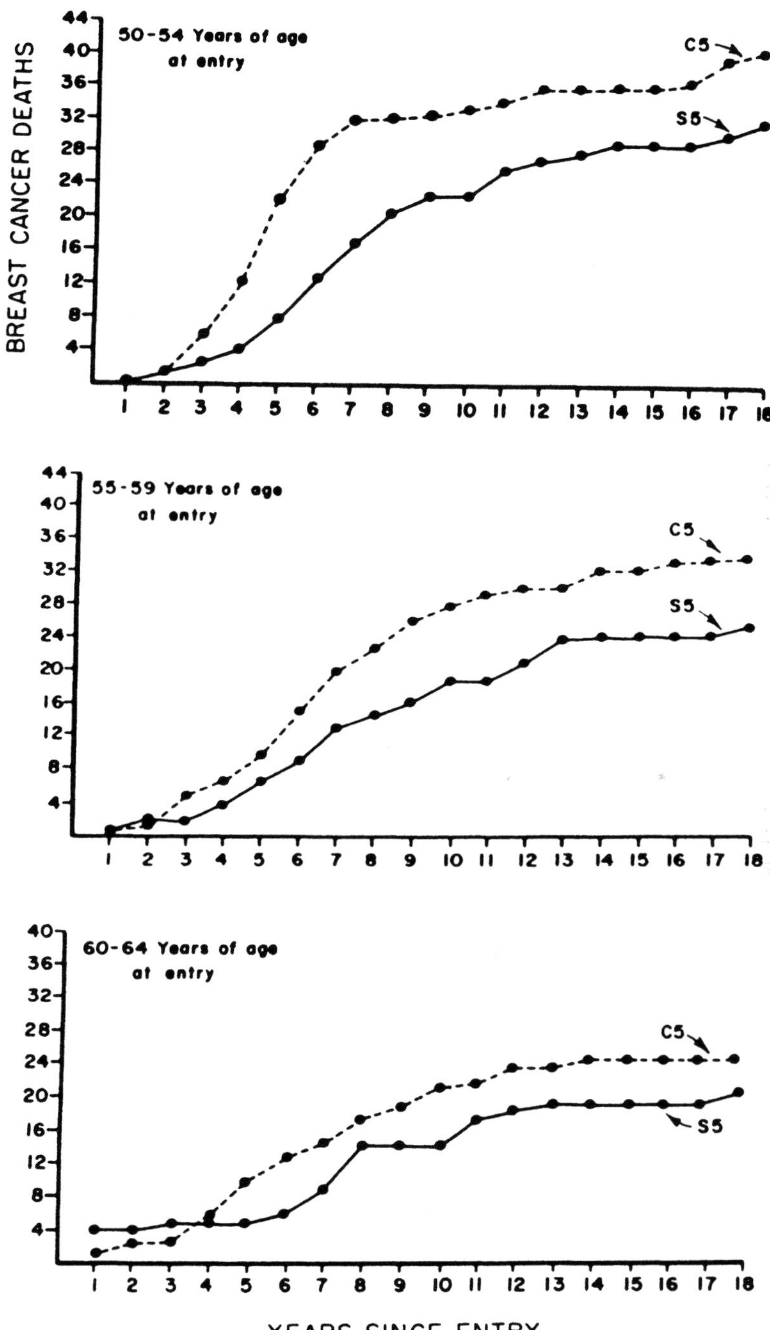

Figure 2: *Cumulative breast cancer deaths from breast cancers diagnosed within 5 years of entry for study (S5) and control group (C5) women aged 50–64 at entry. From Shapiro et al.[17] with permission.*

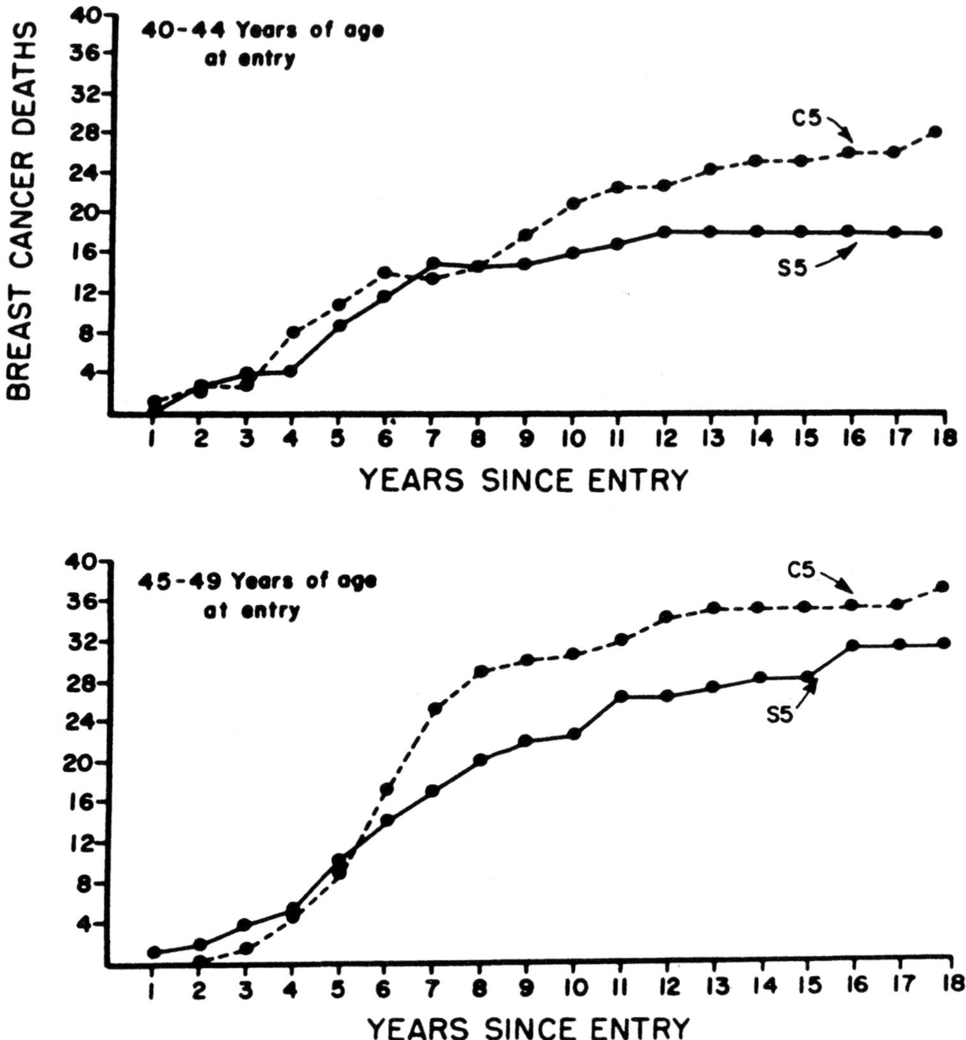

Figure 3: *Cumulative breast cancer deaths from breast cancers diagnosed within 5 years of entry for study (S5) and control group (C5) women aged 40–49 at entry. From Shapiro et al.[17] with permission.*

is similar (24.6% vs. 23.0%) to that found among study women 50–59 years old on entry (Table 3).

Because Habbema et al.[20] found no statistically significant inhomogeneity in mortality reduction across any 5-year age-at-entry class among HIP women between 40 and 64 years old at entry, the authors concluded that the study and control groups should contain the same number of breast cancer cases for each age at entry. Differences in the observed numbers should be due to chance variation. When corrections are made for these differences in the number of

Table 3

Cumulative Number of Breast Cancer Deaths* by 18 Years Follow-Up According to Age at Entry, HIP Study and Control Groups

Age at Entry (yr)	Study	Control	Difference (%)
40–49	49	65	24.6
40–44	18	28	35.7
45–49	31	37	16.2
50–59	57	74	23.0
50–54	32	41	22.0
55–59	25	33	24.2
60–64	20	24	16.7
Total	126	163	22.7

*Deaths from breast cancer diagnosed within 5 years from entry
Source: Shapiro et al.[17] with permission.

breast cancer cases in each age class, an even more homogeneous mortality reduction was shown (Table 4). These data from across all age cohorts present a uniform pattern of benefit.

Comparable benefits for women 40–49 and 50–64 years old at entry may also be obtained using survival data for cancers diagnosed within 6 years from entry.[21] Although use of such survival data (as opposed to counting the number of breast cancer deaths in study and control groups) would ordinarily be subject to possible length bias, this should not occur when the 6-year "catch-up point" is used because it represents the earliest point at which the number of cancers diagnosed in the control group has caught up with the number of cancers diagnosed in the study group. Similarly, Chu et al.[21] precluded lead time bias, another possible consequence of using survival data by measuring survival from time of entry into the trial. Using this method, these investigators found

Table 4

Effect of Correction for Difference in Number of Breast Cancer Cases Between Study and Control Groups on Homogeneity of Mortality Reduction* Across Age Groups

	Mortality Reduction %	
Age at Entry	Before Correction	After Correction
40–44	31	26
45–49	14	19
50–54	22	15
55–59	19	19
60–64	27	13
Total	22	19

*Based on 14-year follow-up.
Source: Habbema et al.[20]

mortality reductions of 24% and 21% for women 40–49 and 50–64 years old on entry, respectively, when compared with their control group cohorts on 19-year follow-up.

Not all investigators are convinced of the significance of these data because the mortality reduction among women age 40–49 on entry can be partially attributed to cases diagnosed after these women had advanced beyond the age of 50 years. When analysis is performed according to cancers diagnosed between ages 40 and 49, mortality reduction is lower (36 deaths in study group women versus 42 in control group women) in contrast to 49 deaths in the study group versus 65 deaths in the control group for the age-at-entry type analysis. Nevertheless, the mortality reduction seen among women between 40 and 44 years old on entry is significant (18 deaths in the study group vs. 28 deaths in the control group) and cannot be explained by cancers diagnosed after age 50.

Moreover, assessment according to age at diagnosis may underestimate the benefit of screening. Some incurable cancers detected in study group women before age 50 would not have surfaced clinically until after age 50 if these women had not been screened. Therefore, analysis according to age at diagnosis, rather than age at entry, would add additional breast cancer deaths to the younger study group and thus underestimate the benefit from screening these women. For these reasons, many screening experts maintain that age at entry is a more appropriate measure than age at diagnosis.[20–25]

The validity of this line of reasoning may be seen in Table 5. For age at entry of 40–44 years, the number of cases in the study and control group cohorts are similar for age 40–44 at diagnosis (17 vs. 15) as well as for study and control

Table 5
Breast Cancer Cases and Deaths* According to Age at Diagnosis, HIP Study and Control
Groups

Age at Diagnosis (yr)	Deaths Due to Breast Cancer		Difference %	Breast Cancer Cases	
	Study/Control			Study/Control	
Age at Entry, 40–44 Years					
40–49	18	28	35.7	49	45
40–44	7	10	30.0	17	15
45–49	11	18	38.9	32	31
Age at Entry, 45–49 Years					
45–54	31	37	16.2	68	68
45–49	18	14	28.6	40	30
50–54	13	23	43.5	28	38

*Breast cancer deaths by 18-year follow-up for cases diagnosed within 5 years of trial entry.
Source: Shapiro et al.[17] with permission.

group cohorts for age 45–49 at diagnosis (32 vs. 31). For age at entry of 45–49 years, the number of cases in the study and control groups are identical (68 vs. 68) for age 45–54 at diagnosis.

This pattern is seen to change when for age at entry 45–49, the two age-at-diagnosis groups are analyzed separately. For the age 45–49 years at diagnosis cohort there are 10 more cases (40 vs. 30) in the study group than in the control group, whereas for the age 50–54 years at diagnosis cohort there are 10 fewer cases (28 vs. 38) in the study group than in the control group.

Thus, there were 10 patients whose ages at diagnosis were moved forward by screening from age 50–54 years to age 45–49 years. If these patients had a poorer prognosis than the 30 women in the corresponding control group cohort diagnosed at age 45–49, then the excess number of breast cancer deaths in the study group cohort (19 vs. 14) would not imply that screening is ineffective between age 45 and 49. Rather, the data for that age-at-diagnosis cohort would seem to be a statistical variation from the general benefit seen throughout all the other age groups screened in the HIP study.

To compensate for the lower estimate of benefit for an age under 50 at diagnosis analysis, the number of deaths in the control group could be increased by the number of deaths in control group women with cancers that surfaced clinically between age 50 and 52 (assuming a 2-year lead time for screening women in their late 40s). When this adjustment is made, there are 36 deaths in the screened group and 48 deaths in the control group, resulting in a 25% reduction in mortality.[26]

Both Eddy et al.[26] and Shapiro et al.[17] have expressed reservations about this approach because the HIP data do not provide clear evidence for lead time at age 45–49.[17] However, the estimated lead time at age 40–44 at entry is 15.8 months, at age 45–49 is indeterminate, at age 50–54 is 25.2 months, at age 55–59 is 18.7 months, and at age 60–64 is indeterminate, suggesting that lack of lead time data for age 45–49 at entry is due to statistical fluctuation.

Although the HIP study seems to indicate that screening under age 50 is beneficial, some observers believe the data are not fully conclusive.[9,27] To them, the HIP results raised the possibility that breast cancer in younger women has a worse prognosis that would vitiate any benefit from screening. However, this possibility seems unlikely since breast cancer survival rates for younger women are as high[28,29] or higher[30,31] than those for older women when similar stage lesions are considered.

Another explanation for the less convincing results in younger women would be that the relatively small number of HIP study and control group women in this age group, along with their lower age-related breast cancer incidence, makes it difficult to demonstrate even sizable differences in mortality. The HIP study was not designed to determine the efficacy of screening separate age groups, but rather a single group of all study women between ages 40 and 65. Attempts to subdivide the study group reduces statistical power, permits a large sampling error, and leads to possibly erroneous conclusions.

It is also possible that the screening potential was restrained by the limited ability of the mammography technology of that era to detect early nonpalpable breast cancers in the denser, more glandular breasts of these younger women. Among cancers detected in women over age 50, 38% were found on mammography alone. For cancers detected under age 50, only 20% were found by mammography alone. Thus, although results from the HIP study support screening all women from 40 to 65 years of age, the case for screening those 40–50 years old could have been more convincing if the study group had been larger and the image quality had not been limited by the mammographic equipment of that era.

BCDDP Study

Unlike the HIP study, the Breast Cancer Detection Demonstration Project (BCDDP) which screened 280,000 women by mammography and physical examination from 1973 to 1981[4–6] was not a randomized trial with study and control groups. However, because newer mammography methods were used, detection rates were approximately twice those of the HIP: 5.54 versus 2.73 cancers/1,000 women on initial screening and 2.65 versus 1.49 cancers/1,000 women on second annual examination. It would seem that these differences were due to improved detection sensitivity rather than differences in screening self-selection, since interval cancer rates for the first 5 years of screening at the BCDDP were actually lower than those in the HIP: 0.78 versus 0.92 cancers/1,000 women screened.[6,32]

Altogether 3,548 cancers were detected at screening during the entire BCDDP. Among these cancers, 39% (1,375) were found by mammography only, 7% (257) by physical examination alone, and 51% (1,805) by both mammography and physical examination.[5]

Minimal cancers (defined here as all invasive cancers less than 1 cm and all in-situ and intraductal cancers) represented 25% (893/3,548) of all screening-detected cancers at the BCDDP compared with 8% at the HIP study. Among the minimal cancers detected at the BCDDP, 54% (484/893) were detected by mammography only, 5% (42/893) by physical examination alone, and 38% (340/893) by both mammography and physical examination.[5]

As another measure of screening sensitivity, only 13% of breast cancers at the BCDDP were found between annual interval screenings[5] compared with 34% at the HIP.[17]

Although the HIP and BCDDP populations are not strictly comparable, these data do indicate that mammography had become a more accurate modality due to improvement in technique and interpretive expertise. The improved sensitivity of mammography was particularly marked for younger women. Among women screened by mammography and physical examination at the BCDDP, 45% of cancers in those aged 40–49 and 47% of cancers in women aged 50–59 were found only by mammography. These results may be compared with those from the HIP project, where following screening by mammography and physical examination, 38% of cancers in women aged 50–59 and 20% of cancers in women aged 40–49 were found only by mammography.[4] This observation that the ability of mammography to detect nonpalpable cancers was now independent of patient age suggested that if the BCDDP had been conducted as a randomized trial, a substantial mortality reduction could have been observed for women age 40 and over.

This conclusion can also be supported by data from a study by Seidman et al.[5] of survival experience at the BCDDP (Table 6). A cumulative relative 8-year survival rate of 83% for all screening-detected cancers may be compared with an expected 8-year rate of 65% for invasive breast cancers among nonscreened women followed in the National Cancer Institute Survival, Epidemiology and End Results (SEER) Program from 1977 to 1982. Although not a true matched concurrent control group for the BCDDP, the SEER Program does provide a comparable historical index for nationwide survival rates among generally nonscreened women. Thus, the BCDDP data suggest that there is an increased survival achievable as a result of screening.

Estimates for breast cancer mortality reduction can also be made from the Seidman data by means of case fatality rates, the complement of relative survival rates. For example, the 8-year case fatality rate would be 17% (100%–83%) for women with breast cancer detected at the BCDDP and 35% (100%–65%) for patients in the SEER Program. These data indicate a 49% (17/35) reduction in breast cancer deaths among the BCDDP screened women.

Five-year survival rates from all screenings of women below and above age 50 at diagnosis were similar, 93% versus 89%, respectively (Table 7). Estimated mortality reductions for each age group were correspondingly similar, 63% versus 58%. Actually, evaluation of the initial screening data as opposed to data from all screenings might represent a better index of the value of mammography in younger women. The radiation risk controversy that occurred in 1975 after the

---

Table 6

Expected Mortality Reduction for Women Screened at the BCDDP Based on Cumulative Relative 8-Year Survival by Age at Diagnosis for Breast Cancers Detected through Screening* and for White Females in the SEER Program

	BCDDP			SEER		
	No. of Women	8-Year Survival	Case Fatality Rate	No. of Women	8-Year Survival	Case Fatality Rate	Expected Mortality Reduction at BCDDP
Total including intraductal and in situ	3,548	83%	17%	NA	NA	NA	51% (18/35)
All invasive	2,934	81%	19%	46,849	65%	35%	46% (16/35)

One year lead time for screening detected cancers.
No lead time allowed for cancers not detected at screening.
*Based on data from Seidman et al.[5]
NA = not applicable.

Table 7

Expected Mortality Reduction for Women Screened at the BCDDP Based on Cumulative Relative 5-Year Survival by Age at Diagnosis for Breast Cancers Detected through Screening* and for White Females in the SEER Program

	BCDDP			SEER			
	No. of Women	5-Year Survival	Case Fatality Rate	No. of Women	5-Year Survival	Case Fatality Rate	Expected Mortality Reduction at BCDDP
Age Under 50 at Diagnosis							
Total including intraductal and in situ (initial screenings)	377	93%	7%	NA	NA	NA	71% (17/24)
Total including intraductal and in situ	999	91%	9%	NA	NA	NA	63% (15/24)
All invasive	802	88%	12%	10,353	76%	24%	50% (12/24)
Age 50 and Over at Diagnosis							
Total including intraductal and in situ (initial screenings)	2,549	89%	11%	NA	NA	NA	58% (15/26)
All invasive	2,132	87%	13%	34,496	74%	26%	50% (13/26)

One year lead time for screening detected cancers.
No lead time allowed for cancers not detected at screening.
*Based on data from Seidman et al.[5]

initial screenings had been completed resulted in restrictions being placed on the use of mammography in women below age 50 and a consequent marked decline in early cancer detection in this age group.[6] Mortality reduction from initial screenings of women below age 50 at diagnosis is estimated at 71%.

Another consideration in assessment of the BCDDP data is the validity of survival rates for in-situ cancers. Critics of screening maintain that these lesions are not "true cancers" and that their inclusion in survival calculations will overestimate benefit. However, even when survival rates and mortality reduction are calculated for invasive cancers only, results are only slightly different from those obtained for invasive and intraductal cancers combined (Tables 6 and 7).

Similarly, although the calculations in Tables 4 and 5 are for screening-detected cancers only, inclusion of other cancers in screened women (interval and postscreening cancers) causes little or no change in results, i.e., the cumulative 5-year relative survival rate for all women is 89%, using either method. Only 16% of cancers were not detected at screening (Table 8). Survival rates for screening-

Table 8
BCDDP End Results: Breast Cancers Detected at Screening and Breast Cancers not
Detected at Screening

	Number of Cases	Percent
Screening-detected	3,548	84
Not screening-detected	692	16
Interval	540	13
Postscreening	152	3
Total	4,240	100

Total included all intraductal, in situ and invasive cancers.
Based on data from Seidman et al.[5]

detected and nonscreening-detected cancers at the BCDDP are fairly similar (Fig. 4), a situation quite different from that at the HIP. The high survival rates for interval and postscreening cancers enhance the success of the BCDDP program.

Neither lead time bias nor length bias, the two main theoretical objections to the use of survival data to demonstrate benefit from a nonrandomized screening trial such as a BCDDP seem to invalidate conclusions from Tables 5 and 6. Length bias seems to have been of little or no importance since survival rates for cancers detected at initial screenings (where presumably slower growing prevalence cancers dominate) were similar to survival rates found at later screenings (where presumably more rapidly growing incidence cancers dominate). Likewise, lead time bias was eliminated by making an adjustment of 1 year in cumulative survival rates for screening-detected cancers, e.g., the 6-year survival rate becomes the 5-year survival rate. If a 2-year time had been assumed, survival rates for screening-detected cancers would have been only slightly lower. Thus, the comparison by Seidman et al.[5] of breast cancer survival rates for BCDDP participants and nonparticipants seems to be a valid index of benefit and strongly suggests substantial mortality reduction for screening women between the ages of 35 and 74.

Using a different approach, Morrison et al.[33] compared population breast cancer mortality among BCDDP participants with the mortality expected among the general female population without diagnosed breast cancer at the start of observation. The expected breast cancer mortality was estimated by the sequential use of incidence and case fatality data from the SEER program. The methods of investigation also differ in that the findings presented by Morrison et al. are the observed results without adjustment for lead time.

The breast cancer incidence at the BCDDP was higher than that found in the population at large, a finding that can be explained by the tendency of women who are at high risk or symptomatic to enroll in a screening program. Morrison et al. found that the breast cancer mortality among BCDDP participants was 20% less than expected from the national data[33] (Table 9). However, among women screened for routine reasons only, the incidence was similar to national data, but
... ... 40% lower than the expected level.

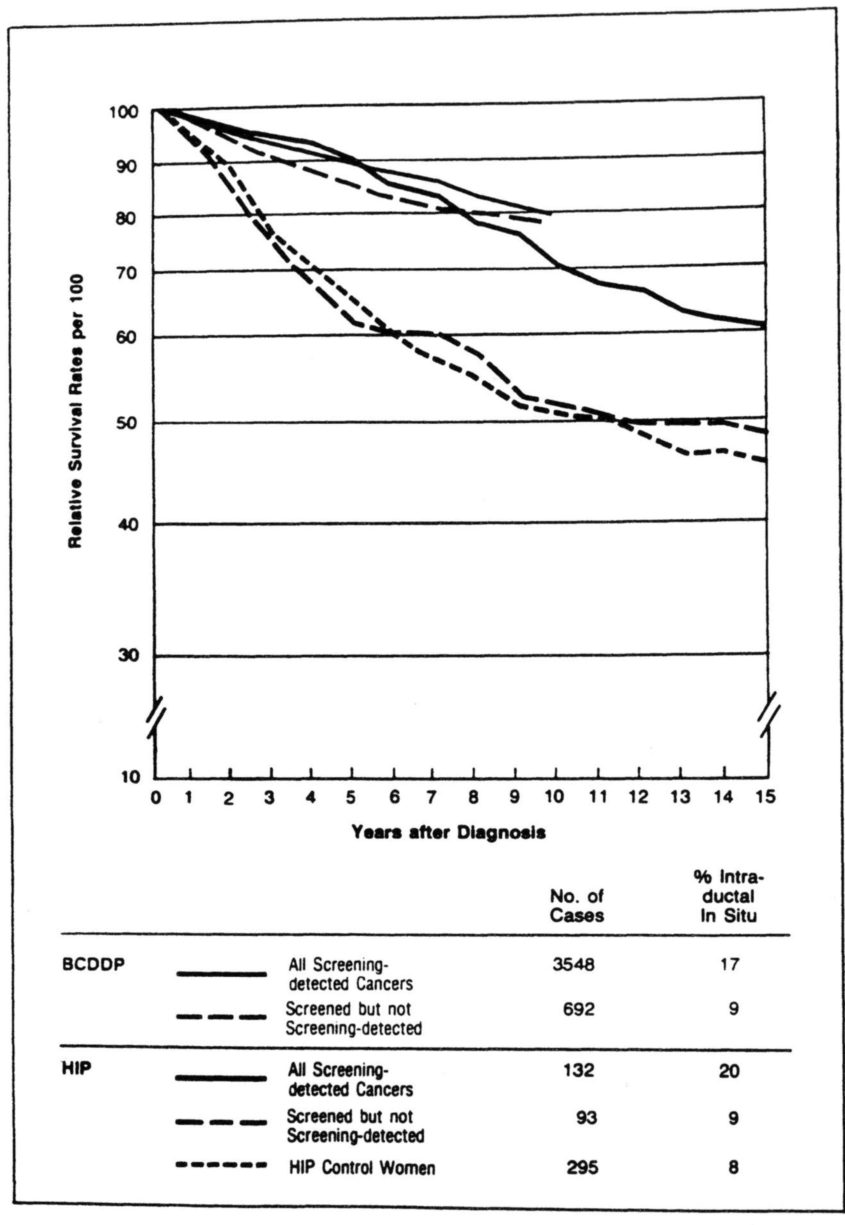

Figure 4: *Relative survival rates for cases in the BCDDP through 10 years of follow-up and in the HIP Screening Program through 15 years of follow-up for all screening-detected cancers and for all cancers screened but not screening-detected. Lead time of 1 year allowed for cancers that were detected at screening. From Seidman et al.[5] with permission.*

Table 9
Nine-Year Cumulative Reduction in Breast Cancer Mortality at the BCDDP According to Age at Entry

	Age at Entry (Years)			
	35–49	*50–59*	*60–74*	*All Ages*
Percent mortality reduction	11	24	26	20

Based on data from Morrison et al.[24]

In summary, analysis of survival rates from the BCDDP seems to be a valid index of benefit and strongly suggests substantial mortality reduction for screening women from age 35 to age 74.

Swedish Two-County Trial (Tabar Trial)

An initial 5–7 year follow-up from a randomized screening trial begun in 1977 in Kopparberg County and in 1978 in Ostergotland County in Sweden has shown a 40% reduction in breast cancer deaths in the 50–74 year age group and a 30% mortality reduction for all women between age 40 and age 74.[34] This mortality reduction persists on the most recent 11-year follow-up.[35] Mortality reduction has not yet been observed in the 40–49 year age group because of the small number of breast cancer deaths seen so far in the study group, i.e., 16 versus 71 among older women. However, the proportion of cancers detected in the in-situ and early invasive stages was similar in both age groups.[36] Among younger women, more cases of advanced disease are already seen in the control group than in the screened group[37] (Fig. 5). Moreover, the reduction in advanced disease among screened women aged 40–49 is similar to that seen among women screened between age 40 to age 69 (Fig. 6). These findings strongly suggest that mortality reduction among younger women will be seen over the longer term. Near-term mortality reduction might have been shown for women screened under age 50 if there had been annual screening by two-view mammography and physical examination.

The only screening modality used for all women was a single mediolateral oblique view mammogram. Women between ages 40 and 49 at entry were screened every 24 months and older women were screened every 33 months. It is likely that the mortality reduction would have been even greater if there had been annual screening by two-view mammography and physical examination. Mortality reduction was calculated using the entire study group, even though the attendance rate was 85%. This would underestimate the actual mortality

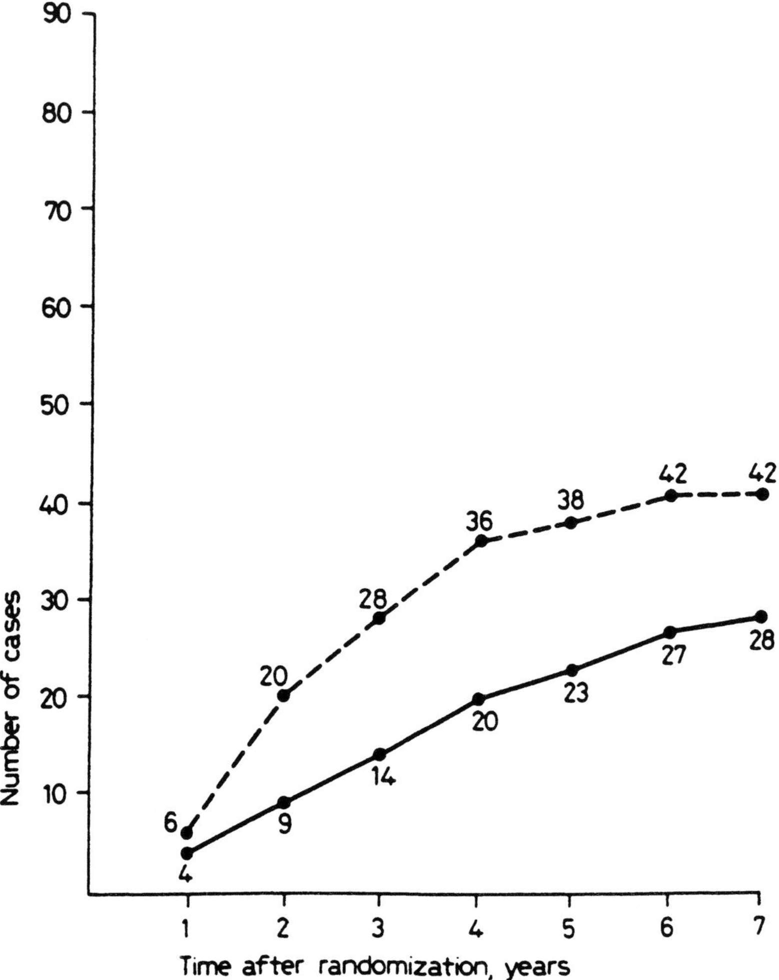

Figure 5: *Cumulative number of women aged 40–49 years with stage II and higher breast cancer among women invited to undergo screening (solid line) and control group (dashed line). From Tabar et al.[37]*

reduction by about 7%. Also, 13% of control group women had mammography during their routine medical care. Any resulting benefit to the control group would diminish the relative mortality reduction in the study group.

Dutch Case-Control Studies

Two case-control studies were begun in 1975 in Holland. Seven-year follow-up was reported in 1984. In Nijmegen, single-view mammography only was performed biannually. Among women aged 35–65, a 50% mortality reduction was found. However, there were too few breast cancer cases in women

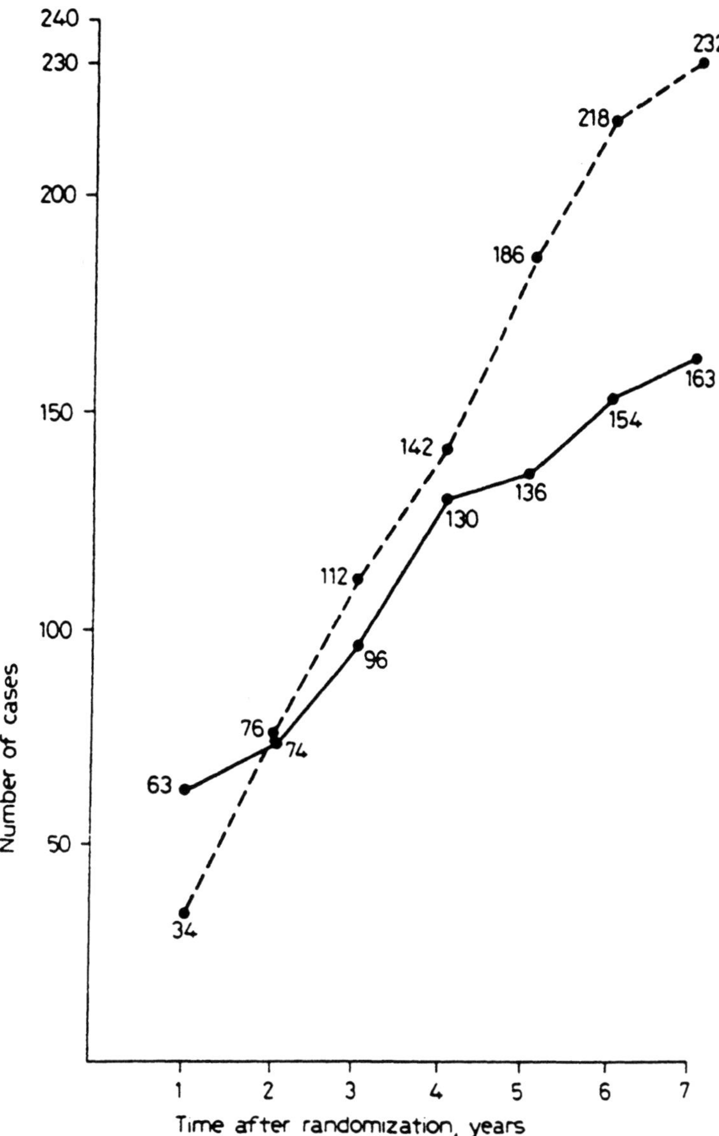

Figure 6: *Cumulative number of women aged 40–69 years with stage II and higher advanced breast cancer among women invited to undergo screening (solid line) and control group (dashed line). From Tabar et al.*[37]

under age 55 to specifically demonstrate a benefit to that age group.[38] In Utrecht, a 70% mortality reduction was found among women aged 50–64, possibly due to more frequent screening (initial, 12, 18, 24 months) by both physical examination and two-view mammography.[39]

Longer-term follow-up will be necessary to confirm these benefits. However, the mortality reductions in the Dutch studies were for screened women only, whereas the mortality reductions for the HIP and Swedish Projects were for the total study population, both screened and nonscreened. Thus, the estimates from the Dutch studies more accurately reflect the benefit to women screened rather than those who are offered screening.

British Screening Trial

The United Kingdom Screening Trial of women aged 45–64 has shown a 22% mortality reduction for the first 6 to 7 years since their entry between 1979 and 1981. The mortality difference between screening centers and comparison centers is still widening so that a 46% mortality reduction has been found for years 6 and 7 alone. Although each participant was offered annual screening by physical examination, the mortality reduction may have been restrained by the use of mammography in alternate years only.[40] Recruitment for a new randomized British trial that will offer screening to 70,000 women aged 40–41 at entry may provide better information on the efficacy of screening these younger women.[41]

Canadian Screening Trial

The Canadian randomized trial[42] was designed to answer two main questions: (1) Will annual mammography and physical examination reduce breast cancer mortality in women aged 40–49? and (2) Does annual mammography and physical examination of women aged 50–59 reduce breast cancer mortality more than annual physical examination alone? Unfortunately, already documented problems with mammographic image quality, interpretation, and study implementation may limit the usefulness of their data.

During the first 6 years of the project, fewer than 50% of the mammograms were judged to be of acceptable quality.[43] An excess of late-stage cancers in the study group compared with the control group[44] was probably attributable to a faulty randomization process.[45] In addition, some surgeons were unwilling to perform a biopsy on a lesion based on mammographic suspicion alone.[46] But unexpectedly, on early follow-up, excess breast cancer deaths were found among women aged 40–49 offered screening[41] and no mortality reduction was seen among those aged 50–59.[47]

Conclusion

The value of mammographic screening has been proven for women above age 50, but there is disagreement among experts as to the benefit in the 40–50 age group. At present, clinical decisions on screening must be based on the best available evidence, a common situation in many clinical problem areas where medicine often involves the art of applying judgment and common sense in dealing with uncertainty.

Documentation of benefit from a screening trial is often difficult. Since breast cancer is a chronic disease, results will not be observed for many years. The lower incidence in younger women requires a much larger study population in this age group. Optimization of screening factors includes high-quality mammographic technique and interpretation, annual screening, two-view rather than one-view mammography, annual physical examination, proper randomization with no significant screening of the control group (which is difficult to achieve), and proper randomization with no advanced cancers channeled into the study group. Conducting such a perfect or even near-perfect trial may not be feasible today. At least for the present, screening guidelines may have to be based on our best judgment.

In the United States, mammographic screening of women aged 40–50 every 1–2 years has been advised in guidelines from the American Cancer Society, National Cancer Institute, American Medical Association, and American College of Radiology.[48] Some organizations have not endorsed screening of this age group,[9] while other experts have advocated screening every year rather than less often.[49,50]

References

1. Wanebo HH, Huvos AG, Urban JA: Treatment of minimal breast cancer. Cancer 1974; 33:349–357.
2. Frazier TG, Copeland EM, Gallager HS, et al: Prognosis and treatment in minimal breast cancer. Am J Surg 1977; 133:697-701.
3. Department of Health, Education and Welfare: Cancer Patient Surveillance, DHEW publication No. (NIH) 77–992. National Technical Information Service, Springfield, VA. 1977.
4. Beahrs OH, Shapiro S, Smart C: Report of the working group to review the National Cancer Institute-American Cancer Society Breast Cancer Detection Demonstration Projects. JNCI 1979; 62:640–709.
5. Seidman H, Gelb SK, Silverberg E, et al: Survival experience in the Breast Cancer Detection Demonstration Project. CA 1987; 37:258–290.
6. Baker LH: Breast Cancer Detection Demonstration Project: five-year summary report. CA 1982; 32:194–226.
7. O'Malley MS, Fletcher SW: Screening for breast cancer with breast self-examination: a critical review. JAMA 1987; 257:2197-2202.
8. Miller AB: Is routine screening mammography appropriate for women 40–49 years of age? Am J Prev Med 1991; 7:55–62.

9. American College of Physicians, Health and Public Policy Committee: The use of diagnostic tests for screening and evaluating breast lesions. Ann Int Med 1985; 103:147–151.
10. Feig SA, Ehrlich SM: Estimation of radiation risk from screening mammography: recent trends and comparison with expected benefits. Radiology 1990; 174:638–647.
11. Zelen M: Theory of early detection of breast cancer in the general population. In: Heuson JC, Mattheiem WH, Rozencweig M (eds.) Breast Cancer Trends in Research and Treatment. Raven Press, New York, pp 287–300, 1976.
12. Feinleib M, Zelen M: Some pitfalls in the evaluation of screening programs. Arch Environ Health 1969; 19:412–419.
13. Nemoto T, Natarajan N, Smart CR, et al: Patterns of breast cancer detection in the United States. J Surg Oncol 1982; 21:183-188.
14. Seidman H, Mushinski MH: Breast cancer incidence, mortality, survival, prognosis. In: Feig SA, McLelland R (eds). Breast Carcinoma: Current Diagnosis and Treatment. Masson, New York, pp 9–46, 1983.
15. Haagensen CD, Lane N, Lattes R, et al: Lobular neoplasia (so-called lobular carcinoma in situ) of the breast. Cancer 1978; 42:737–769.
16. Millis RR, Thynne GSJ: In-situ intraduct carcinoma of the breast: a long-term follow-up study. Br J Surg 1975; 62:957-962.
17. Shapiro S, Venet W, Strax P, et al: Periodic Screening for Breast Cancer: The Health Insurance Plan Project and its Sequelae, 1963–1986. Johns Hopkins University Press, Baltimore, 1988.
18. Strax P, Venet L, Shapiro S: Value of mammography in reduction of mortality from breast cancer in mass screening. AJR 1973; 117:686–689.
19. Shapiro S, Venet W, Strax P, et al: Ten-to-fourteen-year effect of screening on breast cancer mortality. JNCI 1982; 69:349–355.
20. Habbema JDF, Van Oortmarssen GJ, Van Putten DJ, et al: Age-specific reduction in breast cancer mortality by screening: an analysis of results of the Health Insurance Plan of Greater New York Study. JNCI 1986; 77:317–320.
21. Chu KC, Smart CR, Tarone RE: Analysis of breast cancer mortality and stage distribution by age for the Health Insurance Plan clinical trial. JNCI 1988; 80:1125–1132.
22. Tabar L, Dean PB : The control of breast cancer through mammography screening: what is the evidence? Radiol Clin of North Am 1987; 25:993–1006.
23. Day NE, Tabar L, Fagerberg G: Letter to the editor. Lancet 1984; ii:1217–1218.
24. Morrison AS: Screening in Chronic Disease. Oxford University Press, New York, pp 74–80, 1985.
25. Prorok PC, Hankey BF, Bundy BN: Concepts and problems in the evaluation of screening programs. J Chron Dis 1981; 34:159-171.
26. Eddy DM, Hasselblad V, McGivney W, et al: The value of mammography screening under age 50 years. JAMA 1988; 259:1512-1519.
27. Shapiro S: Letter to the editor. Lancet 1985; i:216.
28. Stoll BA: Effect of age on growth pattern. In: Stoll BA (ed). Risk Factors in Breast Cancer. Year Book Medical Publishers, Chicago, pp 129–148, 1976.
29. Mausner JS, Shimkin MKB, Moss NH, et al: Cancer of the breast in Philadelphia hospitals 1951–1964. Cancer 1969; 23:260–274.
30. Adami H-0, Malker B, Holmberg L, et al: The relation between survival and age at diagnosis in breast cancer. N Engl J Med 1986; 315:559–563.
31. Host H, Lund E: Age as a prognostic factor in breast cancer. Cancer 1986; 57:2217–2221.
32. Shapiro S: Evidence of screening for breast cancer from a randomized trial. Cancer 1977; 39:2772–2782.
33. Morrison AS, Brisson J, Khalid N: Breast cancer incidence and mortality in the Breast Cancer Detection Demonstration Project. JNCI 1988; 80:1540–1547.

34. Tabar L, Fagerberg G, Eklund G, et al: Reduction in breast cancer mortality by mass screening with mammography: first results of a randomized trial in two Swedish counties. Lancet 1985; 1:829–832.
35. Tabar L, Fagerberg G, Duffy SW, et al: Update of the Swedish two-county program of mammographic screening for breast cancer. Radiol Clin North Am 1992; 30:187–210.
36. Tabar L, Gad A, Akerlund E, et al: Screening for breast cancer in Sweden. In: Feig SA, McLelland R (eds). Breast Carcinoma: Current Diagnosis and Treatment. Masson, New York, pp 315–326, 1983.
37. Tabar L, Gad A, Holmberg L, et al: Significant reduction in advanced breast cancer: results of the first seven years of mammography screening in Kopparberg, Sweden. Diagn Imag Clin Med 1985; 54:158–164.
38. Verbeek ALM, Hendriks JHCL, Holland R, et al: Reduction of breast cancer mortality through mass screening with modern mammography: first results of the Nijmegen Project, 1975–1981. Lancet 1984; 1:1222–1224.
39. Collette HJA, Day NE, Rombach JJ, et al: Evaluation of screening for breast cancer in a non-randomized study (the DOM Project) by means of a case-control study. Lancet 1984; 1:1224-1226.
40. UK Trial of Early Detection of Breast Cancer Group: First results on mortality reduction in the UK Trial of Early Detection of Breast Cancer. Lancet 1988; 2:411–416.
41. Editorial: Breast cancer screening in women under 50. Lancet 1991; 337:1575–1576.
42. Miller AB, Howe GR, Wall C: The national study of breast cancer screening. Clin Invest Med 1981; 4:227–258.
43. Baines CJ, Miller AB, Kopans DB, et al: Canadian breast screening study: assessment of technical quality by external review. Am J Roentgenol 1990; 155:743–746.
44. Miller AB, Baines CJ, To J, et al: The Canadian National Breast Screening Study. In: Miller AB, Chamberlain J, Day NE, et al. (eds). Cancer Screening. Cambridge University Press, Cambridge, 1992.
45. Day NE, Duffy SW: Breast screening in women under 50. Lancet 1991; 338:113–114.
46. Kopans DB: Breast screening in women under 50. Lancet 1991; 338:447.
47. Miller AB: ACP policy on mammogram in women 40–49 faulted. Internal Med News 1990; 23:35.
48. Vanchieri C: Breast cancer screening, evidence for benefit for women 40 to 49. JNCI 1988; 80:1090–1092.
49. Moskowitz M: Breast cancer age-specific growth rates and screening strategies. Radiology 1966; 161:37–41.
50. Tabar L, Fagerberg G, Day NE, et al: What is the optimum interval between mammographic screening examinations? An analysis based on the latest results of the Swedish two-county breast cancer screening trial. Br J Cancer 1987; 55:547–551.

29

Breast Cancer Screening With Mammography Should be Abandoned

Charles J. Wright

Introduction

Breast cancer is a bad disease. The physical and psychological consequences of having breast cancer, the high mortality, and the persistent and long-term relapse rate, have inevitably led to the thought that earlier diagnosis is essential if the outcome is to be improved. In a very large study of women with breast cancer, unselected for stage of disease, method of therapy, or any other consideration, 8% of the residual population died of breast cancer annually.[1] This rate of dying appears to be continued even out to 20 years from diagnosis, resulting in the fact that 80% to 85% of women who have breast cancer diagnosed eventually die of the disease. These are depressing figures. It is also interesting to note that death from cancer *in the breast* is rare or nonexistent. Death occurs because of the metastatic cancer in the bones, liver, brain, lungs, and elsewhere throughout the body.

The thought that a "cancer control window" may exist in the natural history of breast cancer is extremely attractive, and has led to the philosophy underlying screening. Figure 1 represents a model of the disease from onset to final outcome. It is obvious that detection of the disease by screening must occur before clinical detection is possible, but also before any metastatic disease has occurred. It is also easy to see from Figure 1 how screening for a disease results in increased survival rates without altering the outcome in any way, by allowing earlier diagnosis of the disease and longer disease duration. This will be discussed further below.

It is perhaps self-evident, but worth restating, that for a screening program

From: Wise L, Johnson H Jr (eds): *Breast Cancer: Controversies in Management.* Futura Publishing Company, Inc., Armonk, NY, © 1994.

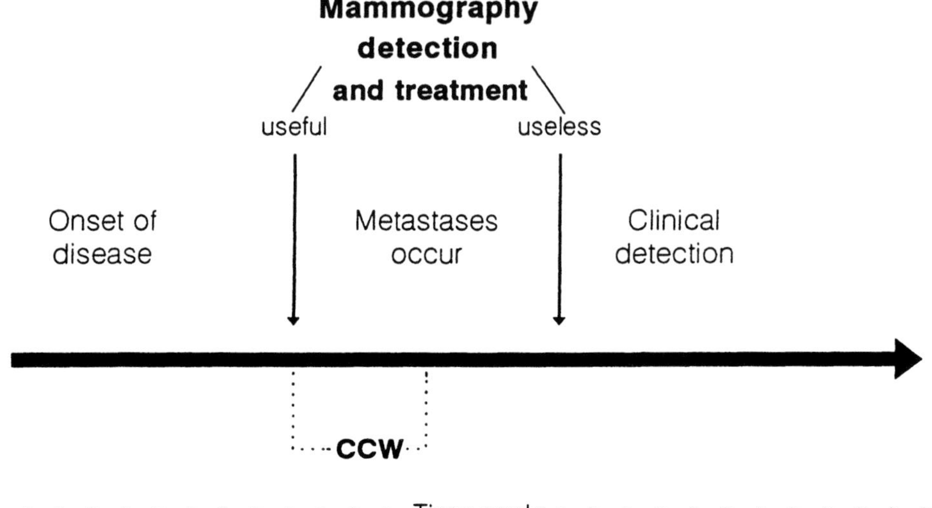

Figure 1: *Diagrammatic model of disease from onset to final outcome. CCW represents the "cancer control window."*

to be justifiable it has to bring demonstrable benefit to patients. Even if benefit is clearly demonstrated, it does not follow automatically that the program should be implemented. Scientific evidence may demonstrate benefit, but a very difficult and entirely subjective process of human judgment must then determine whether the magnitude of the benefit renders the harm caused and the dollar cost generated acceptable. In the case of mammographic screening for breast cancer, the evidence from the earlier trials suggests that there is a small benefit, but the screening enthusiasts have chosen to ignore the necessity for careful analysis of the harm caused before moving to the next step of screening program design implementation. The more recent trials, demonstrating no benefit whatsoever, probably render the cost/benefit issue irrelevant in any case.

Essentials of a Successful Screening Program

Two questions must have a positive answer before even considering implementation of a screening program. First, does it work? That is, does the proposed screening technique really permit earlier diagnosis of the target lesion? The answer is undoubtedly positive in the case of mammography and breast cancer. The Breast Cancer Detection Demonstration Project (BCDDP)[2] demonstrated a 0.5% incidence of breast cancer among over 250,000 women. The data from the first year of the BCDDP are summarized in Table 1. Many of these lesions were clinically undetectable and therefore there is no question that the diagnosis would have been delayed in the absence of screening. Table 2 is also derived from the BCDDP first year data, demonstrating a sensitivity of 87% and

Table 1
Breast Cancer Detection Demonstration Project: First Year Data

	Number	%
Total number of women screened	268,141	100
Positive screening result	14,851	5.54
Biopsy performed	9,602	3.58
Cancer detected*	1,460	0.54
False-positive results	13,391	4.99

*Includes invasive cancer and carcinoma in situ.

Table 2
Breast Cancer Detection Demonstration Project: First Year Data

Screening Result	Breast Cancer*		Total
	+	−	
Positive	1,460	13,391	14,851
Negative	210**	253,080	253,290
Total	1,670	266,471	268,141

*Plus sign indicates proven breast cancer.
**Proven breast cancer developed within 12 months of a negative mammogram.

a specificity of 95% in an overall prevalence of the disease in this population of 0.62%. Mammography works in terms of detecting breast cancer in many cases earlier than would otherwise be possible.

The second and more important question, however, is whether the earlier diagnosis leads to any benefit for the patient. A major problem here is lead-time bias which is the bias introduced by moving the diagnosis to an earlier point on the time scale, thus automatically increasing the case survival rate even when there is no benefit whatsoever. The case survival rate is the proportion of patients still alive at any given time after a diagnosis. Lead-time bias is best understood by thinking of a patient with cancer who is diagnosed by the presence of a breast lump and, for example, who dies 5 years later. If that diagnosis had been made 2 years earlier by mammography, then the patient would have survived 7 years instead of 5 even in the absence of any change whatsoever in the clinical course. Another problem in screening programs is length-bias. There is a large biological range of activity in breast cancer, some being very rapidly growing and some having a very slow progression. A "snapshot" of cases at screening mammography brings to light a higher proportion of the slow-growing type of case which has a better prognosis. This, too, would tend to make the case survival statistics look better without any real benefit to the patient. Both of these biases render case survival data completely irrelevant in outcome evaluation of screening programs, and yet reports of the HIP study, for example, have published impressive looking graphs of the irrelevant "case survival" rates.[3,4]

The only outcome worth evaluating in a breast cancer screening program is the population mortality from the target disease. Other outcomes, such as the proportion of node-positive patients diagnosed or tumor size are of interest only insofar as they reflect on eventual mortality or choice of therapy. The large majority of women with breast cancer now choose treatment plans involving conservative breast surgery in any case.

The Evidence for Screening Benefit

There have now been five randomized prospective controlled clinical trials published on the effect of mammographic screening on breast cancer mortality. These are, in chronological order, the Health Insurance Plan (HIP) study,[3-5] the Swedish National Board of Health Study (SNBH),[6,7] the Malmo Study,[8] the Edinburgh Study,[9] and the Canadian National Breast Screening Study (CNBSS).[10,11] In Figures 2 and 3, the results of these studies are portrayed,

RANDOMIZED CONTROLLED TRIALS
OF MAMMOGRAPHY

	H.I.P. (at 10 yrs)	S.N.B.H. (at 7 yrs)
No.of women screened	31888	78085
Deaths from breast ca		
—study	147	87
—control	192	127 *
Reductn. in mortality relative(%)	23	31
No. of women screened for 1 less death/yr	7086	13665

*adjusted for the different n in study and control groups

Figure 2: *Data from the Health Insurance Plan of New York study (HIP) and the Swedish National Board of Health study (SNBH).*

RANDOMIZED CONTROLLED TRIALS
OF MAMMOGRAPHY

	Edinburgh (at 7 yrs)	Malmo (at 9 yrs)	CNBSS (at 7 yrs)
No.of women screened	23226	21088	44854
Deaths from breast ca			
−study	68	63	76 *
−control	76	66	67
Reductn. in mortality (relative,%)	11	5	Nil
No. of women screened for 1 less death/yr	20322	63264	N/A

*the increased mortality occurred in those aged 40−49 years

Figure 3: *Data from the Edinburgh, Malmo, and Canadian (CNBSS) studies. None of the mortality rate differences is significant.*

showing the number of women screened, the actual number of deaths in the stated follow-up period, the claimed percentage relative reduction in mortality, and finally, the number of women screened in each study for one less death from breast cancer per year. If the data from the earlier studies are accepted at face value (and some of the problems with this are discussed below), then it is apparent that up to 63,000 women must be screened to prevent one death from breast cancer each year.

The Fragility of the Case for Benefit

Of the five randomized prospective controlled clinical studies, the first two demonstrated a significant benefit,[4,6] whereas the last three demonstrated no significant benefit.[8,9] Consistency in successive different trials is important in drawing conclusions about cause and effect. Those who are currently driving the implementation of mass mammography screening programs are clearly doing so on the basis of the results from the first two trials and in spite of the negative results from the latter three trials. This is remarkable in view of the progressive improvement in mammography technique that has occurred over the last 20 years since the first trial was commenced. If there were a cause and effect relationship between mammography and lower mortality from breast cancer, a progressively stronger association would be expected with the progressive improvement in mammographic techniques since the first study. The reverse is true.

It was predictable that an assault would be launched against the most recently published Canadian study (which showed no benefit of screening at any age) by radiology interests, in view of the serious threat to what has become a multi-million dollar industry. At a recent convention, the American College of Radiology reinforced its previous recommendation that women between ages 40–49 should undergo mammography every 1 to 2 years, and every year at age 50 and older for the rest of their lives. This recommendation is currently supported by various other groups of physicians and cancer agencies. It is interesting to note how they prefer to adhere to the results of the oldest studies rather than taking into account all of the evidence now available. The attacks on the Canadian study (which has the most rigorous design of all) claim that the results at 7 years are too early to take any notice, but they were not slow to recommend screening mammography in the first place on the basis of the HIP study results at the same interval.

The quality of the mammography at the beginning of the Canadian study is also under attack, which is bizarre on two counts. First, the mammography in the CNBSS reflected the real world, and improved progressively with time through the 1980s. It is incredible that anyone would criticize the quality of the mammography in the CNBSS in comparison with the more primitive mammography of the HIP study of 20 years ago. Secondly, the criticism is completely invalidated by the fact that the CNBSS cancer detection rate compares favorably with that reported in all other modern studies and was twice the rate in the HIP study, for example. The trial was designed to pick up breast cancers, and it did just that as well as any other study.

The claimed benefits from the HIP and SNBH studies are illustrated in a different perspective in Figure 4. The difference of 25% to 30% relative mortality reduction is seen as a tiny absolute mortality reduction in the population of women screened. This is in exchange for a positive mammogram rate of around 5% with a large number of breast biopsies consequently generated. It is even more troubling to reflect on Figure 5, which demonstrates no significant difference in all-cause mortality between the screened and control populations in the SNBH study. This is the study that has claimed the greatest extent of benefit for screening but it shows that, in the final analysis, not a single life has been "saved" by the program.

The difference in breast cancer mortality is so small in actual numbers that it is necessary to question the accuracy with which the cause of death was classified. It is notoriously difficult to ascribe with certainty the cause of death

BCDDP, HIP and SNBH MAMMOGRAPHY DATA

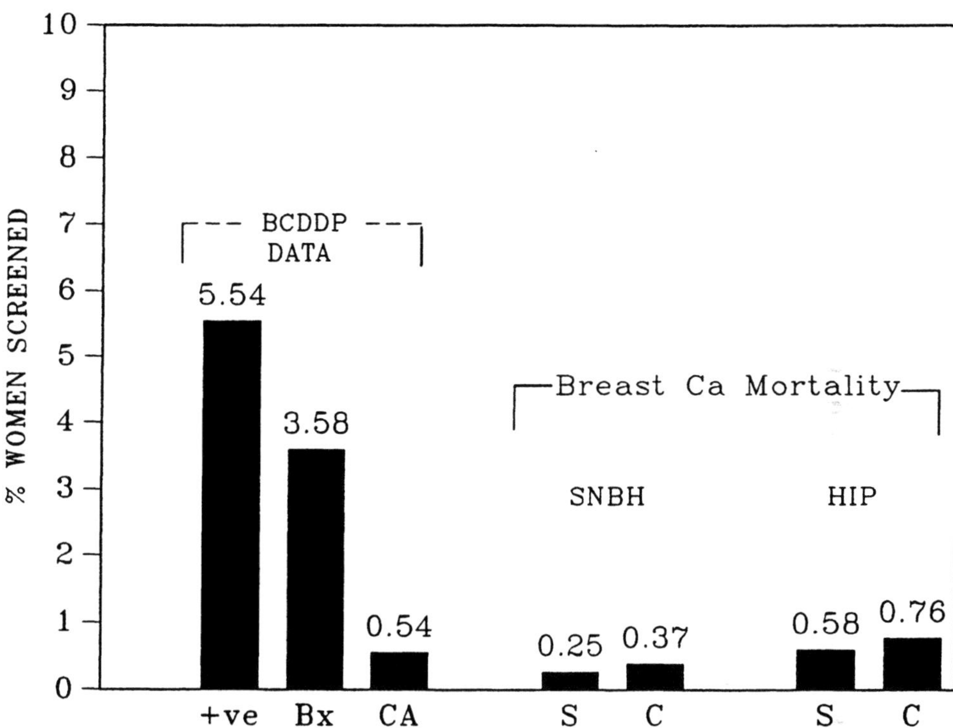

Figure 4: *Rates of positive screening results (+ve), breast biopsy (Bx), cancer detection (CA), and mortality from breast cancer in screened (S) and control (C) populations. BCDDP, HIP, and Swedish study.*

when there are several contributing factors and a very small error in categorization of the cause of death would lead to erroneous conclusions. This must be suspect as a factor in the discrepancy between different studies, as no study has succeeded in demonstrating any overall change in mortality. It is noteworthy that only two of the studies (Malmo and CNBSS) fully investigated and verified the cause of death of study subjects and that these are two of the studies showing no benefit whatsoever for mammography.

In contrast to the earlier results of the HIP study, it has recently been claimed that there is a benefit in women under the age of 50 years,[12,13] although it is even smaller than that claimed in older women. The more recently published studies, however, fail to demonstrate benefit at any age and, in fact, raise suspicion of mortality *increase* in younger screened women.

SCREENING MAMMOGRAPHY
Mortality – of breast cancer and total

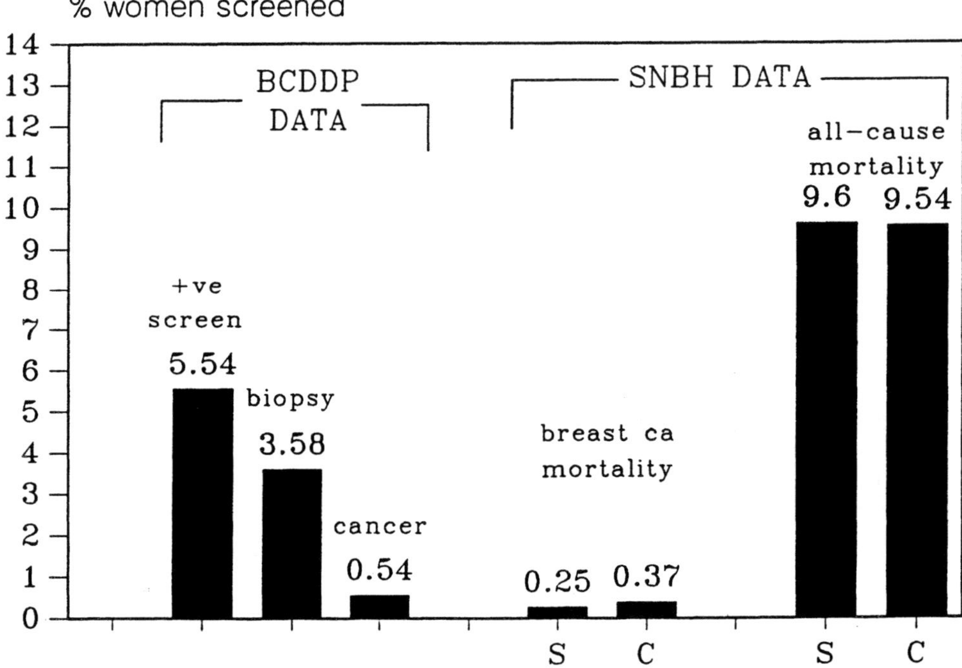

Figure 5: *Rates of positive screening results, breast biopsy, and mortality from breast cancer and all causes in screened (S) and control (C) populations. BCDDP and Swedish study.*

The Harm Caused by Mammography

Unlike the assessment of benefit, the assessment of harm is direct and simple. First, mammography hurts, and it is not unusual in my experience for women to comment that regular mammography would be advocated less enthusiastically if men could experience it. The other aspects of mammography that cause harm are as follows: (1) false-positive mammography causing unnecessary intervention; (2) false-negative mammography causing inappropriate reassurance; (3) false hopes of cure of breast cancer; (4) increased level of anxiety concerning breast cancer; (5) diversion of resources from worthwhile issues; and (6) radiation risk.

The most serious of these, in terms of the impact of a mammography mass screening program, is the generation of false-positive results. In the BCDDP study, approximately 1 in 20 women screened was found to have a mammographic abnormality.[2] The positive predictive value of mammography ranges from

7% to 20%, that is, between 1 out of 5 and 1 out of 14 women with a positive screen and subjected to biopsy will actually be found to have carcinoma.[14,15] A mammogram that is labeled as either "positive" or "suspicious" inevitably leads to intervention, and it is for this reason that fine wire needle localization of breast lesions became a major growth industry of the 1980s. The corollary of the high false-positive rate is that the vast majority of these women should never have been subjected to biopsy or operation in the first place. Mammography, therefore, causes a large number of unnecessary operations to be performed, with consequent scarring and deformity. Physicians without a surgical background do not always realize that operations for nonpalpable mammographic "disease" are more difficult and often more traumatic than operations to remove a palpable lump. As the techniques for less invasive biopsy improve, such as stereotactic needle localization, the number of unncessary open operations that result due to mammographic findings should diminish, but this is an irrelevant argument as these unfortunate women should not be subjected to any procedure whatsoever.

The problem of false-positives is compounded by the inclusion of cases of carcinoma in situ along with the cases of invasive breast cancer. Table 3 demonstrates that in the BCDDP data, for example, 22% of the cases of "cancer" were in fact carcinoma in situ. This is a very disturbing aspect of all the breast cancer screening studies. It is well-known that only 50% of women with ductal carcinoma in situ[16] and 20% of those with the lobular type[17,18] will develop invasive cancer after biopsy alone. In other words, most women with carcinoma in situ of the breast do not subsequently have breast cancer at all. Carcinoma in situ of the breast is not a cancer, and this is more than a semantic issue; it is a high-risk marker for the subsequent development of cancer in a minority of cases.

The false reassurance of a negative mammogram is another serious disadvantage of mammography. In Table 2 it may be seen that only 87% of the breast cancers in the screened population which developed during the first year of the study were diagnosed at the time of mammography screening. Another way of stating these data is that 13% of early breast cancers are missed by mammography. Radiologists may quote one of the advantages of the procedure to be the reassurance that cancer is not present. The data show this argument to be false.

False hope of cure arises because of the "hype" concerning the whole subject to which women are subjected. The headlines state that "there is a 30% reduction in breast cancer mortality with screening." The reality is that screening

---

Table 3
Histologic Features of "Cancers" Detected
Five-Year Breast Cancer Detection Demonstration Project Data (All Women)

	Number	%
Total number of breast cancers	3557	100
Infiltrating breast cancer	2775	78
Carcinoma in situ	782	22

makes no difference to the outcome in the great majority of cases, even if the most favorable trial results are accepted. The general level of anxiety about breast cancer among women is very high in our society and this is accentuated by the constant recommendations for screening. Dr. Maureen Roberts, who was the Director of the Edinburgh Breast Screening Trial, wrote a very poignant article on the subject months before her own unfortunate and untimely death from breast cancer.[19] The negative emotional impact of screening is extremely difficult to quantitate, but it has probably been seriously underestimated.[19,20]

The radiation risk from regular mammography is also impossible to quantitate accurately. The radiation-induced breast cancer risk can only be assessed by mathematical models[21] and no useful data are available. The risk is certainly small, but it does exist and must be included, albeit marginally, in the list of disadvantages.

Financial Cost

Enormous diversion of resources would be necessary to conduct a state or nationwide mammographic screening program. Based on 1986 US statistics, in an area with a population of one million, for example, 580 women every working day would have to be invited to undergo mammography, assuming that there are approximately 250 working days in the year and that the program is limited to those over 50 years of age. If a compliance rate of 70% were achieved, then approximately 98,000 women would have to be screened daily in the United States at a cost of $1.5 to $2.5 billion annually, depending on pricing policy for mammography, which varies greatly. This sum does not include the cost of the large related diagnostic and therapeutic industry that has developed to deal with the results of "positive" mammograms. The implications for other health services would be profound. Surgeons, anesthetists, pathologists, operating room staff, and many others would be very busy indeed. In the Swedish study, for example, the rate of breast operations doubled following implementation of the mammography screening program.[22]

Assessment of Benefit/Harm/Cost

No clinical trial can ever answer the question of whether a screening program should be implemented. Even if there were a small but credible benefit, we have to consider whether the benefit is worth the unnecessary intervention and surgery, the false hopes, the risks, and the enormous costs.

Unfortunately, there is no mathematical formula that enables a consensus decision to be made. Even if the cost for each death delayed is calculated, diametrically opposed reactions are generated. One recent study suggests that the cost per woman benefited is $1.08 million.[12] If a mean figure is accepted from the five randomized prospective clinical trials (Figs. 2 and 3), then at least 26,000 women would have to be screened for one to benefit. At a cost of $75.00 per mammogram, the cost for each woman benefited is $2 million. It is clear that different persons and groups will make different decisions based on identical data on harm, costs, and benefits, and decisions will differ from place to place and from time to time. The current debate concerning mammography in our very wealthy society would be quite ridiculous in most other areas of the world where a much greater benefit to cost ratio would be required even to justify discussing the issue. The American Cancer Society abounds with enthusiasm[23] that has been called "wishful thinking" by others.[24] The American Cancer Society recommends that women age 35 to 39 years have a "baseline" mammogram, women age 40 to 49 years have one every 1 to 2 years, and for women age 50 and over, annual mammograms are recommended.

Perhaps we should look more closely at the harm caused rather than the costs incurred when assessing the negative aspects of mammography.[25] Is it really worth the trauma inflicted by mammography and the resultant surgical intervention in order to benefit one woman in 26,000 per year, at a cost in excess of $2 million each?

Tempering the Propaganda

We certainly need to counter the triumphal propaganda of the American Cancer Society that a mammogram ". . . helps your doctor see breast cancer before there is a lump, when the cure rates are near 100%."[26] There are billboards in the United States recommending the ". . . gift of life for Mother's Day. Give your mother a mammogram today." The extent of the misinformation passed to women on the mammography issue may be seen most remarkably in these comments published in 1989 by one of the principal investigators of the HIP study:[27]

> Most women with breast cancer could be saved by detection of the disease in an early, more curable stage if the physicians would teach their patients to examine their breasts once a month, and, this is most important, to encourage (sic) them to have complete periodic breast examinations to include mammography, according to American Cancer Society guidelines. Perhaps it is now time that concerns over risk in screening women should be allayed.

In view of the facts, this can only be construed as a deliberate attempt to mislead. In claiming that most women with breast cancer would be "saved" by early mammographic diagnosis, the author is presumably ignoring the results of his own study, let alone the other studies that have shown even less benefit or no benefit at all.

Mammography has become big business and the business interests involved are only too willing to promote the message of hope carried by the enthusiasts.

Conclusion

Mammography screening for breast cancer offers, at best, a very small benefit in exchange for great harm and cost, and at worst, no benefit whatsoever. Even if the results of those trials claiming the largest benefit are accepted, the only "benefit" for the large majority of women with breast cancer is extra time spent with the knowledge that they have the disease. As the quality of the mammography and the protocol design has increased in successive studies, the claimed benefit has, unfortunately, fallen progressively to nil.

The value of mammography for the evaluation of breast disease is not in question, but this debate concerns the use of mass mammography for *screening* purposes. The patient with a breast lump has a problem for which she is seeking help; the patient with a positive screening mammogram is, more often than not, given a problem where none existed. For women at high risk of developing breast cancer—for example, those with a family history of premenopausal onset—the harm/benefit scales may tip in favor of screening because of the higher disease prevalence and the consequently higher positive predictive value of an abnormal mammogram in this group.

The current failure to accept and act upon the evidence against screening mammography is fueled by the understandable desperate desire to find something, anything, that might help in this terrible disease, together with the vested interests of the industry. It is foolish, however, to continue pouring resources into the nonsolution to the problem that mammography has turned out to be. On the basis of currently available evidence on mass screening, the benefits, if any at all, are much too small and the harm and cost generated much too great to justify implementation. Mammography as a mass screening procedure should be abandoned.

References

1. Mueller CB, Jeffries W: Cancer of the breast: its outcome as measured by the rate of dying and causes of death. Ann Surg 1975; 182:334–340.
2. Baker LH: Breast cancer detection demonstration project: five-year summary report. Cancer J Clinicians 1982; 32:194–225.
3. Shapiro S, Strax P, Venet L: Periodic breast cancer screening in reducing mortality from breast cancer. JAMA 1971; 215:1777-1785.
4. Shapiro S, Venet W, Strax P, et al: Ten to fourteen year effects of breast cancer screening on mortality. J Natl Cancer Inst 1982; 69:349–355.
5. Shapiro S: Determining the efficacy of breast cancer screening. Cancer 1989; 63:1873–1880.
6. Tabar L, Fagerberg CJ, Gad A, et al: Reduction in mortality from breast cancer after mass screening with mammography. Lancet 1985; 1:829–832.
7. Tabar L, Fagerberg CJ, Day NE: In: Day NE, Miller AB (eds). Screening for Breast Cancer. Huber, Toronto, 1988.
8. Andersson I, Aspegren K, Janzon L, et al: Mammographic screening and mortality from breast cancer: the Malmo mammographic screening trial. Br Med J 1988; 297:943–948.
9. Roberts MM, Alexander FE, Anderson TJ, et al: Edinburgh trial of screening for breast

cancer: mortality at 7 years. Lancet 1990; 335:241–246.

10. Miller AB, Baines CJ, To T, et al: Canadian National Breast Screening Study: 1. Breast cancer detection and death rates among women aged 40 to 49 years. Can Med Assoc J 1992; 147:1459-1476.

11. Miller AB, Baines CJ, To T, et al: Canadian National Breast Screening Study: 2. Breast cancer detection and death rates among women aged 50 to 59 years. Can Med Assoc J 1992; 147:1477-1488.

12. Eddy DM, Hasselblad V, McGivney W, et al: The value of mammography screening in women under age 50 years. JAMA 1988; 259:1512–1519.

13. Chu KC, Smart CR, Tarone RE: Analysis of breast cancer mortality and stage distribution by age for the health insurance plan clinical trial. JNCI 1988; 80:1125–1132.

14. Norton LW, Zeligman BE, Pearlman NW: Accuracy and cost of needle localization breast biopsy. Arch Surg 1988; 123:947-950.

15. Baines CJ, McFarlane DV, Miller AB: Sensitivity and specificity of first screen mammography in 15 NBSS centers. J Can Assoc Radiol 1988; 39:273–276.

16. Page DL, Dupont WD, Rogers LW, et al: Intraductal carcinoma of the breast: follow-up after biopsy only. Cancer 1982; 49:751-758.

17. Rosen PP, Kosloff C, Lieberman PH, et al: Lobular carcinoma in situ of the breast: detailed analysis of 99 patients with average follow-up of 24 years. Am J Surg Pathol 1978; 2:225-251.

18. Haagensen CD, Lane N, Lattes R, et al: Lobular neoplasia (so-called lobular carcinoma in situ) of the breast, Cancer 1978; 42:737–769.

19. Roberts MM, Breast screening: time for a rethink? Br Med J 1989; 299:1153–1155.

20. Marteau T: Psychological costs of screening. Br Med J 1989; 299:527.

21. Howe GR, Sherman GJ, Semenciw RM, et al: Estimated benefits and risks of screening for breast cancer. Can Med Assoc J 1981; 124:399–403.

22. Holmberg DM, Adami HO, Persson I, et al: Demands on surgical inpatient services after mass mammography screening. Br Med J 1986; 293:779–782.

23. American Cancer Society: Mammography guidelines 1983: background statement and update of cancer-related checkup guidelines for breast cancer detection in asymptomatic women age 40 to 49. Cancer J Clinicians 1983; 33:255.

24. Skrabanek P: False premises and false promises of breast cancer screening. Lancet 1985; 2:316–319.

25. Wright CJ: Breast cancer screening: a different look at the evidence. Surgery 1986; 100:594–597.

26. American Cancer Society, 1986, Pamphlet 86 (30 mm), No. 2077-LE.

27. Strax P: Control of breast cancer through mass screening: from research to action. Cancer 1989; 63:1881–1887.

30

Cost-Benefit Analysis of Screening for Breast Cancer in the United Kingdom and the United States

Michael Baum

Introduction

The advocates of screening well-women populations by mammography base their arguments on the seductively appealing notion that the smaller a cancer is at the time of detection, the earlier the disease in its natural history and the greater the likelihood of cure by local surgery alone. This simplistic notion ignores the variable biological nature of the disease and its capacity for dissemination even at a subclinical stage. Furthermore, the use of case fatality statistics showing improvement in length of survival with the smaller detection size of the tumor ignores the well-recognized phenomena of lead time and length bias. Nevertheless, it has been essential to subject the theory of population screening for early breast cancer to the rigors of scientific evaluation through randomized controlled trials, and it should be on the basis of the results from these trials that health policies are determined, not by the a priori reasoning of the screening zealots or those with a cash incentive for marketing annual mammography for well women.

Results of Screening Trials

There is little controversy these days about calculating the benefit of screening for populations of well women based on the results of published randomized controlled trials. A recent overview of the literature of screening trials has suggested that we can anticipate approximately a 20% reduction in cause-specific mortality for an unselected population of women.[1]

Assuming this to be true, Table 1 illustrates the benefits that might be anticipated for two populations under and over the age of 50 to whom screening was made available, based on the most optimistic estimates.[2] It can be seen that taking the upper limit of risk reduction for women over the age of 50, we might expect a little under 1% of the population to benefit over a 20-year period, whereas taking the most optimistic estimate for the women under the age of 50, this can only translate into a benefit for less than 0.15% of the population over a 20-year period, with 99.85% of the total population shouldering the burden of costs (see below). However, these estimates are based on a selection bias favoring the most optimistic estimates. Some trials for screening women under the age of 50 have shown no benefits at all, and two trials (the Malmo Study and the Canadian trial) show a significant detriment for the younger cohort.[3] At the present time, therefore, it is an absurdity to offer screening for women under the age of 50, and advertisements by the American Cancer Society advocating screening from the age of 35 years on would be in breach of the code of our Advertising Standards Authority if they were used in the United Kingdom.

Coming now to the postmenopausal woman, where there is no argument that screening can reduce cause-specific mortality, it is necessary to translate the relative reduction in risk into some description of the absolute gains achieved from this activity. The best case scenario has been described by Tabar and colleagues based on the Swedish Two County Trial.[4] They show how, in years 4 to 9 after the start of the study, among women aged 50 to 69 at entry, approximately one breast cancer death was avoided per year for 4,000 women allocated to screening, with an average screening interval of 33 months and a compliance of 90%. Putting it in another way, one death was prevented per 1,500 mammographic examinations generating 13.5 biopsies, in a program that has one of the highest specificity rates in the world.

Table 1
Proportion of Women Who Benefit from Screening

Age Group	*Age 50–69 Years*	*Age 40–49 Years*
Frequency of breast cancer during the following 20-year period	5%	1.5%
Deaths from breast cancer	2.5%	0.75%
Reduction in deaths anticipated "best-case scenario"	40%	20%
Proportion who benefit	2.5 × 0.4	0.75 × 0.2
Bottom line	1%	0.15%

The Cost of Screening

Against this undoubted benefit must be balanced the cost, both in terms of finance, and psychological or physical morbidity. First of all, the financial costs are very important in the UK and in the Scandinavian countries where there is socialized medicine because money spent on screening could, in theory, be more usefully spent in other areas of the Health Service. For example, I had personal experience of establishing a screening service for the South East of England at a time when there were cuts in the overall Health Service budget. This resulted in the closure of many acute surgical wards with the absurd result that, having detected early breast cancer on mammography, patients were then forced to wait for 3 weeks or more to come in for their biopsy to establish whether or not they had a cancer. At the same time, the waiting list grew for other elective surgery procedures so that women with symptomatic breast cancer were equally well inconvenienced by the knock-on effects of screening the well population. These issues become less relevant in the US, where the majority of screening activities are funded by the clients themselves. In this case, however, it is all the more important to consider the other costs of mammographic screening to the individual apart from dollars so that she can make an informed decision as a consumer whether or not to purchase the service: for example, the psychological morbidity of false alarms,[5] the financial and psychological costs of unnecessary biopsies, and worst of all, the problems for a woman living under the shadow of cancer when she has been diagnosed as having ductal carcinoma in situ which, if left alone, in theory might never have threatened her life.[6] Such a woman lives with a fear of premature death and the problems of health insurance.

I find it paradoxical that if there is a delay in the diagnosis of the breast cancer, a surgeon is subject to litigation which may cost him millions of dollars even though there is no good evidence that the delay in diagnosing symptomatic breast cancer influences the chances of long-term survival. Whereas, if a surgeon is overzealous, performing unnecessary biopsies in women suspected of having abnormalities in the breast, he is never subjected to litigation. This fear of litigation leads American surgeons to practice defensive medicine with a resulting fall in the specificity of the screening technique.

In fact, when considering the individual woman rather than a population of women, it is virtually impossible to identify anyone who would benefit from the screening activity, and thus outside of a socialized health care system, it would be foolish for a consumer to purchase this service. For example, at one extreme, it has already been suggested that the diagnosis of ductal carcinoma in situ does not mean that the screening was of benefit, since if it were left alone, the disease might not progress in a woman's lifetime. A number of postmortem studies have suggested that approximately five times the rate of ductal carcinoma in situ has been detected in women dying of acute illness or trauma than might be expected to have appeared as invasive cancer in the rest of that woman's lifetime at risk.[6]

At the other extreme, having diagnosed a small invasive breast cancer does not confirm that screening was a success because the woman may yet die of her disease in spite of the putative earlier stage of diagnosis. Furthermore, many screening zealots promote the exercise in order to reduce the burden of unnecessary mastectomies on the female population, yet at the same time, many surgeons advocate total mastectomy for the treatment of ductal carcinoma in situ, and many women may be disappointed when their disease is found to be multifocal and they are left without a choice for breast-conserving surgery. A paradox is, therefore, beginning to emerge whereby you are more likely to have breast-conserving surgery for a clinically detected invasive disease than for a screening-detected in-situ or early invasive cancer.[7] The psychological impact on such women is difficult to estimate and is likely to be more profound than that experienced after clinically overt disease. In the former, the woman assumes that she is well until she is being told that she is sick, whereas in the latter, the woman assumes that she has cancer unless she is being reassured.

Cost Versus Benefits of Screening

In countries where there is socialized medicine, the decision to screen is considered a public health measure based on careful cost/benefit analyses ending up with a value judgment. The Forrest recommendation for the UK program for screening all women between the ages of 50 and 64 at three yearly intervals has recently been vindicated following the publication of the Quality Assurance Statistics for the first round of activity.[8] These data demonstrated approximately a 70% compliance rate with less than 8% referral for a second line evaluation and assessment. Approximately 1% were subjected to biopsy with a 1:1 benign to malignant biopsy ratio. These excellent statistics for specificity were not associated with an impaired detection rate, as this has been running at approximately 7 per 1,000 in the prevalance round. At the same time, as a valuable spin-off from the National Screening Programme, there has been the establishment of specialist breast clinics, the upgrading of mammographic equipment, and the improvement in quality of cytopathology and histopathology throughout the country. In contrast, in the US where the individual has to pay and where many centers are operating at a 10:1 benign to malignant biopsy ratio, as a result of the pressures of defensive medicine, it can be fairly deduced that the harm to benefit ratios are excessive and that the current programs of opportunist activity should be seriously reconsidered. I believe that the majority of the clients of the screening programs in the US have been bamboozled into purchasing a product as a result of misguided promotion and wishful thinking. The consumer in the US deserves a better deal that could result only from a more controlled access to screening and a desensitization of the population under the age of 50 to the perceived value of mammography in the symptomless woman.

References

1. Department of Health Advisory Committee: Breast Cancer Screening 1991: Evidence and experience since the Forrest Report, London. January 1991.
2. Miller AB: Screening for cancer: issues and future directions. J Chron Dis 1986; 39:1067–1077.
3. Anderson I, Aspegren K, Janzon K, et al: Mammographic screening and mortality from breast cancer: the Malmo mammographic screening trial. Br Med J 1988; 297:943–948.
4. Tabar L, Fagerburg G, Duffy SW, Day NE: The Swedish Two County Trial of mammographic screening for breast cancer: recent results and calculations of benefit. J Epidemiol Community Health 1989; 43:107–114.
5. Garstin WIH, Kaufman Z, Baum M: False alarms of breast cancer. Lancet 1990; 335:229.
6. Nielsen M, Jensen J, Andersen J: Precancerous and cancerous breast lesions during lifetime and at autopsy. Cancer 1984; 54:612–615.
7. Fisher ER, Leeming R, Anderson S, et al: Conservative management of intraductal carcinoma (DCIS) of the breast. J Surg Oncol 1991; 47:139–147.
8. Department of Health Advisory Committee, London: Audit of the first round of National Health Service Screening Programme. November 1992.

Adjuvant Therapy for Breast Cancer

Editorial Commentary

Chapters 31–33

Chapters 31–33 summarize some of the current thoughts about adjuvant chemotherapy for patients with potentially curable breast cancer. Dr. Holland gives the view of an activist but his data are also supported by the Early Breast Cancer Trialists collaborative group study (Lancet 1992; 339:71,115). This study summarizes the results from 133 randomized trials; adjuvant chemotherapy resulted in a 28% decrease in recurrence rate and a 16% decrease in mortality. It was also found that 6 months of chemotherapy was just as effective as the 12-month regime, and that polychemotherapy was better than single-agent chemotherapy. In addition, between ages 50 and 69 years, chemotherapy with additional tamoxifen gave a better synergistic decrease in mortality rate than chemotherapy alone. The proportional risk reductions were similar for node-positive and node-negative patients, but the absolute improvement in 10-year survival was about twice as good in the former as in the latter.

Professor Blamey and Dr. Galea from the United Kingdom bring out some thoughtful arguments against the routine use of adjuvant chemotherapy in node-negative patients. They feel that apart from the nodes, one should also evaluate the histologic grade and tumor size. Using these criteria, they selected a group of patients who are estrogen receptor-negative and have grade III tumors, and these are the only node-negative patients for whom they advise cytotoxic therapy.

Finally, Dr. Mueller presents an extremely provocative chapter about the ethical issues concerning chemotherapy, which should be read by all clinicians involved in the management of breast cancer.

Chapters 34 and 35

The chapters on tamoxifen as adjuvant therapy by Sir Patrick Forrest and Professor Michael Baum are complementary, and in the British tradition they both advocate its use much more widely than is the current practice in the United States. These views are supported by the Early Breast Cancer Trialists collaborative group (Lancet 1992; 339:71,115). They have shown that tamoxifen caused a 25% decrease in recurrence, a 17% decrease in mortality, and a 39% decrease in the development of contralateral breast cancer. Although tamoxifen had a beneficial effect on both estrogen receptor-positive and estrogen receptor-negative patients, the effect on the estrogen receptor-positive patients was much more significant.

Chapters 36 and 37

Chapters 36 and 37 deal with the controversies regarding irradiation following conservative surgery for breast cancer. Dr. Shank gives an excellent overview and Drs. Moffat and Ketchum provide some good arguments to support the thesis that adjuvant radiotherapy is not always necessary following lumpectomy. Obviously, prospective randomized studies would be needed to come to a final conclusion, but it seems that especially with small tumors (less than 2 cm in diameter) with adequate negative microscopic margins, the role of radiotherapy is questionable.

We don't believe that there is good evidence to support the use of radiotherapy to the axillary nodes following an appropriate level I and II axillary dissection. In our view, radiotherapy to these nodes should be withheld and should be given only in the very rare instance of local occurrence in the axilla. As far as sequencing is concerned, we use a sandwich approach, starting off with chemotherapy, sandwiching irradiation in the middle for about 6 weeks, followed by completion of the chemotherapy schedule.

31

Adjuvant Chemotherapy for Breast Cancer: An Activist's View

James F. Holland

Introduction

Breast cancer is a singular term, representing a group of diseases. I think the sooner we come to recognize that the entity of breast cancer is not a single process, but one of many different kinds characterized by genetic abnormalities in the breast cells, the better we will be.[1] Unfortunately, none of this has been promoted to clinical utility so far, but it is clear that certain breast cancers lack a tumor suppressor gene, P53, which is on chromosome 17.[2] The same loss of P53 function is common to many other kinds of cancer. It has been shown by Stanbridge that in colon cancer, the reintroduction of the P53 gene, by virtue of reintroducing chromosome 17, can eliminate the tumorigenicity of the neoplasm.[3] Others have confirmed this observation in different tumor systems, including ovarian cancer. This makes me think that we are still dealing with primitive approaches to cancer, by using surgery, chemotherapy, and radiotherapy. It may well be that an understanding of the disease in terms of its molecular etiology will allow us either to design other drugs or to reconstitute the normal genetic functioning of the breast. Everything that I present is thus a temporary endorsement of an approach that I think is time-limited. One should look eventually for the molecular chemotherapist to solve the problem without toxic and/or amputative approaches.

After having said that, it has been clear that surgery alone is an inadequate treatment for breast cancer. A wide variety of treatment programs have been introduced for breast cancer using chemotherapeutic agents. The first American controlled trial, Bernard Fisher's demonstration of the effectiveness of a single alkylating agent, phenylalanine mustard versus a placebo in women with breast cancer with positive nodes, caused an increase in disease-free and overall

From: Wise L, Johnson H Jr (eds): *Breast Cancer: Controversies in Management*. Futura Publishing Company, Inc., Armonk, NY, © 1994.

survival at 10 years[4] (Fig. 1). Although this led to a great deal of controversy at the time and to the erroneous concept that it did not work in postmenopausal women, the eventual outcome was positive. Simultaneously, Veronesi and Bonadonna demonstrated that three drugs, cyclophosphamide, methotrexate, and fluorouracil (CMF), after mastectomy demonstrated better 10-year disease-free survival rates than the control treatment of surgery only in node-positive women (Fig. 2). Prior to these reports, Cooper recognized that five drugs were active in combination in metastatic breast cancer, and having seen that patients with four or more metastatic nodes at the time of surgery were nearly all destined to relapse, he used the five, CMFVP (vincristine and prednisone), for 9 months in adjuvant fashion.[5] Cooper's data in 73 women with four or more positive lymph nodes who were treated with CMFVP after surgery were compared with national mortality data at the time and with Fisher's control data (Fig. 3).

There would not appear to be much question that a variety of chemotherapies given after surgery have had an impact on the relapse of node-positive breast cancer. At the time I served as Chairman of the Cancer and Leukemia Group B (CALGB), a national organization that has made substantial contributions in this area. Because Cooper's data had been

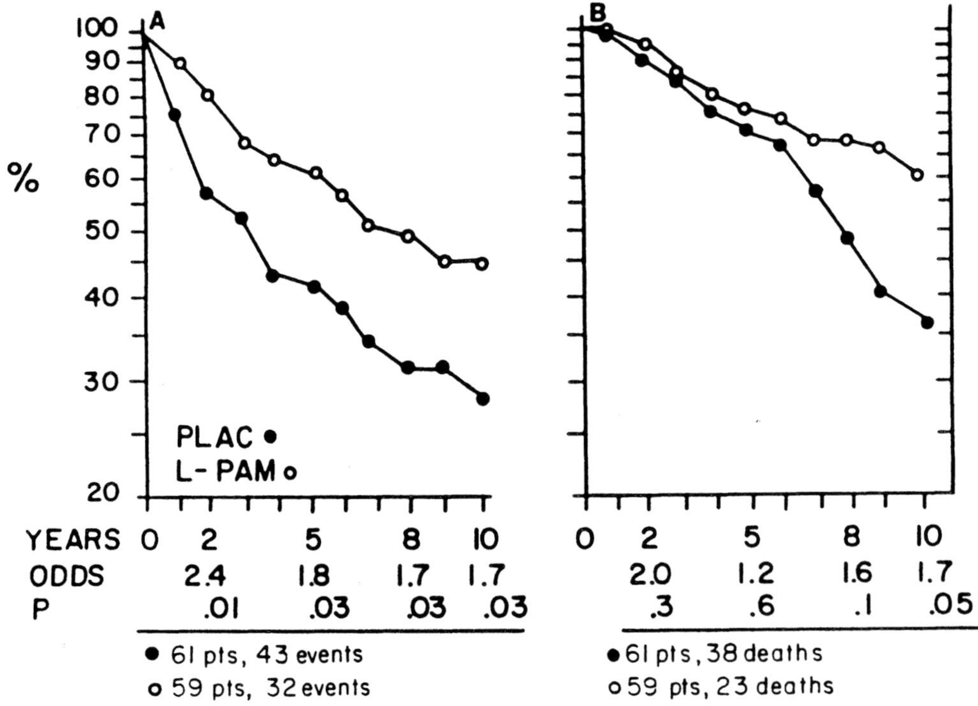

Figure 1: *National Surgical Adjuvant Breast Program (NSABP) data for their first study showing activity of l-phenylalanine mustard (L-PAM) superior to placebo (PLAC) in disease-free survival (left) and survival (right). From Fisher et al.[4]*

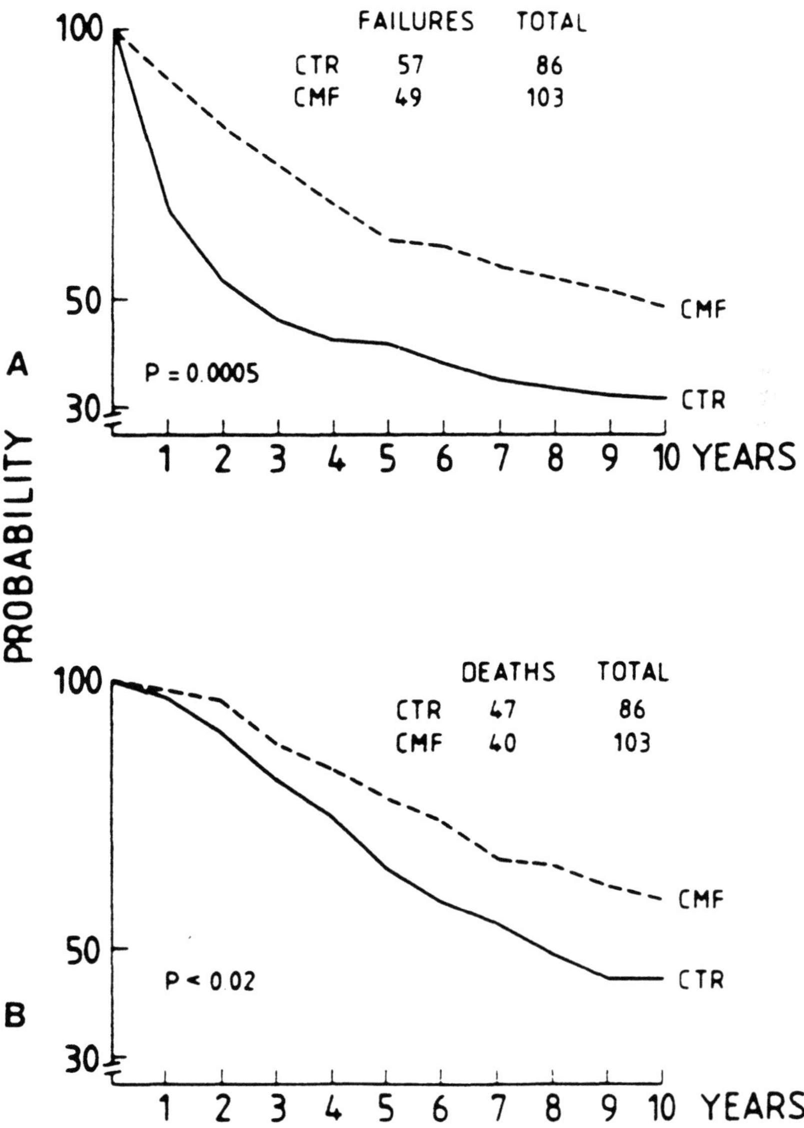

Figure 2: *Data of Bonadonna and Veronesi from the National Cancer Institute in Milan. The combination of cyclophosphamide, methotrexate, and fluorouracil (CMF) is significantly superior to control (CTR) in disease-free survival (top) and survival (bottom). From Fisher et al.*[4]

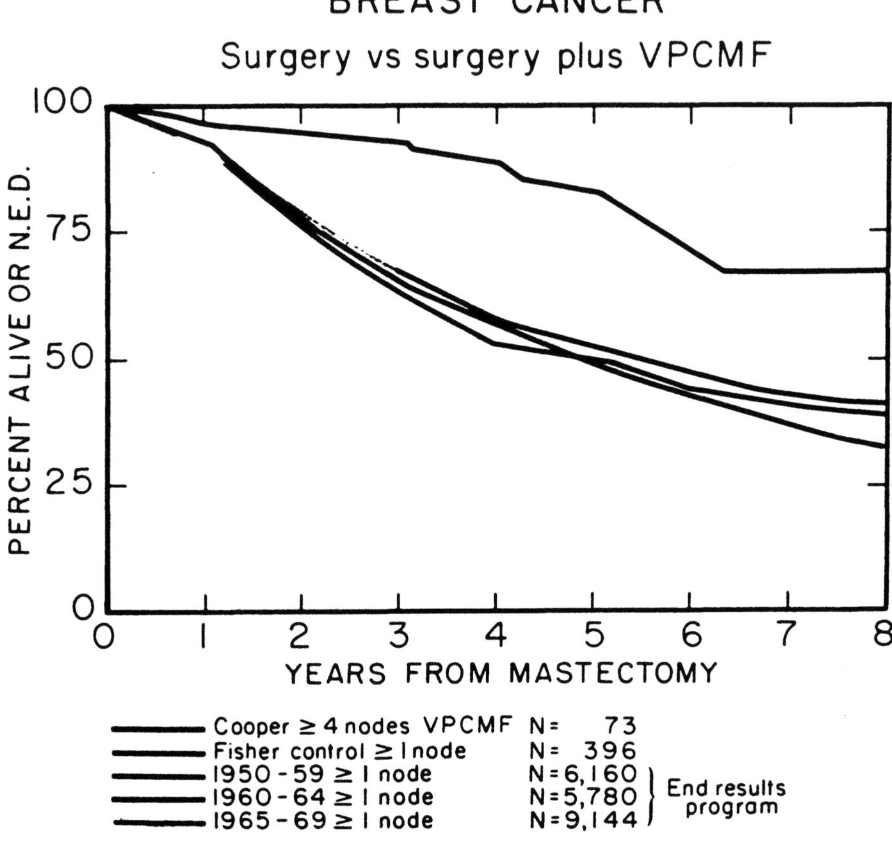

Figure 3: *Disease-free survival of women with ≥4 metastatic axillary nodes who received adjuvant vincristine, prednisone, cyclophosphamide, methotrexate, and fluorouracil (VPCMF) chemotherapy for 9 months (top curve) compared to mortality curves for women with ≥1 metastatic axillary node from NSABP studies and data collected by the National Cancer Institute in the end results program.[5]*

achieved with five drugs (CMFVP) and the three drugs used by Bonadonna and Veronesi (CMF) were derivative of it, we compared the two drug regimen programs. The five drugs proved superior in women with four or more positive nodes (Fig. 4). My colleague Norton, then at Mount Sinai, looked at the data for the five drugs and constructed a mathematical model of what happens when one kills off a sensitive population: a resistant population emerges and accounts for the eventual relapse. The mathematical model predicts that a second treatment could be applied when the cancer cells surviving the first treatment were still small in number. This second hit, in the fashion AAAA BBBB (the Norton-Simon approach) is significantly superior in the model to ABABABAB (the Goldie-Coldman approach).[6] We designed a successor pilot study consisting of the authentic original Cooper regimen and

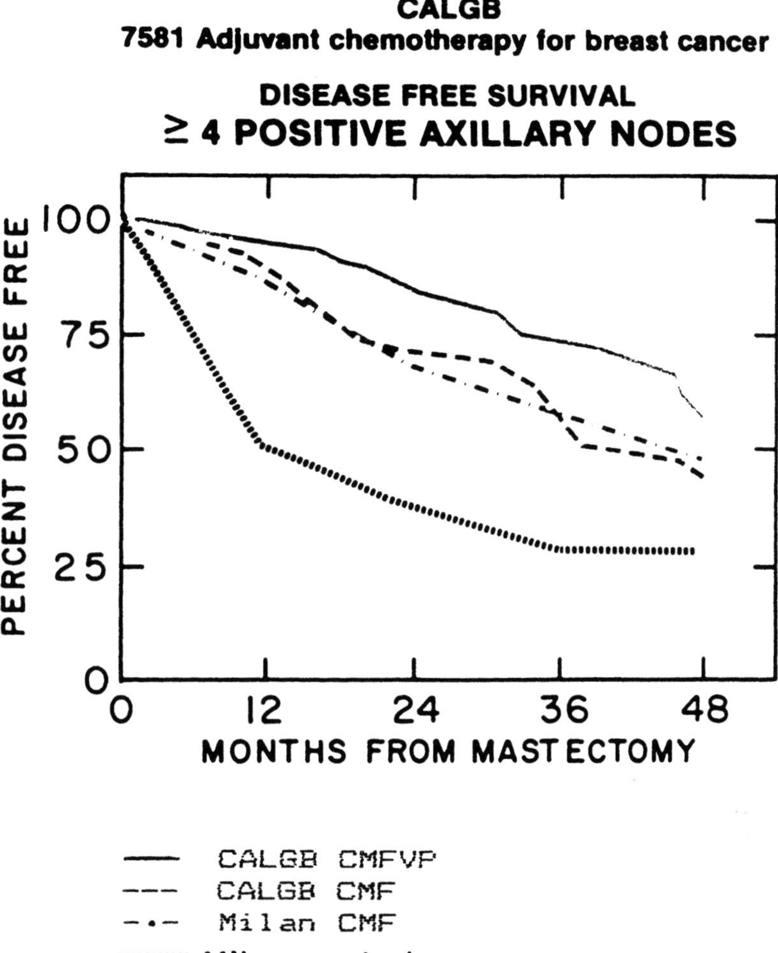

Figure 4: *Comparison of results of Milan data on adjuvant chemotherapy with CMF versus control, and the Cancer and Leukemia Group B (CALGB) data of CMF (superimposed on the Milan data) and CMFVP which is significantly superior in premenopausal women with ≥4 metastatic axillary nodes.*

the intensive use of adriamycin, probably the most active single drug, which we had demonstrated to have high activity in metastatic disease. This 32-week treatment program demonstrated some very satisfactory results at Mount Sinai,[7] and thus was extrapolated to the CALGB. The data there in 29 patients with one to three positive nodes treated with this 4-month induction of the Cooper regimen and then four courses of intensive adriamycin have been analyzed by Bhardwaj and show only a single relapse in observations up to 4 years. Although early, and further relapses may occur, the results are better at this stage than any other prior CALGB or Mount Sinai study.

I don't think that there should be any controversy that women with metastatic breast cancer to the axillary nodes are best helped by chemotherapy with surgery. Whether this should be given before or after surgery is a controversial point. There isn't much controversy anymore concerning age. The initial Fisher data for phenylalanine mustard had a superior result in those under 50. The question arose whether it was inert in those who are over 50. All other studies of the National Surgical Adjuvant Breast and Bowel Program (NSABBP), Milan, and CALGB after the original two have also shown chemotherapeutic activity in older or postmenopausal women. This fact has been broadly confirmed in the meta-analysis of the early trialists.[8]

Data from the NSABBP on tamoxifen versus adriamycin and cyclophosphamide plus tamoxifen show that the combination treatment is superior in terms of disease-free survival, distant disease-free survival (relapse outside of the breast), and survival in women over the age of 50, both estrogen receptor (ER)-positive and ER-negative (except for one small subgroup of women under the age of 60 who were progesterone receptor-negative and not included in the study)[4] (Fig. 5). There are obviously older women who are unsuitable medical risks for surgery, chemotherapy, or any other procedure; their medical problems should be taken into account when considering a chemotherapy regimen. On the other hand, their breast cancer, which may not be their most serious problem, may well be helped by attention not only to endocrine therapy, but to chemotherapy as well.

The real controversy relates to women who don't have node metastases. The data of the Early Breast Cancer Trialists, Peto and colleagues, in node-negative patients compare surgery only with surgery plus polychemotherapy.[8] Several thousand women were included in the meta-analysis. At 5 years, about 30% relapsed who were node-negative[8] (Fig. 6). There is a subset of node-negative women who may be at low risk, but most are at high risk. By 5 years, to have a 30% relapse rate among all node-negative women is an unnecessary chance if it is possible to mitigate this by therapy. It is possible in the more adverse circumstance of node-positivity to diminish the relapse rate. It is possible to mitigate relapse among node-negative women by polychemotherapy.[8] I offer another example from the NSABBP of women who are node-negative.[4] Using methotrexate and fluorouracil only, without cyclophosphamide, the disease-free survival rate is considerably better in the treated women (Fig. 7) by a factor of about one third. The benefit extended to women of all ages (Fig. 8). Node-negative women are at high enough risk to justify treatment. This early attempt by the NSABP placed emphasis on the fact that chemotherapy with cyclophosphamide can be toxic, so it was omitted. But the women who have recurrent breast cancer have already sustained a very major late toxicity. In this context, the CALGB and other investigators are now studying the combination of CMF (with the cyclophosphamide) versus CAF (with adriamycin). It is probable that these will prove not to be the ultimate chemotherapies. They are steps on the way, however.

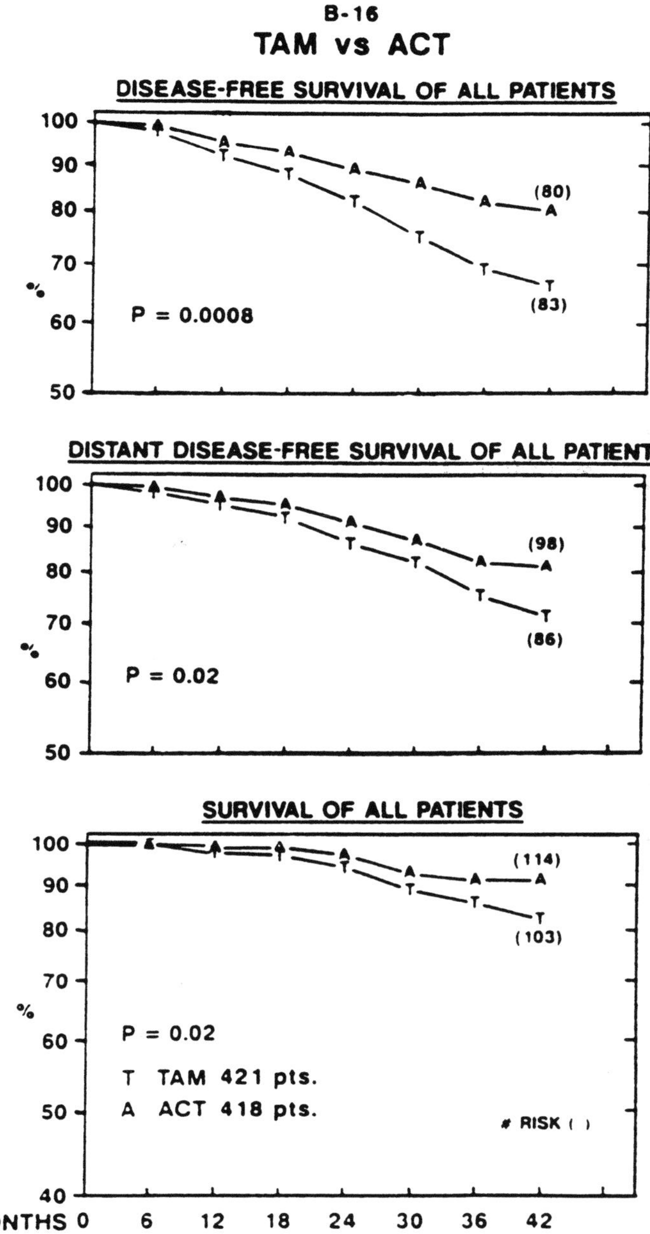

Figure 5: *Data of the NSABBP comparing tamoxifen alone (T) versus adriamycin, cyclophosphamide, and tamoxifen (A) as adjuvant therapy for women over 50, independent of estrogen receptor status. (One small group of women from age 50 to 60 who were progesterone receptor-negative was studied in another protocol and are not included). From Fisher et al.[4]*

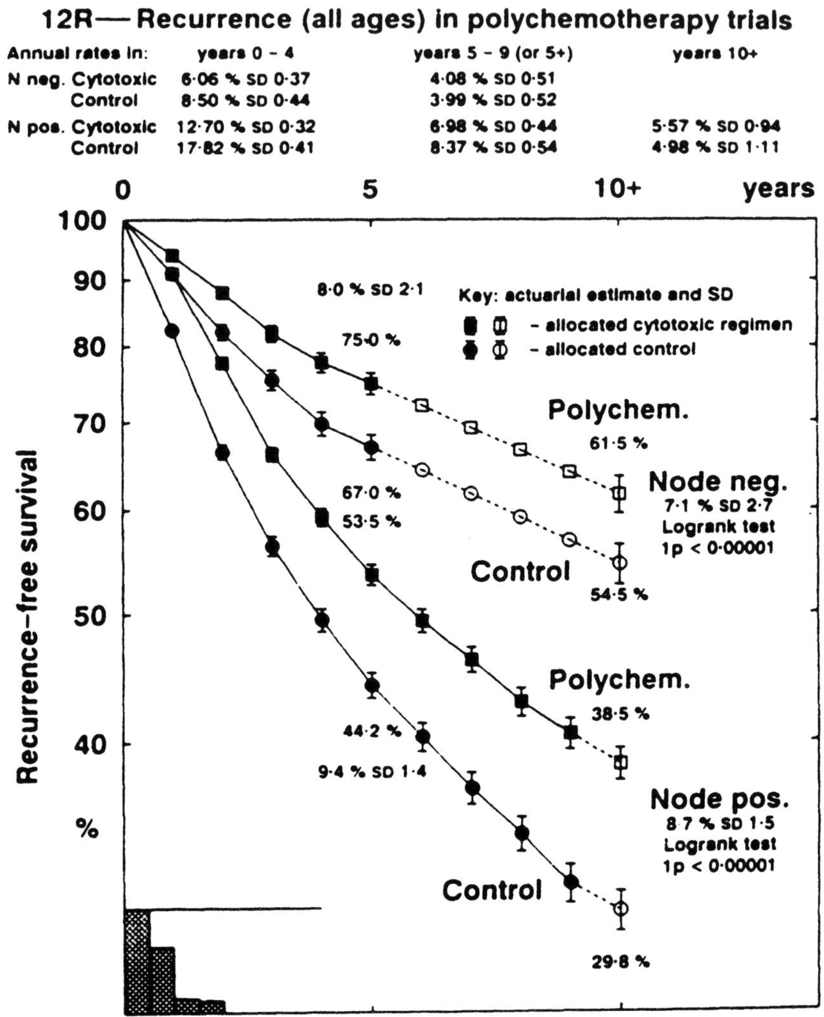

Figure 6: *Meta-analysis of the effects of surgery or surgery plus polychemotherapy on recurrences in women, irrespective of age, with node-negative and node-positive breast cancer. From the Early Breast Cancer Trialists Group.[8]*

I think that the design of more intensive, shorter course, higher dose chemotherapies, even for node-negative women, is highly likely. The dilemma is that 70% of the women at 5 years are still disease-free (Figs. 6 and 7), and therefore one is treating 70% of the women, perhaps without necessity, in order to help the 30% of the women who are affected. This 2:1 ratio, treating three although two might not need the treatment, means that therapy must be tolerable and safe. That is possible through chemotherapy given in a much more imaginative and intensive way than we had used previously at the time that CMF, MF, phenylalanine mustard, and other such chemotherapy regimens were

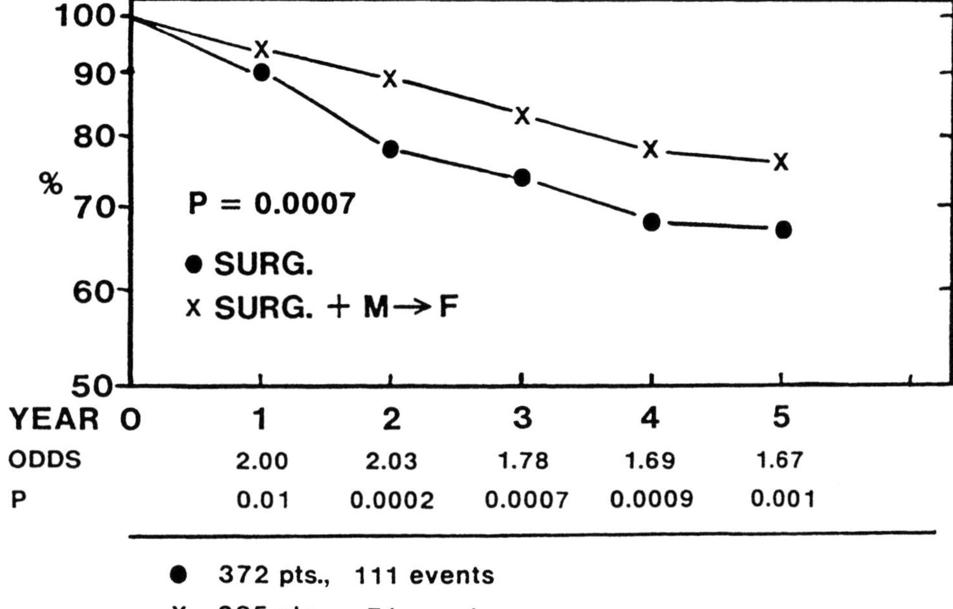

Figure 7: *Disease-free survival in node-negative women randomly allocated to surgery (surg) alone or to surgery plus adjuvant methotrexate followed by fluorouracil (Surg + M → F) data of NSABBP from Fisher et al.[4]*

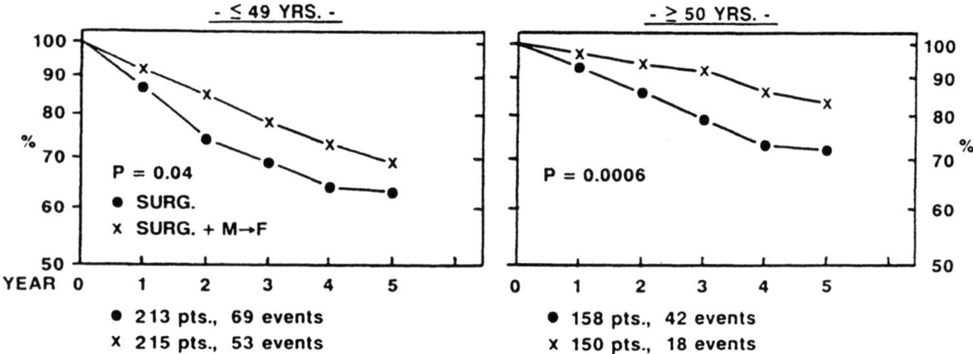

Figure 8: *Data from Figure 7 analyzed by age: methotrexate and fluorouracil delay recurrence in node-negative women with breast cancer. From Fisher et al.[4]*

designed. The arrival of a whole armamentarium of genetically engineered colony-stimulating factors, and good antibiotics, makes it possible now to take patients to levels of marrow toxicity that no longer are of major concern, and to propose more intensive treatments for breast cancer that will more likely have greater effect. Some of this perspective must be taken on faith, because it takes

5 years at minimum and perhaps 10 years to tell the outcome of intensive chemotherapies of women who have negative nodes. But many do have micrometastatic disease and are susceptible to chemotherapeutic improvement, as already demonstrated. I believe we should aim toward eradication of the tumor rather than consider the safety of the host as the prime driving force. This change in emphasis is now possible.

I would invite all surgeons to participate in the research, since the crux of the issue is that there are enough women in this country to answer these questions in short time if more of them were entered in the study programs. To adopt into practice a chemotherapeutic program that is old enough to show data is to adopt something that is not modern enough to be related to the current research thrust.

Chemotherapeutic effects are real. It is necessary to continue this research in chemotherapy, since it is the systemic aspects of breast cancer that determine the outcome. We seek cure. Surgery alone won't do it, radiotherapy alone won't do it, and the chemotherapy we have today won't do it. But the chemotherapy available is indeed active. We must keep a clinical trials apparatus intact so that we are ready for the next generation of rationally designed chemotherapeutic agents. We are all waiting to reap the research benefits of molecular chemotherapy. Understanding the importance of oncogenes, of tumor suppressor genes, and of the potential availability of their gene products gives us major hope for the future.

References

1. Chen L, Kurisu W, Ljung B, Goldman E, et al: Heterogeneity for allelic loss in human breast cancer. J National Cancer Institute 1992; 84:506–510.
2. Coles C, Thompson AM, Elder PA, Cohen BB, et al: Evidence implicating at least two genes on chromosome 17p in breast carcinogenesis. Lancet 1990; 336:763–765.
3. Stanbridge E: Personal communication, 1992.
4. Fisher B, Osborne K, Bloomer W, Margolese R: Breast cancer. In: Holland JF, Frei E III, Bast RC Jr, et al (eds). Cancer Medicine, 3rd edition. Lea and Febiger, Philadelphia, 1992.
5. Cooper RG, Holland JF, Glidewell O: Adjuvant chemotherapy of breast cancer. Cancer 1979; 44:793.
6. Norton L: Cytokinetics. In: Holland JF, Frei E III, Bast RC Jr, et al (eds). Cancer Medicine, 3rd edition. Lea and Febiger, Philadelphia, 1992.
7. Bhardwaj S, Holland JF, Norton L: An intensive sequenced adjuvant chemotherapy regimen for breast cancer. Cancer Invest 1993; 11:6–9.
8. Early Breast Cancer Trialists Collaborative Group: Systemic treatment of early breast cancer by hormonal, cytotoxic or immune therapy. Lancet 1992; 339:1–15,71–85.

32

Routine Use of Adjuvant Chemotherapy in Node-Negative Patients With Breast Cancer Is not Indicated

Roger W. Blamey, Marcus H. Galea

Introduction

The arguments for the use of adjuvant treatment in breast cancer are that (1) the patient is likely to have her life span shortened by breast cancer and (2) chemotherapy early in the course of the disease can delay the appearance of distant metastases and lengthen survival. On the other hand, the argument against routine adjuvant chemotherapy is that total potential benefit does not match the total side effects.

Prognostic factors are now well established in our center. At the time of diagnosis and treatment of the primary lesion, a group of women can be identified in whom long-term survival is little short of that of a group of age-matched women who do not suffer from breast cancer; in this chapter we will demonstrate this. Such a group can gain very little benefit from adjuvant therapy; 5% at most could benefit, assuming that all women who are likely to die from breast cancer over a 15-year period benefit; 95% of women would receive treatment for no advantage whatever. Since the side effects of cytotoxic chemotherapy are not inconsiderable, it seems quite clear that this group should not receive such treatment.

Our other contention is that the concept of node negativity in the estimation of prognosis should now be redundant. Nodal status alone is not a good enough indicator of prognosis. In clinical use, it does not select a group with a high probability of cure nor one with a high probability of early recurrence (Fig. 1); like

From: Wise L, Johnson H Jr (eds): *Breast Cancer: Controversies in Management.* Futura Publishing Company, Inc., Armonk, NY, © 1994.

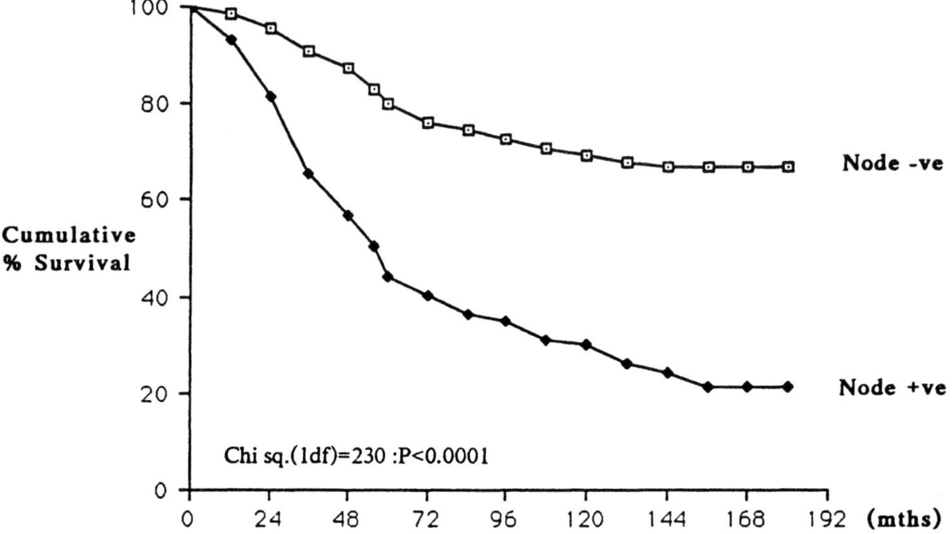

Figure 1: *Patient survival: lymph node-negative vs. lymph node-positive, Nottingham Breast Cancer Series: 1976–1988.*

tumor size, it is a time-dependent factor. Rather, prognosis should be estimated using a combination of intrinsic biological tumor factors with time-dependent factors. In this chapter we will demonstrate that a group of patients with good prognosis can be defined and that these patients account for 25–35% of the patient population depending on whether or not breast cancer screening is available. We will then go on to discuss the maximum possible benefits that could be achieved in this group using cytotoxic chemotherapy.

Nottingham Prognostic Index

In 1973 we began a study of prognosis in the patient series which we were then accumulating. In a comparatively short time it became obvious to us that patients who had poorly differentiated tumors and had nodal involvement had a very poor prognosis, with early distant recurrence of their disease. After sufficient time had elapsed, we carried out multivariate analysis of nine factors in our series which we thought might have a bearing on prognosis. Two factors—histological grade and lymph node stage—were shown to be the most powerful, with tumor size also making a contribution. The other factors did not add to estimation of survival once these three had been included. An easily calculable prognostic index for each patient was derived. This index indicates:

1. the size of the tumor in centimeters,

2. the histologic grade of the tumor, using a method[1] that relies on assigning scores to mitotic index, tubule formation, and nuclear pleomorphism, and

3. lymph node stage, which relies upon the Nottingham triple biopsy method, estimating lymph node involvement and its level.

The latter two factors are allocated scores of 1 to 3, histologic grading 1 to 3 from well-differentiated through moderate to poor differentiation, lymph node stage, with no lymph node involvement scoring 1, low lymph node (low axillary) involvement scoring 2, and high lymph node involvement (second intercostal space internal mammary node or a node at the apex of the axilla alongside the axillary vein) scoring 3. An index (I) for each patient is then calculated as:

$$I = grade + stage + (size \times 0.2).$$

The index scores range from 2.2 to 7.0. The very best type of tumor would be a grade 1 tumor with no lymph node involvement, measuring approximately 1 cm (tumors that are frequently seen from breast cancer screening programs) scoring 2.2, whereas a large tumor of 3 cm with high lymph node involvement and poor differentiation would score 6.6. The cut-off levels found most useful for clinical practice were less than or equal to 3.4, 3.41 to 5.4 and greater than 5.4. This splits off a group of patients I ≤3.4, good prognostic group (GPG), in whom the survival chance is never far short of an age-matched normal female population group (calculated from insurance statistics) (Fig. 2). In the poor prognostic group (PPG) with a score of 5.4 or more, 80% have distant recurrence apparent within 5 years. These account for, respectively, 28% and 20% of the patient population in a series without breast cancer screening.

The initial description of the index[2] was derived from retrospective examination of a patient series. It has since been prospectively applied in a new series of

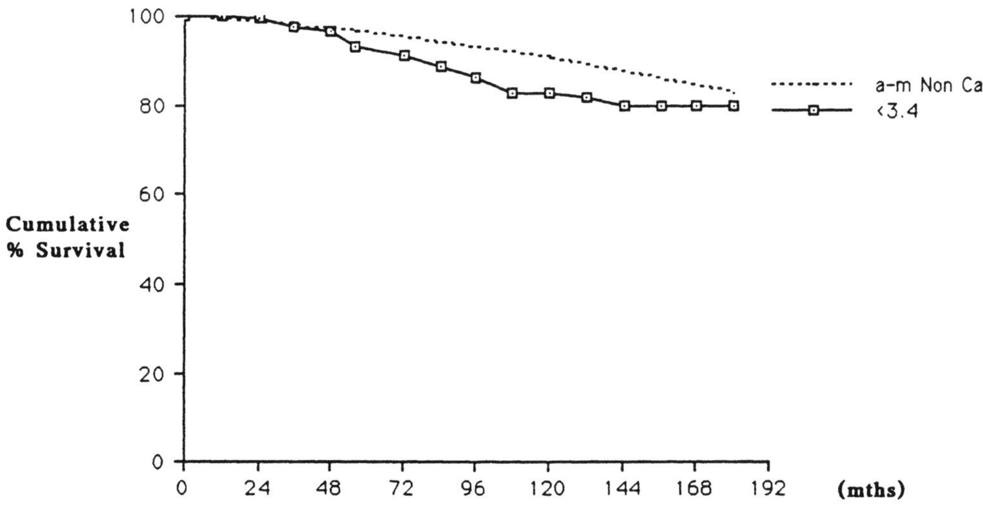

Figure 2: *Patient survival: Nottingham prognostic index, good prognosis group (NPI ≤3.4) vs age-matched non-breast cancer population*

patients.[3] It can be seen in Figure 3 that there is a very close fit in the graphs of the retrospective and prospective series. This confirmed the reproducibility of the index. Observations have now been extended over a period of up to 15 years and the differences between the three prognostic groups, if anything, widen with time; also with time, the contribution of each of the components to the index has remained constant.

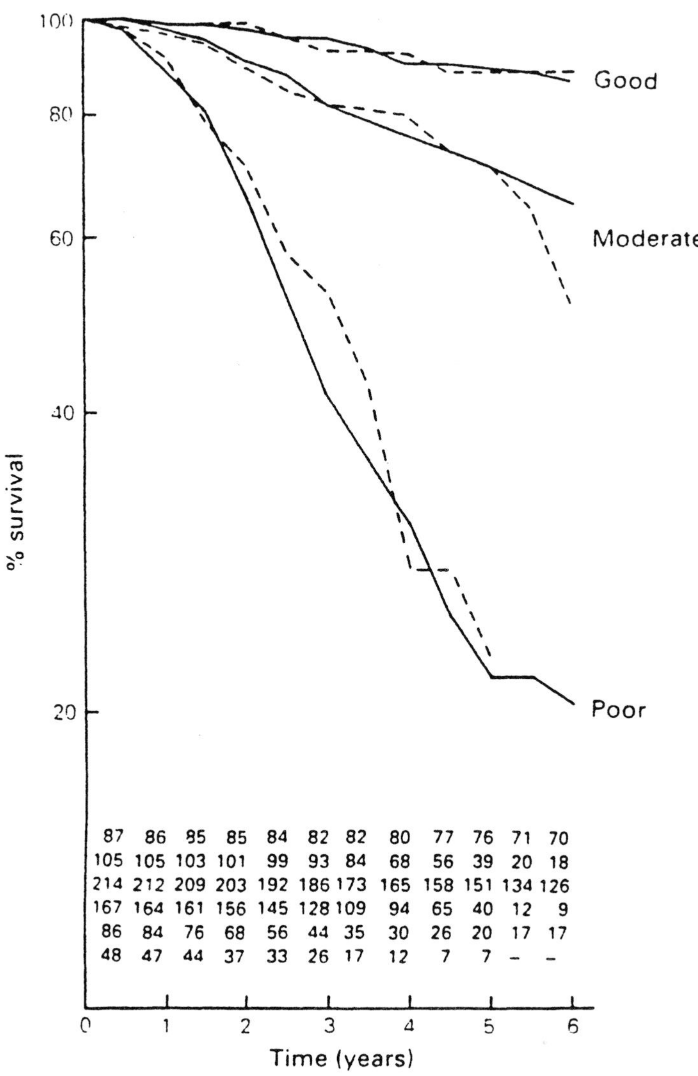

Figure 3: *Patient survival: comparison of survival in the original Nottingham series (whole lines) and prospective Nottingham series (dotted lines) within each of the three prognostic index groups.[3]*

The Good Prognostic Group (GPG)

Here then, is a situation in which only approximately 10% of patients are likely to die from distant metastases over the next 10 years. The very best results so far achieved by adjuvant chemotherapy (Early Breast Cancer Trialists' Collaborative Group, 1992[4]) show that around 30% of women benefit from such treatment. This may be the wrong interpretation, since it may alternatively be suggested that graphs should be read horizontally, showing a lengthening of survival rather than overall cure; adopting this interpretation and saying the duration of survival is lengthened in those who die, this works out at a median prolongation of survival of around 1 year. The maximum benefit in the good prognostic group would be a prolongation of life of 1 year, in 10 women, over a period of 10 years; around 100 months in a total number of life months at risk of 12,000! The maximum possible gain in this group is ludicrously small. This would be bought at the expense of 6 months of chemotherapy for all 100 women, with side effects for a total of 600 months. With these figures in mind, surely no one could suggest giving cytotoxic chemotherapy to the good prognostic group.

Should, then, the good prognostic group have adjuvant systemic therapy at all? Tamoxifen is a drug with little or no side effects in postmenopausal women. When given to premenopausal women, it has marked side effects, including those of an early menopause. We therefore think that the very small possible benefit is definitely not worthwhile in premenopausal women.

In postmenopausal women, the side effects are lower but the gain remains negligible. Also, the good prognostic group often has grade 1 tumors and a long tumor-free interval; this is the group most likely to benefit from the use of tamoxifen if it ever has to be given at a late stage.[5] We prefer to hold tamoxifen in reserve for those few women who will need it for the treatment of distant metastases.

In summary, our recommendation for the good prognostic group is no adjuvant cytotoxic or hormonal systemic therapy.

The Impact of Breast Cancer Screening

The Super-Good Prognostic Group (GPG)

Breast cancer screening brings to light many cancers with an extremely good prognosis. Fifteen percent to 17% of cancers detected in a prevalence (first) screen are ductal carcinoma in situ and over 30% are grade I, special histologic types (tubular and tubular mixed), lymph node-negative, and less than 1.5 cm.

The remarks on the inappropriateness of adjuvant systemic therapy in the GPG apply even more strongly to this group.

Poor Prognostic Group: (PPG)

Patients in the poor prognostic group are highly likely to suffer recurrence and death within years of the diagnosis of breast cancer. By definition, all patients in this group must be node-positive and they are therefore outside the scope of the present argument. Their median survival is 2.5 years and is akin to that of patients with locally advanced (stage III) disease; several centers are now investigating the use of intensive chemotherapeutic regimes in stage III. It may be that such intensive chemotherapy will be the way forward in this group of patients in the future.

Moderate Prognostic Group (MPG)

Women in this group have a 70% chance of surviving for 5 years. The interval probabilities of recurrence and death from breast cancer continue much the same for the next 10 years, so that only 50% are alive at 15 years. Some form of adjuvant systemic therapy seems worthwhile but, with this moderate outlook, one is less likely to give aggressive treatment. Where suitable, hormonal therapy is the best choice.

The Oxford overview has demonstrated that adjuvant hormone therapies have a significantly greater effect in patients with estrogen receptor (ER)-positive tumors.[4] There is a strong association between ER status and histologic grade.

The moderate prognostic group is composed of lymph node-negative grade III tumors and lymph node-positive grade II tumors. The former are the subject of this chapter. As they are grade III, the great majority are ER-negative and unlikely to gain benefit from adjuvant endocrine therapy. In lymph node-negative grade III tumors, we advise *considering* adjuvant cytotoxic therapy, taking into account patient age and general fitness. Premenopausal women in this group are advised to have cytotoxic chemotherapy, as are the younger, fitter women in their 50s. A woman in her late 60s, however, has a good chance of remaining free of the symptoms of distant spread until the end of her natural life. To these patients, we give tamoxifen as there is a small chance of response.

The Best Prognostic Factors for Regular Use

Most would agree that nodal status is a useful prognostic factor and we, of course, take it into account in our index (see above); but for useful prognostication, it must be combined with a measure of the tumor's intrinsic biological aggressiveness. The question that is frequently addressed in the medical literature is what should be combined with nodal status to achieve powerful prognostic prediction of survival. A great number of factors have been advanced. In Nottingham, we have studied DNA ploidy and proliferative index measured by flow cytometry, estrogen receptor, *c-erb* B-2, EFG receptor, epithelial mucin antibodies, lectin binding, oncogenes such as *c-myc*, other biological features such as vascular invasion and morphometry studied by image analysis. Histologic grade, however, consistently emerges as the most powerful histologic prognostic variable: this is, of course, not entirely surprising as it is itself a biological index contributed to by three components. It seems that the ability of the pathologist to estimate these three components—mitoses, tubule formation, and nuclear pleomorphism—overrides any one of these other single factors. It is possible, however, by the estimation of proliferative index in flow cytometry and of pleomorphism in image analysis, to simulate histologic grade to some degree.[6]

It has been stated that histologic grade is difficult to reproduce in other centers. Our answer to this is that we have demonstrated its prognostic power prospectively in our own center and we have demonstrated its reproducibility. If histologic grade can be reliably estimated in our center, then it can be similarly estimated in other centers.

The Other Breast

We have not addressed the question of the management of the opposite breast. Any woman with breast cancer has an approximate incidence of breast cancer in the opposite breast of 7 per 1,000 per year. The trials of adjuvant systemic hormone therapy[4] show that opposite-breast cancer occurrence is considerably lower at 5 years in women receiving tamoxifen and may remain lower at 10 years. The subject of tamoxifen prevention of breast cancer is being investigated in large multicenter trials of women at high risk both in the United States and in the United Kingdom.

Cytotoxic chemotherapy does not avoid tumors in the opposite breast.

Conclusion

The question that we were asked to address was whether node-negative breast cancer patients should receive adjuvant chemotherapy. In summarizing, we would first note that patients with medial tumors may well be axillary node-negative yet have involvement of their internal mammary nodes; they should undergo biopsy of these nodes.[7]

However, we do not find node negativity by itself to be a useful prognostic concept. Node-negative patients with well-differentiated tumors have an 85% survival chance at 15 years whereas node-negative patients with poorly differentiated tumors have only a 53% chance of surviving 15 years. We have demonstrated the power of histologic grade in separating these node-negative patients with an additional contribution from tumor size. The Nottingham Prognostic Index thus formed can identify a group of patients with an excellent prognosis in whom a strong case for the avoidance of adjuvant systemic therapy is made.

Women in the moderate prognostic group who are node-negative must be poorly differentiated and are likely to be ER-negative. They may be considered for adjuvant chemotherapy, depending on their age and health.

The protocol for recommending adjuvant systemic therapy at our center as it applies to women with node-negative tumors is shown in Table 1.

Table 1
Protocol for Recommending Adjuvant Systemic Therapy to Node-Negative Patients

Group	Grade/ER	Adjuvant Systemic Therapy Recommendation
Good prognostic group (GPG)	Grades I & II	NIL
Moderate prognostic group (MPG)	Grade III/ER- Grade III/ER +	Consider cytotoxic Endocrine

References

1. Elston CW: In: Page DL, Anderson TJ (eds). Diagnostic Histopathology of the Breast. Churchill Livingstone, Edinburgh, pp 300–311, 1987.
2. Haybittle JL, Blamey RW, Elston CW, Johnson J, et al: A prognostic index in primary breast cancer. Br J Cancer 1982; 45:361–366.
3. Todd JH, Dowle C, Williams MR, Elston CW, Ellis IO, Hinton CP, et al: Confirmation of a prognostic index in primary breast cancer. Br J Cancer 1987; 56:489–492.
4. Early Breast Cancer Trialists' Collaborative Group: Systemic treatment of early breast cancer by hormonal, cytotoxic or immunotherapy. Lancet 1992; 339:1–15, 71–84.
5. Williams MR, Todd JH, Nicholson RI, Elston CW, Blamey RW, Griffiths K: Survival patterns in hormone treated advanced breast cancer. Br J Surg 1986; 73:752–755.
6. Galea MH, Dilks B, Gilmour A, Ellis IO, Elston CW, Blamey RW: Image analysis and flow cytometry in the automated analysis of histological grade. Breast Cancer Res Treat 1991; 19:213.
7. du Toit RS, Locker AP, Ellis IO, Elston CW, Blamey RW: Evaluation of the prognostic value of triple node biopsy in early breast cancer. Br J Surg 1990; 77; 163–167.

33

Ethical Concerns Surrounding Adjuvant Chemotherapy

C. Barber Mueller

The decade of the nineties began with overwhelming enthusiasm to treat subgroups of women with breast cancer by postoperative adjuvant medical therapy, either chemical or hormonal. In many respects, this raises problems not unlike those that were present when oophorectomy was promoted as an adjunct to surgical management. Many women lost their ovaries, a few benefited by a delay in recurrence but survival benefits were never shown. Today the huge multi-center effort of the National Surgical Adjuvant Breast Project (NSABP), which is conducted across the United States and Canada, encourages many women to enter clinical trials in an attempt to determine if adjuvant chemotherapy will produce significant survival benefits. Lay and scientific publications and publicity surrounding the reports are such that many oncologists, rather than looking for reasons to give chemotherapy, now look for reasons not to give it. A consensus conference has recommended it as standard therapy, particularly for premenopausal node-positive women,[1] and fear of litigation drives the system towards treatment rather than withholding it.

The evidence for adjuvant chemotherapy comes from clinical trials that compare one drug regimen against another or a drug regimen versus no therapy. Unfortunately, early closure has made it impossible to determine if any of the current adjuvant regimens are of any benefit over a similar sample of breast cancer women not so treated. The last stage II untreated group studied by NSABP was entered in 1971 in the study known as B-05.[2] The conclusion that benefits were achieved in the subgroup of node-positive premenopausal women now seems invalid, because NSABP produced sufficient data in the next four trials to indicate that their adjuvant chemotherapy regimen did *not* produce a survival difference better than the placebo.[3] Subsequent efforts to determine whether or not benefits would occur in node-negative women were carried out.

Four articles published in the *New England Journal of Medicine* suggested that prolongation of the disease-free interval without a benefit in survival was possible by the use of adjuvant chemotherapy.[4-7] This led to a clinical alert from the National Cancer Institute advocating that the "bias of physicians not deny the benefits of adjuvant chemotherapy" to estrogen receptor (ER)-negative premenopausal node-negative women.[8a]

In 1990 a major report that collected the world-wide experience from clinical trials of adjuvant chemotherapy was published using a statistical procedure—meta-analysis—to coalesce many clinical trials into one analysis despite different entrance criteria and drug regimens.[8b] These results probably describe the maximum possible obtainable benefit. "Publication bias" is an unknown feature of such analyses for it is suspected that trials which fail to show a benefit in the experimental arm during their early period are aborted and never achieve publication. The results of these meta-analyses have not only been published in book form but also in two articles in *Lancet*.[9] One section is devoted to the administration of adjuvant chemotherapy to node-positive women. This shows a benefit of 5.7 ± 1.7% in the treated women and is reported as an 11.6% reduction in mortality at 5 years.

When two groups are compared by constructing life table survival curves, it is customary to use a single point in time—fixed time—for a comparison between the two groups. This gives a difference in percent alive. It is also possible to use a fixed percent survival as the comparison point and report the difference in terms of time, e.g., how long it takes each group to reach a 70% survival, thus describing the benefit as a delay in time rather than, or in addition to, percent survival.

The multitude of trials reported in the meta-analysis show that adjuvant chemotherapy may benefit approximately 6.3 ± 1.4 percent at 10 years by a delay in death of approximately 20 months. This changes the expected 10-year mortality of 55% in the controls to 48.7% in the polychemotherapy group.

Stage II premenopausal women constitute the subgroup most frequently reported to have received the greatest benefit from adjuvant chemotherapy, and at 5 years there is approximately a 14-month delay in death for 5% of the women. Conversely, 95% of women who receive the adjuvant treatment do so without benefit, and it is impossible to tell which women received benefit and which did not.

The administration of toxic drugs to well women for no personal identifiable benefit raises many issues. The cost/benefit issue has been raised by Hillner.[10] Harm/benefit was discussed by McGuire,[11] and ethical issues surrounding the physician in the role of the clinical investigator have been discussed by Hellman.[12]

A review of the medical statutes of several states and a couple of provinces fails to clearly identify specific activities, knowledge, skills, and behavior that define the physician. Broad statements in these statutes suggest that the license to practice medicine conveys the privilege or responsibility to diagnose and treat illness, alleviate suffering, and permit invasion of the body, its corporeal as well as its mental aspect, but this must be done *only* for the diagnosis or treatment of illness or the relief of suffering of an individual who has become a patient in a

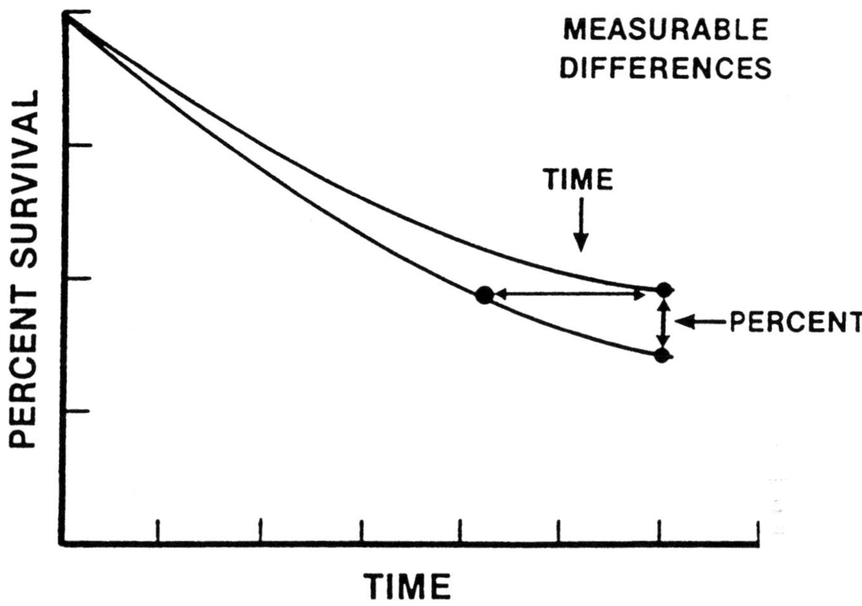

Figure 1: *Theoretical life table analyses showing the decreasing survival of two groups under study. The curves may be compared at a fixed time, producing percentage differences, or at a fixed percent, producing time differences. The use of both indices is the complete way in which to express differences between two groups under comparison. From Mueller CB.[19]*

special relationship. The license to practice medicine thus carries with it the ability to produce harm to individuals, to commit physical and mental assault, to invade the body, to administer drugs, and to perform acts prohibited to individuals not so licensed. During the last 2,500 years, a series of statements regarding the expected behavior of physicians have been developed and these ethical constraints define the role of the physician in the doctor/patient relationship—a trust covenant. They are uniquely individual. They found early expression in the Oath of Hippocrates and the prayer of Maimonides, and currently they may be seen as ethical statements produced by the American Medical Association, the World Health Organization, the Geneva Convention, and almost all medical organizations.[13-15] The central regulatory themes include "do no harm," "maintain confidentiality," and contain a pledge to "come for the benefit of the sick, remain free of intentional injustice" and to "act solely for the benefit of the patient." These reflect the current moral theory of many philosophers who assert that human beings, by virtue of their unique capacity for rational thought, are bearers of dignity and as such ought not to be treated as a means to an end for other purposes, but treated as an end in themselves. Traditionally, the physician treats an individual and rarely, if ever, accepts group responsibilities. He deals with one patient in a singularly individual setting, a very privileged trust relationship in which the doctor possesses

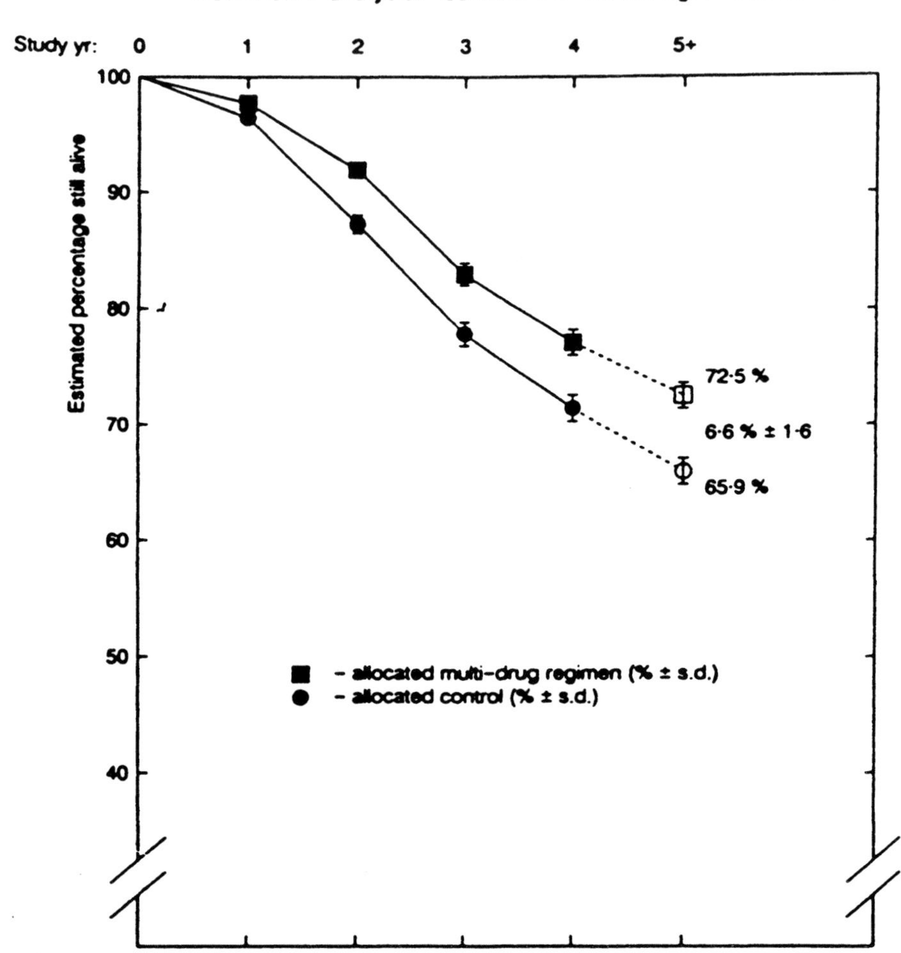

Figure 2: *Survival curves created by meta-analysis for all available trials of multiple versus no/single agent cytotoxic adjuvant therapy in women under 50 years of age. From Early Breast Cancer Trialists' Collaborative Group.[8b]*

extraordinary powers. It requires the physician to hold the interests of the individual patient as primary and compelling, for patients possess rights that cannot be given up or used for the good of humanity, particularly if they are accompanied by detriment to that patient. Education, observations, the results of prior actions, peers, clinical trials, and ethical beliefs all influence the actions, choices, or options that any physician may offer any patient at a specific moment, and with adjuvant chemotherapy there arises a central question: "Is it ethical, is it in the best interest of the patient to offer or suggest a treatment that will carry cost, morbidity, time, and suffering, but never have a measurable benefit to that patient?"

Ethical constraints that play upon researchers who conduct clinical trials are not expressed in the Hippocratic deontologic tradition. They are governed by the utilitarian (consequentialistic) ethic which defines what is right as that which produces the greatest good to the greatest number, i.e., that which produces the greatest aggregate net benefit over harm. The morally correct act is the one that produces the most pleasure and the least pain. Bentham[16] and Mill[17] express this as the means whereby one may determine the right course by choosing one that, on balance, will produce maximum social utility without concern for distributive justice, without concern for the individual. This ethic is concerned with net benefit over net cost or net harm. The quantity of harms and benefits may be designated in the aggregate, but who gains and who loses cannot, and the quality of benefit generally cannot be balanced against the type of harm. It is this ethic that must underpin the adjuvant chemotherapy research on human subjects for the research is neither designed nor expected to produce a benefit to any specific subject in any trial, for trials are set up to determine net benefit in one group over another. There is the expectation that trial results will ultimately produce changes in therapy for the benefit of someone else. If this ethic were transferred to the patient/doctor setting, it would lead logically to the conclusion that a physician could be justified in or expected to compromise the interests of his patient in order to benefit some individual in the future, one who is not yet a patient.

Clinical trials must operate with the utilitarian ethic, wherein benefits and harms to individual subjects are lost in group outcome. Even though clinical trials may examine facets of the practice of medicine or a proposed new treatment, they are *not* the practice of medicine. They are experiments with human subjects who happen to be patients in another setting. Individuals in clinical trials are subjects and, by definition, not patients of the trial organizer. Those who conduct the trials are researchers constrained by research ethical guidelines, not physicians functioning under their set of ethical constraints, even though the researcher may hold the M.D. degree. This experimenter/subject relationship has been defined in several codes of ethics on research with human beings that have been established since World War II. First expressed in the Nuremberg Code, it was followed by the Declaration of Helsinki, American Medical Association Guidelines and Department of Health, Education and Welfare (DHEW) Guidelines. In addition, other organizations have adopted standards for the ethical behavior expected from experimenters who do research on human subjects. These codes contain several themes: voluntary participation of the subject, no duress, freedom to withdraw, implicit assurance that there will be minimal harm when compared to expected benefit, informed consent, and confidentiality. There is no explicit statement or implicit expectation that the study will be in the best interests of the subject, or that the subject will not be harmed without benefit.[15]

The utilitarian ethic and these statements are not only acceptable but required in the clinical trial setting for the primary concern of the trial organizer is not that of patient care, but scientific information. Since trials investigate groups and measure benefits by using group statistics, the researcher is not responsible for individual patient management or the individual's good, and as such he loses individuals as people. When a woman newly diagnosed with breast cancer is approached to become a subject in a trial, such terms as voluntary, informed, confidential, and free to withdraw can hardly be comprehended in a way that permits a clear decision as to her willingness to participate in a clinical trial as a subject rather than be treated as a patient. Her illness constitutes duress upon which it is easy to capitalize.

This author has heard many statements to the effect that once a statistically significant difference between two groups is identified, it is no longer ethical to continue the study. If there is an untreated control group, it is "not ethical to withhold treatment." This position leads to early closure in clinical trials and results in a lack of scientific rigor. The ethical foundations for such statements are not clear and are not easy to find in the many documents that underpin the ethical behavior of either physician or researcher. One trial, regardless of P values, should probably be repeated to ensure a firmly established scientific base before thousands of women are treated—the harm to those who are not benefited should be sufficiently small and not outweigh marginal benefits that might be achieved. Statistical significance does not confer clinical significance. In premenopausal stage II women, benefits of chemotherapy are in the neighborhood of a delay in death of between 1 and 1½ years for 5% of the women. Harm versus benefit is easily visible in the study of estrogen receptor-negative, node-negative premenopausal women reported from the B-14 study.[6,18] The claimed benefit is a delay in time to recurrence (lengthened disease-free survival) of 14 months in 9% of the women without any benefit in survival. This is 9 × 14 or 126 months of benefit achieved by treating 100 women with 12 cycles of methotrexate, fluorouracil, and leucovorin—one cycle per month for a year. With an estimated 1 week of illness per month, 12 weeks (3 months) per woman, there results a total of 300 months of illness. If so, 126 months of net benefit is fairly difficult to justify when balanced against 300 months of net illness—for no gain in survival. Hillner[10] used similar material, reduced the harm time by half, and estimated that the 9% of women achieved these 14 months at a cost of $16,000 each. A profound "social" ethical question then arises: "Is this a result of sufficient magnitude that it is *ethical* to treat 18 or 19 women for the one who benefits, particularly when the benefited woman cannot be identified?"[19]

These two sets of ethical considerations, the deontological and the utilitarian, bring into extreme positions possible changes in the upcoming roles of the physician, particularly in those societies in which the physician is increasingly being seen as an agent of the state rather than as an independent practitioner. Does the physician function as an agent of society with his value measured by social outcomes independent of individual patient demands or is he a partner in a special trust convenant—someone who acts primarily and solely in the patient's best interest, independent of social overtones?

Veatch[20] recognizes the changing social role of the physician and has attempted to provide integration between the traditional role of the independent physician, not responsible or necessarily responsive to social demands, and some newer concepts of the role of the physician as an agent of society to keep it well. Jonsen[21] provides a thoughtful dissection of the physician role—as an individual attempting to serve both patients and society simultaneously.

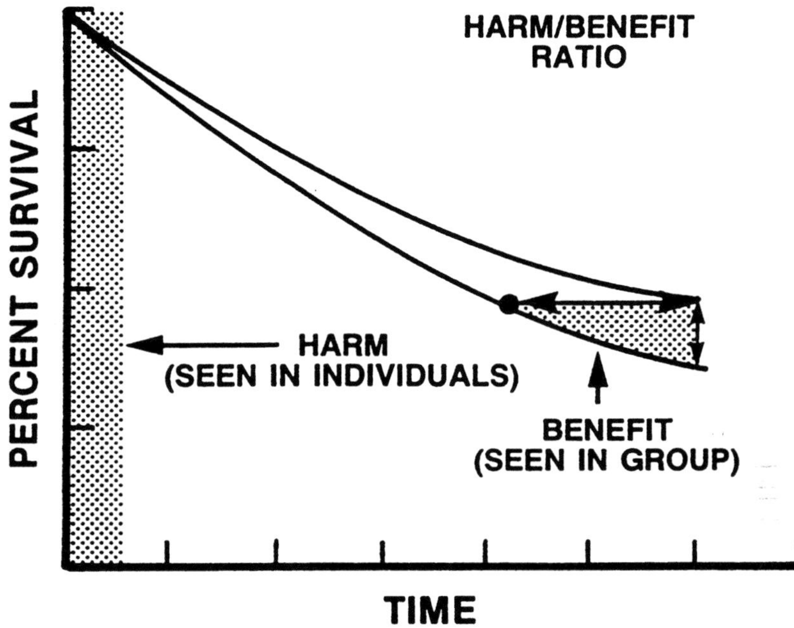

Figure 3: *Theoretical pair of life table curves showing the possibility of assessing harm to benefit. The shaded areas represent illness incurred as a result of the adjuvant chemotherapy versus the benefit achieved by that illness. From Mueller CB.*[22]

Clinical trials are important, but minimal trial benefits do not of themselves create standard therapy; it requires more than numbers since harms are individual and gains are social. It requires sober clinical and ethical compromise. The issues are more than money, more than morbidity or even death. They are ethical issues that transcend adjuvant chemotherapy and become concerned with the relationship of a physician to a patient and the trust implicit in that convenant. Until the benefits of adjuvant treatment are self-evident with benefits that may be seen in individual patients, it strains ethical credibility to recommend adjuvant chemotherapy as standard therapy, particularly when the benefits are marginal at best (seen only in group comparisons), and the cost in dollars, time, and suffering is visible and significant (always seen in individuals). Adjuvant chemotherapy, with its harm balanced against marginal or minimal benefit, can hardly be seen to be in the classic traditions of medicine and it is difficult to see it as an ethically acceptable proposal, even in the group in which it is supposedly of greatest benefit, i.e., stage II premenopausal women with breast cancer.

Author's Note

Many societies and organizations have produced statements of ethical principles that constrain the doctor/patient and the researcher/subject relationships. These statements form the substantive base for commonly agreed upon ethical policy. They have been collected into one volume and are easily available to anyone interested in formal positions of authority and custom rather than idiosyncratic interpretations.

Encyclopedia of Biomedical Ethics, Vol 4, pp 1721–1815.

Doctor/patient

Oath of Hippocrates, 6th century B.C.
Prayer of Maimonides, 1793
Declaration of Geneva, W.M.A., 1948
Am. Med. Assoc. Ethical Principles, 1957

Researcher/subject
Nuremberg Code, 1946
Declaration of Helsinki, 1964, 1975
Am. Med. Assoc. Guidelines, 1966
DHEW Guidelines, 1971

References

1. Consensus Conference: Adjuvant chemotherapy for breast cancer. JAMA 1985; 254:3461–3463.
2. Fisher B, Fisher ER, Redmond C, et al: Ten year results from the National Surgical Adjuvant Breast and Bowel Project (NSABP) clinical trial evaluating the use of L-phenylalanine mustard (L-PAM) in the management of primary breast cancer. J Clin Oncol 1986; 4:929–941.
3. Mueller CB, Lesperance ML: NSABP trials of adjuvant chemotherapy for breast cancer: a further look at the evidence. Annals Surg 1991; 214:206–212.
4. Ludwig Breast Cancer Study Group: Prolonged disease-free survival after one course of perioperative adjuvant chemotherapy for node-negative breast cancer. N Engl J Med 1989; 320:491–496.
5. Mansour EG, Gray R, Shatilor AH, et al: Efficacy of adjuvant chemotherapy in high risk node negative breast cancer: an intergroup study. N Engl J Med 1989; 320:485–490.
6. Fisher B, Redmond C, Dimitrov NV, et al: A randomized clinical trial evaluating sequential methotrexate and fluorouracil in the treatment of patients with node-negative breast cancer who have estrogen-receptor negative tumors. N Engl J Med 1989; 320:473–478.
7. Fisher B, Constantine J, Redmond C, et al: A randomized clinical trial evaluating Tamoxifen in the treatment of patients with node-negative breast cancer who have estrogen-receptor positive tumors. N Eng J Med 1989; 320:479–484.
8a. National Cancer Institute: Clinical Alert. Bethesda, MD; May 16, 1988.
8b. The Treatment of Early Breast Cancer, Vol I, Worldwide Evidence 1985–1990. Early Breast Cancer Trialist Collaborative Group Oxford University Press, New York, 1990.
9. Early Breast Cancer Trialists Collaborative Group: Systemic treatment of early breast cancer by hormonal cytotoxic or immune therapy. Lancet 1992; 339:1–15, 71–86.
10. Hillner BE, Smith TJ: Efficacy and cost effectiveness of adjuvant chemotherapy in women with node negative breast cancer. N Engl J Med 1991; 324:160–168.
11. McGuire W: Adjuvant therapy of node negative breast cancer. N Engl J Med 1989; 320:525–527.

12. Hellman S, Hellman D: Of mice but not men. N Engl J Med 1991; 324:1585–1589.
13. Edelstein L: The Hippocratic oath: text translation and interpretation. (Suppl. to Bulletin of History of Medicine). Johns Hopkins Press, Baltimore, MD, 1943.
14. Etziony MB: The Physician's Creed. Charles C. Thomas, Springfield, IL, 1973.
15. Reich WT: Encyclopedia of Bioethics, Vol. 4. The Free Press, MacMillan, New York, pp 1721–1815, 1978.
16. Bentham J: An Introduction to the Principles of Morals and Legislation. Athlone Press, London, 1970.
17. Mill JS: Utilitarianism. Bobbs Merrill Co., Indianapolis, 1975.
18. Mueller CB: The disease-free interval in breast cancer trials: scientific or spurious. Surgery 1991; 110:629–635.
19. Mueller CB: Adjuvant chemotherapy for breast cancer: ethical considerations. Bull Am Coll Surg 1989; 74:9–12.
20. Veatch RM: A Theory of Medical Ethics. Basic Books, Inc., New York, 1981.
21. Jonsen AR: New Medicine and the Old Ethics, 2nd ed. Harvard University Press, Cambridge, MA, 1991.
22. Mueller CB: Statistical, clinical and ethical concerns. In: Najarian JS, Delaney JP (eds). Progress in Cancer Surgery. Mosby Year Book, Chicago, pp 338–348, 1991.

34

Tamoxifen as Adjuvant Therapy

Sir Patrick M. Forrest

Introduction

The "surgical" management of operable breast cancer has the objective of removing all clinically apparent disease in the breast and axillary lymph nodes. But a fatal outcome is not due to lack of control of the malignant mass in the breast, but instead it is due to failure to eradicate microscopic metastases in locoregional and distant sites. These ultimately cause clinically evident metastases and organ failure. The aim of adding radical radiotherapy to surgery was to destroy microscopic deposits of tumor in the regional lymphatics and lymph nodes; but although this reduces the incidence of local relapse, there is no evidence that it benefits survival. To the contrary, an overview of trials in which surgery alone (by "radical" or "simple" mastectomy) has been compared with the same surgery followed by radical radiotherapy indicated that long-term survival might even be reduced.[1-3]

It is not surprising that extension of local therapy fails to increase rates of cure. Systemic micrometastatic disease can be eradicated only by systemic treatment.

Adjuvant Therapy

Patients with symptomatic breast cancer normally consult a surgeon first. Their concern is directed to the breast mass and in general wish that this be removed. Although logically it is more rational to treat systemic disease by systemic therapy first so that its effect on its clinical manifestations (in this case the primary tumor) can be observed, the conventional primary treatment of

From: Wise L, Johnson H Jr (eds): *Breast Cancer: Controversies in Management.* Futura Publishing Company, Inc., Armonk, NY, © 1994.

breast cancer is first to eradicate the clinically apparent disease by local therapy, to which systemic treatment is regarded as an "adjuvant."

Methods of adjuvant treatment include antiestrogens and chemotherapy. Under consideration in this paper is the synthetic antiestrogen tamoxifen.

Tamoxifen

This synthetic triphenylethylene hydrocarbon was first synthesized as a potential antifertility drug. Recognizing that it had antiestrogen effects,[4] Walpole suggested that it might be useful as a therapeutic agent in breast cancer and in clinical trials in patients with advanced breast cancer.[5,6] A recent review of 86 major clinical studies involving 5,353 patients with locally advanced and metastatic breast cancer indicated that the overall objective response to tamoxifen was 34%, with disease stabilization in a further 19%.[7] The clinical use of two other drugs, chlomiphene and nafoxidene, was also being explored at that time, but their side effects, which included blurring of vision, ichthyosis, and photosensitivity, precluded further studies. On the other hand, tamoxifen has minimal side effects (Table 1).[8] It was this low morbidity that encouraged European investigators to explore its efficacy as adjuvant therapy.

Table 1
Principal Side Effects of Tamoxifen Therapy

Side Effects	(% Incidence)		
	20 mg/day	30 mg/day	40 mg/day
Gastrointestinal upset	9.8	7.9	6.6
Hot flushes	7.6	4.2	6.9
Transient leucopenia and thrombocytopenia	3.1	2.3	2.5
Vaginal bleeding/discharge	1.4	1.0	0
Pruritus vulvae	0.3	0.5	0
Edema	1.4	2.4	0
Withdrawn from therapy	1.4	1.6	1.1

From ref. 8 with permission.

Action of Tamoxifen

The ability of tamoxifen to suppress the growth of breast cancer is due to its competition with estrogen for binding to the estrogen receptor protein, which is a necessary intermediate in estrogen action. This receptor, which normally resides within the nucleus, is a member of the steroid receptor family. It contains DNA and steroid-binding domains, the latter at the carboxy-terminal end of the receptor protein. Following the binding of estrogen, the receptor undergoes dimerization and binds to a specific site on DNA to trigger transcriptional activation of estrogen-responsive genes. Tamoxifen also binds to the ligand-binding domain of the receptor and promotes binding of the receptor to DNA. But as a result of conformational changes in the receptor complex, it no longer activates transcription of estrogen-responsive genes.[9] The effect of tamoxifen is tissue-specific, and at some sites it does not act as an antagonist to estrogen, but as an estrogen agonist, an action of considerable importance when considering its potential role as a chemosuppressive preventative agent. Unlike tamoxifen, the new class of C7 substituted estradiol analogs would appear to be pure antiestrogens at all sites.[10] From this brief description, it is apparent that tamoxifen acts primarily through the estrogen receptor. But a direct inhibitory action has also been described, possibly by stimulating the expression of TGFβ, which is a known inhibitor of growth of certain breast cancer cell lines.[11]

Tamoxifen as Adjuvant Therapy

The Overview

The recent publication of the report of the 1990 overview of the Early Breast Cancer Trialists Collaborative Group has firmly established the role of tamoxifen as adjuvant therapy for operable breast cancer.[12] This overview includes 40 randomized trials (which include 42 therapeutic comparisons) of tamoxifen given with or without chemotherapy versus the same regime without tamoxifen. These include a total of some 30,000 women, of whom 22,000 had taken tamoxifen for 2 years or more, and 8,000 for 1 year. In addition, there were 2,000 women included in five trials in whom shorter-and longer-term tamoxifen administrations were compared. Entry to these trials and the numbers of deaths and relapsed patients available for analysis are given in Table 2. These 42 trials included all such trials carried out before 1985 throughout the world, except for eight trials consisting of 1,400 women, the results of which were not yet available for inclusion in the analysis. The analysis was initiated and performed by Richard Peto and his colleagues in the ICRF/MRC Clinical Trials Service Unit in Oxford. As all the trials had commenced before 1985, the effect of tamoxifen on mortality at 10 years could be predicted with confidence.

The method of analysis of mortality and of relapse-free survival has been described in detail.[13] This involved estimating the log-rank of observed minus expected events (relapse or death) and its variance. Relapse is defined as recurrence of disease, death, or both. The observed events were the number recorded in the treated arm of a trial; expected events were the number that would have been expected if the event rate for a particular year was equal to that occurring in both treated and control arms, i.e., total events in the whole population randomized. By adding the values for individual trials, overall effects were assessed. In addition, the annual probability of death between treated and control groups was calculated as an odds ratio, for which the 95% confidence limits provided an estimate of the significance of change from a null effect. This ratio, expressed as the percentage reduction in each year, was used to predict absolute benefit at different stages of the disease and different ages of patients.

Table 2
Randomized Trials (That Began Before 1985) of Tamoxifen Therapy as Adjuvant to the
Surgical Treatment of "Operable" Cancer of the Breast

| | | Available for Analysis | | |
Treatment Comparison	No. of Trials	Women	Deaths	Recurrences
Tamoxifen vs. same without tamoxifen	42	29,892	8,219	11,055
Mean scheduled duration ≥5 years	4	4,551	667	1,030
Mean scheduled duration 3 years	3	1,847	371	536
Mean scheduled duration 2 years	23	15,284	4,196	5,698
Mean scheduled duration ≤1 year	12	8,210	2,985	3,791
Longer vs. shorter tamoxifen	5	2,319	317	492

From ref. 12 with permission.

The results indicate that when tamoxifen is given to patients with operable cancer of the breast for a median duration of 2 years, relapse-free survival is increased and deaths are reduced at a level of significance that allows no possible doubt of benefit. These are illustrated in Figures 1 and 2 (redrawn from the original publication). Reductions in annual odds of death and in overall and relapse-free survivals at 5 and 10 years are also highly significant (Table 3).

The pattern of change is notable. For relapse-free survival, the main divergence takes place during the first 5 years, following which the curves run parallel between 5 and 10 years. But for mortality, the divergence between tamoxifen and control arms, again noted to commence during years 0 to 5, increases steadily up to 10 years. The difference in overall survival at 10 years is greater than that at 5 years.

These differences are apparent in patients with positive axillary nodes as well as in patients with negative axillary nodes (Figs. 3 and 4). Outcomes, in terms of overall survival and relapse-free survival for different subsets of patients, are given in Tables 4 and 5.

Annual odds (risks) of relapse and death are summarized in Table 5, subdivided according to duration of tamoxifen dosage, age, menstrual status, and estrogen-receptor (ER) concentrations in the tumor.

From these data, it can be concluded that:

1. Tamoxifen has a greater effect on mortality and relapse when schedules of longer duration are used, a significant effect on mortality being evident only when tamoxifen is taken for at least 2 years.

2. While the effect of tamoxifen is less apparent in younger women, it still has a significant effect in delaying relapse in women under 50 and in premenopausal women under 60 years of age. The effect on overall survival is less pronounced. But not only were the numbers of young and premenopausal

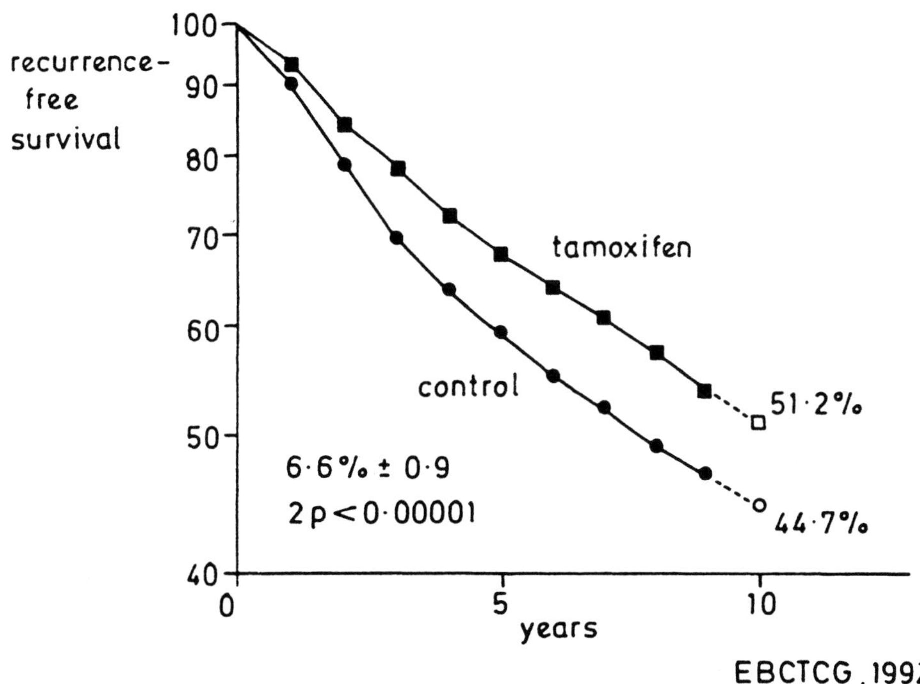

Figure 1: *Ten-year relapse-free survival among 30,000 women of all ages randomized to receive tamoxifen or not. From reference 12 with permission.*

women fewer, but a larger proportion was given chemotherapy in both arms of the trials than for older postmenopausal women.

3. Benefit from tamoxifen is greater in those women with ER-rich tumors. But relapse rates were still reduced significantly in those women whose tumors were receptor-poor, as defined by a concentration of receptor of less than 10 f moles per mg cytosol protein.

Comparison with Chemotherapy

In the overview, chemotherapy of multiple drug types was shown to effect reductions in death and relapse similar to those for tamoxifen. But the effects of polychemotherapy were more pronounced in younger (<50 years) women. Ovarian ablation also effected highly significant reductions in both relapses and deaths in the young age-group, these being equal to those achieved with polychemotherapy (Figs. 5 and 6).

In women over 50 years of age, the benefit achieved by tamoxifen on relapse and survival was no less than that of polychemotherapy (Table 6). On grounds of

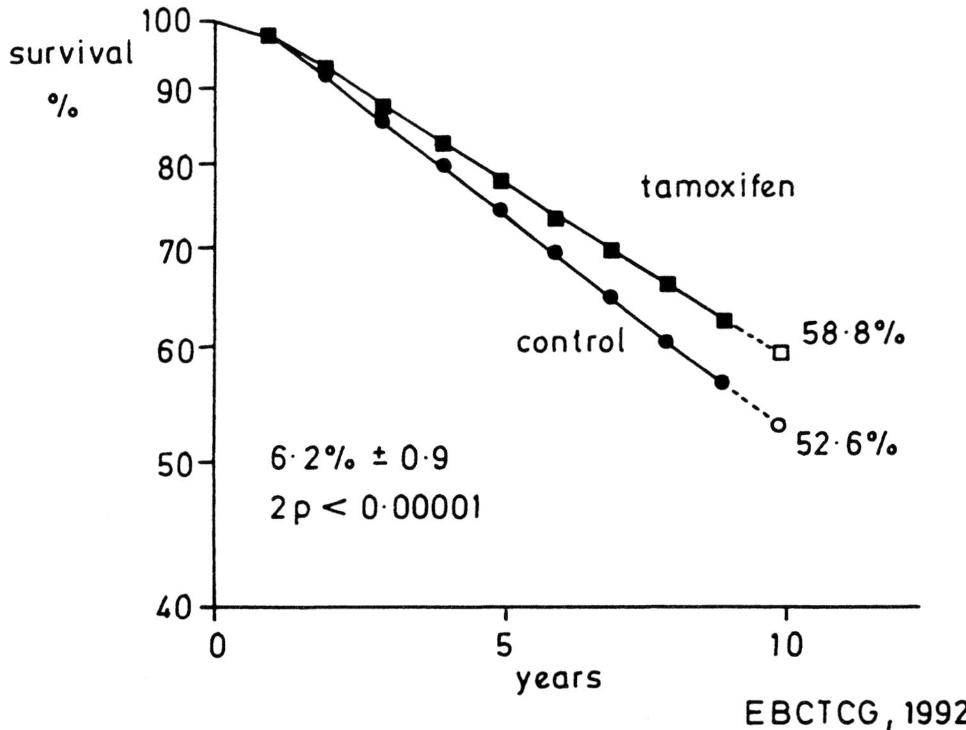

Figure 2: *Ten-year mortality (overall survival) among women of all ages in tamoxifen trials. From reference 12 with permission.*

Table 3
Five- and Ten-Year Outcome in Tamoxifen Trials (± SD)

Outcome	Tamoxifen	Control	Difference
Overall survival (%)			
(all ages)			
5 years	73.9	77.5	3.6 ± 0.6
10 years	52.6	58.8	6.2 ± 0.9
Relapse-free survival (%)			
(all ages)			
5 years	59.6	67.9	8.3 ± 0.6
10 years	44.7	51.2	6.6 ± 0.9

From ref. 12 with permission.

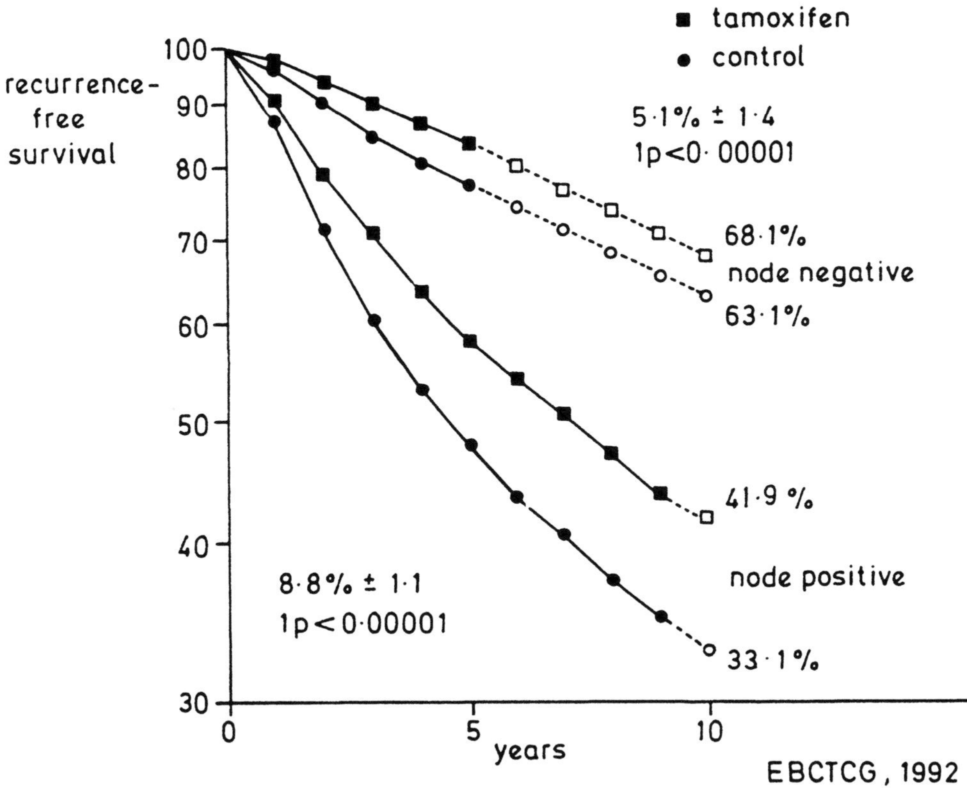

Figure 3: *Ten-year relapse-free survival among women of all ages included in tamoxifen trials subdivided by node status. From reference 12 with permission.*

morbidity, it is therefore preferable to chemotherapy alone. But the question that must be addressed is whether the combination of tamoxifen plus chemotherapy is better than either alone. That this is so is apparent from those trials included in the overview which have compared tamoxifen with tamoxifen plus chemotherapy, and chemotherapy with chemotherapy plus tamoxifen; but compared to those in the total overview, the numbers are small (Table 7). But greater numbers will be contributed by more recent trials of similar construction, the results of which will become available with time.

A direct comparison of tamoxifen plus chemotherapy with no adjuvant therapy cannot come from the overview. But in postmenopausal patients, there is assumptive evidence that the combination of tamoxifen plus chemotherapy would, compared to no adjuvant therapy, produce an annual risk reduction of about 45% ± 3 in relapse and 30% ± 4 in mortality. Since in the current

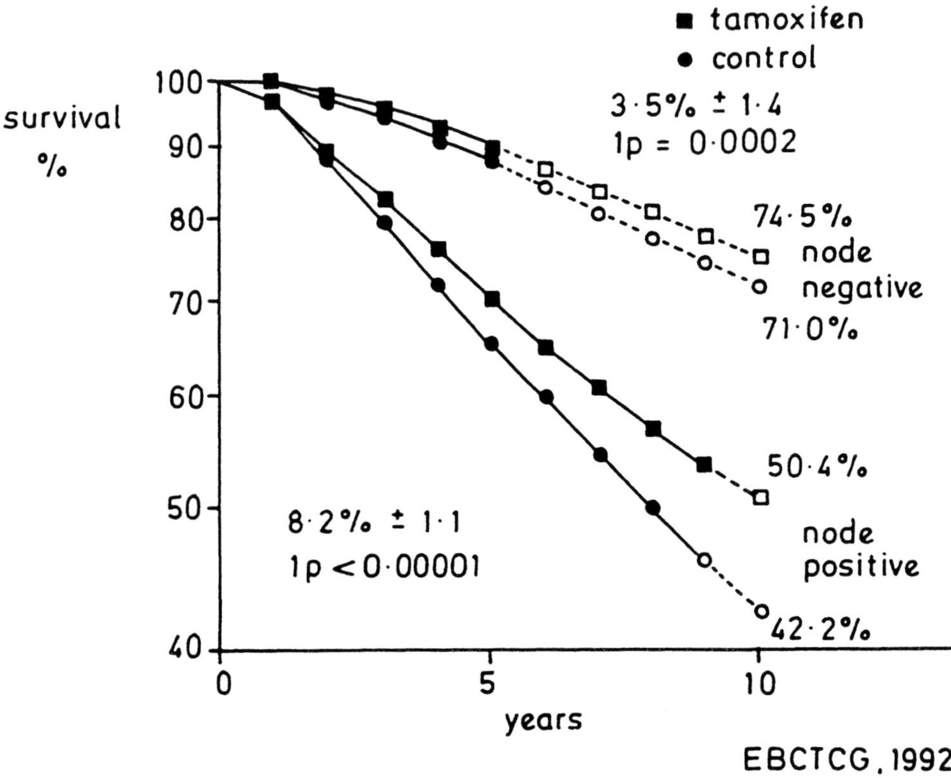

Figure 4: *Ten-year mortality (overall survival) among women of all ages in tamoxifen trials subdivided by node status. From reference 12 with permission.*

Table 4
Effect of Node Status on Tamoxifen Effect (10-Year Outcome)

Outcome	Tamoxifen	Control	Difference
Overall survival (%)			
(all ages)			
node-negative	74.5	71.0	3.5 ± 1.4
node-positive	50.4	42.2	8.2 ± 1.1
Relapse-free survival (%)			
(all ages)			
node-negative	68.1	63.1	5.1 ± 1.4
node-positive	41.9	33.1	8.8 ± 1.1

From ref. 12 with permission.

Table 5
Annual Hazard of Death in Tamoxifen Trials

Subset	Annual Odds Ratio	
	Reduction Relapse-Free Survival	*Reduction All Deaths*
Tamoxifen		
less than 2 years	16% ± 3	11% ± 4
average 2 years	27% ± 2	18% ± 3
average more than 2 years	38% ± 4	24% ± 6
Total	25% ± 2	17% ± 2
Premenopausal		
<50 years	12% ± 4	6% ± 5
50–59 years	33% ± 7	23% ± 9
Postmenopausal		
50–59 years	28% ± 3	19% ± 4
60–69 years	29% ± 3	17% ± 4
70 + years	28% ± 5	21% ± 6
Total	25% ± 2	16% ± 2
ER poor (<10 f. mol/mg cytosol protein)	13% ± 4	11% ± 5
ER positive	32% ± 3	21% ± 3
ER unknown	22% ± 3	15% ± 3

From ref. 12 with permission.

generation of trials there are no "no-treatment" control arms, such a direct comparison can no longer be made.

There is no evidence from these and other studies that a dose of tamoxifen in excess of 20 mg confers any additional advantage.

UK Trials

The input into the overview from the UK included four large trials: Christie Hospital (1 year tamoxifen), NATO (2 years tamoxifen), the Cancer Research Campaign (2 years tamoxifen), and Scottish trials (5 years tamoxifen).[14-17] In that reported from Scotland, a total of 1,312 women with operable disease of stages I and II (242 premenopausal axillary node-negative or unknown and 1,070 postmenopausal axillary node-negative and positive or unknown), following mastectomy and an axillary dissection (node sampling or clearance) were randomly allocated to receive tamoxifen 20 mg daily immediately or to reserve tamoxifen therapy until the first evidence of relapse of disease (Table 8). This was a unique objective that has been achieved in 93% of relapsed patients in the control arm who have received tamoxifen as first-stage treatment for their recurrence.

In addition, a secondary randomization procedure has been carried out at 5 years allocating women who were then still free of relapse to stop tamoxifen or

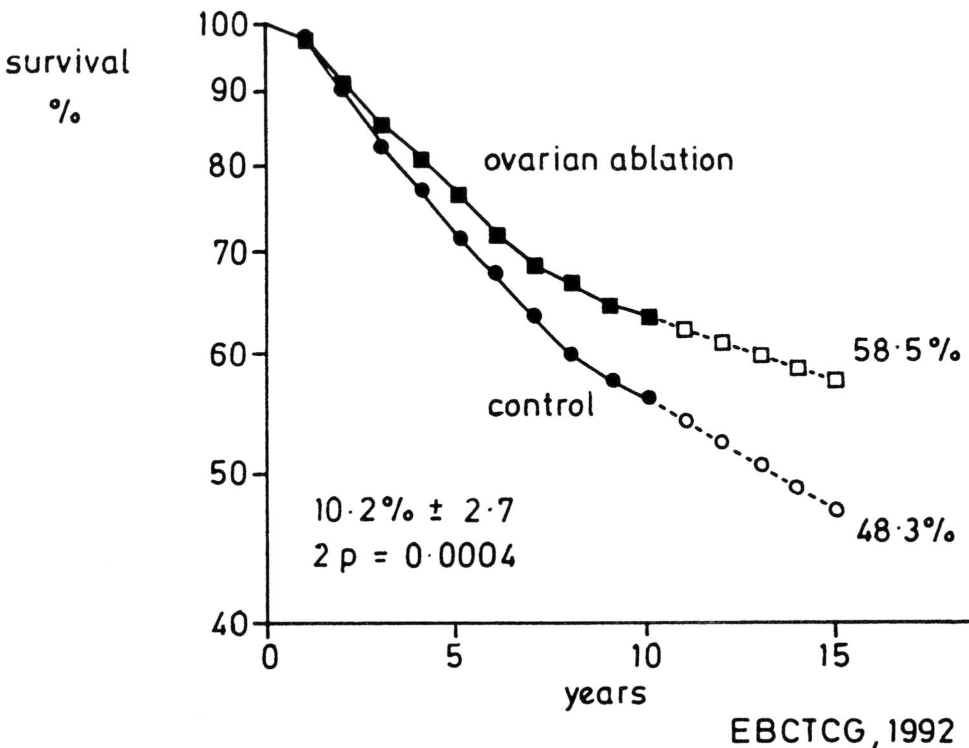

Figure 5: *Fifteen-year mortality (overall survival) for 2,000 women aged less than 50 years randomized for ovarian ablation or not. From reference 12 with permission.*

to continue it indefinitely. This has now been completed in 341 women. Those women who did not agree to participate in this further randomization have opted either to continue (40) or to stop tamoxifen therapy (10).

The results of the Scottish trial are in keeping with those from the overview, there being an overall reduction in relapse and death which was highly significant. Although there is a similar trend in the premenopausal patients included in the trial (node-negative and unknown), this reached significant proportions only for disease-free survival. Significant reductions in relapse but not death were apparent for pre-and postmenopausal node-negative (and unknown) patients combined, and for both relapse and deaths in postmenopausal node-positive patients. Although the duration of survival *following* relapse has proven longer in the control group who received tamoxifen at the time of relapse than those who had tamoxifen as adjuvant, the significance of the difference of overall survival from the time of entry to the trial is maintained. Therefore, the administration of tamoxifen as first-line treatment to relapsed patients who have not received the

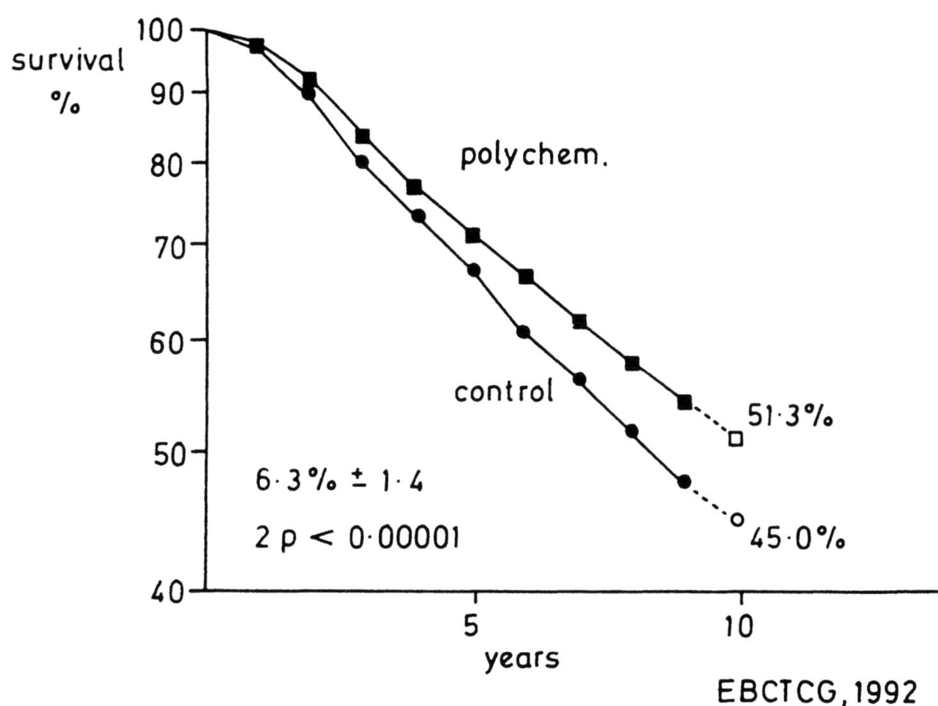

Figure 6: *Ten-year mortality (overall survival) for 11,000 women of all ages randomized to receive polychemotherapy or not. From reference 12 with permission.*

Table 6
Effects of Tamoxifen and Chemotherapy (Indirect Estimation) in age ≥50

		Reduction Annual Odds %	
	No.	Relapse Prior Death	Death
(Chemotherapy + tamoxifen) vs. (chemotherapy alone)	8,148	28% ± 3	20% ± 4
(Tamoxifen + chemotherapy) vs. (tamoxifen alone)	3,932	26% ± 5	10% ± 7

drug previously as adjuvant therapy does not replace the benefit of adjuvant tamoxifen.

In the Scottish trial, estrogen-receptor assays were performed in 56% of participants. Assays by dextran-charcoal saturation analysis were performed in two laboratories with strict quality control. As in the overview, the main benefit from tamoxifen occurred in women with receptor-rich tumors, but the data were

Table 7
Patients Included in Scottish Tamoxifen Trial

Subset of Patients	Immediate Tamoxifen	Tamoxifen on Relapse
Premenopausal		
node-negative	107	105
node-positive	0	0
unknown	15	15
Postmenopausal		
node-negative	270	269
node-positive	230	236
unknown	39	36
Total	661	651

Table 8
Regressions of Large Tumors Achieved by Antiestrogen and Chemotherapy

Treatment	Number of Patients	Significant Regression (Complete)	No Change	Progression
Antiestrogen Therapy				
ER <20 f moles/mg	15	0	5	10
ER ≥20 f moles/mg	46	24	16	6
Chemotherapy				
primary (ER <20 f moles/mg)	27	23 (8)*	4	0
following failed antiestrogens	20	11 (5)*	9	0

( )* = regression complete.
ER = estrogen receptor.
From ref. 21 with permission.

consistent with benefit of adjuvant tamoxifen at all levels of receptor concentration.

At the present time, there seems little justification for limiting adjuvant tamoxifen therapy to those with receptor-rich tumors, but the question remains open.

Primary Tamoxifen Therapy

Because of the uncertainty in selecting those patients whose disease is responsive to antiestrogen therapy by ER-receptor assays, studies are being carried out in Edinburgh and in the Royal Marsden Hospital, London, in which the primary tumor is being used as a biological marker for the effectiveness of the antiestrogen treatment.[18,19] This approach was reported first by Thomlinson, who monitored, by precise clinical measurements, the response of primary disease to a variety of treatments including tamoxifen.[20]

We have reported the use of a similar method of measurement to study the response to both antiestrogen and chemotherapy treatment in 88 patients with tumors greater than 4 cm in diameter, all of whom were suitable for conventional treatment by mastectomy.[18,21]

Following the institution of systemic treatment, tumors were measured at weekly intervals, the response being assessed from the slope of a regression line fitted to sequential estimates of tumor volume between 4 and 12 weeks (Fig. 7). Local therapy was carried out between 3 and 6 months once the response to antiestrogen and/or chemotherapy was known—usually from the start of treatment.

In this study, tamoxifen was but one of a number of forms of antiestrogen treatment used. Initially these were given to all patients, but with the finding that none of these tumors with ER concentrations of less than 20 f mole/mg cytosol protein (estimated on an incisional biopsy) regressed, antiestrogens were reserved for those with ER-rich tumors. In 46 patients with receptor concentrations of 20 f mole/mg or more, approximately half had objective regression of the tumor, while in a further third, the primary tumor remained static. In this study, patients continued on long-term tamoxifen (or if premenopausal, were treated by oophorectomy) following mastectomy.

TOTAL SURVIVAL

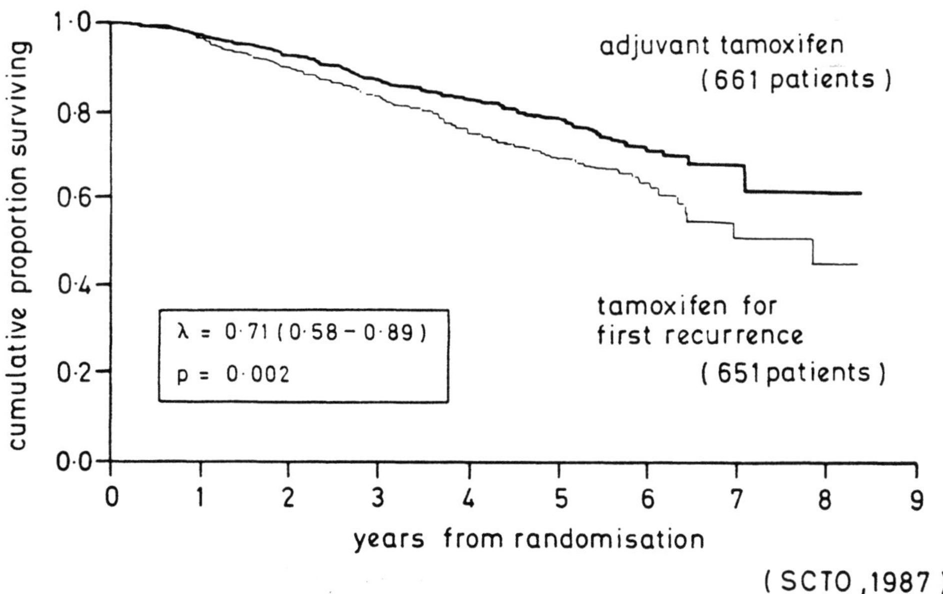

Figure 7: *Overall survival in Scottish trial in which 1,312 women were randomized to receive tamoxifen as adjuvant therapy or to delay its use to treat relapse. From reference 17 with permission.*

Forty-seven of the 88 patients received chemotherapy [four cycles of 28 days with cyclophosphamide (1 g/m^2), doxorubicin (50 mg/m^2), and vincristine (1.4 mg/m^2) on day 1, prednisone 40 mg on days 1 to 5]. Significant regression was observed in 33, in 13 of whom it was clinically (and in 8, pathologically) complete. These findings are detailed in a recent report and summarized in Table 8.[21]

The value of this selective approach to systemic therapy for operable disease is currently being compared with conventional treatment in a controlled randomized trial initiated in Edinburgh, using tamoxifen as the only antiestrogen.

Conclusions

There is no doubt that tamoxifen has an important role in the management of "curable" breast cancer. Because of the relatively low incidence of side effects that accompany its use, it can be given as adjuvant therapy to both node-negative and node-positive patients. However, further information is required about the potential additive benefit of chemotherapy before ideal regimes can be developed. And if the use of resources is to be distributed logically, it is also critical to know which tumors will be influenced by the suppression of estrogens.

Acknowledgments: I am grateful to Dr. Helen Stewart, Director, Scottish Cancer Trials Office (MRC) for providing information on the Scottish tamoxifen trial, and for her assistance in preparation of this manuscript.

References

1. Cuzick J, Stewart HJ, Peto R, Fisher N, et al: Overview of randomized trials comparing radical mastectomy without radiotherapy against simple mastectomy with radiotherapy in breast cancer. Cancer Treatment Rpts 1987; 71:7-14.
2. Cuzick J, Stewart HJ, Peto R, Baum M, et al: Overview of randomized trials of postoperative adjuvant radiotherapy in breast cancer. Cancer Treatment Rpts 1987; 71:15–29.
3. Haybittle JL, Brinkley D, Houghton J, A'Hern RP, et al: Postoperative radiotherapy and late mortality: evidence from the Cancer Research Campaign trial for early breast cancer. Br Med J 1989; 298:1611–1614.
4. Harper MJ, Walpole AL: Contrasting endocrine activities of cis-and trans-isomers in a series of substituted triphenyl ethylenes. Nature (London) 1966; 212:87.
5. Cole MB, Jones DTA, Todd IDH: A new antioestrogen agent in late breast cancer: an early appraisal of ICI 46474. Br J Cancer 1971; 25:270–275.
6. Ward HWC: Antiestrogen therapy for breast cancer: a trial of tamoxifen at two dose levels. Br Med J 1973; 1:13–14.
7. Litherland S, Jackson IM: Antioestrogens in the management of hormone-dependent cancer: a review. Cancer Treatment Rev 1988; 15:183–194.
8. Jackson IM, Lowery C: Clinical rise of anti-oestrogens. In: Furr BJA, Wakeling AE (eds). Pharmacology and Clinical Uses of Inhibitors of Hormone Secretion and Action. Builiere, Tindall and Cox, London, pp 87–105, 1987.
9. King RJB: Oestrogen receptors: an overview of recent advances in their structure and function. Proc Royal Soc Edinb 1989; 95B:133–144.
10. Wakeling AE, Bowler J: Novel antiestrogens. Proc Royal Soc Edinb 1989; 95B:247–254.
11. Thompson AM, Kerr DJ, Steel CM: Transforming growth factor β is implicated in the failure of tamoxifen therapy in human breast cancer. Br J Cancer 1991; 63:609–614.

12. Early Breast Cancer Trialists' Collaborative Group: Systemic treatment of early breast cancer by hormonal cytotoxic or immune therapy: 133 randomized trials involving 31,000 recurrences and 24,000 deaths among 75,000 women. Lancet 1992; 339:1–15,71–85.
13. Early Breast Cancer Trialists' Collaborative Group: Treatment of early breast cancer. Volume 1, World-wide Evidence 1985–1990. Oxford University Press, Oxford, 1990.
14. Ribiero G, Swindells R: The Christie Hospital Tamoxifen (Novaldex) Adjuvant Trial status at 10 years. Br J Cancer 1988; 57:601–603.
15. Novaldex Adjuvant Trial Organisation: Controlled trial of tamoxifen as a single adjuvant agent in the management of early breast cancer. Br J Cancer 1988; 57:608–611.
16. Baum M, Ebbs SR, Houghton J, A'Hern RP, et al: The Cancer Research Campaign trials of adjuvant therapy for early breast cancer. Acta Oncologica 1989; 28:907–912.
17. Breast Cancer Trials Committee: Scottish Cancer Trials Office (MRC) Edinburgh: Adjuvant tamoxifen in the management of operable breast cancer: the Scottish trial. Lancet 1987; 11:171–175.
18. Forrest APM, Chetty U, Levack PA, Miller WR, et al: A human tumor model. Lancet 1986; ii:840–842.
19. Mansi JL, Smith IA, Walsh G: Primary medical treatment for operable breast cancer. Eur J Clin Oncol 1989; 25:1623.
20. Thomlinson RH: Measurement and management of carcinoma of the breast. Clin Radiol 1982; 33:481–493.
21. Anderson EDC, Forrest APM, Hawkins RA, Anderson TJ, et al: Primary systemic therapy for operable breast cancer. Br J Cancer 1991; 63:561–566.

35

The Role of Adjuvant Tamoxifen in the Treatment of Early Breast Cancer

Michael Baum

Introduction

The publication of the 10-year follow-up World Overview of Adjuvant Systemic Therapy for Early Breast Cancer[1,2] is a historic event representing three remarkable achievements. First, the success of the World Overview process was dependent on achieving world-wide collaboration between fiercely independent national groups, each of which is organized on feudal rather than on democratic principles! Persuading such groups from as far afield as the USA, the USSR, Sweden, and Australia to pool their data and forget their differences should set an example for the United Nations in working together for the benefit of mankind.

The World Overview also represents a bravura statistical achievement by the Oxford Clinical Trials Service Unit. The detective work alone necessary to identify approximately 150 trials from the four corners of the earth is worthy of acknowledgment. Then to collate and check individual patient data referring to more than 70,000 women followed up at intervals between 5 and 15 years pushed statistical and computing capacity to its limits. In other words, this study is likely to be a model for the evaluation of any intervention that is likely to produce modest benefits for common diseases.

Last but not least, the data themselves vindicate the conceptual and biological revolution concerning the nature of breast cancer that emerged in the

From: Wise L, Johnson H Jr (eds): *Breast Cancer: Controversies in Management.* Futura Publishing Company, Inc., Armonk, NY, © 1994.

1960s and 1970s following the seminal studies of the Fishers in Pittsburgh.[3] These new data suggest that hundreds of thousands of women's lives can be saved worldwide over the next decade.

The Bottom Line

An accountant wishing to read the bottom line of this audit would conclude that the appropriate use of adjuvant systemic therapy following surgical treatment of early breast cancer will lead to an approximately 25% reduction in the relative risk of death at a constant rate over a period of at least 10 years. This can be translated into absolute gains according to a relatively simple formula. Say that for an average prognosis of women with early breast cancer the annual risk of death is 8%, then in each year this will lead to a gain of 2% among those still alive at the beginning of that year. This then translates to an approximately 10% net gain after an interval of 10 years. In the UK alone we expect 150,000 deaths over this period, thus we can anticipate the net salvage of 15,000 lives before the year 2000. However, this is not the only way of interpreting the bottom line. Even among those who are ultimately doomed to die, it is likely that there will be a prolongation of life, with the median survival extended by approximately 2 to 3 years. Furthermore, as the relative risk reduction following the use of adjuvant systemic therapy appears to be fairly constant across all clinicopathological subgroups, it is likely that these extra years of life will be shared among all groups.

With the exception of ovarian ablation for the premenopausal group, there do not appear to be any qualitative interactions between treatment and outcome across these clinicopathological subgroups, although it is likely that some will benefit quantitatively more than others.

The Question of Choice

What then is the "appropriate" use of adjuvant systemic therapy for different patients with early breast cancer? The Overview process is not intended to tell us how to treat individual patients, but is intended to provide hard objective data based on powerful statistical inferences upon which doctors and patients can make sensible value judgements on the benefits and costs of a particular intervention. Furthermore, any advice or commentary based on the data will inevitably reflect either the prejudice or the intellectual investment of the individual clinician. For that reason, I am sensibly cautious in avoiding precise recommendations.

For example, collaborative groups in the USA, Italy, and Japan have a major intellectual investment in the investigation of adjuvant systemic chemotherapy, whereas the rest of the world, in particular the UK, Canada, and the Scandinavian countries, has been more interested in the endocrine approach to this disease. This variety of approach, in retrospect, has been scientifically rewarding and of enormous clinical value, allowing some choice for doctors and their patients, particularly in the developing world where they may not have access to or confidence in complex polychemotherapy regimens. However, this variety of approach also has its inbuilt hazard for the Overview process which is dependent on certain assumptions concerning interaction between treatments. For example, the "main effect" analysis for endocrine therapy summates the trials that are confounded by concomitant chemotherapy with those unconfounded studies that compared the endocrine regimen versus an untreated control group. As will be seen later, indirect comparisons of the results from confounded and unconfounded trials produce evidence suggestive of a negative interaction between the cytotoxic and the endocrine approaches.

Putting that aside for the moment, individual clinicians now have to grapple with some rather complex concepts if they are to make intelligent recommendations for their patients. This could be approached at two levels of understanding. Even a most simplistic approach to these data demands an understanding of the difference between relative risk reductions and absolute benefits and also how these statistics enable sensible cost/benefit analyses to be calculated. Thus the greater the risk of relapse calculated from the clinicopathological details of the patient, the greater the absolute benefit. Looking at it another way, the smaller the risk of relapse for the individual patient, then the smaller the absolute benefit of adjuvant therapy and the greater the significance of the toxic side effects of that therapy. With these principles in mind, some simple guidelines might emerge. For example, a premenopausal woman judged to have a poor prognosis, based either on the nodal status or on a variety of biological variables decoded from the primary tumor, would benefit from six cycles of polychemotherapy or some form of ovarian ablation, whereas for a postmenopausal woman who appears to have a preferential benefit from tamoxifen compared with chemotherapy, one might consider adjuvant tamoxifen for 2 years or more even if she has a relatively good prognosis because of the low toxicity of that approach.

Biological 'Fallout' From Trials

Many readers may safely and wisely stop at this point, comfortable with these simple recommendations, but a more sophisticated understanding of the Overview process points to some interesting paradoxes. Adjuvant chemotherapy does indeed appear to have some long-term benefit in postmenopausal women, although with a relative risk reduction approximately half of that achieved by tamoxifen; indirect comparisons might suggest that the addition of chemotherapy to tamoxifen will produce a greater net benefit. At the same time there does appear to be a quantitative interaction between adjuvant tamoxifen and the estrogen-receptor (ER) status of the primary tumor, with almost twice the benefit for the ER-positive compared to ER-negative cases. Yet the ER status itself does not identify a subgroup of women who are wholly unresponsive to adjuvant tamoxifen, leading to the observation that the relative risk reduction for polychemotherapy in the ER-negative postmenopausal women is slightly less than that achieved by tamoxifen in the same group! Furthermore, looking at the unconfounded studies of tamoxifen, there is no doubt that the relative risk reductions are more or less identical in premenopausal women as in postmenopausal women, and this is in spite of the fact that tamoxifen induces very high levels of unopposed estradiol in premenopausal women,[4] once again throwing into doubt the comfortable notion that tamoxifen exerts its effect purely as an antiestrogen.

In fact, it can be stated categorically that far from being an antiestrogen, tamoxifen is a weak estrogen on most tissues, such as the endometrium, the liver, and the skeleton, while mediating some of its biological effects through the estrogen receptor of the breast cancer cell. For some time now it has been suspected that tamoxifen mediates its effect as an adjuvant therapy through alternative mechanisms independent of the estrogen-receptor pathway; these include immunomodulation and central effects on the production of insulin-like growth factor. Of particular interest to my group has been the possibility of tamoxifen influencing stromal epithelial interaction. We have published studies that show that tamoxifen can induce the production of the epithelial growth inhibitory polypeptide, transforming growth factor beta (TGF beta) from fibroblasts with undetectable levels of estrogen receptor. Recently, using immunocytochemistry, we have demonstrated that the fibroblasts within the stroma of the breast cancer of patients treated with tamoxifen stain deeply for the presence of TGF beta-1 with no staining of the epithelial cells themselves. There is thus a very plausible explanation as to why tamoxifen could exert an adjuvant effect on the micrometastases shed from a tumor whose cells were predominantly ER-negative.[5] Therefore, to ignore the data of the benefits of tamoxifen on ER-negative patients based on a priori reasoning is both unscientific and inhumane.

This last set of observations demonstrates that randomized controlled trials and their overviews provide powerful biological insights into the nature of the disease under study, which then indirectly suggest directions for the next generation of trials. The surprising observation that long-term follow-up of the early ovarian ablation trials demonstrates an advantage of the same order as that achieved by polychemotherapy once again raises the question of whether chemotherapy in premenopausal women exerts its influence via an indirect chemical castration.[6]

Apparent negative interactions between polychemotherapy and tamoxifen and the surprising benefit of tamoxifen in premenopausal women provide certain clues as to the mechanism of action of this enigmatic drug. The fact that the benefits of either approach persist or improve with time is in itself a remarkable observation that cannot be explained adequately on conventional biological models.

From these speculations, the next generation or two of clinical trials suggest themselves. For premenopausal women, polychemotherapy needs to be compared directly with ovarian ablation, but, in addition, it is also necessary to determine whether any additional benefit is obtained by ovarian ablation in patients pretreated with polychemotherapy. For postmenopausal women, it is necessary to define the optimum duration of tamoxifen, comparing 2-year regimens with those where the drug is given for longer periods or until relapse. Furthermore, the benefits of adding polychemotherapy to 2 years or more of tamoxifen need to be clearly defined. The chance observation that tamoxifen produces about a 40% reduction in the risk of contralateral breast cancers has already spurred the UKCCCR and the NSABP into large-scale trials to investigate the chemoprevention of breast cancer.[7]

References

1. Early Breast Cancer Trialists' Collaborative Group: Systemic treatment of early breast cancer by hormonal, cytotoxic or immune therapy. Lancet 1992; 339:1–15.
2. Early Breast Cancer Trialists' Collaborative Group: Systemic treatment of early breast cancer by hormonal, cytotoxic or immune therapy. Lancet 1992; 339:71–85.
3. Fisher B: Laboratory and clinical research in breast cancer: a personal adventure: the David Kasnofsky Memorial Lecture. Cancer Res 1980; 40:3863–3881.
4. Sunderland MC, Osbourne CK: Tamoxifen in premenopausal patients with metastatic breast cancer: a review. J Clin Oncol 1991; 9:1283–1297.
5. Colletta AA, Wakefield LM, Howell FV, van Roozendaal KEP, et al: Anti-oestrogens induce the secretion of active transforming growth factor beta from human fetal fibroblasts. Br J Cancer 1990; 62:405–409.
6. Bianco AR, Del Mastro L, Gallo C, Perrone F, et al: Prognostic role of amenorrhea induced by adjuvant chemotherapy in premenopausal patients with early breast cancer. Br J Cancer 1991; 63:799–803.
7. Baum M, Ziv Y, Colletta AA: Can we prevent breast cancer? Br J Cancer 1991; 64:205–207.

36

Controversies Regarding Irradiation after Preservative Surgery for Breast Cancer

Brenda Shank

Introduction

Although irradiation following preservative surgery has become established not only as an alternative method of treating breast cancer, but as a preferred method in many early breast cancers, there are still controversies remaining in several areas. The major questions may be summarized as follows: (1) Is adjuvant irradiation always necessary? (2) Is a "boost" always required to the primary site? (3) What are the indications for irradiating regional lymph nodes? (4) What is the optimal sequencing of chemotherapy and radiation therapy?

Methods

A review of the literature regarding the local pathology and natural spread of breast cancer, recurrence pattern, and results of the treatment interventions described in the Introduction was done. The results of this review will be presented along with recommendations for treatment. Each one of the questions enumerated above will be addressed separately in the Results and Discussion to follow.

From: Wise L, Johnson H Jr (eds): *Breast Cancer: Controversies in Management.* Futura Publishing Company, Inc., Armonk, NY, © 1994.

Results and Discussion

Is Adjuvant Irradiation Always Necessary?

In order to address this issue, one has to understand the basic "geographic" pathology of breast cancer, i.e., where is the tumor likely to be located? When a primary site is discovered, is the cancer truly multicentric and likely to be located anywhere in the rest of the breast? Or does it extend radially some distance from the clinically palpable or mammographically visible primary? Is multicentricity in some cases really a result of contiguous extension along ducts, as suggested by Holland?[1] Multicentricity has been considered to be high by many authors[2,3] as shown in Table 1, but in ductal carcinoma in situ (DCIS), true multicentricity was shown to be only 1%[1] when the tumor was examined by careful serial subgross sectioning with radiological and histologic correlation; comedo-type carcinomas frequently showed contiguous growth along the ductal system.

Table 1
Multicentricity of Breast Cancer

Study/Reference No.	No. of Multicentric/No. of Cases (%)
Lagios[2]	18/85 (21%)
Schwartz et al.[3]	
(nonpalpable Ca)	
Invasive	10/25 (40%)
Microinvasive	4/7
Noninvasive	5/11 (46%)
Overall	19/43 (44%)
Holland et al.[1]*	1/82 (1%)
(DCIS)	

*Serial subgross sectioning with radiological/histologic correlation.

In invasive TI, T2 primaries, foci of tumor have been found to extend >2 cm from the clinically and radiologically unifocal primary site in 43% of cases.[4] Only 37% had no foci around the primary mass. Extension beyond the primary site was an even greater problem when extensive intraductal carcinoma (EIC) was found histologically in an invasive tumor;[5] 20% had invasive foci and 58% had intraductal foci at >2 cm from the primary tumor. When EIC was not present, 12% had invasive foci and 19% had intraductal foci at >2 cm.

Breast recurrences have been shown to be less in several prospective trials[6-8] when adjuvant irradiation has been done (Table 2), but overall survival has not been significantly improved. One could certainly argue, however, that it would be far better not to have a recurrence, which necessitates further treatment (often mastectomy), and its attendant morbidity, both physical and psychological. Looking at the National Surgical Adjuvant Breast Project (NSABP) B-06 trial[6] in

Table 2
Breast Recurrence and Survival in Prospective Trials of Preservative Surgery (PS) ±
Irradiation (RT)

Study/Reference No.	% Breast Recurrence			Difference in Overall Survival	F/U (y)
	PS		PS + RT		
Node-Negative					
NSABP[6]	37	[Sig]	12	[NS]	8
Uppsala-Orebro[7]	10	[NS]	3*	[NS]	5
Ontario COG[8]	14	[Sig]	2	[NS]	3
Node-Positive					
NSABP[6]	43	[Sig]	6	[NS]	8

particular, we can conclude that chemotherapy alone did not prevent breast recurrences after preservative surgery, but that irradiation did.

It is important, however, to determine if there are any subsets of patients who may *not* need breast irradiation. One recent study[9] has suggested that one may not need to treat patients who have tumors <1 cm, since none of 20 patients had recurred at a median follow-up of 4 years without breast irradiation compared with 23/102 (23%) who had tumors ≥1 cm and had not received irradiation. Also in that same study, only 1/31 (3%) of patients ≥70 years old had recurrences compared with 22/91 (24%) who were <70 years old, when irradiation was not done. Fewer recurrences in an older age group is also supported by data from the Royal Marsden Hospital;[10] 50 postmenopausal and 10 perimenopausal women had a 12% incidence of recurrences compared with 24% in 21 premenopausal women.

One randomized study (NSABP B-21[11]) has been designed to answer the question as to whether breast irradiation is needed in women with <1 cm invasive node-negative tumors who are receiving tamoxifen (TMX). There are three arms after lumpectomy and axillary dissection: TMX only, breast irradiation + TMX, and breast irradiation + placebo.

In DCIS, breast recurrences with irradiation after lumpectomy range from 2% to 16%.[12–18] When the DCIS patients from the NSABP B-06 trial were analyzed separately,[13] the recurrence rate was 23% (5/22), but one must keep in mind that tumor size in this trial was <4 cm. When DCIS patients were carefully selected, with <2.5 cm tumors, in a study by Lagios,[19] the recurrence rate was only 10% (8/79). The need for breast irradiation in DCIS patients is being addressed in the NSABP B-17 trial[11] which randomizes patients with DCIS to breast irradiation or no further treatment after lumpectomy and only until June 1987 axillary dissection.

Clearly, all of the answers are not yet available on the need for breast irradiation, but in selected subgroups, it may be possible to avoid irradiation. The results of the randomized trials discussed are eagerly awaited.

Is a "Boost" Always Required to the Primary Site?

From the detailed pathological studies of Holland,[4] we know that, even in small (≤2 cm) tumors, there are invasive foci of tumor extending beyond 2 cm from the tumor, even ≥4 cm from the tumor in 5% of these cases. Conversely, in the vast majority of patients, tumor foci are within 3 cm of the primary tumor. For this reason, a higher dose, achieved by adding a "boost" to the primary site, is logical. The percent of cases with prominent intraductal carcinoma extending various distances radially from the tumor is considerably higher when EIC is present,[5] yielding further rationale for adding a "boost" to this subgroup.

In the NSABP B-06 study, 100% of the breast recurrences (at 39 months) were close to or in the original quadrant when no boost was given to the irradiated group.[13] Schnitt et al.[20] also noted that after preservative surgery and irradiation, 88% of breast relapses were in the area of the original tumor, with an average time to recurrence of 33 months. The remainder (12%), which occurred in distinctly separate sites, had an average time to recurrence of 75 months.

Since (1) most residual tumor pathologically is near the primary site, (2) most recurrences are at or close to the primary site, and (3) the morbidity of boost treatment is generally minimal, it is logical to use a "boost" to the primary site. What is the evidence that such a "boost" is of value in preventing recurrence?

One study from the Joint Center[21] demonstrated a significant difference ($P = 0.002$) in the probability of local recurrence when patients who received a "boost" were compared to those without it. A study from the City of Hope Medical Center in California[22] showed that with clear surgical margins, local control was 100% without any "boost," which was better than that for patients who had uncertain surgical margins *with* a "boost." Bedwinek et al.[23] also showed that when the biopsy was ≥excisional, local recurrence was low (5%), regardless of whether an implant "boost" was done or not. However, when the biopsy was <excisional, the implant decreased the local recurrence rate to 7% from 28% without it.

Finally, another study from the Joint Center[24] statistically showed no significant difference in local failure as a function of either total dose to the primary site or the number of radioactive seeds used (a measure of implant volume) in either EIC patients or in all patients.

The EORTC is running a randomized trial comparing "boost" versus no "boost" in patients who have tumors that measure ≤3 cm with negative margins. Only after such trials are completed will we have a definitive answer to this question, but at present it would appear that it would be better to "boost" when irradiation is done unless there is truly a "surgical boost" (large specimen excised with good margins around a small tumor).

What Are the Indications for Irradiating Regional Lymphatics?

Data regarding the frequency of nodal involvement in initial surgical specimens and the frequency of nodal recurrences after treatment for various primary tumor sizes and locations are difficult to find and are often widely disparate from study to study.

For example, Dewar et al.[25] reported on axillary recurrences with and without axillary irradiation after a low axillary dissection. There were no recurrences in the 56 node-positive (N+) patients in whom irradiation was given and one recurrence in the nine N+ patients in whom it was not given. If axillary levels I and II were cleared, there were no recurrences regardless of whether irradiation was given. When nodes were negative (N-) after a low axillary dissection, irradiation was not given to any of 302 patients; two patients in this group had recurrences. Clearly, one can see the difficulty of analyzing data with so few events.

A couple of studies[26,27] have suggested that the axillary dissection may be therapeutic in itself in terms of axillary recurrence, since the probability of recurrence in the axilla decreased with the number of lymph nodes taken.

Nodal failures as a function of treatment after axillary dissection were analysed by Recht et al.[28] If their data for N+ and N-patients are examined for axillary recurrences based on treatment of the axilla or supraclavicular recurrences based on treatment of this area (Table 3), it can be seen that although the number of events is small, in all but one nodal grouping there were fewer recurrences to a nodal region when that region was irradiated. The only exception were supraclavicular recurrences in the axillary N+ groups; there were no recurrences here, irrespective of whether the area was or was not irradiated. The lack of recurrences without irradiation to this area could reflect the fact that chemotherapy was given to 80% of N+ patients.

Table 3
Supraclavicular and Axillary Failure After Axillary Dissection

		No. Failures/No. Cases	(%)	Axilla RT
Axilla:	n−*	3/244	(1.2)	−
		0/45	(0)	+
	1–3 nodes +	2/121	(1.7)	−
		2/202	(1.0)	+
	≥ 4 nodes +	2/21	(9.5)	−
		0/87	(0)	+
				SCL RT
SCL:	N−	8/420	(1.9)	−
		2/342	(0.6)	+
	N+	0/57	(0)	−
		0/374	(0)	+

*Note: Chemo to <2% of N− cases and in >80% of N+ cases.
Recht et al., 1991[28]

The internal mammary nodes (IMN) have frequently been found to be positive[29,30] when they have been removed as part of an extended radical mastectomy (Table 4), especially in medial and central tumors and when the

Table 4
Incidence of + IMN in Patients with Extended Radical Mastectomy

| | % Positive IMN | | | | | |
| | Lateral Lesions | | | Med./Central Lesions | | |
Primary	No.	N+*	N−	No.	N+	N−
T1–2	182	22	8	120	35	9
T3	15	64	25	25	43	18
	[Veronesi & Valagussa, 1981][30]					
TX	34	42	13	691	53	16
	[Urban & Marjani, 1971][29]					

*N+ and N− refer to axillary nodes.

axillary nodes are positive. However, the value of treating these nodes, either surgically or with irradiation, has been quite controversial.

In a multi-institution study from France,[31] surgical dissection of these nodes significantly decreased locoregional recurrences from 24% to 14% at 10 years (P = 0.05). Overall survival was improved with statistical significance only in the group with medial tumors, although a later report from the same group[32] described no survival benefit.

A report from the Institut Gustave-Roussy,[33] which included some of the same patients, noted a decrease in locoregional recurrence with IMN treatment, from 32% without any treatment to 22% for surgery, 6% for irradiation, and 8% for both. Survival was improved with statistical significance in patients with medial tumors. A follow-up study[34] reported that in patients with medial tumors, there was a statistically significant decrease in distant metastases, with IMN treatment, 40% versus 56% (P = 0.02) and in contralateral breast cancers, 20% versus 8% (P = 0.01). IMN treatment again was either surgery, irradiation, or both. There was no difference in either distant metastases or contralateral cancer in patients with lateral tumors.

The risks of nodal recurrence (without treatment) for the axilla, supraclavicular area, and IMN are estimated in Table 5 for N+ and N-tumors, with a further breakdown by medial and lateral tumors for the IMN node risk. Chemotherapy regimens may alter some of these risks, e.g., a decreased risk for the supraclavicular area when chemotherapy is given as noted by Recht et al.[28]

Although all of the answers are not in, if a patient has had an adequate level I–II axillary dissection, and nodes are negative, it would be logical to consider treatment of the IMNs in patients with medial tumors. If the nodes are positive, then one may consider treatment not only of the IMNs, but also the supraclavicular area, especially if ≥4 nodes are positive. One may consider treating the axilla if (1) no nodes were identified, (2) there is extracapsular extension, and (3) ≥4 nodes were positive.

Table 5
Risks of Nodal Recurrence* By Axillary Status and Quadrant

Axilla Status	Predicted Recurrence Rate (%)		
	Axilla	SCL	IMN
N−	<2	<2	5–10—medial <2—lateral
N+	<5 (1–3 nodes) 5–10 (≥4 nodes)	10	5–10—medial <2—lateral

What Is the Optimal Sequencing of Chemotherapy and Radiation Therapy?

The optimal sequencing of chemotherapy and irradiation is the most difficult question to answer. When adjuvant chemotherapy has been given in addition to irradiation, overall cosmesis has not been as good as when irradiation alone is given.[35] From separate studies from the Joint Center, we have also learned that if chemotherapy (CMF) is given sequentially, cosmesis is better,[36] and there is less interstitial pneumonitis,[37] i.e., 1% (3/284) versus 8% (8/95), compared with concomitant treatment.

If chemotherapy is delayed, there is concern that disease-free survival (DFS) may be compromised. In a study from the Arizona Cancer Center[38] using Adriamycin and cyclophosphamide ± radiation therapy (RT) between courses 3 and 4, there was a statistically significant decrease in percent DFS at 5 years in patients with 1–3 positive nodes when treatment was delayed more than 4 weeks, 52% versus 73% when treatment was begun in <4 weeks. There was no difference in DFS for patients with ≥4 positive nodes. In a study from the M.D. Anderson Cancer Center,[39] a decrease in DFS that was statistically significant was found only in poor prognosis patients, when initiation of adjuvant FAC (5-fluorouracil, Adriamycin, and cyclophosphamide) was delayed >14 weeks.

Delaying RT until the end of chemotherapy resulted in a statistically significant increase in percent local failure at 5 years (41%) when compared with RT first (4%), a "sandwich" chemotherapy-RT regimen (8%), and concurrent treatment (6%), in a retrospective study.[40] On further analysis, actuarial local failure was only 5% at 5 years when irradiation was initiated ≤16 weeks from surgery, but was 35% when irradiation was delayed >16 weeks from surgery.

Such findings on DFS and local failures need to be analyzed in prospective randomized studies, but the data do suggest that when both chemotherapy and irradiation are indicated, both should probably be initiated early (<16 weeks?), but not concomitantly. Possible schedules include irradiation first (which lasts only for about 6 weeks), a "sandwich" schedule with irradiation after 1–2 cycles of chemotherapy, or perhaps an untested, but theoretically beneficial, schedule of alternating chemotherapy and irradiation.[41]

Summary

Irradiation to the breast may not be necessary in carefully selected early tumors for which recurrence rates may be expected to be ≤10%, such as (1) small DCIS (<2.5 cm), (2) very small invasive tumors (<1 cm) with no other bad prognostic features, or in (3) older women (≥70 years). Randomized studies are in progress to test the first two possibilities and are needed to test the latter.

A "boost" may not be required in some situations, such as in patients who have negative margins with a "generous" excision relative to tumor size, i.e., in patients who have had, in effect, a "surgical boost." This may be especially valid when EIC is not present. The EORTC trial randomizing "boost" treatment in patients with tumors ≤3 cm and negative margins should shed additional light on this issue.

Regional nodes should be considered for treatment when their likelihood for involvement and/or recurrence is high (~10%), as discussed. The best data available are for the IMNs, which now strongly suggest that there is value to treating these nodes when the primary tumor is a medial or central tumor.

Optimal sequencing of chemotherapy and irradiation is still unclear, although both should probably be given early after surgery, but not concomitantly. Randomized, prospective studies are needed in order to sort out this issue in different patient groups.

References

1. Holland R, Hendricks JHCL, Verbeek ALM, Mravunac M, et al: Extent, distribution, and mammographic/histologic correlations of breast ductal carcinoma in situ. Lancet 1990; 335:519–522.
2. Lagios MD: Multicentricity of breast carcinoma demonstrated by routine correlated serial subgross and radiographic examination. Cancer 1977; 40:1726–1734.
3. Schwartz GF, Patchesfsky AS, Feig SA, Shaber GS, et al: Multicentricity of non-palpable breast cancer. Cancer 1980; 45:2913–2916.
4. Holland R, Veling SHJ, Mravunac M, Hendricks JHCL: Histologic multifocality of Tis, T1–2 breast carcinomas: implications for clinical trials of breast-conserving surgery. Cancer 1985; 56:979–990.
5. Holland R, Connolly JL, Gelman R, Mravunac M, et al: The presence of an extensive intraductal component following a limited excision correlates with prominent residual disease in the remainder of the breast. J Clin Oncol 1990; 8:113–118.
6. Fisher B, Redmond C, Poisson R, Margolese R, et al: Eight-year results of a randomized clinical trial comparing total mastectomy and lumpectomy with or without irradiation in the treatment of breast cancer. N Engl J Med 1989; 320:822–828.
7. The Uppsala-Orebro Breast Cancer Study Group: Sector resection with or without postoperative radiotherapy for stage I breast cancer: a randomized trial. J Natl Cancer Inst 1990; 82:277-282.
8. Clark R, McCulloch P, Levine M, Lipa M, et al., Ontario Clinical Oncology Group: A randomized clinical trial to assess the effectiveness of breast irradiation following

lumpectomy and axillary dissection for node-negative breast cancer. Proc ASCO 1990; 9:21(abstract).

9. Nemoto T, Patel JK, Rosner D, Dao TL, et al: Factors affecting recurrence in lumpectomy without irradiation for breast cancer. Cancer 1991; 67:2079–2082.

10. Greening WP, Montgomery ACV, Gordon AB, Gowing NFC: Quadrantic excision and axillary node dissection without radiation therapy: the long-term results of a selective policy in the treatment of stage I breast cancer. Eur J Surg Oncol 1988; 14:221–225.

11. Wolmark N: 1989: the year of adjuvant therapy in node-negative breast cancer. PPO Updates 1989; 3:1–10.

12. Bornstein BA, Recht A, Connolly JL, Schnitt SJ, et al: Results of treating ductal carcinoma in situ of the breast with conservative surgery and radiation therapy. Cancer 1991; 67:7–13.

13. Fisher ER, Sass R, Fisher B, Wickerham L, et al., collaborating NSABP investigators: Pathologic findings from the National Surgical Adjuvant Breast Project (protocol 6): I. Intraductal carcinoma (DCIS). Cancer 1986; 57:197–208.

14. Recht A, Danoff B, Solin LJ, Schnitt S, et al: Intraductal carcinoma of the breast: results of treatment with excisional biopsy and irradiation. J Clin Oncol 1985; 3:1339–1343.

15. Silverstein MJ, Waisman JR, Gamagami P, Gierson ED, et al: Intraductal carcinoma of the breast (208 cases): clinical factors influencing treatment choice. Cancer 1990; 66:102–108.

16. Montague ED: Conservation surgery and radiation therapy in the treatment of operable breast cancer. Cancer 1984; 53:700–704.

17. Zafrani B, Fourquet A, Vilcoq JR, Legal M, et al: Conservative management of intraductal breast carcinoma with tumorectomy and radiation therapy. Cancer 1986; 57:1299–1301.

18. Solin LJ, Recht A, Fourquet A, Kurtz J, et al: Ten-year results of breast-conserving surgery and definitive irradiation for intraductal carcinoma (ductal carcinoma in situ) of the breast. Cancer 1991; 68:2337–2344.

19. Lagios MD, Margolin FR, Westdahl PR, Rose MR: Mammographically detected duct carcinoma in situ: frequency of local recurrence following tylectomy and prognostic effect of nuclear grade on local recurrence. Cancer 1989; 63:618–624.

20. Schnitt SJ, Connolly JL, Harris JR, Hellman S, et al: Pathologic predictors of early local recurrence in stage I and II breast cancer treated by primary radiation therapy. Cancer 1984; 53:1049–1057.

21. Ryoo MC, Kagan AR, Wollin M, Tome MA, et al: Prognostic factors for recurrence and cosmesis in 393 patients after radiation therapy for early mammary carcinoma. Radiology 1989; 172:555–559.

22. Pezner RD, Lipsett JA, Desai K, Vora N, et al: To boost or not to boost: decreasing radiation therapy in conservative breast cancer treatment when "inked" tumor resection margins are pathologically free of cancer. Int J Rad Oncol Biol Phys 1988; 14:873–877.

23. Bedwinek JM, Perez CA, Kramer S, Brady L, et al: Irradiation as the primary management of stage I and II adenocarcinoma of the breast: analysis of the RTOG breast registry. Cancer Clin Trials 1980; 3:11–18.

24. Boyages J, Recht A, Connolly JL, Schnitt SJ, et al: Early breast cancer: predictors of breast recurrence for patients treated with conservative surgery and radiation therapy. Radiother Oncol 1990; 19:29–41.

25. Dewar JA, Sarrazin D, Benhamou E, Petit J-Y, et al: Management of the axilla in conservatively treated breast cancer: 592 patients treated at Institut Gustave-Roussy. Int J Rad Oncol Biol Phys 1987; 13:475–481.

26. Fisher B, Slack NH: Number of lymph nodes examined and prognosis of breast cancer. Surg Gynecol Obst 1970; 131:79–88.

27. Fowble B, Solin LJ, Schultz DJ, Goodman RL: Frequency, sites of relapse, and

outcome of regional node failures following conservative surgery and radiation for early breast cancer. Int J Rad Oncol Biol Phys 1989; 17:703–710.

28. Recht A, Pierce SM, Abner A, Vicini F, et al: Regional nodal failure after conservative surgery and radiotherapy for early-stage breast carcinoma. J Clin Oncol 1991; 9:988–996.

29. Urban JA, Marjani MA: Significance of internal mammary lymph node metastases in breast cancer. Am J Roentgenol 1971; 3:130-136.

30. Veronesi U, Valagussa P: Inefficacy of internal mammary nodes dissection in breast cancer surgery. Cancer 1981; 47:170–175.

31. Lacour J, Bucalossi P, Caceres E, Jacobelli G, et al: Radical mastectomy versus radical mastectomy plus internal mammary dissection: five-year results of an international cooperative study. Cancer 1976; 37:206–214.

32. Lacour J, Le M, Caceres E, Koszarowski T, et al: Radical mastectomy versus radical mastectomy plus internal mammary dissection: ten-year results of an international cooperative trial in breast cancer. Cancer 1983; 51:1941–1943.

33. Arriagada R, Le MG, Mouriesse H, Fontaine F, et al: Long-term effect of internal mammary chain treatment: results of a multivariate analysis of 1195 patients with operable breast cancer and positive axillary nodes. Radiother Oncol 1988; 11:213-222.

34. Le MG, Arriagada R, deVathaire F, Dewar J, et al: Can internal mammary chain treatment decrease the risk of death for patients with medial breast cancers and positive axillary lymph nodes? Cancer 1990; 66:2313–2318.

35. Beadle GF, Come S, Henderson IC, Silver B, et al: The effect of adjuvant chemotherapy on the cosmetic results after primary radiation treatment for early stage breast cancer. Int J Rad Oncol Biol Phys 1984; 10:2131–2137.

36. Abner AL, Recht A, Vicini FA, Silver B, et al: Cosmetic results after surgery, chemotherapy, and radiation therapy for early breast cancer. Int J Rad Oncol Biol Phys 1991; 21:331-338.

37. Lingos TI, Recht A, Vicini F, Abner A, et al: Radiation pneumonitis in breast cancer patients treated with conservative surgery and radiation therapy. Int J Rad Oncol Biol Phys 1991; 21:355–360.

38. Dalton WS, Brooks RJ, Jones SE, Salmon SE, et al: Breast cancer adjuvant therapy trials at the Arizona Cancer Center using Adriamycin and cyclophosphamide. In: Salmon SE (ed). Adjuvant Therapy of Cancer. 5th ed. Grune & Stratton, Philadelphia, pp 263–269, 1987.

39. Buzdar AU, Smith TL, Powell KC, Blumenschein GR, et al: Effect of timing of initiation of adjuvant chemotherapy on disease-free survival in breast cancer. Breast Cancer Res Treat 1982; 2:163–169.

40. Recht A, Come SE, Gelman RS, Goldstein M, et al: Integration of conservative surgery, radiotherapy, and chemotherapy for the treatment of early-stage, node-positive breast cancer: sequencing, timing, and outcome. J Clin Oncol 1991; 9:1662-1667.

41. Looney WB, Hopkins HA: Rationale for different chemotherapeutic and radiation therapy strategies in cancer management. Cancer 1991; 67:1471–1483.

Adjuvant Radiotherapy Is Not Always Necessary Following Conservative Surgery for Early Breast Cancer

Frederick L. Moffat, Jr., Alfred S. Ketcham

Introduction

That breast-conserving surgery (BCS) is as effective therapy as modified radical mastectomy for early breast cancer has been established beyond reasonable doubt.[1-13] In particular, the National Surgical Adjuvant Breast Project (NSABP) B-06 trial comparing total mastectomy (TM), segmental mastectomy (SM), and SM plus radiotherapy (RT) to the affected breast has to date shown no significant differences in survival between these three treatment arms.[3,9,10] This trial did show that in patients with primary cancers of up to 4 cm in diameter who underwent SM with tumor-free margins, tumor recurrence in the ipsilateral breast at 9 years was seen in 12% of those who received RT and in 43% of those who did not. This almost fourfold higher incidence of local (breast) recurrence for SM as compared to SM + RT had no apparent effect on overall or distant disease-free survival.

The B-06 trial and other studies have also proven beyond question that postoperative adjuvant radiotherapy (RT) significantly reduces, but does not eliminate, the problem of local tumor recurrence in the residual ipsilateral breast in patients undergoing BCS.[3-7,9,10,12] B-06 was not designed to identify independent variables associated with excess risk for local recurrence, although risk

From: Wise L, Johnson H Jr (eds): *Breast Cancer: Controversies in Management.* Futura Publishing Company, Inc., Armonk, NY, © 1994.

factors were examined as the study matured.[14] Rather, its purpose was to assess only "the effectiveness of SM for breast conservation, whether radiation therapy reduces the incidence of tumor in the ipsilateral breast after SM, whether breast conservation results in a higher risk of distant disease and death than does mastectomy, and the clinical importance of tumor multicentricity."[3] The results to date suggest that the first two questions will be answered in the affirmative and the latter two in the negative.

While the findings of B-06 continue to show no overall or distant disease-free survival differences between the three treatment arms, analysis at nine years has shown for the first time that ipsilateral breast tumor recurrence is associated with a threefold increase in risk for dissemination of disease.[10] However, while local recurrence is a highly significant predictor of distant metastasis, it is only a marker of risk, and is not the cause of subsequent presentation of distant disease. The absence of any significant survival differences in this trial confirms that, while total mastectomy or adjuvant radiotherapy may ablate or decrease the frequency of expression of the local recurrence risk marker, these therapies do not modify the underlying risk for disseminated breast cancer. This new finding may provide a rationale for administering adjuvant systemic therapy following ipsilateral breast tumor relapse.[10]

NSABP B-06 is frequently misconstrued or overinterpreted as definitive proof that postoperative adjuvant RT must always be administered whenever BCS is performed for early breast cancer. Such a conclusion goes beyond the objectives of the B-06 trial and what the results have thus far shown. It does not necessarily follow that because postoperative breast RT reduces the incidence of local recurrence in breast cancer patients undergoing BCS, RT must always be given. Fisher and Wolmark noted that "it remains to be defined which women do or do not need breast radiation."[15] In the absence of such information, they recommended that all patients undergoing SM be treated with breast RT whenever high-quality radiotherapy is available. They also felt that patients should not be denied SM or coerced into accepting TM simply because of inaccessibility of radiotherapy. In these particular circumstances, SM alone (without RT) was deemed to be an acceptable, even preferable, alternative to TM.[15,16]

There is now a substantial and rapidly expanding literature on the clinicopathological variables that influence the risk of local recurrence following SM. There are also a few series in which SM has been used without RT in selected patients with early breast cancer. These data call into question the emerging dogma that patients having conservative surgery for breast cancer must always submit to postoperative adjuvant RT. There are some breast cancer patients amenable to SM who can safely forego RT and thereby be spared the added expense, inconvenience, and infrequent excess morbidity associated with combined surgery and radiotherapy.

In articulating the case for selective radiotherapy, the published results with SM alone in unselected patients will be reviewed. The drawbacks of SM + RT as compared to SM alone will be discussed. The known risk factors for local recurrence following SM or SM + RT will be enumerated and put into perspective. Finally, recent results with SM alone in patients at low risk for local recurrence will be reviewed.

Breast-Conserving Surgery Without Radiotherapy in Unselected Patients

The experience with local recurrence following BCS alone in unselected patients is summarized in Table 1.

A series of 31 patients with clinical T1-T2 N0 breast cancer who, for various reasons, were "treated" only by excisional biopsy at the Royal Marsden Hospital, were reported by Montgomery et al.[17] None of these patients had any evidence of systemic disease at the time of biopsy. The "biopsy excision" used in these patients consisted of gross tumor excision with no attempt to obtain histologically tumor-free margins; this was in essence inadequate surgery for definitive conservative therapy. Of 28 patients followed 3 or more years, two died of intercurrent disease and one was lost to follow-up. Seven of the remaining 25 patients (28%) had experienced locoregional recurrence by 3 years.

Lagios et al.[18] reported 43 patients treated by SM, 36 without RT. At an average of 24 months of follow-up (range 6–48 months), tumor had recurred in the ipsilateral breast in 19%. Clark et al.[12] from the University of Toronto reported 1,504 patients with clinically node-negative breast cancer treated between 1958 and 1984 by BCS with or without RT. Of these, 374 patients were treated by SM alone and the remainder by SM + RT. Primary tumor stage was pT1 in 730 patients (49%), pT2 in 404 patients (27%), undocumented (pTx) in 260 patients (17%), and in the remainder was pT3, pT4, multifocal or synchronous bilateral. Of those undergoing SM alone, 40% had pT1 and 20% had pT2 tumors. The local recurrence rate at 5 years for those who had SM alone was 25%. Ipsilateral breast relapse in patients undergoing SM alone and SM + RT occurred

Table 1
Conservative Surgery Without Postoperative Adjuvant Radiotherapy in Unselected Patients

Author/Reference No.	No. of Patients	Follow-up (Years)	Local Recurrence Rate
Montgomery[17]*	28	3	28%
Lagios[18]	36	2	19%
Clark[12]	374	5	25%
		10	28%
Nemoto[19]	122	4	18%
Fisher[3,9,10]	632	5	28%
		8	39%
		9	43%

*These patients underwent excisional biopsy only, with no attempt to obtain tumor-free margins of resection.

in 28% and 14%, respectively, at 10 years follow-up. Breast relapses usually occurred within the original primary tumor site. Despite their higher local failure rate, survival of the nonirradiated patients was not compromised. RT to the axilla did not influence axillary recurrence rate.

Nemoto et al.[19] reported 122 breast cancer patients treated by BCS without RT at Roswell Park Memorial Institute. At a median follow-up of 4 years, there were 22 ipsilateral breast recurrences (18%). These were significantly more frequent in younger patients and those with primary breast cancers of over 1 cm in diameter.

The NSABP B-06 trial[3,9,10,14–16,20] included 632 patients randomized to the SM without RT treatment arm. Of these, 565 patients were found to have tumor-free margins at SM, the remainder requiring completion TM as stipulated by the study protocol. SM consisted of a local excision removing enough normal tissue adjacent to the tumor to afford histologically tumor-free margins; there was no defined "minimum" margin in this study. As already noted, local recurrence developed in 28% at 5 years, 39% at 8 years, and 43% at 9 years follow-up. Clinicopathological analysis of the SM treatment arm at 5 years identified primary tumor size of 2 cm or greater, high nuclear or histological tumor grade, and invasion of the intramammary lymphatics by tumor as significant risk factors for local failure. In the SM + RT patients, only intralymphatic extension of tumor within the breast was found to augment the risk of local recurrence significantly.[14,20] Almost all breast recurrences were situated within the SM site or within the quadrant of the breast in which the primary tumor arose.

Thus, SM without RT results in local recurrence in approximately 25% to 30% of unselected breast cancer patients within 5 years of surgery, and in 30% to 45% by 8 to 10 years.

These recurrences are usually in or close to the original site of the primary tumor, suggesting that multicentricity in breast cancer patients amenable to BCS is of little clinical importance, certainly within the first 5 years of follow-up.[3,9,10,12]

Drawbacks of Combined Breast-Conserving Surgery and Radiotherapy

Cost-Benefit Considerations

It is difficult to calculate with precision the relative costs of the various locoregional treatment options for early breast cancer. First, some (but by no means all) patients treated by modified radical mastectomy will elect to have, and incur the additional costs of, breast reconstruction. Second, adjuvant RT regimens vary substantially between institutions with respect to dose, fields, and the use of boost doses to the tumor bed, as reflected in our series[21]; this variation persists despite the NSABP B-06 results that demonstrate that 5,000 cGy external beam RT to the breast only, without a boost, is sufficient. The cost of postoperative adjuvant RT is therefore quite variable. Third, patients who relapse in the breast following breast-conserving therapy may be salvaged by a second partial mastectomy or by completion total mastectomy with or without reconstruction. The costs of reconstruction undertaken following completion mastectomy for recurrence are usually substantially greater when adjuvant RT has previously been administered; in these patients, complex multistage surgery involving myocutaneous flaps and tissue transfers is necessary.[22,23] The costs of salvage surgery for local failure are therefore far from uniform.

It is clear, however, that replacement of total mastectomy (with only some patients electing to be reconstructed) by BCS plus *routine* RT amounts to the addition of an extra modality to the management of *every* patient. This would almost certainly result in a substantial increment in the overall expense of locoregional therapy for stage I and II breast cancer. In this era of health care cost-containment, the cost-benefit analysis of such indiscriminant use of adjuvant therapy deserves consideration. As there are no survival differences between BCS alone and BCS + RT, and the risk of breast relapse among patients opting for breast-conserving therapy is not homogeneous, omission of RT from the treatment of selected low-risk patients undergoing breast-conserving therapy is medically justifiable and economically advantageous.

Inconvenience to Patients

Modified radical mastectomy or segmental mastectomy plus axillary lymphadenectomy necessitate a relatively brief interruption in the normal routines and activities of patients' lives, amounting to a 2-to 3-day hospital stay and 2 to 3 weeks' convalescence. Radiotherapy imposes an additional demand of five daily treatments per week for at least 5 weeks, starting about 4 weeks after surgery. While this is not an onerous burden for many patients, it can be a significant inconvenience for full-time mothers, the elderly, the infirm, and those in the work force. Moreover, such protracted treatment is occasionally problematic from the standpoint of patient compliance. It is therefore important to ascertain that the individual patient's risk of ipsilateral breast relapse is of sufficient magnitude to warrant this inconvenience. Radiotherapy should be reserved for such patients.

Surveillance of the Treated Breast

In some patients, the combination of breast surgery and RT may give rise to accentuated dermal and parenchymal edema and fibrosis throughout the treated breast, as well as at the SM site.[22,24-30] These changes may compromise or even confound the clinician's and radiologist's ability to detect locally recurrent or new primary neoplasia in the affected breast. The increased cicatricial reaction and fat necrosis caused by BCS + RT in some patients can force the surgeon to resort to biopsy more often than he or she otherwise might.[28,31] Such biopsies further hinder surveillance, may be complicated by wound healing problems, and have a detrimental effect on cosmesis. Completion total mastectomy even in the absence of breast relapse may eventually prove unavoidable.[28] In these patients, breast-conserving therapy eventuates in the radical surgery it was supposed to replace.

Cosmetic Considerations

Most breast cancer patients treated by SM + RT are quite pleased with their cosmetic results. Good to excellent cosmetic outcomes, as measured by physicians, are generally achieved in 80% to 90% of cases.[22,24–27,30,33–36] It is acknowledged, however, that physician-assessed cosmesis tends to deteriorate over at least the first 3 years of follow-up[25,30,33,34] and that women who are obese or have large, fatty breasts are at greater risk of having an adverse cosmetic outcome.[27] In patients with fair or poor cosmetic results, breast retraction, fibrosis, and cutaneous telangiectasia are the most significant detrimental factors.[25,27,32,34,37] Breast retraction and nipple deviation are the consequence of the excessive fibrosis incited by combined surgery and RT. While selective use of RT following BCS would not affect the proportion of fair or poor results in patients treated with both modalities, the absolute number of patients with suboptimal or disappointing cosmetic outcomes following conservative therapy could be minimized.

As already noted, breast reconstruction following completion of total mastectomy for local failure or treatment complications is substantially more complex and expensive in patients originally treated by SM + RT, and less likely to result in a good cosmetic outcome.[22,23] Some of these vexing clinical problems would be avoided by selective use of RT.

Concerns About Carcinogenesis

There is a substantial literature on this contentious issue. These concerns include possible associations between RT and leukemia, soft tissue sarcomas in the irradiated tissue volume, and new primary adenocarcinomas in the contralateral breast.

The NSABP reported a significant increase in relative risk for acute myelogenous leukemia following RT for breast cancer, as compared to nonirradiated study patients.[38] This association has recently been confirmed in a case-control study conducted in over 80,000 breast cancer patients treated between 1973 and 1985.[39]

There are a number of reports of soft tissue sarcomas arising in treated tissue volumes many years after irradiation for breast cancer.[40–44] The incidence of these lesions is low, but they tend be highly malignant and difficult to treat.

An association between exposure to ionizing radiation and the development of breast cancer many years to decades later has been made in women irradiated for medical indications and in Japanese survivors of the atomic bomb.[45–52] This association is strongest when radiation exposure occurs at a young age.[45,46,48,49,51] When adjuvant RT is administered for breast cancer, the contralateral breast is unavoidably exposed to low but carcinogenic doses of ionizing radiation.[53-55] Even with meticulous radiotherapeutic technique, the opposite breast still receives at least 50 cGy of radiation.[53]

The association of ipsilateral breast or chest wall RT with excess risk for metachronous contralateral breast cancer is controversial. There are numerous series of relatively modest numbers of patients that purport to demonstrate or eschew such an association. Affirmative conclusions[54,56] have been challenged because of potential biases in studied patient cohorts, whereas negative studies[57-62] may be discounted on grounds of inadequate statistical power. Three large (27,000 to 56,300 patients) population-based studies from Connecticut and Denmark have reported that adjuvant breast or chest wall irradiation for breast cancer augments relative risk for a second (contralateral) breast cancer by up to 39%.[63-66] That this difference is only significant in such large numbers of patients suggests that the magnitude of the carcinogenic effect is not great.

A recent case-control study in 41,000 breast cancer patients demonstrated a significantly increased risk for metachronous contralateral breast cancer among those who were 45 years of age or younger at the time their first tumors were treated with BCS + RT. The carcinogenesis issue is of greatest potential significance to young breast cancer patients and those with prognostically favorable breast cancer (and therefore a long life expectancy). Thoughtful oncologists of all disciplines would concur that even a small potential for therapy-related carcinogenesis would make selective rather than routine application of that therapy desirable, provided such an approach is otherwise medically acceptable.

Radiation-Related Cardiac Complications

An association between the use of postoperative adjuvant RT in breast cancer patients and late excess mortality due to cardiac disease has been documented in several long-term European studies.[56,62,67,68] This association applies not only to older orthovoltage radiotherapy but also to more recent [60]Cobalt and supervoltage technology.[56,62] While avoidance of certain high-risk RT treatment ports[62,69] might mitigate the risk of accelerated coronary atherosclerosis and fatal myocardial infarction, conventional tangential pectoral fields do not fully protect the heart, particularly when the left breast or chest wall is irradiated.[56] Once again, patients at greatest potential risk of RT-related long-term cardiac morbidity and mortality include the young and those with a good prognosis. As with the other disadvantages of SM + RT, these complications should temper enthusiasm for a blanket policy of routine postoperative RT in patients undergoing conservative surgery for breast cancer.

Risk Factors for Local Recurrence
Following Conservative Surgery

Variables that influence the risk of local recurrence in conservatively treated breast cancer patients have been the focus of much interest in the recent literature. A number of risk factors for tumor relapse in the ipsilateral breast have been identified, and the effect of several of these on the incidence of local recurrence has been corroborated in multiple series.

Surgical Margins

It is an axiom of oncological surgery that complete resection of primary neoplasia with a margin of adjacent normal tissue is crucial for locoregional disease control. Recent series underscore the veracity of this principle as applied to breast-conserving therapy.[18,70–78] Incomplete surgical excision of primary breast cancer eventuates in a more than fourfold increase in the incidence of ipsilateral breast relapse even in the face of adjuvant RT.[70] It is therefore incumbent on the surgeon to carefully orient and mark the margins of the segmental mastectomy specimen in the operating room for the pathologist. The pathologist should immediately examine the specimen grossly in the fresh state, measure the minimum gross surgical margin, and examine samples from the margins microscopically to verify that they are free of tumor. These samples may be taken directly from the specimen or by the surgeon from the SM wound in the patient.

Multifocality and multicentricity in breast cancer are at the root of the controversy over what constitutes a satisfactory margin of resection.[79,80] Recognizing that the incidence of histological multicentricity is far in excess of the frequency of local recurrence, we believe that the minimum acceptable gross margin for tumors less than 2.5 cm in diameter should be 1 cm, and the margins should be microscopically clear on frozen section; a close margin is defined as microscopic disease less than 0.5 cm from a cut margin on permanent sections. The resection margin is one of our criteria for deciding whether adjuvant RT should be presented to individual patients as optional or mandatory.[21,81]

Primary Tumor Size

Primary tumor size affects margins of resection, survival,[82] and correlates directly with multicentricity.[83] In the NSABP B-06 trial, primary tumors of 2 cm diameter or greater relapsed in the breast significantly more often than smaller lesions in patients treated by SM alone, but not in patients randomized to the SM + RT treatment arm.[14,20] The effect of tumor size on local recurrence rate following breast-conserving therapy has been corroborated by some series[40,75,78,81,84] but not by others[12,70,71,73,85–88]; in these latter studies, patients were generally treated by SM + RT.

Extensive Associated Ductal Carcinoma In Situ

Extensive in-situ carcinoma related to the primary tumor, dubbed "extensive intraductal component" (EIC), has been defined as "intraductal carcinoma comprising 25% or more of the area of the primary mass, and intraductal carcinoma clearly extending beyond the infiltrating margin of the tumor or present in sections of grossly normal adjacent breast tissue."[89] The presence of EIC implies a high likelihood of multicentricity[72,83,90] and is a strong risk factor for local recurrence following breast-conserving therapy.[18,70–74,78,85,91–98] Two groups have defined constellations of variables including EIC (EIC plus high nuclear grade,[93] and EIC plus peritumor mononuclear cell reaction in premenopausal patients[78]) that connote very high risk of breast relapse. However, EIC was not found to be a significant factor in local failures in the NSABP B-06 trial at 5 years' follow-up.[14]

Tumor Grade

Poorly differentiated or high-grade breast cancers (usually as defined by Bloom and Richardson[99]) have a relatively poor prognosis. Recent studies suggest that high tumor grade is also a risk factor for local recurrence following conservative management.[14,20,21,70,71,78,86,93,95,100] Tumor necrosis as a separate variable was identified as a risk factor for local failure by some[78,101] but not by the NSABP[14] or Kurtz et al.[71]

Lymphatic or Vascular Invasion Within the Breast

Invasion of the breast lymphatics or blood vessels by the primary tumor correlated significantly with primary tumor multicentricity in the analysis of the NSABP B-04 trial.[83] The NSABP B-06 5-year analysis revealed that lymphatic or vascular permeation by tumor connoted an excess risk for local recurrence in both SM and SM + RT-treated patients. This association has been corroborated by two European groups[74,78] but not by others.[101,102]

Mononuclear Cell Reaction

Mononuclear cell infiltration into and around the tumor can be semiquantitatively measured; intense mononuclear cell reaction (MCR) correlates well with several variables associated with poor prognosis.[71,78] MCR consists predominantly of T-lymphocytes, and the fraction that is in direct contact with tumor cells consists mainly of suppressor T-cells. MCR appears to be a histological marker for unfavorable host-tumor interaction. This variable has recently been demonstrated as a risk factor for local recurrence, particularly in young breast cancer patients.[71,78,103]

Other Risk Factors for Local Recurrence

Axillary nodal involvement by tumor has been cited by some as a risk factor for ipsilateral breast relapse.[40,75,78,102,104] In two studies, the excess risk was confined to patients with clinical axillary disease[75,104] and in one series was seen only in postmenopausal patients.[78] However, the NSABP[14,20] and other studies of larger numbers of patients[71,85,86,91] failed to find any association between local failure rate and presence or absence of axillary metastases. The influence of nodal disease on risk for breast relapse is questionable.

Young age (less than 35 or 40 years of age) has been identified in some series as a risk factor,[12,40,73,74,81,87,96,105,106] while Clarke et al.[86] failed to find any such association. More recent studies have shown that much or all of the apparent excess risk in young breast cancer patients can be ascribed to other factors, specifically EIC, MCR, and/or tumor grade.[71,75,78,92,94,97,103] Age per se may not be a strong risk factor for local recurrence following conservative therapy for breast cancer.

Other variables reported as risk factors for local relapse include gross multicentricity (a rather uncommon feature in early breast cancers),[78,85] hormone receptor status,[78,88] premenopausal status,[74,87,105] and lobular histology.[101] Hormone receptor negativity has been identified as a significant risk factor in one study,[78] a borderline risk factor in another,[88] and of no importance in the NSABP analysis[14] and the Princess Margaret Hospital experience.[12] The significance of premenopausal status may well be attributable to other influences as that of young age has been.[86] Invasive lobular carcinomas were not disproportionately multicentric or multifocal in NSABP B-04 patients,[107,108] and were not associated with excess risk for breast relapse in the B-06 trial.[14] On balance, hormone receptors, menopausal status, and lobular histology probably have little influence on risk for local recurrence following breast-conserving therapy.

Breast-Conserving Surgery Without Radiotherapy in Selected Patients

Recently published experience with conservative surgery alone in carefully selected patients is summarized in Table 2.

Hermann et al.[102,109] published a series of 1,593 breast cancer patients treated at the Cleveland Clinic between 1957 and 1975, of whom 291 were selectively treated by partial mastectomy without adjuvant RT. These patients had breast cancers of 2 cm or less which were usually peripherally situated, and clinically negative axillary nodes. Ipsilateral breast relapses occurred in 11% at 5 years, in 15% at 10 years, and in 16% at 15 years, and did not affect survival. These recurrences were managed by completion total mastectomy.

Greening et al.[105] reported 81 patients selectively treated at the Royal Marsden Hospital since 1972 by partial mastectomy and axillary lymphadenectomy without RT. Eligibility criteria included tumor size of 2 cm or less, primary tumor site at least 2 cm away from the nipple, clinically negative axillary nodes, no distant metastases, and generous margins of resection (2.5 cm; in essence, the operation was a quadrantectomy). At the time of publication, patients had been followed for 5 to 14 years. Local recurrence rate at 5 years was 10%, and 11% for the entire follow-up period.

Table 2
Conservative Surgery Without Adjuvant Radiotherapy in Selected Patients

Institution/Reference No.	No. of Patients	Selection Criteria	Follow-up (Years)	Local Recurrence Rate
Cleveland Clinic[102,109]	291	Peripheral tumours	5	11%
		Tumours ≤ 2 cm	10	15%
		Clear margins	15	16%
		Clinical NO axilla		
Royal Marsden Hospital[105]	81	Peripheral tumours	5	10%
		Tumours ≤ 2 cm	5–14*	11%
		Wide margins		
		Clinical NO axilla		
University of Miami[21,81]	67	Tumours ≤ 2.5 cm	5	6.4%
		Margins ≥ 1.0 cm		
		No EIC		
		No lymphatic/vascular invasion		
Uppsala-Örebro Study Group[110]	192	Unifocal, ≤ 2 cm tumors	3	7.6%
		Wide margins		
		Pathological NO axilla		

*The follow-up period for the entire series at the time of publication.

We have reported the experience with SM at the University of Miami, in which postoperative adjuvant RT was offered as optional or mandatory on the basis of four pathological criteria.[21,81] These criteria were tumor size of 2.5 cm or less, minimum resection margins of approximately 1 cm, no invasion by tumor of the intramammary lymphatics or blood vessels, and little (less than 25% of the tumor area) or no associated in-situ cancer. We initially reported on 111 private patients treated by conservative surgery between 1975 and 1986. All four criteria were met in 64; 51 of these patients elected to be followed and 13 chose RT. RT was presented to the other 47 patients as mandatory; 38 patients complied and 9 refused radiation. At a median follow-up of 72 months,[21] only three local recurrences had occurred in the 51 patients for whom RT was considered optional and who decided not to have this adjuvant therapy (5-year local recurrence rate of 6%; 95% confidence interval 0% to 13.5%). It was found retrospectively that seven of the eight local recurrences in this series occurred in patients with high-grade breast cancers. These results have recently been updated to June 1990.[81] There has been one further local recurrence among the 67 patients who met all four selection criteria and were not irradiated by choice (median follow-up 80 months).

The Uppsala-Örebro Breast Cancer Study Group has reported the results at 3 years of a randomized trial comparing partial mastectomy to partial mastectomy plus RT in selected patients with early breast cancer.[110] Criteria for admission to the study included tumor size of 2 cm or less (as measured on the preoperative mammogram), unifocal primary tumor, tumor-free resection margins and histopathologically negative axillary lymph nodes. At a median follow-up time of 33 months, the 3-year local recurrence rate in the 194 patients undergoing surgery alone was 7.6%, as compared to 2.9% in the 187 patients randomized to BCS + RT. The incidence of breast relapse for surgery alone compares quite favorably to that of the NSABP B-06 trial (20.6% at 3 years). While these results are early,[111] it is increasingly apparent from this and the other reports of BCS with selective RT that the incidence of ipsilateral breast relapse can be mitigated by careful patient selection, and that RT reduces but does not prevent recurrence even in low-risk patients. It is quite likely that further follow-up will demonstrate that the local recurrence rate following surgery alone in selected patients remains at an acceptable level, and that adjuvant RT is therefore not cost-effective in such patients.

Conclusion

The advent of breast-conserving therapy for breast cancer represents significant progress in our concern for patients' quality of life and our understanding of the biology of this disease. Credit for this belongs to the early pioneers of conservative locoregional therapy and to the Milan,[1,2] Guy's Hospital,[8] and NSABP[3,9,10,14–16,20] prospective randomized trials which proved the effectiveness of conservative treatment. Recent data demonstrating that risk for ipsilateral breast relapse is variable in patients amenable to conservative treatment suggest that such therapy need not be the same for all patients. The rationale for selective use of BCS without RT is sound, as confirmed by the results published to date (5% to 11% local recurrence rate at 5 years with appropriate patient selection, as compared to 25% to 30% in unselected patients).

Regardless of the place of RT in breast-conserving therapy, it is critically important to the long-term success of conservative breast cancer treatment that surgeons and pathologists are compulsive in pursuit and verification of complete excision of primary breast cancers and in assessment of the various clinicopathological parameters discussed above. The importance of microscopically tumor-free resection margins cannot be overstated; even large doses of ionizing radiation will not prevent local relapse when excision has been incomplete. The pathologist must assess the SM specimen in the fresh state for minimum gross resection margin and gross tumor size. The final pathology report must include specific information about tumor grade, histological subtype, and the presence or absence of EIC, MCR, and lymphatic or vascular invasion within and around the primary cancer. Axillary nodal status and hormone receptor data are of critical therapeutic importance. The surgeon must insist that all of this information be available for every patient prior to making any recommendations about adjuvant therapy.

That postoperative adjuvant RT reduces the incidence of local recurrence is a very significant therapeutic observation. However, it is not valid to conclude from this that RT must always be given with BCS. By far the most important contribution of adjuvant RT to breast-conserving therapy is that it permits the use of BCS in a larger number of patients than would otherwise be prudent. The proportion of candidates for BCS that is at sufficiently small risk of local recurrence to permit omission of RT is not yet clear and will ultimately be determined by what comes to be considered an acceptable incidence of local recurrence at 5 or 10 years' follow-up. Currently available data strongly suggest that routine RT with BCS would constitute overtreatment for at least some patients. As it is now possible to identify many of these individuals prospectively, rigid treatment guidelines mandating the use of RT in every patient undergoing conservative surgery are increasingly difficult to justify.

References

1. Veronesi U, Saccozzi R, Del Vecchio M, et al: Comparing radical mastectomy with quadrantectomy, axillary dissection and radiotherapy in patients with small cancers of the breast. N Engl J Med 1981; 305:6–11.
2. Veronesi U, Salvadori B, Luini A, et al: Conservative treatment of early breast cancer: long-term results of 1232 cases treated with quadrantectomy, axillary dissection and radiotherapy. Ann Surg 1990; 211:250–259.
3. Fisher B, Bauer M, Margolese R, et al: Five-year results of a randomized clinical trial comparing total mastectomy and segmental mastectomy with or without radiation in the treatment of breast cancer. N Engl J Med 1985; 312:665–673.
4. Calle R, Pilleron JP, Schlienger P, Vilcoq JR: Conservative management of early breast cancer: ten years experience at the Foundation Curie. Cancer 1978; 42:2045–2053.
5. Hellmann S, Harris JR, Levene MB: Radiation therapy of early carcinoma of the breast without mastectomy. Cancer 1980; 46:988-994.
6. Clark RM, Wilkinson RH, Mahoney LJ, Reid JG, et al: Breast cancer: a 21 year experience with conservative surgery and radiation. Int J Radiat Oncol Biol Phys 1982; 8:967–975.
7. Clark RM, Wilkinson RH, Mahoney LJ, Reid JG, et al: Breast cancer: a 22 year study of the conservative approach. Rev Endocrine-Related Cancer 1984; 14(Suppl):227–232.
8. Hayward JL: The Guy's trial of treatments of "early" breast cancer. World J Surg 1977; 1:314–316.
9. Fisher B, Redmond C, Poisson R, et al: Eight-year results of a randomized clinical trial comparing total mastectomy and lumpectomy with and without irradiation in the treatment of breast cancer. N Engl J Med 1989; 320:822–828.
10. Fisher B, Anderson S, Fisher ER, et al: Significance of ipsilateral breast tumour recurrence after lumpectomy. Lancet 1991; 338:327–331.
11. Kurtz JM, Amalric R, Brandone H, et al: Local recurrence after breast-conserving surgery and radiotherapy: frequency, time course and prognosis. Cancer 1989; 63:1912–1917.
12. Clark RM, Wilkinson RH, Miceli PN, MacDonald WD: Breast cancer: experiences with conservation therapy. Am J Clin Oncol 1987; 10:461–468.
13. Lichter AS, Lippman ME, Danforth DN Jr, et al: Mastectomy versus breast-conserving therapy in the treatment of stage I and II carcinoma of the breast: a randomized trial at the National Cancer Institute. J Clin Oncol 1992; 10:976–983.
14. Fisher ER, Sass R, Fisher B, et al: Pathologic findings from the National Surgical Adjuvant Breast Project (Protocol No. 6). II. Relation of local recurrence to multicentricity. Cancer 1986; 57:1717–1724.
15. Fisher B, Wolmark N: Limited surgical management for primary breast cancer: a commentary on the NSABP reports. World J Surg 1985; 9:682–691.

16. Fisher B, Wolmark N, Fisher ER, Deutsch M: Lumpectomy and axillary dissection for breast cancer: surgical, pathological and radiation considerations. World J Surg 1985; 9:692–698.
17. Montgomery ACV, Greening WP, Levene AL: Clinical study of recurrence rate and survival time of patients with carcinoma of the breast treated by biopsy excision without any other therapy. J Royal Soc Med 1978; 71:339–342.
18. Lagios MD, Richards VE, Rose MR, Yee E: Segmental mastectomy without radiotherapy: short-term follow-up. Cancer 1983; 52:2173-2179.
19. Nemoto T, Patel JK, Rosner D, Dao TL, et al: Factors affecting recurrence in lumpectomy without irradiation for breast cancer. Cancer 1991; 67:2079–2082.
20. Fisher B, Wolmark N: Conservative surgery: the American experience. Semin Oncol 1986; 13:425–433.
21. Moffat FL, Ketcham AS, Robinson DS, Legaspi A, et al: Segmental mastectomy without radiotherapy for T1 and small T2 breast carcinomas. Arch Surg 1990; 125:364–369.
22. Bostwick J, Stevenson TR, Nahai F, Hester TR, et al: Radiation to the breast: complications amenable to surgical treatment. Ann Surg 1984; 200:543–553.
23. Bostwick J, Paletta C, Hartrampf CR: Conservative treatment for breast cancer: complications requiring reconstructive surgery. Ann Surg 1986; 203:481–490.
24. Welch JS: The postirradiated breast. Mayo Clin Proc 1986; 61:392–395.
25. Beadle GF, Silver B, Botnick L, Hellmann S, et al: Cosmetic results following primary radiation for early breast cancer. Cancer 1984; 54:2911–2918.
26. Clarke D, Martinez A, Cox RS, Goffinet DR: Breast edema following staging axillary node dissection in patients with breast carcinoma treated by radical radiotherapy. Cancer 1982; 49:2295–2299.
27. Clarke D, Martinez A, Cox RS: Analysis of cosmetic results and complications in patients with stage I and II breast cancer treated by biopsy and irradiation. Int J Radiat Oncol Biol Phys 1983; 9:1807–1813.
28. Clarke D, Curtis JL, Martinez A, Fajardo L, et al: Fat necrosis of the breast simulating recurrent carcinoma after primary radiotherapy in the management of early stage breast carcinoma. Cancer 1983; 52:442–445.
29. Harris JR, Recht A, Amalric R, et al: Time course and prognosis of local recurrence following primary radiation therapy for early breast cancer. J Clin Oncol 1984; 2:37–41.
30. Lipsztein R, Dalton JF, Bloomer WD: Sequelae of breast irradiation. J Am Med Assoc 1985; 253:3582–3584.
31. El-Deeb NA: Fat necrosis of the breast: an unusual complication of lumpectomy and radiotherapy in breast cancer: review of literature and report of four new cases. Eur J Surg Oncol 1990; 16:248–250.
32. Harris JR, Recht A, Schnitt S, et al: Current status of conservative surgery and radiotherapy as primary local treatment for early carcinoma of the breast. Breast Cancer Res Treat 1985; 5:245–255.
33. Danoff BF, Pajak TF, Solin LJ, Goodman RL: Excisional biopsy, axillary node dissection and definitive radiotherapy for stages I and II breast cancer. Int J Radiat Oncol Biol Phys 1985; 11:479-483.
34. Rose MA, Olivotto I, Cady B, et al: Conservative surgery and radiation therapy for early breast cancer. Arch Surg 1989; 124:153–157.
35. Amalric R, Santamaria F, Robert F, et al: Radiation therapy with or without primary limited surgery for operable breast cancer. Cancer 1982; 49:30–34.
36. Harris JR, Hellmann S, Kinne DW: Limited surgery and radiotherapy for early breast cancer. N Engl J Med 1985; 313:1365–1368.
37. Pezner RD, Patterson MP, Hill LR: Breast retraction assessment: an objective evaluation of cosmetic results of patients treated conservatively for breast cancer. Int J Radiat Oncol Biol Phys 1985; 11:575–578.
38. Fisher B, Rockette H, Fisher ER, Wickerham DL, et al: Leukemia in breast cancer

patients following adjuvant chemotherapy or postoperative radiation: the NSABP experience. J Clin Oncol 1985; 3:1640–1658.

39. Curtis RE, Boice JD Jr, Stovall M, et al: Risk of leukemia after chemotherapy and radiation treatment for breast cancer. N Engl J Med 1992; 326:1745–1751.

40. Delouche G, Bachelot F, Premont M, Kurtz JM: Conservation treatment of early breast cancer: long-term results and complications. Int J Radiat Oncol Biol Phys 1987; 13:29–34.

41. Kuten A, Sapir D, Cohen Y, Borovik R, et al: Postirradiation soft tissue sarcoma occurring in breast cancer patients: report of seven cases and results of combination chemotherapy. J Surg Oncol 1985; 28:168–171.

42. Hardy TJ, An T, Brown PW, Terz JJ: Postirradiation sarcoma (malignant fibrous histiocytoma) of axilla. Cancer 1978; 42:118-124.

43. Stokkel MPM, Peterse HL: Angiosarcoma of the breast after lumpectomy and radiation therapy for adenocarcinoma. Cancer 1992; 69:2965–2968.

44. Otis CN, Peschel R, McKhann C, Merino MJ, et al: The rapid onset of cutaneous angiosarcoma after radiotherapy for breast carcinoma. Cancer 1986; 57:2130–2134.

45. Baral E, Larsson L-E, Mattson B: Breast cancer following irradiation of the breast. Cancer 1977; 40:2905–2910.

46. Li FP, Corkery J, Vawter G, Fine W, et al: Breast carcinoma after cancer therapy in childhood. Cancer 1983; 51:521–523.

47. McGregor DH, Land CE, Choi K, et al: Breast cancer incidence among atomic bomb survivors, Hiroshima and Nagasaki, 1950–69. J Natl Cancer Inst 1977; 59:799–811.

48. Shore RE, Hempelmann LH, Kowaluk E, et al: Breast neoplasms in women treated with X-rays for acute postpartum mastitis. J Natl Cancer Inst 1977; 59:813–822.

49. Boice JD, Monson RR: Breast cancer in women after repeated fluoroscopic examinations of the chest. J Natl Cancer Inst 1977; 59:823–832.

50. Tokunaga M, Norman JE, Asano M, et al: Malignant breast tumors among atomic bomb survivors, Hiroshima and Nagasaki, 1950-1974. J Natl Cancer Inst 1979; 62:1347–1359.

51. Land CE, Boice JD, Shore RE, Norman JE, et al: Breast cancer risk from low-dose exposures to ionizing radiation: results of parallel analysis of three exposed populations of women. J Natl Cancer Inst 1980; 65:353–376.

52. Hoffman DA, Lonstein JE, Morin MM, et al: Breast cancer in women with scoliosis exposed to multiple diagnostic X-rays. J Natl Cancer Inst 1989; 81:307–312.

53. Fraas BA, Roberson PL, Lichter AS: Dose to the contralateral breast due to primary breast irradiation. Int J Radiat Oncol Biol Phys 1985; 11:485–497.

54. Brinkley D, Haybittle JL: A 15-year follow-up study of patients treated for carcinoma of the breast. Br J Radiol 1968; 41:215–221.

55. Svensson GK, Kase KR, Chin LM, Harris JR: Dose to the opposite breast as a result of primary radiation therapy for carcinoma of the breast. Int J Radiat Oncol Biol Phys 1981; 7:1209(abstr).

56. Haybittle JL, Brinkley D, Houghton J, A'Hern RP, et al: Postoperative radiotherapy and late mortality: evidence from the Cancer Research Campaign trial for early breast cancer. Br Med J 1989; 298:1611–1614.

57. McCredie JA, Inch WR, Alderson M: Consecutive primary carcinomas of the breast. Cancer 1975; 35:1472–1477.

58. Basco VE, Coldman AJ, Elwood JM, Young MEJ: Radiation dose and second breast cancer. Br J Cancer 1985; 52:319–325.

59. Kurtz JM, Amalric R, Delouche G, Pierquin B, et al: The second ten years: long-term risks of breast conservation in early breast cancer. Int J Radiat Oncol Biol Phys 1987; 13:1327-1332.

60. Kurtz JM, Amalric R, Brandone H, Ayme Y, et al: Contralateral breast cancer and other second malignancies in patients treated by breast-conserving therapy with radiation. Int J Radiat Oncol Biol Phys 1988; 15:277–284.

61. Lavey RS, Eby NL, Prosnitz LR: Impact of radiation therapy and/or chemotherapy on the risk for a second malignancy after breast cancer. Cancer 1990; 66:874–881.
62. Host H, Brennhovd IO, Loeb M: Postoperative radiotherapy in breast cancer: long-term results from the Oslo study. Int J Radiat Oncol Biol Phys 1986; 12:727–732.
63. Storm HH, Jensen OM: Risk of contralateral breast cancer in Denmark 1943–80. Br J Cancer 1986; 54:483–492.
64. Hankey BF, Curtis RE, Naughton MD, Boice JD, et al: A retrospective cohort analysis of second breast cancer risk for primary breast cancer patients with an assessment of the effect of radiation therapy. J Natl Cancer Inst 1983; 70:797–804.
65. Harvey EB, Brinton LA: Second cancer following cancer of the breast in Connecticut, 1935–1982. Natl Cancer Inst Monogr 1985; 68:99–112.
66. Boice JD Jr, Harvey EB, Blettner M, Stovall M, et al: Cancer in the contralateral breast after radiotherapy for breast cancer. N Engl J Med 1992; 326:781–785.
67. Cuzick J, Stewart H, Peto R, et al: Overview of randomized trials of postoperative adjuvant radiotherapy in breast cancer. Cancer Treat Rep 1987; 71:15–29.
68. Jones JM, Ribeiro GG: Mortality patterns over 34 years of breast cancer patients in a clinical trial of postoperative radiotherapy. Clin Radiol 1989; 40:204–208.
69. Harris JR, Hellmann S: Put the "hockey stick" on ice. Int J Radiat Oncol Biol Phys 1988; 15:497–499.
70. Schnitt SJ, Connolly JL, Harris JR, Hellmann S, et al: Pathologic predictors of early local recurrence in stage I and II breast cancer treated by primary radiation therapy. Cancer 1984; 53:1049–1057.
71. Kurtz JM, Jacquemier J, Amalric R, et al: Why are local recurrences after breast-conserving therapy more frequent in younger patients? J Clin Oncol 1990; 8:591–598.
72. Kurtz JM, Jacquemier J, Amalric R, et al: Breast-conserving therapy for macroscopically multiple cancers. Ann Surg 1990; 212:38–44.
73. Bartelink H, Borger JH, van Dongen JA, Peterse JL: The impact of tumor size and histology on local control after breast-conserving therapy. Radiother Oncol 1988; 11:297–303.
74. Fourquet A, Vilcoq JR, Zafrani B, Durand JC, et al: Early stage breast cancer: a multivariate analysis of the risk of local recurrence following conservative treatment: long-term results. Int J Radiat Oncol Biol Phys 1988; 15(Suppl 1):181(abstr).
75. van Limbergen E, van den Bogaert W, van der Schueren E, Rijnders A: Tumor excision and radiotherapy as primary treatment of breast cancer: analysis of patient and treatment parameters and local control. Radiother Oncol 1987; 8:1–9.
76. Solin LJ, Fowble B, Martz K, Pajak TF, et al: Results of re-excisional biopsy of the primary tumor in preparation for definitive irradiation of patients with early stage breast cancer. Int J Radiat Oncol Biol Phys 1986; 12:721–725.
77. Recht A, Silver B, Schnitt S, Connolly J, et al: Breast relapse following primary radiation therapy for early breast cancer. I. Classification, frequency and salvage. Int J Radiat Oncol Biol Phys 1985; 11:1271–1276.
78. Kurtz JM, Jacquemier J, Amalric R, et al: Risk factors for breast recurrence in premenopausal and postmenopausal patients with ductal cancers treated by conservation therapy. Cancer 1990; 65:1867–1878.
79. Frazier TG, Wong RWY, Rose D: Implications of accurate pathologic margins in the treatment of primary breast cancer. Arch Surg 1989; 124:37–38.
80. Carter D: Margins of "lumpectomy" for breast cancer. Human Pathol 1986; 17:330–332.
81. Moffat FL, Ketcham AS: Breast-conserving surgery and selective adjuvant radiation therapy for stage I and II breast cancer. Semin Surg Oncol 1992; 8:172–176.
82. Cutler SJ, Myers MH: Clinical classification of extent of disease in cancer of the breast. J Natl Cancer Inst 1967; 39:193-207.
83. Fisher ER, Gregorio R, Redmond C, Vellios F, et al: Pathologic findings from the National Surgical Adjuvant Breast Project (Protocol No. 4). I. Observations concerning the multicentricity of mammary cancer. Cancer 1975; 35:247–254.

84. Leung S, Otmezguine Y, Calitchi E, et al: Locoregional recurrences following radical external beam irradiation and interstitial implantation for operable breast cancer: a twenty-three year experience. Radiother Oncol 1986; 5:1–10.
85. Osteen RT, Connolly JL, Recht A, Silver B, et al: Identification of patients at high risk for local recurrence after conservative surgery and radiation therapy for stage I and II breast cancer. Arch Surg 1987; 122:1248–1252.
86. Clarke DH, Le MG, Sarrazin D, et al: Analysis of local-regional relapses in patients with early breast cancers treated by excision and radiotherapy: experience of the Institut Gustave-Roussy. Int J Radiat Oncol Biol Phys 1985; 11:137–145.
87. Calle R, Vilcoq JR, Zafrani B, Vielh P, et al: Local control and survival of breast cancer treated by limited surgery followed by irradiation. Int J Radiat Oncol Biol Phys 1986; 12:873–878.
88. Kurtz JM, Spitalier J-M, Amalric R, et al: Mammary recurrences in women younger than forty. Int J Radiat Oncol Biol Phys 1988; 15:271–276.
89. Recht A, Connolly JL, Schnitt SJ, et al: Conservative surgery and radiation therapy for early breast cancer: results, controversies, and unsolved problems. Semin Oncol 1986; 13:434-449.
90. Lagios MD: Multicentricity of breast carcinoma demonstrated by routine correlated serial subgross and radiographic examination. Cancer 1977; 40:1726–1734.
91. Recht A, Silen W, Schnitt SJ, et al: Time-course of local recurrence following conservative surgery and radiotherapy for early stage breast cancer. Int J Radiat Oncol Biol Phys 1988; 15:255–261.
92. Peterse JL, van Dongen JA, Bartelink H: Recurrence of breast carcinoma after breast conserving therapy. Eur J Surg Oncol 1988; 14:123–126.
93. Harris JR, Connolly JL, Schnitt SJ, et al: The use of pathologic features in selecting the extent of surgical resection necessary for breast cancer patients treated by primary radiation therapy. Ann Surg 1985; 201:164–169.
94. Recht A, Connolly JL, Schnitt SJ, et al: The effect of young age on tumor recurrence in the treated breast after conservative surgery and radiotherapy. Int J Radiat Oncol Biol Phys 1988; 14:3–10.
95. Harris JR, Connolly JL, Schnitt SJ, Cohen RB, et al: Clinical-pathologic study of early breast cancer treated by primary radiation therapy. J Clin Oncol 1983; 1:184–189.
96. Boyages J, Recht A, Connolly J, et al: Factors associated with local recurrence as a first site of failure following the conservative treatment of early breast cancer. Int J Radiat Oncol Biol Phys 1988; 15(Suppl 1):181–182(abstr).
97. Recht A, Connolly J, Schnitt S, Silver B, et al: Conservative surgery and radiotherapy for early breast cancer: the effect of age on breast recurrence. Int J Radiat Oncol Biol Phys 1986; 12(Suppl 1):93(abstr).
98. Schnitt SJ, Connolly JL, Khettry U, et al: Pathologic findings on re-excision of the primary site in breast cancer patients considered for treatment by primary radiation therapy. Cancer 1987; 59:675–681.
99. Bloom HJG, Richardson WW: Histological grading and prognosis in breast cancer. Br J Cancer 1957; 11:359–377.
100. Kurtz JM, Amalric R, Brandone H, et al: Local recurrence after breast-conserving surgery and radiotherapy. Cancer 1989; 63:1912–1917.
101. Mate TP, Carter D, Fischer DB, et al: A clinical and histopathologic analysis of the results of conservation surgery and radiation therapy in stage I and II breast carcinoma. Cancer 1986; 58:1995–2002.
102. Hermann RE, Esselstyn CB, Crile G, Cooperman AM, et al: Results of conservative operations for breast cancer. Arch Surg 1985; 120:746–751.
103. Jacquemier J, Seradour B, Hassoun J, et al: Special morphologic features of invasive mammary carcinomas in women under 40 years of age. Breast Dis 1985; 1:119–122.
104. Osborne MP, Ormiston N, Harmer CL, McKinna JA, et al: Breast conservation in the treatment of early breast cancer: a 20-year follow-up. Cancer 1984; 53:349–355.
105. Greening WP, Montgomery ACV, Gordon AB, Gowing NFC: Quadrantic excision

and axillary node dissection without radiation therapy: the long-term results of a selective policy in the treatment of stage I breast cancer. Eur J Surg Oncol 1988; 14:221–225.

106. Vilcoq JR, Calle R, Stacey P, Ghossein NA: The outcome of treatment by tumorectomy and radiotherapy of patients with operable breast cancer. Int J Radiat Oncol Biol Phys 1981; 7:1327–1332.

107. Fisher ER, Gregorio RM, Fisher B: The pathology of invasive breast cancer: a syllabus derived from the National Surgical Adjuvant Breast Project (Protocol No. 4). Cancer 1975; 36:1-85.

108. Fisher ER, Fisher B: Lobular carcinoma of the breast: an overview. Ann Surg 1977; 185:377–385.

109. Hermann RE, Esselstyn CB, Cooperman AM, Crile G: Partial mastectomy without radiation therapy. Surg Clin North Am 1984; 64:1103–1113.

110. The Uppsala-Örebro Breast Cancer Study Group: Sector resection with or without postoperative radiotherapy for stage I breast cancer: a randomized trial. J Natl Cancer Inst 1990; 82:277–282.

111. Hellmann S: It's too soon to know. J Natl Cancer Inst 1990; 82:250–251.

The Management of Advanced Breast Cancer

Editorial Commentary

Chapter 38

While many surgeons believe that there is no role for radical mastectomy, we agree with Dr. Rush that there are some specific situations where radical mastectomy is still indicated and these situations are well described in this chapter. We feel that many of these patients should be treated by preoperative chemotherapy as discussed in Chapter 39.

Chapter 39

Dr. Hortobagyi's work has revolutionized the management of locally advanced breast cancer. When such patients are treated aggressively with chemotherapy prior to local therapy, there is significant improvement in both disease-free and overall survival compared to other approaches. This work represents one of the major contributions over the past two decades to the management of breast cancer. For stage III-A disease (resectable stage) 80% and 64% and for stage III-B disease (unresectable stage) 45% and 28%, 5- and 10-year survivals, respectively, have been achieved with neoadjuvant chemotherapy. Before this, the average 5-year survival for stage III disease was in the 30% range.

Chapter 40

The chapter by Drs. Aisner and Abrams is a state-of-the-art summary of the treatment of metastatic breast cancer and points out some of the issues that are still begging to be addressed.

It may be of value, however, to re-emphasize a few points. Bone radiation is extremely useful in the management of *localized bony metastases* with complete response rates in the range of 50% and some response rates in the region of 80%. The duration to the response is usually rapid; of the patients who respond, 60% will do so within 7 days after the beginning of treatment and almost all of those who respond will respond within 4 weeks. The duration of response varies, but in about 70% of patients who respond, the treated area will not relapse before death. Since radiation interferes with the bone healing mechanism, in patients at risk for a pathological fracture, surgical intervention is best performed prophylactically prior to radiation. Features that suggest a high risk of fracture include lytic lesions greater than 2 cm in diameter on either the AP or lateral view or destruction of more than 50% of the cortex.

Brain metastases are a fairly common indication for palliative radiation therapy. The response rate is approximately 60% and the median duration of survival after radiation is 5 months. The general consensus is that if there is a solitary intracranial lesion and the metastases are located in an accessible location then surgical resection followed by postoperative radiotherapy is the best method of therapy.

Spinal cord compression is probably best treated using steroids and radiation. Only those patients whose neurological signs progress during the course of radiation should be treated by decompressive laminectomy.

Malignant pleural effusions should be treated systemically and local treatment should be reserved only for relief of the symptoms of the effusion. Repeated accumulation of malignant pleural fluid is probably best treated by tetracycline administered via a chest tube.

Chapter 41

Dr. Peters is one of the pioneers of bone marrow transplantation for breast cancer and gives an excellent overview of this subject.

Surgery Plays a Major Role in the Primary Management of Advanced Breast Cancer

Benjamin F. Rush, Jr.

Introduction

In recent years, there has been an increasing incidence of the diagnosis of breast cancer at a very early stage. This is a most favorable development since there is an indirect correlation between the size of a malignant tumor and the prospective survival of patients, i.e., the smaller the cancer when found, the better the prognosis. At the same time, management of the patient with advanced breast cancer has received considerably less attention. Unfortunately, there are still many patients who because of fear, ignorance, or denial do not present themselves for treatment until late in the course of their disease. While the results of treating such patients are clearly inferior to those obtained in patients in the early stages of breast cancer, some patients can be rescued and it is important that the oncologist understands the options that are available for their treatment. What can be accomplished for the patient with advanced disease can best be appreciated by an understanding of the natural history of untreated cancer of the breast.

The Natural History of Advanced Breast Cancer

Prior to this century, women with breast cancer rarely, if ever, presented themselves for treatment until their lesions were advanced. It was only when the

From: Wise L, Johnson H Jr (eds): *Breast Cancer: Controversies in Management.* Futura Publishing Company, Inc., Armonk, NY, © 1994.

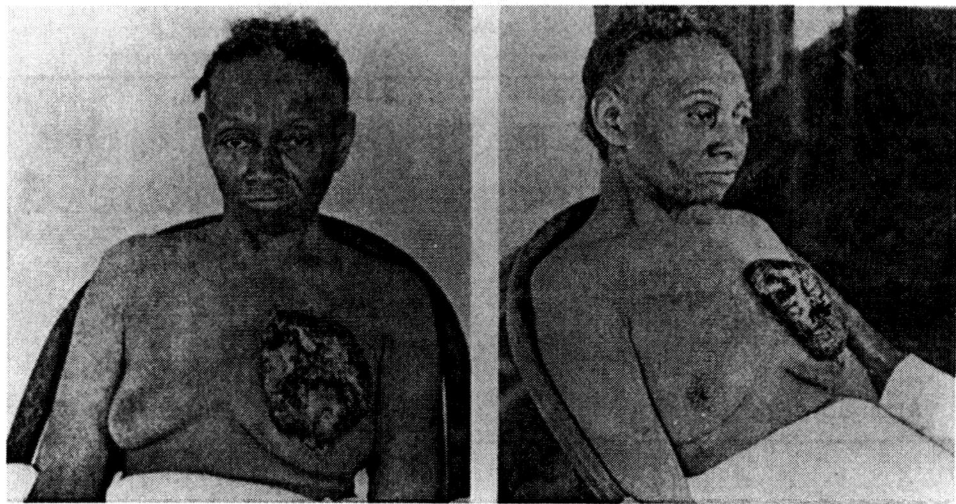

Figure 1: *One of Halsted's patients subsequently healed by radical mastectomy.*[3]

patient was inflicted with ulceration and malodorous drainage or when involvement of nerves had created great pain that women were forced to seek medical aid. Surgical treatment in this era was usually directed solely towards the elimination of the local disease in the hope of eradicating ulcerated lesions or eliminating the source of pain, and was often called a "toilet" mastectomy. As might be imagined, the results of such interventions were often worse than the problem with which the patient presented. The surgical wounds were usually left open to granulate, and these granulating beds were often found to be filled with new and rapidly advancing cancer. It was expected that the patient would ultimately die of the cancer and this is what usually happened. In these circumstances, there were many surgeons who refused to treat these advanced lesions operatively and advised therapies directed towards the use of narcotics and various potions to alleviate the odor and drainage from the ulcerating cancer.

Observations on the untreated patient indicated that the mean survival from time of onset of symptoms was approximately 3 years. Fifty percent of the patients were dead by 2.7 years, 18% survived for 5 years, and 3.6% survived for 10 years. Three-quarters of the patients had advanced ulcerations of the breast at death and almost a quarter had lesions excavating the chest wall with direct invasion of the pleural space and empyema.[1] It was in this setting that the radical operations for breast cancer were developed in the late 1800s.

The great achievement of the Halsted radical mastectomy was the control of local disease in patients with advanced cancer. There have been previous reports of local recurrence rates of 50% to 75% following total mastectomy.[2] Halsted reported a local recurrence rate of only 5% over a 3-year period of follow-up.[3] It was during this early period at the turn of the century, when almost all of the breast tumors presenting were advanced, that the Halsted radical mastectomy became the standard treatment for all cancers of the breast (Fig. 1). Over the intervening decades until the present time, patients began to present with smaller and smaller lesions. In the latter half of this century, it was recognized that the classic radical procedure constituted much more surgery than was required to obtain favorable results. For a small lesion of the breast, segmental resection together with radiation therapy of the remaining breast will produce a long-term result as effective as the Halstedian resection.[4]

The Indications for Halsted Radical Mastectomy in Primary Management

In view of the decreasing extent of surgery now used in the treatment of breast cancer, it is useful to examine the exceptional situations in which radical

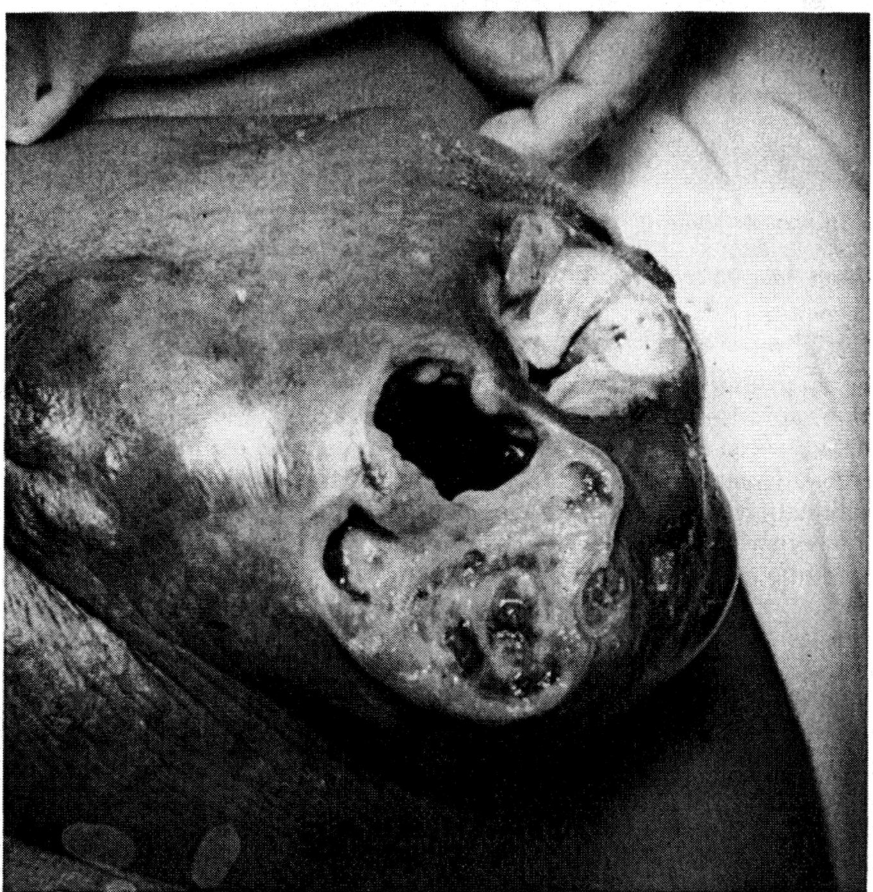

Figure 2: *Stage III lesion of an extent requiring radical mastectomy. This is a colloid adenocarcinoma which tends to grow slowly to massive size with late metastasis.*

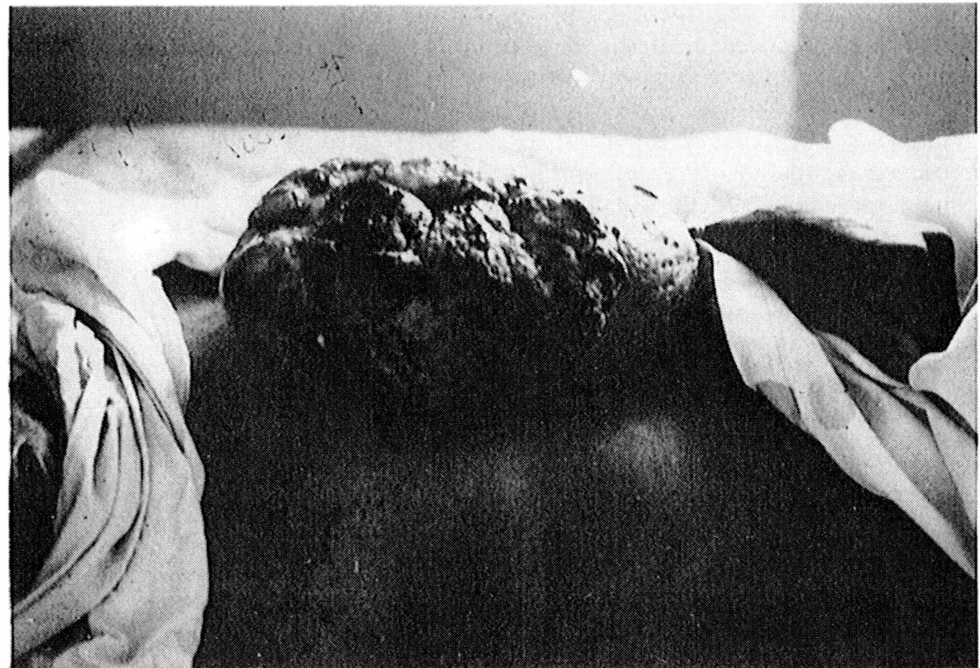

Figure 3: *Another stage III lesion, a conventional scirrhous adenocarcinoma. Radical mastectomy in this patient offers an increased chance for locoregional control even though subsequent distant disease is almost inevitable.*

surgery is indicated. It is no surprise that the main indication for a larger operation is precisely the lesion for which the operation was originally designed, i.e., the advanced lesion (Figs. 2 and 3). The developed countries of the world with access to mammography and effective patient education concerning breast self-examination have harvested the rewards of early diagnosis. The advanced lesion is seen with increasing rarity. There are increasing numbers of surgical residents who are completing their training having never seen a Halsted radical mastectomy, and the numbers of surgeons familiar with the technique are gradually dwindling. Nevertheless, the operation is still the best approach when (1) the underlying muscles of the chest wall have been invaded, or (2) bulky disease of the axilla is so advanced that the pectoralis major and minor must be resected in order to approach the tumor at the chest wall.

Occasionally the claim is made that advanced local disease may be controlled by radiation therapy alone, and if the patient is ultimately incurable, radiation therapy should be adopted as the only treatment. The advanced lesion of the breast will be substantially ameliorated by radiation therapy but it is uncommon for very bulky disease to disappear completely, and in due course such residual disease will remain and begin to grow again (Fig. 4). The object of treatment of the advanced lesion is to totally eliminate local disease even though

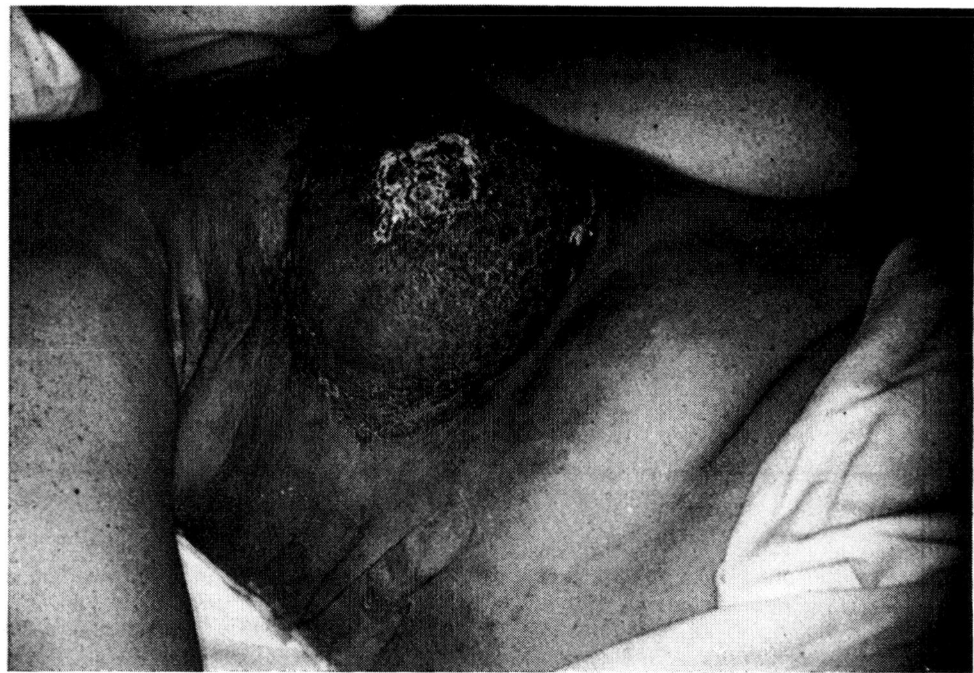

Figure 4: *Large carcinoma of the breast following heavy radiation therapy. Biopsy of this breast revealed persistent carcinoma. Operative removal would be indicated to ensure locoregional control.*

metastatic disease will appear elsewhere. For lesions of these advanced dimensions, the appropriate prevention of local recurrence involves not only the use of radical mastectomy but postoperative radiation therapy as well. The literature is replete with data demonstrating that the combination of radical mastectomy plus radiation therapy does not change survival,[5] but by the same token, this combination is the best guarantee to prevent the appearance of local recurrence. For certain selected groups[6] of advanced lesions, the combination of operation and radiation may prolong survival as well (Fig. 5).

A second indication for the use of radical mastectomy is inflammatory carcinoma of the breast. If used alone, operation will serve only to make the local lesion worse, but if used together with radiation and chemotherapy, a remarkable improvement in local control can be achieved and, surprisingly, an increase in long-term survival as well.[6] Inflammatory carcinoma of the breast was once regarded as uniformly and rapidly fatal with a mean survival between 1 and 2 years. If the lesion is treated with appropriate chemotherapy, either simultaneously with or followed by radiation therapy, a marked regression and sometimes complete responses can be obtained. There has been some debate as to whether adding radical surgery is worthwhile in these circumstances, but

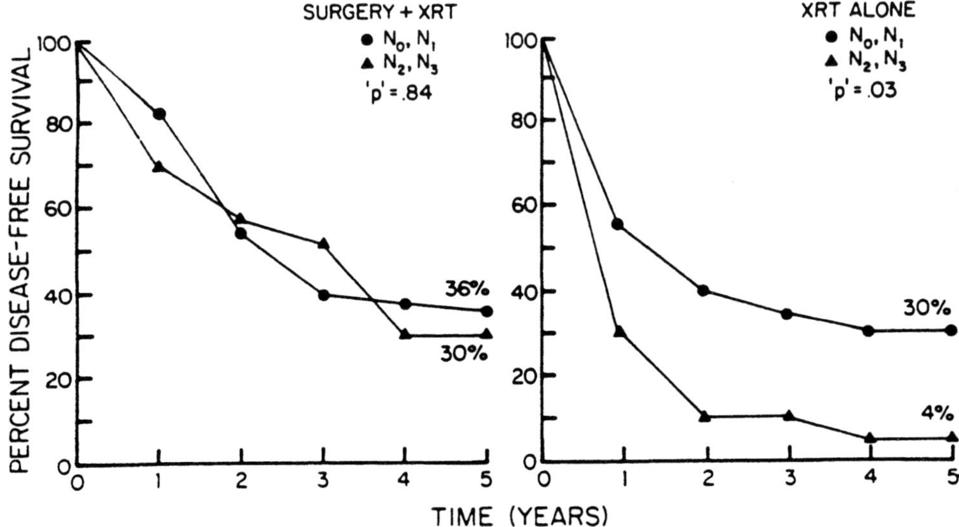

Figure 5: *Data showing difference in disease-free survival in patients treated by radiation alone (XRT) versus radiation plus operation (surgery and XRT). Adding operation was most effective in prolonging survival in patients with the most advanced nodal disease and the largest tumors. From Rao et al. by permission.[19]*

reports from MD Anderson and other institutions indicate that the use of all three modalities gives the best ultimate result.[7–11]

Current thinking reserves radical mastectomy and, occasionally, modified radical mastectomy for patients with stage III and stage IV disease. There are some who have suggested that selected patients with stage I and stage II disease may also be candidates.[9] The various prospective randomized trials of segmental resection and radiation have demonstrated a local recurrence rate of 10% to 15%. An average of 90% of these recurrences are operable and can be treated by total mastectomy. Unfortunately, some 10% to 20% (depending on the series) of these recurrences are inoperable when first found. The question is whether one can select from the much larger group of stage I and stage II tumors, a very small group of no more than 2% to 3% who will ultimately develop inoperable recurrences following the conventional segmental resections. Also, if they can be identified beforehand, would radical mastectomy reduce the incidence of local failure in this group? Kurtz et al.[12] noted that in their group of 586 patients treated by segmental resection and radiation, there were 70 local recurrences of which 13 were inoperable, an incidence of 2.2% of inoperable recurrences. They noted that in those patients with inoperable recurrences, the previous lesions were uniformly invasive ductal carcinomas with a high frequency of unfavorable prognostic features. Ten of the 13 patients had T2 tumors, 11 had pathologically documented positive nodes, five had four or more positive nodes, nine had histologic findings of grade 3 tumors, eight had vascular invasion, and nine had moderate to marked lymphocytic stromal reactions. A somewhat larger percent had negative estrogen receptors compared to patients who did not have inoperable recurrences. Identification of this special subgroup for radical mastectomy would obviously have great advantages for this small number of patients. Appropriate trial as to the effectiveness of this approach would be very difficult because of the small number of patients involved.

Cancer of the Male Breast

Male patients presenting with cancer of the breast often have advanced lesions. In a recent report, 61% of patients seen were stage IV. Presumably, men are less aware that they may be victims of this rare lesion and come for treatment much later than women. Radical mastectomy is still the operation of choice recommended in most reports. This is because (1) the loss of the breast is of little consequence to a man, (2) there is a more advanced stage of most lesions, and (3) the small size of the male breast allows rapid invasion of the underlying pectoral fascia and muscle.[13,14]

The Indication for Chest Wall Resection

The 1950s were probably the peak period for the philosophy of the largest possible operation for the smallest possible tumor. At this time, Urban[15] introduced the extended radical mastectomy to include resection of the internal mammary lymph nodes and a portion of the overlying chest wall. This was proposed primarily for lesions involving the medial breast and subareolar area. The initial retrospective reports suggested that this procedure was an improvement for selected lesions and, interestingly, two prospective randomized trials showed a marginal statistical advantage when the operation was applied to central and medial tumors of the breast, particularly when there was evidence of axillary lymph node involvement.[16,17] In view of the overwhelming success of more limited operations together with radiation for stage I and stage II lesions, application of chest wall resection to such lesions has long been abandoned. One principal indication remains: the direct invasion of the chest wall by tumor. The current philosophy is that surgeons and radiation therapists can have no effect on systemic disease but their major role is in control of local problems. For the rare lesion that has been so neglected that it has begun to penetrate the chest wall, excision of the chest wall in the area of invasion has great value (Fig. 6). Closure of even large chest wall defects today is a relatively simple matter because of the availability of musculocutaneous flaps.

Some Thoughts About Secondary Management

As has been noted, a certain percentage of patients with segmental resections will have local recurrence in the remaining breast. The current findings suggest that such recurrences do not necessarily coincide with treatment failure

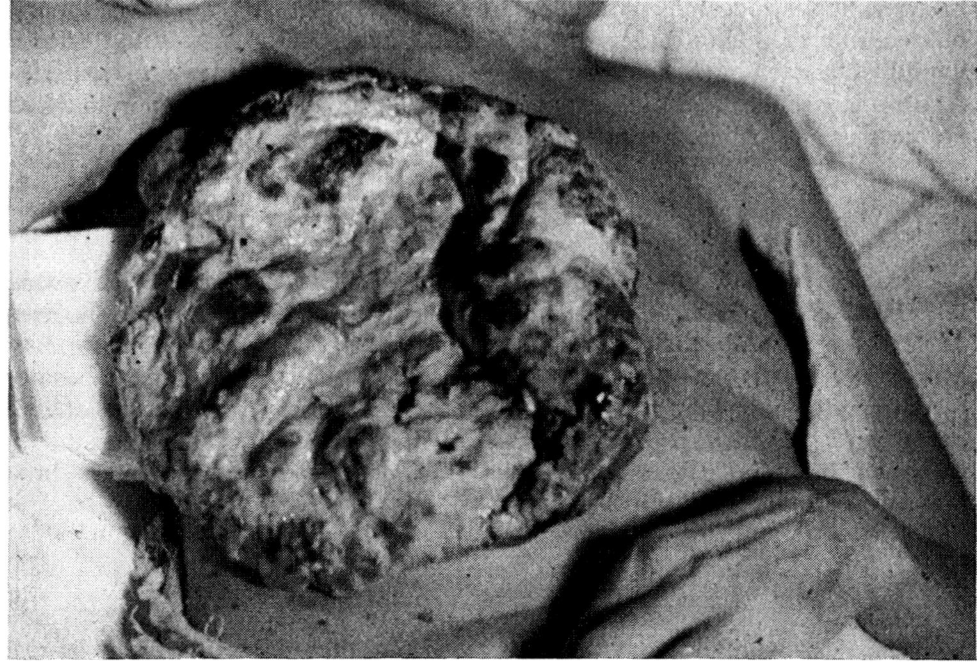

Figure 6: *This neglected untreated lesion formed a mushroomlike growth over the chest wall. The base of the lesion is much smaller than the area of overlying growth but had infiltrated the chest wall, involving intercostal muscles and ribs by direct invasion over a 6–8 cm area. Removal of the lesion with chest wall resection and closure by myocutaneous flap had great value in relieving the symptoms of the lesion even if long-term prognosis was dismal.*

and that total mastectomy will eliminate the majority of these lesions successfully. A few cases may progress so rapidly and be so extensive in their recurrence that they are inoperable and the only local resolution of such lesions would be a larger operation done at an earlier period. The surgeon confronted by recurrence in the remaining breast should be aggressive, and if the lesion involves the underlying muscle, this should be resected. The same applies to the chest wall. Such patients will already have had radiation therapy as part of their original operative treatment so that it may be necessary to bring in fresh tissue by the use of a latissimus dorsi or rectus musculocutaneous flap. In view of the torture that can be inflicted on patients as the result of uncontrolled local disease, such efforts are very worthwhile.[18]

Conclusion

Classic radical mastectomy still has a place in the treatment of cancer of the breast although the indications for its use are now limited. Circumstances where the operation will be indicated are: (1) direct invasion of the pectoralis major or minor muscles; (2) extensive axillary disease infringing on the pectoralis muscles and requiring their removal in order to eliminate bulky disease from the axilla; (3) inflammatory carcinoma of the breast together with radiation and chemotherapy; (4) in highly selected stage I and stage II cases in which there is a high probability of postoperative recurrences following segmental resection and radiation; (5) recurrent cancer in the breast after segmental resection and radiation in which the recurrence has been neglected and is extensive; (6) cancer of the male breast.

References

1. Bloom H, Richardson W, Harries E: Natural history of untreated breast cancer (1805–1933). Br Med J 1962; 52:199–213.
2. Halsted W: The results of operations for the cure of cancer of the breast performed at the Johns Hopkins Hospital from June 1889 to January 1894. Ann Surg 1894; 20:497–555.
3. Halsted W: The results of radical operations for the cure of cancer of the breast. Ann Surg 1907; 26:1–19.
4. Fisher B, Redmond C, Poisson R, et al: Eight-year results of a randomized clinical trial comparing total mastectomy and lumpectomy with or without radiation in the treatment of breast cancer. N Engl J Med 1989; 320:822–828.
5. Fisher B, Slack N, Cavanaugh D, et al: Postoperative radiotherapy in the treatment of breast cancer: results of the NSABP clinical trial. Ann Surg 1970; 172:711.
6. Ackland S, Bilran J, Dowlatshashi K: Management of locally advanced and inflammatory carcinoma of the breast. Surg Gyncol Obstet 1985; 161:399–408.
7. Schifer P, Alberto P, Formi M, et al: Surgery as part of a combined modality approach for inflammatory breast cancer. Cancer 1987; 59:1063–1067.
8. Wiseman C, Jessup JM, Smith TL, et al: Inflammatory breast cancer treated with surgery, chemotherapy and allogenic tumor cell/BCG immunotherapy. Cancer 1982; 49:1266–1271.
9. Brun B, Otmezguine Y, Feuilhade, Julien M, et al: Treatment of inflammatory breast cancer with combination chemotherapy and mastectomy versus breast conservation. Cancer 1988; 61:1096-1103.
10. Shinzaburo N, Miyauchi K, Nishizawa Y, et al: Management of inflammatory carcinoma of the breast with combined modality therapy including intraarterial infusion chemotherapy as an induction therapy. Cancer 1988; 61:1483–1491.
11. Morris DM: Mastectomy in the management of patients with inflammatory breast cancer. J Surg Oncol 1983; 23:255–258.
12. Kurtz J, Brandone H, Ayme Y, et al: Inoperable recurrence after breast conserving surgical treatment and radiotherapy. Surg Gynecol Obstet 1991; 172:357–361.
13. Siddiqui T, Weiner R, Moreb J, et al: Cancer of the male breast with prolonged survival. Cancer 1988; 6:1632–1636.
14. Kinne DW: Management of male breast cancer. Oncology 1991; 5:45–47.
15. Urban J, Baker H: Radical mastectomy in continuity with en bloc resection of the internal mammary lymph node chain. Cancer 1952; 5:992.
16. Lacour J, Bucalosse P, Cacers E, et al: Radical mastectomy versus radical mastectomy plus internal mammary dissection: five-year results of an international cooperative study. Cancer 1976; 37:206–214.
17. Meier P, Ferguson D, Karreson T: A controlled trial of extended radical versus radical mastectomy: ten-year results. Cancer 1989; 63:188–195.
18. Scanlon EF: Local recurrence in the pectoralis muscles following modified radical mastectomy for carcinoma. J Surg Oncol 1985; 30:149–151.
19. Rao DV, Bedwinek J, Perez C, et al: Prognostic indicators in stage III and localized stage IV breast cancer. Cancer 1982; 50:2037.

39

The Importance of Chemotherapy in the Primary Management of Locally Advanced Breast Cancer

Paul A.C. Greenberg, Gabriel N. Hortobagyi

Introduction

Chemotherapy plays a key role in the primary management of locally advanced breast cancer, particularly when used in conjunction with other treatment modalities. This chapter reviews the most recent treatments for this disease and their efficacy, and the reasons that treatment of locally advanced breast cancer should incorporate preoperative chemotherapy with other modalities.

By definition, locally advanced breast cancer excludes the presence of any known distant metastases. For this discussion, it is also defined as cancer limited to stage III of TNM classification[1] and stage IV with M1 limited to ipsilateral supraclavicular nodes (see Table 1). Stage III disease can be divided into resectable stage IIIa disease (without T4, N2, or M1 lesions) and unresectable stage IIIb disease (with T4, N4, or M1 lesions). With all the possible T and N and M combinations, stage III disease can be manifested in a variety of forms, each with its own prognosis and biological behavior.

Inflammatory breast cancer can be considered a separate entity within the category of locally advanced disease because of its unique features [2–6]: rapid onset and evolution (usually less than 3 months); diffuse breast involvement, often without underlying mass; and erythematous, inflammatory changes, with peau d'orange and ridging of the skin. In addition, dermal lymphatic invasion by cancer cells is often present. Locally advanced breast cancer with these second-

---

Table 1
TNM Staging for Breast Cancer

DEFINITION OF TNM
Primary Tumor (T)
Definitions for classifying the primary tumor (T) are the same for clinical and for pathological classification. The telescoping method of classification can be applied. If the measurement is made by physical examination, the examiner will use the major heading (T1, T2, or T3). If other measurements, such as mammographic or pathological, are used, the telescoped subsets of T1 can be used.

TX   Primary tumor cannot be assessed
TO   No evidence of primary tumor
Tis   Carcinoma in situ: Intraductal carcinoma, lobular carcinoma in situ, or Paget's disease
  of the nipple with no tumor.
T1   Tumor 2 cm or less in greatest dimension
   T1a   0.5 cm or less in greatest dimension
   T1b   More than 0.5 cm but not more than 1 cm in greatest dimension
   T1c   More than 1 cm but not more than 2 cm in greatest dimension
T2   Tumor more than 2 cm but not more than 5 cm in greatest dimension
T3   Tumor more than 5 cm in greatest dimension
T4   Tumor of any size with direct extension to chest wall or skin
   T4a   Extension to chest wall
   T4b   Edema (including peau d'orange) or ulceration of the skin of the breast or satellite
    skin nodules confined to the same breast
   T4c   Both (T4a and T4b)
   T4d   Inflammatory carcinoma

Regional Lymph Nodes (N)
NX   Regional lymph nodes cannot be assessed (e.g., previously removed)
N0   No regional lymph node metastasis
N1   Metastasis to movable ipsilateral axillary lymph node(s)
N2   Metastasis to ipsilateral axillary lymph node(s) fixed to one another or to other
  structures
N3   Metastasis to ipsilateral internal mammary lymph node(s)
Distant Metastasis (M)
MX   Presence of distant metastasis cannot be assessed
M0   No distant metastasis
M1   Distant metastasis (includes metastasis to ipsilateral supraclavicular lymph node(s))

STAGING GROUPING

Stage 0	Tis	NO	MO
Stage 1	T1	NO	MO
Stage IIA	TO	N1	MO
	T1	N1*	MO
	T2	NO	MO
Stage IIB	T2	N1	MO
	T3	NO	MO
Stage IIIA	TO	N2	MO
	T1	N2	MO
	T2	N2	MO
	T3	N1, N2	MO
Stage IIIB	T4	Any N	MO
	Any T	N3	MO
Stage IV	Any T	Any N	M1

---

ary inflammatory changes is different from primary inflammatory breast can cer[7,8] because the former often does not have the same aggressiveness and poor prognosis as primary inflammatory breast carcinoma.

An Overview of the Treatments Used to Manage Locally Advanced Breast Cancer

The various therapies employed to manage locally advanced breast cancer can be divided into the two broad categories of locoregional therapy and systemic therapy. Locoregional includes surgery and radiation therapy, while systemic includes hormonal, chemo-, and biological therapies.

Locoregional Therapies

Until the early 1970s stage III breast cancer was managed with locoregional therapy alone, without the addition of systemic treatments, until local recurrence or distant metastases occurred. Only a minority of these localized breast cancers were cured using this strategy.

Surgery

The 5-year overall survival rate for stage IIIa (resectable) breast cancer treated by radical mastectomy alone varied between 30% and 45%, and the 10-year overall survival rates varied from 20% to 30% (Table 2). The survival data for similar treatment of stage IIIb (unresectable) breast cancer were considerably worse, with 5-year survival rates ranging from 2% to 28%[9-13] and 10-year survival rates ranging from 0% to 10%,[11,12,14,15] depending on the series examined. The local recurrence rate for stage III breast cancer patients treated with surgery alone has been reported to be as high as 60%.[12] Based on these data, surgical therapy should not be considered the only treatment for stage IIIb breast cancer.[12,16]

Radiotherapy

When the data are examined for radiotherapy as treatment for locally advanced breast cancer, the 5-year survival rates range from 10% to 30% and local recurrence rates range from 25% to 72%. An accurate comparison between surgery and radiotherapy as treatment for stage III breast cancer is difficult, because the inclusion criteria for surgical trials were often much more selective than were those for radiotherapy trials. Therefore, since the surgical trials often included a better prognostic group than did the early radiotherapy trials, radiotherapy series often led to less favorable outcomes (Table 2). Another consideration is the dose-response correlation that occurs for radiotherapy.[17-19] Still another consideration in the high-dose radiotherapy for locally advanced

Table 2
Five-Year Survival in Stage III Breast Cancer after Locoregional Therapy

Reference No./Authors	No. of Patients	% Survival at 5 Years	at 10 Years
Surgery Alone			
13 Atkins	43	16	—
9 MacKay	587	32	—
10 Sicher	604	29	—
82 Lacouri[1,2,3,4]	449	61	—
15 Fracchia[3,5,6]	207	43	27
11 Garcia[7,8]	454	35	15
12 Haagensen	109	3	0
63 Veronesi[1,2,3]	83	—	42
Radiotherapy Alone			
83 Nohrman	123	1	—
21 Baclesse	85	—	9
21 Baclesse	159	19	—
99 Langlands	165	14	—
20 Zucali	321	21	—
84 Rubens	184	13	0
85 Spitalier[1,2,3]	104	42	—
22 Calle[1,2,3]	191	59	30
23 Amalric[1,2,3]	341	45	33
86 Balwajder[5]	108	40	14
18 Harris[5,6]	137	30	—
24 Pierquin[1,2,3]	69	66	44
87 Zaharia[4]	484	22	—
Surgery + Radiotherapy			
88 McWhirter[1,3,4]	546	30	—
94 Schottenfeld	62	53	34
95 Arnold	228	33	22
89 Nemoto[1,2,3]	1020	35	—
90 Ferguson[1,3,5]	339	39	48
91 Donegan[5,9]	121	38	20
92 Toonkel[6]	509	41	26
15 Fracchia[3,5,6]	281	34	13
13 Atkins	79	21	—
93 Delarue	299	28	—
93 Delarue[1]	204	—	14
19 Fletcher	226	28	—
26 Pearlman	305	12	—
10 Zucali	133	45	—
37 Terez[1,2,3]	35	17	—
14 Zucali[2,3,4]	66	44	—
TOTAL	**9460**	**32%**	**23%**

[1]T$_4$ excluded; [2]N$_2$ excluded; [3]SCLN excluded; [4]Inflammatory breast cancer excluded; [5]Some patients had chemotherapy; [6]Some patients had hormone therapy; [7]Axillary extranodal disease was called N$_2$; [8]Histological dermal invasion was called T$_4$b; [9]Disease-free survival.

tumors was the fact that while there were reports of good local control and a few reports of long-term survivals,[20-24] there were also considerable toxic effects and unacceptable long-term side effects.[25]

Surgery with Radiotherapy

Another step in the progression of treatments for locally advanced breast cancer has been combination locoregional therapy or, more specifically, the combination of surgery plus either preoperative or postoperative radiotherapy. Although this combination of locoregional therapies has led to better local control than either surgery or radiotherapy alone, the overall survival rates were not significantly improved. Most of the deaths that occurred were a consequence of distant metastases and, therefore, locoregional therapies were unlikely to influence survival substantially.

Systemic Therapies

Systemic therapies can be divided into two main groups: hormonal therapy and chemotherapy. A third, biological therapy, has not yet played a major role in breast cancer, so it is beyond the scope of this discussion.

Table 3
Hormonal Therapy of Stage III Breast Cancer

Reference No./ Authors	Treatment	No. of Patients	Response Rate	Survival Mean (months)	Survival 5 Years (%)
Hormonal Therapy Alone					
26 Pearlman	AbH	18	NA	12	10
26 Pearlman	AddH	7	NA	6	0
84 Rubens	Estrogens	23	NA	14	13
86 Burn	Hypophysectomy	20	60	NA	NA
	Oophorectomy	12	58	NA	NA
	Tamoxifen	35	46	NA	NA
	Estrogen	3	100	NA	NA
97 Blamey	Tamoxifen	53	45	32[1]	NA
98 Bradbeer	Tamoxifen	59[2]	59[2]	28[3]	62[2]
Hormonal Therapy as Adjuvant					
26 Pearlman	RT + AbH	18	NA	14[1]	10[1]
	RT + AddH	11	NA	18[1]	8[1]
27 Bruckman	RT + AbH	12	NA	NA	25
	RT + Estrogen	3	NA	NA	25
28 Bland	S + RT + AbH	13	NA	68	54
15 Fracchia	S + RT + AbH	8	NA	42[1]	38[1]

NA = Not available; AbH = Ablative hormone therapy; AddH = Additive hormone therapy; S = Surgery; RT = Radiotherapy.
[1]Estimated from graph.
[2]Included T_1 and T_2.
[3]Mean response duration in months.

Hormonal Therapy

Hormonal therapy has been used alone, and in combination with local therapies for locally advanced breast cancer (Table 3). Used alone, it has achieved objective regression of breast tumors in up to 50% of patients with locally advanced breast cancer; however, the durations of these responses and overall survival rates have not been substantially different from those achieved by local therapies alone. When hormonal therapy has been used as adjuvant therapy after locoregional treatment for stage III breast cancer, it has not improved local control of tumors or survival rates.[2,6,26–28] This lack of improvement has led to investigations involving the use of cytotoxic chemotherapy.

Chemotherapy

Chemotherapy has been used in the treatment of breast cancer only since the mid-1960s. Initially, single-agent chemotherapy was used, but this led only to brief partial responses in patients with metastatic cancer and did not change

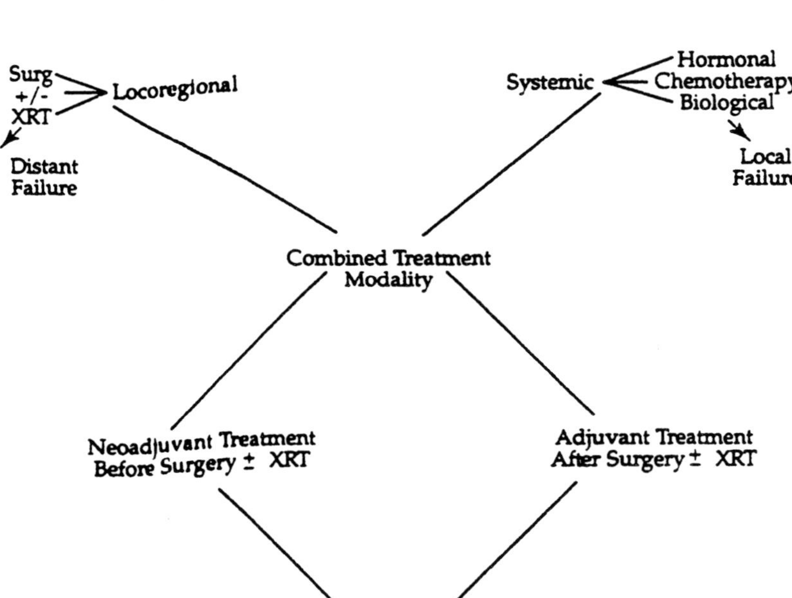

Figure 1: *Schematic representation of the evolution of treatment for locally advanced breast cancer.*

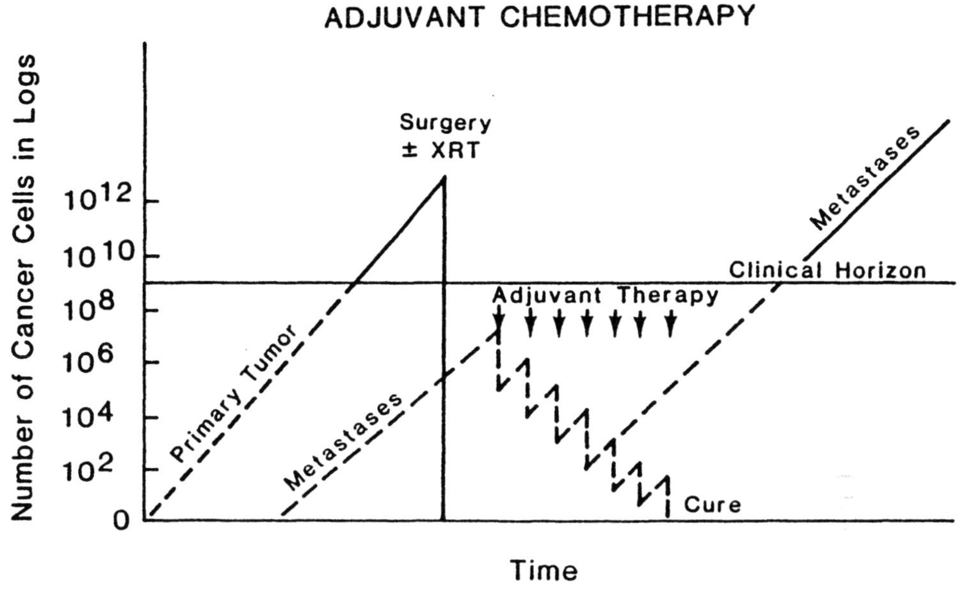

Figure 2: *Graphic representation of postoperative adjuvant systemic therapy. The vertical axis shows the magnitude of tumor burden expressed in logs of the number of cancer cells. Interrupted lines represent subclinical changes in tumor burden with time while the continuous lines demonstrate clinically apparent or measurable changes in tumor burden. Reproduced from ref. 100 by permission.*

overall survival rates. Combination chemotherapy, however, has been shown to induce complete remissions, which have exceeded, on average, 18 months.

Combined Modality Therapies (Locoregional Plus Systemic Therapy)

This success led to trials of combined modality treatment whereby chemotherapy and locoregional therapies were used together with and without hormonal therapies in an effort to obtain better local control of tumors and to eradicate any as-yet-undetected micrometastases. Two scheduling strategies have developed (Fig. 1): adjuvant chemotherapy (Fig. 2), in which chemotherapy is given following locoregional therapy,[29-34] and neoadjuvant (induction) chemotherapy, in which chemotherapy is given before locoregional therapy and may be continued afterward (Fig. 3).

Theoretical Basis for Neoadjuvant Systemic Therapy[35,36]

Cancer results from a single cell mutation that proliferates. Approximately 30 doublings of the original, single malignant cell must occur before the resulting detectable tumor reaches a size of 1 cubic centimeter. Almost all patients with stage III breast cancers harbor micrometastases that can eventually lead to their

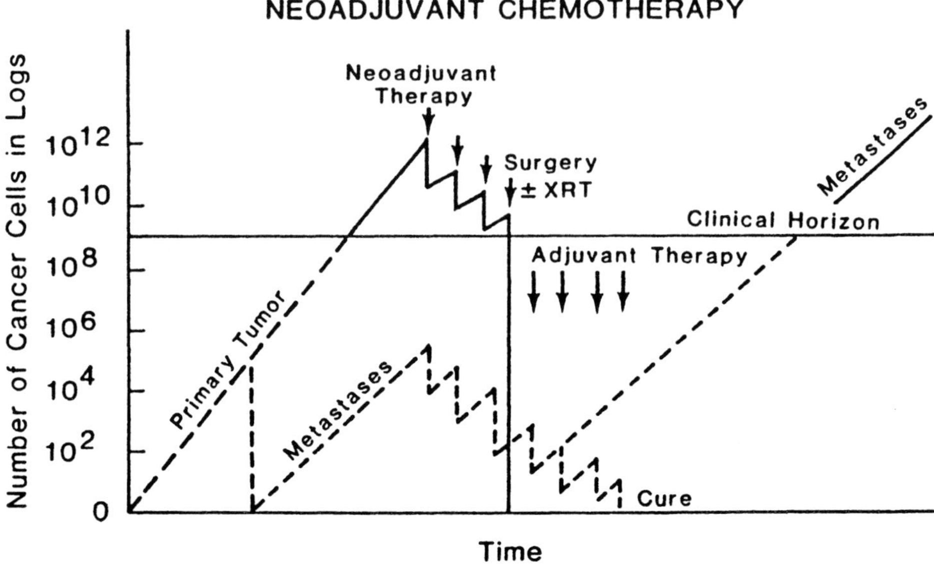

Figure 3: *Graphic representation of neoadjuvant systemic therapy demonstrating changes in tumor burden in response to treatment. See legend for Figure 2.*

death.[26,37–39] As the tumor grows, the proliferation rate of individual cells within it decreases, and the doubling time of the tumor as a whole increases.

Following noncurative resection of various tumors, there is an increase in the proliferative activity of the remaining tumor cells.[34,40–44,100] The same phenomenon has been seen when the primary tumor is damaged by irradiation.[45–47]

In experimental animals, this change in the tumor cell proliferation rate occurs within 24 hours of primary tumor injury and can no longer be detected after 7 days.[34] Exactly what causes the enhancement of micrometastases in the immediate postoperative period is unclear, although humoral factors have been implicated.[29]

The growth of micrometastases is known to be stimulated by noncurative resection of the tumor. An open biopsy can be considered a form of noncurative surgery in the case of locally advanced breast cancer. Thus, from the standpoint of tumor kinetics, fine-needle aspiration may be a better, quicker, and simpler procedure not involving the same amount of tissue manipulation and trauma.

The above argument illustrates why the practice of locoregional therapy alone may be flawed. The following discussion will demonstrate why earlier systemic therapy has at least a theoretical advantage for the successful treatment of locally advanced breast cancer.

Primary tumors contain cell variants destined to form metastases.[48] If these intact cells are forced into circulation by local perturbation of the primary tumor, as would occur during surgery, they may then establish micrometastases elsewhere in the body. Surgery performed after effective chemotherapy would greatly reduce the chances of these clonogenic cells being disseminated in significant quantities.

Until recently, there was no way of knowing how tumor cells would react to a drug after it was administered, as in the case of adjuvant chemotherapy. Chemoresistance was evidenced by a recurrence of disease. Preoperative chemotherapy, on the other hand, provides a very simple and effective means of measuring chemosensitivity in vivo.

Ragaz et al.[36] have suggested, based on the Goldie-Coldman mathematical model,[50] that a 35-day delay in instituting chemotherapy after surgery can decrease the potential for cure. Earlier systemic therapy has the advantage of treating a smaller tumor burden. If the average doubling time of breast cancer at the time of diagnosis is 90 days,[43] then a delay of 1 month from diagnosis in instituting chemotherapy will result in approximately a 30% increase in the microscopic tumor burden.

The elaboration of substances suppressing macrophage function or chemotaxis is one of several mechanisms that tumors use to evade immunological destruction by the host.[51,52] Chemotherapy given perioperatively may help counteract the stimulation of the growth of micrometastases by these tumor substances released into the circulation as a result of surgery. Preoperative chemotherapy ensures better delivery of anticancer agents to the tumor because of intact vasculature. Also, earlier systemic treatment of the tumor, when it is still small, allows chemotherapy to be more efficacious and makes maximal use of tumor kinetics by attacking tumor cells when their proliferative activity is at the highest level.[53] This is also the stage when micrometastases may be synchronizable and more vulnerable to cell cycle specific drugs.[54]

Recent Data on Neoadjuvant Therapies

Studies at the National Cancer Institute of Milan

From 1978 to 1983, the National Cancer Institute of Milan conducted several trials using combined modality treatment that included chemotherapy followed by locoregional treatment, followed by systemic drug treatments.[55–57] Results of these studies showed that most patients with stage III breast cancer could be rendered disease-free by the combination of local and systemic therapies and that this approach also improved disease-free and overall survival rates.[55] The results suggested that the combination of surgery and radiation therapy for local treatment was more effective than either alone. When combined with other forms of treatment, surgical resection appeared to give results equivalent to radiation therapy[56,58]; in other trials where both therapies were combined,[59–62] however, the local recurrence rate was lower than those in the Milan trials. Jacquillat et al.[63] reported that in a multimodality trial using aggressive neoadjuvant chemotherapy and radiotherapy, all of the patients were initially rendered disease-free. No surgery was used except in the case of a local recurrence. Although the median time for follow-up evaluation was short, the local recurrence rates and 3-year survival rates were excellent. Considering its implication for breast conservation, this approach seems very advantageous.

Table 4
Survival Data From Combined Modality Treatment of 174 Patients Treated at the University of Texas M.D. Anderson Cancer Center

Stage	Median Disease-Free Survival	5-Year Disease-Free Survival	10-Year Disease-Free Survival	Median Overall Survival	5-Year Overall Survival	10-Year Overall Survival
IIIA	NA	66%	47%[1]	NA	80%	64%
IIIB	30 months	32%	31%	48 months	45%	28%

[1]Projected survival.
NA = not available.

The University of Texas M.D. Anderson Cancer Center has studied combined modality treatments for locally advanced breast cancer since 1974.[64] Results from these trials, which involved 174 women, are shown in Tables 4 and 5. The initial response to neoadjuvant chemotherapy correlated with disease-free and overall survival rates.[65] All patients who could not be rendered free of disease eventually died of progressive breast cancer. Table 6 gives the breakdown of treatment failures.

The rates for local control of tumors, and the 10-year survival rates for stage III, were substantially improved by this combined modality regimen when compared with historical controls at the institution.

Inflammatory Breast Cancer

Another series at M.D. Anderson Cancer Center, which ran from 1974 to 1981, involved 63 patients with inflammatory breast cancer. They were treated with neoadjuvant 5-fluorouracil, Adriamycin, and Cytoxan (FAC) followed by

Table 5
Response Rates From Combined Modality Treatment of 174 Patients at University of Texas M.D. Anderson Cancer Center

	After Three Cycles of Induction Chemotherapy		After Induction Chemotherapy + Initial Local Therapy	
Complete response	29/174	16.6%	168/174	96.5%
Partial Response	123/174	70.6%	6/174	3.5%

Table 6
Patterns of Failure of Combined Modality Treatment of 174 Patients Treated at the
University of Texas M.D. Anderson Cancer Center

	N	%
Overall Treatment Failures	103	59%
Local Treatment Failure	22	13%
Distant Metastases	81	46.5%

local therapy and more chemotherapy. An overall response rate of 68% was reported with 20% of the patients achieving complete remissions. One patient experienced disease progression during neoadjuvant chemotherapy. The remaining 62 (92%) were rendered disease-free after neoadjuvant and local therapy. The median overall survival rate was 24 months. Patients who achieved a greater than 50% reduction in tumor burden with neoadjuvant 5-fluorouracil, Adriamycin, and Cytoxan had a disease-free and overall survival rate well in excess of that for nonresponders (the median follow-up was more than 72 months).

In a subsequent study at M.D. Anderson, 43 patients with inflammatory breast cancer were treated with a different combined modality program. Neoadjuvant chemotherapy was followed by total mastectomy, axillary dissection, and adjuvant chemotherapy and then later, at the end of all chemotherapy, by radiation therapy.[66] At the conclusion of the neoadjuvant chemotherapy and surgery, 95% of the patients were rendered disease-free, four with pathologically confirmed complete remissions. After 2 years of follow-up, 65% of the patients remained disease-free, and 82% were still alive. The main prognostic factor appeared to be a good objective response to the primary induction chemotherapy.

Neoadjuvant chemotherapy has been shown to be highly efficacious in producing major objective responses (Table 7) and when incorporated into a program of combined modality treatment, has resulted in the complete elimination of all detectable tumor in more than 90% of the patients with locally advanced breast cancer, including primary inflammatory cancer. Long-term, disease-free survival rates of 5 to 14 years from diagnosis have been achieved.[26,37,39] Before combined modality treatment was used, fewer than 5% of the patients with inflammatory breast cancer survived 5 years from diagnosis[66–73] (Table 8).

Studies on Other Important Issues

Despite the improved survival rates clearly evident in these studies, there is still considerable disagreement on the type and sequence of local therapies and the duration of chemotherapy.

Table 7
Results of Combined Modality Treatment with Neoadjuvant Chemotherapy (Locally Advanced and Inflammatory Breast Cancer)

Author/ Reference No.	Treatment	No. of Patients	Maximum % Disease Free	Median Survival (Mos)	3 Years	(%) Survival 5 Years	10 Years
Rubens[103]	CR-RT-CT	12	67	36	50	NA	NA
	RT-CT	12	75	36	50	NA	NA
Bedwinek[107]	CT-RT-CT	22	78	28	40	NA	NA
Valagussa[57]	CT-RT	72	64	30	43	20	NA
	CT-RT-CT	126	75	42	60	36	NA
	CT-S-CT	79	85	58	64	49	NA
Balawajder[104]	CT-RT	23	NA	NA	NA	46	NA
	CT-RT-S	30	NA	NA	NA	38	NA
Shaake-Koning[105]	RT	45	75	42	59	37	NA
	RT-CT	34	71	45	59	37	NA
	CT-RT-CT	39	71	50	61	37	NA
Olson[106]	RT-CT	119	42	24	NA	32	NA
	CT-RT-CT		51	34	NA	33	NA
Lesnick[74]	CT-S-CT	105	100	43	65	39	NA
	CT-RT-CT		52	40	47	39	NA
Pouillart[67]	CT-S-RT	82	100	NA	85	NA	NA
	CT-RT-CT						
Jacquillat[63,118]	CT-RT-CT	98	66IIIa[1] 64IIIb[1]	NA	68IIIa 74IIIb	60IIIa 58IIIb	NA
Hortobagyi[118]	CT-RT/S-CT	174	96	66	65	44IIIb	26IIIb
Swain[107]	CT-RT/S-CT	75	100	39	42	NA	NA
Hobar[108]	CT-S-CT ± RT	40	71[2] 43[3]	NA	NA	46	NA
Ragaz[109]	CT-RT-S-CT	47	71[1]	NA	73	NA	NA
	CT-RT-CT	28	34[1]		72		
Montrocoli[110]	CT-S-CT	129	NA	NA	NA	NA	8.5
Tran[111]	CT-S	95	NA	NA	92	80	NA
Chauvergne[112]	CT-RT-S-CT	270	25.9	Not reached[7]	NA	NA	NA
Israel[113]	CT-S	25[4]	NA	53+	NA	NA	NA
Schwartz[114]	CT-S-RT-CT	100	67[5]	NA	NA	85[5]	NA
Namer[115]	CT-S-RT-CT	170	50[6]	80	NA	NA	NA
Feldman[116]	CT-S	90	NA	NA	NA	93	NA
Koyama[117]	Intra-art-CT-S	55	NA	NA	NA	57	41

[1]at 3 years; [2]in CT responders; [3]in CT non-responders; [4]inflammatory breast cancer; [5]projected for responders at 5 years; [6]at 65 months; [7]at 70 months.
CT = Chemotherapy.
RT = Radiotherapy.
  S = Surgery.

Table 8
Five-Year Survival of Patients with Inflammatory Breast Cancer after Locoregional
Treatment

Number of Patients	Treatment	% 5-Year Survival
398	Surgery	2
334	Radiotherapy	3
142	Surgery + Radiotherapy	5
874	All Variants	3

Data from Hortobagyi.[102]

Type and Sequence of Local Therapies

Many noncontrolled studies have been conducted to study the efficacy of
the types and sequences of local therapies including surgery alone, radiotherapy
alone, and combinations of both in a combined modality setting. The results of
these studies are difficult to compare because of the differences in patient
selection, chemotherapy regimens, and definitions of response and local control.
In contrast, however, a few prospective, randomized trials have been reported
using local therapy as the variable.[57,74,75] Their results suggest that when surgery
follows chemotherapy, it is equivalent to radiotherapy in achieving local control.
Interestingly, although local control rates for this strategy, which varied from
60% to 70%, were quite good, they were inferior to the rates of 80% to 90%
reported by some studies that used surgery plus radiotherapy for local treatment.[39] Undoubtedly, additional studies are needed to further define the best
approach for administering local therapies.

The results from neoadjuvant trials have already shown how the response of
tumors to preoperative chemotherapy may result in more extensive control.
Additional studies will probably show the combination of preoperative and
postoperative chemotherapy to be more active than either alone.[55] With the
development of better agents, techniques, and scheduling, the need for locoregional therapies may diminish or be eliminated.

Duration of Chemotherapy

During the last decade, the trend for postoperative adjuvant chemotherapy
has been a shorter duration of therapy. This trend has been supported by certain
randomized studies[76–78] that have suggested that shorter, more intensive courses
of adjuvant chemotherapy were just as effective as long-term adjuvant chemotherapy. A short course of neoadjuvant chemotherapy may therefore be possible. At least one other study, however, suggested that patients who received
neoadjuvant chemotherapy benefited from continued chemotherapy after the
completion of their local treatment.[57] Additional studies are necessary to evalu-

ate the most effective duration of chemotherapy as well as the most effective type, intensity, and sequencing.

The Effect of Combined Modality Therapies on Survival

It is unclear whether regimens for treating locally advanced breast cancer that use neoadjuvant chemotherapy are superior to those that consist of local therapies followed by adjuvant chemotherapy. What is clear, however, is that combined modality regimens improve survival for patients with locally advanced breast cancer.[79-81] Furthermore, ongoing phase II trials of neoadjuvant chemotherapy suggest that the survival rates of patients with locally advanced breast cancer may be improved and that neoadjuvant chemotherapy clearly is superior to local therapy for patients with inflammatory breast cancer.[42,69] From the available data, however, there does not seem to be a definite survival advantage of neoadjuvant chemotherapy over postoperative adjuvant chemotherapy although one can be inferred. Even if there is no survival benefit, neoadjuvant chemotherapy can make breast conservation possible for many patients with locally advanced disease,[39,63] and it does have the potential for using the response to neoadjuvant chemotherapy as a prognostic factor in designing consolidation (post-regional therapy) systemic treatment. These are two very good reasons for choosing this treatment option.

Conclusion

From the literature, then, it is clear that no substantial progress in the treatment of locally advanced breast cancer was made in the decades preceding the advent of chemotherapy. The importance of chemotherapy in the treatment of locally advanced breast cancer is evidenced by the following points:

1. Multimodality treatments incorporating the use of chemotherapy have resulted in very high overall response rates, in addition to substantial clinically and pathologically complete responses.

2. Chemotherapy has resulted in longer overall and disease-free survival rates than those obtainable before the addition of chemotherapy.

3. Chemotherapy has provided the opportunity both for treatment using lower doses of radiotherapy and less radical surgery and, in many instances, for breast conservation.

4. It offers the possibility of local control and long-term survival to patients with unresectable lesions advanced beyond the scope of radiotherapy.

5. In the case of neoadjuvant chemotherapy, the ability to assess the response to therapy in vivo helps in appropriate treatment planning: deletion of ineffective chemotherapy or substitution with non-cross-resistant regimens.

6. Finally, combined modality treatments that include neoadjuvant chemotherapy provide an excellent model for the study of tumor biology through the evaluation of easily accessible tumor samples before and after chemotherapy,

thus paving the road for the development of more innovative treatment strategies.

Acknowledgment: The authors wish to thank Ms. Dean Anthony for her secretarial assistance in the preparation of this paper and Ms. Gayle Nesom for her expertise in the editing of this paper.

References

1. Beahrs OH, et al (eds), American Joint Committee on Cancer: Manual for Staging of Cancer (3rd ed). JB Lippincott, Philadelphia, 1988.
2. Haagensen CD: Inflammatory carcinoma. In: Haagensen CD (ed). Disease of the Breast. WB Saunders Company, Philadelphia, pp 808–814, 1986.
3. Saltzstein SL: Clinical occult inflammatory carcinoma of the breast. Cancer 1974;34:382–388.
4. Droulias CA, Swell CW, McSweeney MB, Powell RW: Inflammatory carcinoma of the breast: a correlation of clinical, radiologic and pathologic findings. Ann Surg 1976;184:217–222.
5. Camp E: Inflammatory carcinoma of the breast: the case for conservatism. Am J Surg 1976;131:583–586.
6. Lucas FV, Perez-Mesa C: Inflammatory carcinoma of the breast. Cancer 1978;41:1595–1605.
7. Donnelly BA: Primary inflammatory carcinoma of the breast: a report of five cases and a review of the literature. Ann Surg 1948;128:918–930.
8. McBride CM, Hortobagyi GN: Primary inflammatory carcinoma of the female breast: staging and treatment possibilities. Surgery 1985;98:792–797.
9. MacKay EN, Sellers AH: A prospective trial of the TNM classification of breast cancer by the Regional Cancer Treatment Centres in Ontario, 1960–1964. Int J Cancer 1970;6:517–528.
10. Sicher K, Waterhouse JAH: Evaluation of TNM classification of carcinoma of the breast. Br J Cancer 1973;28:580–588.
11. Garcia A, Company RA, Fuster E, Checa F, Trullenque R, Garcia-Vilanova A: Sistema TNM 1978 en cancer de mama: propuesta de modificacion. Rev Esp Oncol 1985;32:95–108.
12. Haagensen CD: Clinical classification of the stage of advancement of breast carcinoma. In: Haagensen CD (ed). Disease of the Breast. WB Saunders Company, Philadelphia, pp 851–863, 1986.
13. Atkins HL, Hoorigan WD: Treatment of locally advanced carcinoma of the breast with roentgen therapy and simple mastectomy. Am J Roentgenol 1961;85:860–865.
14. Zucali R, Kenda R: Small size T4 breast cancer: natural history and prognosis. Tumori 1981;67:225–230.
15. Fracchia AA, Evans JF, Eisenberg BL: Stage III carcinoma of the breast: a detailed analysis. Ann Surg 1980;192:705–710.
16. Wilson RE: Surgical management of locally advanced and recurrent breast cancer. Cancer 1984;53:752–757.
17. Davila E, Vogel CL: Management of locally advanced breast cancer (stage III): a review. Int Adv Surg Oncol 1984;7:297–327.
18. Harris JR, Sawicka J, Gelman R, Hellman S: Management of locally advanced carcinoma of the breast by primary radiation therapy. Int J Radiat Oncol Biol Phys 1983;9:345–349.
19. Fletcher GH, Montague ED: Radical irradiation of advanced breast cancer. Am J Roentgenol 1965;93:573–584.
20. Zucali R, Uslenghi C, Kenda R, Bonadonna G: Natural history and survival of

inoperable breast cancer treated with radiotherapy and radiotherapy followed by radical mastectomy. Cancer 1976;37:1422–1431.

21. Baclesse F: Roentgentherapy alone in the cancer of the breast. Acta Unio Internat Contra Cancrum 1959;15:1023–1026.

22. Calle R, Pilleron JP, Schlienger P, Vilcoq JR: Conservative management of operable breast cancer: ten-year experience at the Foundation Curie. Cancer 1978;42:2045–2053.

23. Amalric R, Santamaria F, Robert F, et al: Radiation therapy with or without primary limited surgery for operable breast cancer: a 20-year experience at the Marseilles Cancer Institute. Cancer 1982;49:30–34.

24. Pierquin B, Rynal M, Otmezguine Y, et al: Le traitement conservateur des cancers du sein: resultats a 10 ans. Presse Med 1986;15:375–377.

25. Spanos WJ, Montague ED, Fletcher FH: Late complications of radiation only for advanced breast cancer. Int J Radiat Oncol Biol Phys 1980;6:1473–1476.

26. Pearlman NW, Guerra O, Fracchia AA: Primary inoperable cancer of the breast. Surg Gynecol Obstet 1976;143:909–913.

27. Bruckman JE, Harris JR, Levene MB, Chaffey JT, Hellman S: Results of treating stage III carcinoma of the breast by primary radiation therapy. Cancer 1979;43:985–993.

28. Bland KI, O'Leary JP, Woodward ER, Dragstedt LR: Immediate oophorectomy and adrenalectomy in the treatment of stage III breast carcinoma: a ten-year follow-up study. Am J Surg 1975;129:277–285.

29. Fisher B: Laboratory and clinical research in breast cancer: a personal adventure. The David A. Karnofsky Memorial Lecture. Cancer Res 1980;40:3863–3874.

30. Schabel FM: Concepts for systemic treatment of micrometastases. Cancer 1975;35:15–24.

31. Bonadonna G, Brusamolino E, Valagussa P, et al: Combination chemotherapy as an adjuvant treatment in operable breast cancer. N Engl J Med 1976;294:405–410.

32. Buzdar AU, Gutterman JU, Blumenschein GR, et al: Intensive postoperative chemoimmunotherapy for patients with stage II and III breast cancer. Cancer 1978;41:1064–1075.

33. Simpson-Herren L, Sanford AH, Holmquist JP: Effects of surgery on the cell kinetics of residual tumor. Cancer Treatment Rep 1976;60:1749–1760.

34. Gundoz N, Fisher B, Saffer EA: Effect of surgical removal on the growth and kinetics of residual tumor. Cancer Res 1979;39:3861–3865.

35. Papaioannou AN: Preoperative chemotherapy: advantages and clinical application in stage III breast cancer. In: Recent Results in Cancer Research, Vol 98. Springer-Verlag, Berlin, Heidelberg, pp 65–90, 1985.

36. Ragaz JR, Baird R, Rebbeck R, Goldie A, et al: Preoperative adjuvant chemotherapy (neo-adjuvant) for carcinoma of the breast: rationale and safety report. In: Recent Results in Cancer Research, Vol 98. Springer-Verlag Berlin, Heidelberg, pp 99–105, 1985.

37. Terz JJ, Romero CA, Kay S, Brown PW, et al: Preoperative radiotherapy for stage III carcinoma of the breast. Surg Gynecol Obstet 1978;147:497–502.

38. Osteen RT, Chaffey JT, Moore FD, Wilson RE: An aggressive multimodality approach to locally advanced carcinoma of the breast. Surg Gynecol Obstet 1978;147:75–79.

39. Papaioannou AN, Urban J: Scalene node biopsy in locally advanced primary cancer of the breast of questionable operability. Cancer 1964;17:1006–1011.

40. DeWys WD: Studies correlating the growth rate of a tumor and its metastases and providing evidence for tumor-related systemic growth-retarding factors. Cancer Res 1972;32:374–379.

41. Gorelik E, Segal S, Feldman M: Growth of a local tumor exerts a specific inhibitory effect on progression of lung metastases. Int J Cancer 1978;21:617–625.

42. Ketcham AS, Eexler H, Mantel N: The effect of removal of a primary tumor on the development of spontaneous metastases. I. Development of a standardized experimental technique. Cancer Res 1959;19:940–944.

43. Steel GG: Growth Kinetics of Tumors. Glarendon, Oxford, 1977.

44. Simpson-Heren L: Effects of surgery on the cell kinetics of residual tumor. Cancer Treat Rep 60:1749–1760.

45. Kaplan HS, Murphy ED: The effect of local roentgen irradiation on the biological behavior of a transplantable mouse carcinoma. I. Increased frequency of pulmonary metastasis. J Natl Cancer Inst 1948;407–413.
46. Sheldon PW, Fowler JF: The effect of irradiating a transplanted murine lymphosarcoma on the subsequent development of metastases. Br J Cancer 1973;28:508–514.
47. Van den Brenk HAS, Sharpington C: Effect of local x-irradiation of a primary sarcoma in the rat on dissemination and growth of metastases: dose-response characteristics. Br J Cancer 1971;25:812–830.
48. Fidler JJ, Kripke ML: Metastasis results from pre-existing variant cells within a malignant tumor. Science 1977;197:893–895.
49. Schottenfeld D, Nash AG, Robbins GF, Beattie EJ: Ten-year results of the treatment of primary operable breast carcinoma: a summary of 304 patients evaluated by the TNM system. Cancer 1976;38:1001–1007.
50. Goldie JH, Coldman AJ: A mathematical model for relating the drug sensitivity of tumors to their spontaneous mutation rate. Cancer Treat Reports 1979;63:1727–1733.
51. Pike MC, Synderman R: Depression of macrophage function by a factor produced by neoplasms: a mechanism for abrogation in immune surveillance. J Immunol 1976;117:1243–1249.
52. North RJ, Kirstein DP, Tuttle RL: Subversion of host defense mechanisms by murine tumors. I. A circulating factor that suppresses macrophage-mediated resistance to infection. J Exp Med 1976;143:559–573.
53. Norton L, Simon R: Tumor size, sensitivity to therapy and design of treatment schedules. Cancer Treat Rep 1977;61:1307–1317.
54. Schabel FM Jr: Rationale for adjuvant chemotherapy. Cancer 1977;39:2875–2882.
55. DeLena M, Zucali R, Viganotti G, Valagussa P, Bonadonna G: Combined chemotherapy-radiotherapy approach in locally advanced (T_{3b}-T_4) breast cancer. Cancer Chemother Pharmacol 1978;1:53–59.
56. DeLena M, Varini M, Zuca, et al: Multimodal treatment for locally advanced cancer: results of chemotherapy-radiotherapy versus chemotherapy-surgery. Cancer Clin Trials 1981;4:229–236.
57. Valagussa P, Zambetti M, Bignami P, et al: T_{3b}-T_4 breast cancer: factors affecting results in combined modality treatments. Clin Exp Metastasis 1983;1:191–202.
58. Lesnick G, Perloff M, Korzun A, Chu F, et al: Combination chemotherapy prior to surgery or radiotherapy in locally advanced breast cancer. In: Jacquillat C, Weil M, Khayat D (eds). Neo-adjuvant Chemotherapy. Colloque INSERM, John Libbey Eurotext Ltd, Paris, 1986;137:207–211.
59. Loprinzi CL, Carbone PP, Tormey DC, et al: Aggressive combined modality therapy for advanced loco-regional breast carcinoma. J Clin Oncol 1984;2:157–163.
60. Hortobagyi GN, Blumenschein GR, Spanos W, et al: Multimodal treatment of locoregionally advanced breast cancer. Cancer 1983;51:763–768.
61. Pawlicki M, Skolyszewski J, Brandys A: Results of combined treatment of patients with locally advanced breast cancer. Tumori 1983;69:249–253.
62. Balawajder I, Antich PP, Boland J: An analysis of the role of radiotherapy alone and in combination with chemotherapy and surgery in the management of advanced breast cancer. Cancer 1983;51:574–580.
63. Jacquillat C, Weil M, Baillet, et al: Results of neoadjuvant chemotherapy (NEOAD CHEM) with or without hormonotherapy and external and interstitial radiation in 98 locally advanced breast cancer (LABC). Proc Am Soc Clin Oncol 1987;6:A257.
64. Hortobagyi GN, Spanos W, Montague ED, et al: Treatment of locoregionally advanced breast cancer with surgery, radiotherapy, and combination chemoimmunotherapy. Int J Radiat Oncol Biol Phys 1983;9:643–650.
65. Hortobagyi GN, Kau SW, Buzdar AU, et al: Induction chemotherapy for stage III primary breast cancer. In: Salmon SE (ed). Adjuvant Therapy of Cancer. Grune & Stratton, Orlando, pp 419–428, 1987.
66. Buzdar A, Marcus C, Hortobagyi G, Ames F, et al: Combined modality approach in

inflammatory carcinoma of the breast: preliminary results of a prospective study. 15th International Congress of Chemotherapy, July 19–24, Istanbul, Turkey, p 169 (Abst 378), 1987.
67. Pouillart P, Palangie T, Jouve M, et al: Cancer inflammatoirs du sein traits par une association de chimiotherapie et d'irradiation: resultats d'un essai randomise etudiant le role d'une immunotherapie par le BCG. Masson, Paris, pp 171–186, 1981.
68. Zylberberg B, Salat-Baroux J, Ravina JH, et al: Initial chemoimmunotherapy in inflammatory carcinoma of the breast. Cancer 1982;49:1537–1543.
69. Fastenberg NA, Buzdar AU, Montague ED, et al: Management of inflammatory carcinoma of the breast: a combined modality approach. Am J Clin Oncol 1985;8:134–141.
70. Jacquillat C, Weil M, Auclerc G, et al: Neo-adjuvant chemotherapy in the conservative management of breast cancers: study of 205 patients. In: Jacquillat C, Weil M, Khayat D (eds). Neo-Adjuvant Chemotherapy. Colloque INSERM, John Libbey Eurotext Ltd, Paris, 1986;137:197–206.
71. Keiling R, Guiochet N, Calderoli H, et al: Preoperative chemotherapy in the treatment of inflammatory breast cancer. In: Wagner DJT, Blijham GH, Smeets JBE, Wils JA (eds). Primary Chemotherapy in Cancer Medicine. Alan R. Liss, New York, pp 95–104, 1985.
72. Ferriere JP, Bignon YJ, Legros M, et al: Resultats du traitment des cancers inflammatoires du sein par une association therapeutique comportant une chimiotherapie initiale. In: Jacquillat C, Weil M, Khayat D, eds. Neo-Adjuvant Chemotherapy. Colloque INSERM, John Libbey Eurotext Ltd, Paris, 1986;137:271–277.
73. Rouesse J, Friedman S, Sarrazin D, et al: Primary chemotherapy in the treatment of inflammatory breast carcinoma: a study of 230 cases from the Institute Gustave-Roussy. J Clin Oncol 1986;4:1765–1771.
74. Lesnick G, Perloff M, Korzun A, et al: Neo-adjuvant chemotherapy for stage III breast cancer: 5-year report of CALGB 7784. In: Jacquillat C, Weil M, Khayat D (eds). Neo-Adjuvant Chemotherapy. Colloque INSERM, John Libbey Eurotext Ltd, Paris, 1988;169:185–188.
75. Pouillart P, Palangie T, Jouve M, et al: Essai pilote de chimiotherapie neo-adjuvant dans le cancer. In: Jacquillat C, Weil M, Khayat D (eds). Neo-Adjuvant Chemotherapy. Colloque INSERM, John Libbey Eurotext Ltd, Paris, 1986;137:257–267.
76. Tancini G, Bonadonna G, Valagussa P, Marchini S, et al: Adjuvant CMF in breast cancer: comparative 5-year results of 12 versus 6 cycle. J Clin Oncol 1983;1:2–10.
77. Velez-Garcia E, Moore M, Vogel CL, et al: Postmastectomy adjuvant chemotherapy with or without radiation therapy in women with operable breast cancer and positive axillary lymph nodes. The Southeastern Cancer Study Group Experience. Breast Cancer Res Treat 1983;3(Suppl 1):49–60.
78. Early Breast Cancer Trialists Collaborative Group: Effects of adjuvant tamoxifen and of cytotoxic therapy on mortality in early breast cancer. N Engl J Med 1988;319:1681–1692.
79. Caceres B, Zaharia M, Lingan M, et al: Combined therapy of stage III adenocarcinoma of the breast (abstr). Proc Am Assoc Cancer Res 1980;21:199.
80. Knight WA III, Rivkin SE, Glucksberg H, et al: Adjuvant therapy of breast cancer. The Southwest Oncology Group Experience. Breast Cancer Res Treat 1983;3(Suppl 1):27–33.
81. Buzdar AU, Kau SW, Smith TL, Hortobagyi GN: Ten-year results of FAC adjuvant chemotherapy trial in breast cancer. Am J Clin Oncol 1989;12(2):123–128.
82. Lacour J, Bucalossi P, Caceres E, et al: Radical mastectomy versus radical mastectomy plus internal mammary dissection. Cancer 1976;37:206–214.
83. Nohrman BA: Cancer of breast: clinical study of 1042 cases treated at Radiumhemmet. Acta Radiol (Oncol) 1949;77(Suppl):62–63.
84. Rubens RD, Armitage P, Winter PJ, Tong D, et al: Prognosis in inoperable stage III carcinoma of the breast. Eur J Cancer 1977;13:805–811.
85. Spitalier J, Brandone H, Ayme Y, Amalric R, et al: Cesium therapy of breast cancer: a

five-year report on 400 consecutive patients. Int J Radiat Oncol Biol Phys 1977;2:231–235.

86. Balawajder I, Antich PP, Boland J: The management of breast carcinoma by primary radiotherapy at Mount Sinai Hospital from 1962–1979. Cancer 1982;49:1587–1596.

87. Zaharia M, Caceres E, Valdivia S, Moscol A, et al: Radiotherapy in the management of locally advanced breast cancer. Int J Radiat Oncol Biol Phys 1987;13:1179–1182.

88. McWhirter R: Treatment of cancer of breast by simple mastectomy and roentgeno-therapy. Arch Surg 1949;59:830–842.

89. Nemoto T, Vana J, Bedwani RN: Management and survival of female breast cancer: results of a national survey by the American College of Surgeons. Cancer 1980;45:2917–2924.

90. Ferguson DJ, Meier P, Karrison T, Dawson PJ, et al: Staging of breast cancer and survival rates: an assessment based on 50 years of experience with radical mastectomy. JAMA 1982;284:1337–1341.

91. Donegan WL, Skibba JL: Patterns of survival and disease recurrence after mastectomy for carcinoma of the breast. Cancer Treatment Symposia 1983;2:107–116.

92. Toonkel LM, Fix I, Jacobson LH, Bambert N, et al: Locally advanced breast carcinoma: results with combined regional therapy. Int J Radiat Oncol Biol Phys 1986;12:1583–1587.

93. Delarue N, Ash CL, Peters V, Fielden R: Preoperative irradiation in mangement of locally advanced breast cancer. Arch Surg 1965;91:136–154.

94. Schottenfeld D, Nash AG, Robbins GF, Beattie EJ: Ten-year results of the treatment of primary operable breast carcinoma: a summary of 304 patients evaluated by the TNM system. Cancer 1976;38:1001–1007.

95. Arnold DJ, Lesnick GJ: Survival following mastectomy for stage III breast cancer. Am J Surg 1979;137:362–366.

96. Burn I: Session 1. Primary endocrine therapy of advanced local breast cancer. Review of Endocrine-Related Cancer 1985;16(Suppl):5–8.

97. Blamey RW: Session 1. Primary treatment of the advanced disease. Review of Endocrine-Related Cancer 1985;16(Suppl):9–12.

98. Bradbeer JW: Session 1. Treatment of primary breast cancer in the elderly with "Nolvadex" alone. Review of Endocrine-Related Cancer 1985;16(Suppl):39–42.

99. Langlands AO, Kerr GR, Shaw S: The management of locally advanced breast cancer by x-ray therapy. Clin Oncol 1976;2:365–371.

100. Tyzzer EE: Factors in the production and growth of tumor metastases. J Med Res 1913;28:309–332.

101. Hortobagyi GN, Buzdar AU: High risk breast cancer II. In: Ragaz J, Ariel IM (eds). Locally Advanced Breast Cancer. Springer Verlag, Heidelberg, pp 382–415, 1990.

102. Hortobagyi GN: Factores pronosticos en el cancer de mama. In: Garcia-Conde J (ed). Tratamiento del Cancer de Mama, Ediciones Doyma, Barcelona, Spain. pp 9–30, 1989.

103. Rubens RD, Sexton S, Tong D, Winter PJ, et al: Combined chemotherapy and radiotherapy for locally advanced breast cancer. Eur J Cancer 1980;6:351–356.

104. Baldawajder I, Antich PP, Boland J: An analysis of the role of radiotherapy alone and in combination with chemotherapy and surgery in the management of advanced breast cancer. Cancer 1983;51:574–580.

105. Schaake-Koning C, van der Linden EH, Hart G, Engelsman E: Adjuvant chemo- and hormonal therapy in locally advanced breast cancer: a randomized clinical study. Int J Radiat Oncol Biol Phys 1985;11:1759–1763.

106. Olson JE, Gray R, Sponzo RW, et al: Management of nonresectable locally advanced (stage III) breast cancer: an ECOG trial. Breast Cancer Res Treat 1986;8:109.

107. Swain S, Lippman M, Bagley C: Treatment of locally advanced breast cancer (LABC) using primary induction chemotherapy, with hormonal synchronization followed by radiation therapy with or without debulking surgery (abstr). Proc Am Soc Clin Oncol 1987;6:192.

108. Hobar PC, Jones RC, Schouten J, Leitch AM, et al: Multimodality treatment of locally advanced breast carcinoma. Arch Surg 1988;123(8):951–955.
109. Ragaz J, Manji M, Plenderleith IH, Knowling M, et al: Analysis of the British Columbia study of pre-operative (neo-adjuvant) therapy of breast cancer in stage III disease. In: Jacquillat C, Weil M, Khayat D (eds). Neo-Adjuvant chemotherapy. Colloque INSERM, John Libbey Eurotext Ltd, Paris 1988;169:249–256.
110. Montruccoli GC, d'Errico A, Barnabe D, Montruccoli-Salmi D, et al: Pre-operative chemotherapy and differentiated surgery in the treatment of breast cancer. In: Jacquillat C, Weil M, Khayat D (eds). Neo-Adjuvant Chemotherapy. Colloque INSERM, John Libbey Eurotext Ltd, Paris 1988;169:245–247.
111. Tran TM, Guittard T, Duchatelle V, Bertrand-Desvages G, et al: Pre-operative chemotherapy as a treatment of breast cancer: analysis of 95 cases. In: Jacquillat C, Weil M, Khayat D (eds). Neo-Adjuvant Chemotherapy. Colloque INSERM, John Libbey Eurotext Ltd, Paris, 1988;169:237–240.
112. Chauvergne M, Durand M, Mauriac L, David M, et al: Traitement combine de 270 cancers mammaries localement entendus: resultats d'un programme therapeutique controle. In: Jacquillat C, Weil M, Khayat D (eds). Neo-Adjuvant Chemotherapy. Colloque INSERM, John Libbey Eurotext Ltd, Paris, 1988; 169:225–230.
113. Israel L, Breau JL, Morere JF: Neo-adjuvant chemotherapy without radiation therapy in inflammatory breast carcinoma. In: Jacquillat C, Weil M, Khayat D (eds). Neo-Adjuvant Chemotherapy. Colloque INSERM, John Libbey Eurotext Ltd, Paris, 1988;169:207–210.
114. Schwartz FG, Cantor RI, Biermann WA: Neo-adjuvant chemotherapy prior to definitive treatment for stage III carcinoma of the breast. In: Jacquillat C, Weil M, Khayat D (eds). Neo-Adjuvant Chemotherapy. Colloque INSERM, John Libbey Eurotext Ltd, Paris, 1988;169:201–206.
115. Namer M, Hery M, Abbes M, Frenay M, Ramaioli A: Influence of the response rate obtained by neo-adjuvant chemotherapy on the survival of patients with locally advanced breast cancer. In: Jacquillat C, Weil M, Khayat D (eds). Neo-Adjuvant Chemotherapy. Colloque INSERM, John Libbey Eurotext Ltd, Paris, 1988;169:177–181.
116. Feldman LD, Hortobagyi GN, Buzdar AU, Ames FC, et al: Pathological assessment of response to induction chemotherapy in breast cancer. Cancer Res 1986;41(5):2578.
117. Koyama H, Nishizawa Y, Wada T, Kabuto T, et al: Intra-arterial infusion chemotherapy as an induction therapy in multidisciplinary treatment for locally advanced breast cancer: a long-term follow-up study. Cancer 1985;56(4):725–729.
118. Hortobagyi GN, Ames FC, Buzdar AU, et al: Management of stage III primary breast cancer with primary chemotherapy, surgery, and radiation therapy. Cancer 1988;62:2507–2516.

The Treatment of Metastatic Breast Cancer

Joseph Aisner, Jeffrey S. Abrams

Introduction

Despite advances in early detection and increasing public awareness of the problem, the mortality from breast cancer continues to be fairly constant. Breast cancer is still the most common type of cancer, and the second leading cause of cancer death in women.[1] Nearly 10% of all women with breast cancer present initially with metastatic disease, and another nearly 40% have recurrence of their disease after initial treatments.[2,3] Thus, recurrent or metastatic breast cancer is an enormous medical and social problem for treatment and supportive care. The vast majority of women who develop recurrent or metastatic disease eventually die of their metastases, with a median duration of survival that ranges from 12 to 24 months, depending in part on the sites of metastases, duration of disease-free period from initial diagnosis, prior treatments, and responsiveness to hormonal therapies.[2,4,5] In a series of Cancer and Leukemia Group B (CALGB) chemotherapy studies in stage IV disease, the median duration of survival ranged from about 9 to 24 months and depended, in part, on patient characteristics and treatments. Less than 5% of all the patients were still alive at 5 years.[6–9] In a review of their long-term results in more than 1,400 women, investigators at M.D. Anderson Hospital found that less than 2% of their patients with metastatic disease were still alive at 10 years.[10] Even patients with so-called local recurrences, such as in the chest wall, have a very high cancer-related mortality and less than 10% are alive and free of disease beyond 10 years.[11,12] Although the reasons why a few patients remain alive after 5 to 10 years with metastatic disease can be very instructive in our understanding of the treatment, at the present time one must consider recurrent and stage IV breast cancer as a widely disseminated and practically incurable disease. The purpose of this review will be to consider the approach to conventional treatments of metastatic disease.

Initial Assessment and Goals of Treatment

Given the recognition that cure is not a realistic expectation for stage IV disease with conventional treatments, the patient and her physician should then define the goals and expectations of therapy. These goals could then help to define the philosophical approach to staging and treatment priorities. One would logically assume that the order of the priorities would most likely be: (1) comfort, (2) function, and (3) longevity. Most patients and physicians would likely agree that achieving survival longevity without comfort and function would not be worthwhile.

Following the priorities outlined above, the initial assessment of the woman who presents with recurrent or metastatic disease would first focus on the symptomatic or potentially symptomatic sites of disease involvement. For example, such an approach would focus on: painful or unstable weight-bearing bone, hypercalcemia, epidural spinal cord compression, neurological changes, retinal or choroid involvement, etc. A careful history and physical examination would thus be coupled with serum blood tests for liver function, including alkaline phosphatase, renal function, calcium, and electrolytes, and an isotopic bone scintigram and chest X-ray. Abnormalities on these screening tests would then lead to further investigations to define any potential need for immediate intervention. An abnormal bone scan, for example, should lead to conventional X-ray of the involved area(s). Any radiolucency felt to represent a reasonable chance of fracture or collapse in an area of weight-bearing skeleton would undergo appropriate radiation therapy or orthopedic procedure as the first therapeutic intervention. Similarly, the finding of hypercalcemia would define interventions to reduce the serum calcium as the initial approach,[13] and the finding of vertebral involvement on X-ray corresponding to a painful area would define the need for resolving the potential epidural spinal cord compression[14] as the initial therapeutic maneuver. This approach is illustrated in Figure 1.

Visceral Crisis

The next level of assessment needs to define the presence or absence of visceral crisis. The term "visceral crisis" has been used by different investigators to define a broad range of visceral organ involvement. However, in this stepwise assessment, visceral crisis is used to define potentially life-threatening involvement of visceral organs, wherein rapid progression of disease in this site could result in organ failure and the woman's demise. Examples of such visceral crisis would include lymphangitic lung metastases, myelophthisic bone marrow metastases (wherein the peripheral blood counts are low or unstable), and liver

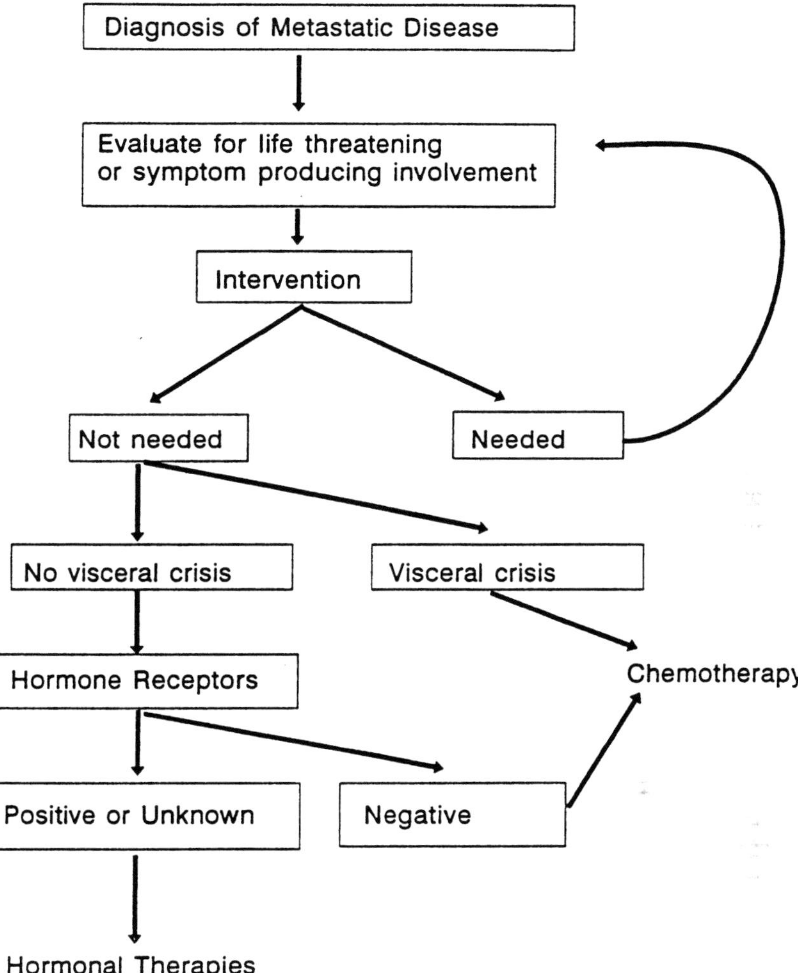

Figure 1: *A diagram illustrating the initial approach to diagnosis, defining life-threatening states (visceral crisis), potential symptom-producing problems, and receptor status.*

metastases with changes in liver function (usually large volume or multiple lesions on ultrasonography, CT, or isotopic scans). Lymphangitic pulmonary metastases are distinguished from discrete nodular (cannonball-like) lesions, and myelophthisic marrow metastases with changes in the peripheral blood are distinguished from cortical bone metastases with extension into the bone marrow. Both nodular lung metastases and cortical bone (+ marrow) metastases have the potential for both slow progression and response to hormonal therapies (see below). The definition of visceral crisis with liver metastases can often be considerably more subjective but is an important distinction since many investigators suggest a lower response to hormonal therapies for liver involvement.[15] Given the clinical need for more immediate response in the presence of visceral

Table 1
Hormone Therapy Options for Advanced Breast Cancer

| | | | Treatment Sequence | |
Therapy	Menopausal Status	Initial	Secondary	Subsequent
Ablative				
Oophorectomy (OOX)	Pre	+ + +	+ +	—
LHRH analogues (medical OO)	Pre	+ + +	+ +	+ +
Adrenalectomy*	Pre/Post	—	—	—
Aromatase inhibitors	Post	+	+ +	+ + +
(medical adrenalectomy)	Pre	—	+	+
Additive				
Progestins	Pre	—	+	+ +
	Post	+ +	+ + +	+ +
Estrogens	Post	—	+	+ +
Androgens†	Post	—	+	+
Antagonists				
Antiestrogens	Pre	+ + +	+ + +	+ + +
	Post	+ + +	+ +	+ +
Antiprogestins	Pre	ND	ND	ND
	Post	ND	ND	

*Adrenalectomy and hypophysectomy have been replaced by medical management to avoid surgery(aromatase inhibitors and LHRH agonists, respectively).
†Androgens may have some desirability over estrogens when fluid retention is a problem.
ND = Appropriate application not well defined.
+ + + Preferred in stated sequence.
+ + Useful but less preferred in sequence.
+ Useful but not currently preferred in sequence.
— Indicates not used in stated sequence.

crisis, the identification of such visceral crisis would most likely then dictate the need for combination chemotherapy. In contrast, those women without visceral crisis could then have their disease evaluated for potential treatment with hormonal manipulations as shown in Figure 1.

Hormonal Therapies

Breast cancer can often be responsive to various hormonal therapies or maneuvers. The various hormonal therapy options are shown in Table 1. There can be a variety of advantages to hormonal therapies as the initial treatment approach. In general, hormonal therapies are less toxic, more easily tolerated, and require less interruption of daily living routine than chemotherapy or radiotherapy. There are several predictors of potential response to the various hormonal therapies. The most powerful predictors are the presence of estrogen receptor proteins, and prior response to hormonal therapies.[15–18]

Predictors of Response

The presence of a sufficient quantity of estrogen or progesterone receptor proteins in the tumor tends to predict for a response to hormonal therapies.[15–20] Since the metastases from a primary source have concordance of receptors in the vast majority of cases, it can often be assumed that the metastatic sites have the same receptor status as the primary tumor. This assumption may be of considerable importance when the metastatic site is difficult to biopsy at the time of recurrence. There have been several suggestions that the absolute value expressed as femtamoles (fmole) of receptor protein per mg of tumor has the greatest degree of predictability for hormone responsiveness.[16–19] Another suggestion is that the simultaneous presence in sufficient quantities of both estrogen and progesterone receptors has a positive predictive value for response to hormonal therapies.[18] The thermolability of the receptor proteins, however, sometimes makes such quantification correlations difficult and the subject of some debate. The greatest degree of prediction for hormone responsiveness does, however, arise from the absence of or very low levels of such hormone receptors. Thus tumors with "negative" estrogen receptor proteins (usually <7 fmole/mg, which can vary with individual laboratory standards) rarely respond to hormonal therapies. Patients with such tumors can usually be spared the delay in more appropriate therapies (i.e., chemotherapy), and the emotional trauma of experiencing disease progression in the face of therapeutic maneuvers. Another highly predictive factor for potential response to hormonal therapies is the failure of the tumor to respond to a prior hormonal manipulation. With the possible exception of high-dose progestins as described below, those tumors which fail to respond to one hormonal therapy are very unlikely to respond to a subsequent hormonal therapy. Patients in this circumstance are also more likely to benefit from change in their treatment to chemotherapy.

When the initial selection criteria are used as shown in Figure 1, those women with visceral crisis and those with estrogen receptor-negative tumors will have been excluded from hormonal therapies. All other women with advanced disease can then be appropriately considered for hormonal therapies. This includes those women whose tumor has unknown estrogen or progesterone receptors. Since it is not always practical, although desirable, to obtain tissue for receptor analysis, such cases can still be included in the treatment with hormonal modalities especially if there is no visceral crisis, and the 8-to 12-week period for assessing the hormonal therapy most likely does not pose a life-threatening delay in the initiation of other treatments.

Flare Reactions

For women with bone metastases, hormonal therapies can occasionally produce a "flare" reaction. This flare is most often characterized by an increase in bone pain seen during the first 8 to 12 weeks of therapy.[20] Such self-limited pain flares, in contrast to progressively increasing pain seen after many months of therapy, often signify a response. With close scrutiny, analgesics can be continued until the response is evident. Early hypercalcemia can also sometimes be a manifestation of such a flare[21] but often requires more complicated medical management. Neither the early pain nor calcium flare should by themselves be an indication to discontinue the hormonal therapy. Similarly, the isotopic bone scan measures osteoblast activity, and an increase in the bone scan may represent healing. Thus an early increase (3–6 months) in the isotopic activity in bone should not by itself be an indication of progression of disease but rather a "flare" that should not be an indication to stop the hormonal therapy.

Selecting the Hormonal Therapy

In general, the various options shown in Table 1 are approximately equal as first-, second-, or third-line therapies.[22,23] For this reason, the choice of initial hormonal therapy rests in part on the menopausal status of the woman and in part on the side effects and potential morbidities of the various choices. For example, oophorectomy might be a very good initial approach to the premeno-pausal woman since it permits the addition of another level of hormonal therapy. After oophorectomy, such women can be considered for hormonal therapy at the initial point of therapy for postmenopausal women. In contrast, however, oophorectomy has the morbidity of a surgical procedure, and several investiga-tors have argued that initial tamoxifen can be equally efficacious.[24,25] At the University of Maryland Cancer Center, we have preferred to use oophorectomy as the initial approach for the premenopausal woman because of the potentially greater number of women who might respond to this sequence and the possibility of an additional layer of hormonal treatments. Recently, LHRH analogues have been tested in premenopausal women with results similar to oophorectomy,[26] but sparing the surgical trauma and complication possibilities.

A potential sequence for hormonal manipulations is shown in Figure 2. The choice of initial treatments may vary, but a logical and systematic approach proceeding from one to another hormonal therapy can sometimes allow a few women with responsive tumors to enjoy responses on hormonal therapy for years.

Antiestrogens: Tamoxifen

Generally, the initial choice for hormonal therapy is the antiestrogen tamoxifen. Ten milligrams of tamoxifen given twice daily has been accepted as a reasonable standard approach for hormone-responsive advanced breast can-cer.[22,27] Many clinical trials involving thousands of women have shown the safety and efficacy of this agent. With the exception of rare idiosyncratic reactions, tamoxifen is virtually free of any toxic reactions. Hot flashes, vaginal secretions, and menstrual irregularities can all be seen due to tamoxifen's action

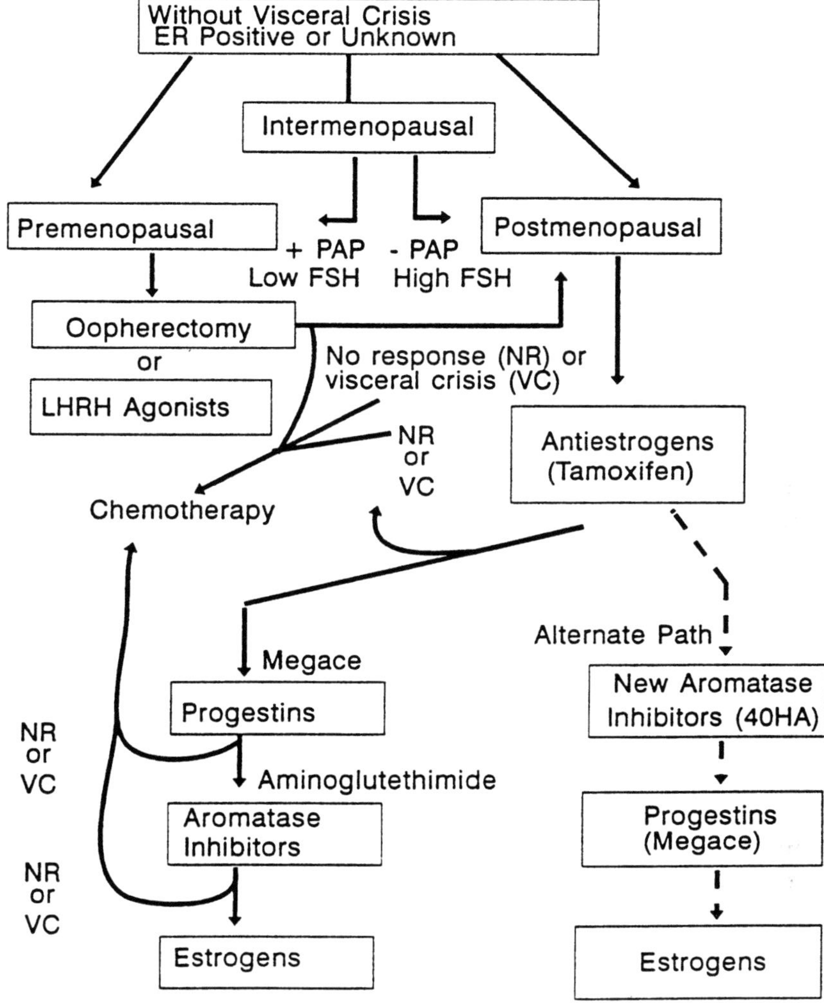

Figure 2: *A diagram illustrating flow of sequential hormonal therapies. Several different paths could be used, and one alternate pathway is illustrated in dotted lines.*

as both an antiestrogen and as a weak estrogen. Other rare <2%) side effects include nausea, rash, headache, fatigue, and blood count depression. The response frequency varies from about 30% to nearly 75% according to sites of disease involvement (soft tissue > bone > viscera), disease-free period from time of diagnosis (more than 2 years > more than 1 year > less 1 year), and absolute value of hormone receptors.[10,11,15–19] With the increasing use of tamoxifen as an adjuvant therapy, its use in advanced disease may become less desirable. In clinical circumstances where the woman has been off tamoxifen for 2 or more years at the time of disease recurrence, tamoxifen may still be an excellent initial choice of hormonal therapy. However, many clinicians now administer tamoxifen for prolonged periods of time so that other alternatives may be more desirable. This situation is likely to become even more complex with the introduction of tamoxifen as a chemopreventive agent among large groups of women. In this latter situation, other alternatives will also likely be more desirable choices.

Following successful therapy with an initial hormonal therapy and subsequent disease regrowth (progression or recurrence), the woman with advanced disease should be considered for a second-line hormonal therapy as shown in Figure 2. There are many choices for second-line therapy as illustrated, but there is often a very important advantage to delaying the initiation of the second-line therapy to evaluate the possibility of a withdrawal response.[28] Although such withdrawal response is more often seen following the discontinuation of an additive hormonal treatment, such responses have been reported following tamoxifen and other manipulations.[28] Such waiting periods can also be important in assessing the pace of the disease, allowing the prior therapy (e.g., tamoxifen) to be cleared from the system and providing for a possible prolongation of the use of the hormonal therapies by stretching the hormonal treatment period. If the disease progression was to a form of visceral crisis, however, then the treatment should proceed to chemotherapy.

Megestrol Acetate

Progestins (e.g., medroxyprogesterone acetate and megestrol acetate) are good second-line agents.[23,29–31] Megestrol acetate (MA) is more bioavailable as an oral agent and is thus currently an excellent choice for second-line therapy of hormone-sensitive advanced breast cancer. Randomized trials of tamoxifen versus megestrol acetate have shown them to be approximately equal as first-and second-line therapies.[23,30] MA, however, has some greater side effects, particularly weight gain. Compared to other current choices, it is an excellent second-line therapy. When women have experienced a recurrence of breast cancer after adjuvant tamoxifen, then MA is currently the most likely first-line agent. MA is usually administered as 160 mg daily in divided doses and results in a response frequency that varies from 18% to 60%, depending on prior therapy as well as the other prognostic factors as listed above. Recently, we observed a possible dose-related activity for MA based on the observation that some women's tumors responded to high-dose MA after the tumors failed to respond to conventional-dose MA.[32] A similar dose-dependent effect has been reported for medroxyprogesterone acetate.[31,33] These observations led to a randomized study by the CALGB of three MA dose levels: 160, 800, and 1600 mg/day. This study did not show an enhanced effect for the MA at higher doses.[34] The CALGB study did not, however, address the possible role of high-dose MA following failure of conventional dose. Another interesting aspect of our pilot study was the observation that women experienced a response to high-dose MA after their tumor failed to respond to first-line tamoxifen with about the same frequency as those who previously responded to the tamoxifen.[32] This observation suggests that high-dose MA may have a unique role as salvage hormonal therapy, but further study of this hypothesis is needed.

Aromatase Inhibitors: Aminoglutethimide

A reasonable third-line choice for hormonal therapy of metastatic breast cancer is an aromatase inhibitor. The use of an aromatase inhibitor has virtually eliminated surgical adrenalectomy as a treatment choice for metastatic breast cancer.[35,36] Currently, the aromatase inhibitor that is commercially available in the US is aminoglutethimide (AMG). AMG inhibits the aromatization of the first ring of the steroid molecule preventing the formation of estrogen from androgenic precursors.[37] AMG also blocks the cholesterol side chain cleavage reaction, resulting in a total suppression of adrenal steroids, thereby affecting a medical adrenalectomy. At the full dose of 250 mg four times daily, treatment with AMG thus requires replacement doses of corticosteroids.[35,36] Rashes are sometimes seen at this dose and are usually self-limiting despite continuation of therapy. At full doses, response frequencies appear about equivalent to other hormonal therapies. Several investigators have suggested that lower doses of AMG such as 250 mg twice daily have nearly the same or equivalent response with considerably less toxicity without the requirement for replacement corticosteroids.[38] Recently, new aromatase inhibitors have been described and introduced into clinical trials. Four-hydroxy-androstenedione (4-OHA) is one such aromatase inhibitor.[37,39] The advantage of 4-OHA rests in its inhibition of the aromatase step without cleavage of the side chain. Subsequently, the women are not corticosteroid-deficient, do not require steroid replacement, and clinical trials in Europe suggest at least equal response to other hormonal agents but with very few side effects.[39] A new analogue of 4-OHA, Fadrozol, is currently undergoing clinical trials in the US and preliminary data suggest that it is active with very few side effects.[40] The role of Fadrozol as a possible second-line agent is currently being tested in a randomized trial in comparison with MA at conventional doses.

Estrogens and Androgens

Estrogens and androgens are currently reserved for the postmenopausal woman who has previously received prior hormonal therapy options. Estrogens are preferred over androgens because of the virilizing effect of the androgens and because of the better response profile in comparative trials.[41,42] Estrogens may have a steep dose-response profile for response,[43] and the usual approach is to start with a moderate dose, e.g., 10–15 mg of diethylstilbestrol (or its equivalent) and escalate to the woman's tolerance. There are multiple and frequent (>20%) side effects with estrogens that can include anorexia, nausea, vomiting, vaginal bleeding, breast engorgement and tenderness, fluid retention, and urinary incontinence. In the elderly woman with congestive heart failure or marginal cardiac status, androgens may be preferred because of less fluid retention.

New Hormonal Therapies

Several newer hormonal agents are currently under clinical investigation throughout the world and offer the possibility of further increasing the armamentarium of hormonal treatment options. For example, several new antiprogestins, originally developed as antifertility agents, have been shown to have activity in breast cancer.[44] Newer antiestrogens that may not be cross-reactive to tamoxifen,[45] biological methods of enhancing hormone receptor protein expression,[46] and antibodies or inhibitors directed against tumor growth factors[47] are

Table 2
Single Agents with Activity in Advanced Breast Cancer[+]

Agent	Approximate % Response
Anthracyclines	
doxorubicin	35
epirubicin*	35
mitoxantrone	30
Alkylating agents	
cyclophosphamide	35
ifosphamide	35
nitrogen mustard	35
thio-tepa	30
phenylalanine mustard	25
melphalan	25
chlorambucil	20
cisplatin	20
prednimustine	25
Antimetabolites	
methotrexate	30
trimetrexate	25
5-fluorouracil	30
Plant alkaloids	
vincristine	15
vinblastine	30
vindesine*	25
Miscellaneous	
mitomycin-c	30
elliptinium*	25
mitolactol*	20
carmustine	20
hexamethylmelamine	20
dibromodulcitol*	30

[+]Compiled in part from Carter,[48] Henderson,[22] and Aisner et al.[62]
*Not commercially available in the USA.

Table 3
New Agents with Promising Antitumor Activity

Agent/Reference No.	Approximate Response %
Taxol[50]	35
Camptothecin; CPT-11[51]	35
Navelbine[52]	35
Elliptinium[49]	20

also interesting and exciting possibilities that suggest that hormonal therapy options will continue to improve. Currently, however, the choices for hormonal therapy remain limited to those discussed above, and occasionally the options for hormonal therapy can be exhausted despite judicious use of rests between the application of hormonal therapies. In this circumstance, there is little advantage to returning to previously tried and failed therapies. As suggested in Figure 2, treatment at this time should probably be to move to chemotherapy.

Chemotherapy

A number of chemotherapeutic agents have been identified with antitumor activity in breast cancer.[48,49] A partial list of these active agents is shown in Table 2. These agents have formed the basis of the combination chemotherapy regimens used for advanced disease as well as adjuvant postoperative therapy. There has been a relative paucity of new active agents identified in the near recent past years. In general, chemotherapy agents produce a greater percentage of response in previously untreated disease than in previously treated disease. For this reason, the CALGB elected to test new antitumor agents first, before the use of combination chemotherapy, as part of a randomized trial of this approach versus conventional combination chemotherapy first (then different new agents if practical). Recently, however, several new agents such as taxol, navelbine, and others have shown promising antitumor activity for advanced breast cancer; these agents are listed in Table 3.[49-52] The identification of new active agents is of critical importance in the identification of better treatments for advanced and early disease.

Initial Combination Chemotherapy

Combinations of active agents with differing mechanisms of action and nonoverlapping or partially overlapping toxicities have been developed for the treatment of metastatic disease.[48,53] A partial list of some of these combinations is shown in Table 4. Greenspan et al.[54] began combination chemotherapy with the sequential addition of active single agents. Cooper et al.[55] subsequently described a combination of five active agents (cyclophosphamide, methotrexate,

Table 4
Combination Chemotherapy Regimens for Advanced Breast Cancer*

Combination	% Range Total Response (CR + PR)	% Range of CR	Range of Response Duration (Months)
TMF	75	ns	7
CMP	44	4	7
CMV	33	7	8
CMF	40–70	8–15	6–10
CMF ± V ± P	30–80	7–25	6–14
CAF ± V ± P	40–80	8–20	8–16
CAMFVP	46	11	9
CAFM	50	10	11
CA	41–78	2–22	10–12
CAV	56–72	16–28	12, 22
AV	52–53	0–8	7–8
MISC+	42–63	2–6	4–8

*Ignores dose, schedule, prior treatment, and other prognostic factors.
+ Includes: VFP, CFP, CFP-V, CFV.
Description of drugs used in combination regimens: T = thiotepa; M = methotrexate; F = 5-fluorouracil; C = cyclophosphamide; N = mitoxantrone; P = prednisone; V = vincristine; A = doxorubicin.

5-fluorouracil, vincristine, and prednisone) with a very high response frequency. Subsequent combination chemotherapy studies have attempted to define the role of the components of this regimen.[6–9,49,53–63] The prognostic indicators for response to chemotherapy include: sites of metastases (soft tissue > bone > viscera), disease-free interval from diagnosis (2 years > 1 > less than 1 year), performance status, and prior therapies.[4,5,10,11,49] The introduction of doxorubicin, a highly active single agent, produced a series of further permutations of the CMF ± V ± P regimens[6,7,9,53,59,61–65] as shown in Table 4. The total response

Table 5
Selected Salvage Chemotherapy Regimens

Regimen	Approximate Response %
AV	25
AMc	40
FAVMc	54
VbMc	7,40
VbATH	49,52
VAPt	42
VACMLe	78
HxVM	45

A = doxorubicin; V = vincristine; Mc = mitomycin-C; F = 5-fluorouracil; Vb = vinblastine; T = thio-tepa; H = halotestin; Pt = cisplatin; M = methotrexate; Le = leucovorin; Hx = hexamethylmelamine.

frequencies vary between 40% and 80%, and the complete response varies between 10% and 25%. When corrected for the prognostic factors, there would appear to be only minor differences in the chemotherapy regimens, at least as applied to advanced metastatic disease. In addition to the established chemotherapy regimens used as first-line therapy, several salvage or second-line regimens have been described as shown in Table 5.[49,56,62,66–76] The minor variations in the first-line regimens and the availability of second-line or salvage regimens have raised several important questions regarding the use of combination chemotherapy regimens. These include the definition of an optimal regimen, the role of doxorubicin as part of initial therapy, the role of fluorouracil in CAF, the dose of chemotherapy, the duration of therapy, and the use of salvage regimens.

Choice of Regimens

Two sequential randomized studies conducted by the CALGB posed a direct comparison of similar combination chemotherapy regimens CAFVP versus CMFVP in one study and CMF versus CAF versus CAFVP in the successor study.[6,7] In both studies, the substitution of doxorubicin produced a greater response and longer survival than the comparable methotrexate-containing combination. A subsequent study compared CAF with VATH and an alternation of VATH with CMFVP.[8] The VATH combination appeared to be similar to the CAF regimen, suggesting the important role of doxorubicin as part of an initial combination. Nevertheless, many clinicians still choose to start with CMF in part to reduce a minor degree of toxicity, and in part to save doxorubicin for so-called salvage chemotherapy. Unfortunately, the use of doxorubicin + vincristine, a reasonably active first-line combination, has only minor activity as a salvage combination with a response frequency no better than doxorubicin used alone in this setting. Thus, at present, there appears to be little justification for withholding doxorubicin for salvage or second-line therapy. Given the minor differences in response and outcome for the various combinations, there can be no "standard" regimen, although CAF is the most commonly used combination for metastatic disease and has entered many adjuvant therapy programs.

Optimal Dose

The optimal dose for CAF (or other combinations) has not been well established. In general, chemotherapy is administered with a philosophy of maximally tolerable dose and highest dose rate.[77,78] Several investigators have argued that reduction of doses below those tested in clinical trials possibly compromises the woman's chance for response and survival. Although not well studied in advanced disease, a dose intensity study of CAF as adjuvant therapy recently showed a statistically significant advantage to the higher dose compared to lower doses.[79] More aggressive treatment with much higher doses of CAF at

M.D. Anderson produced a somewhat higher complete response rate but a much greater level of both hematologic and nonhematologic toxicities, and no significant difference in survival.[80] Even more aggressive chemotherapy with autologous bone marrow transplant as well as cytokines and peripheral stem cells is currently under study with very interesting preliminary data.[81] The overall data would suggest that a doxorubicin-containing regimen is most likely the best initial choice for combination chemotherapy and the regimen should be given at full dose unless the woman has a contraindication to the use of an anthracycline. The use of more aggressive doses along with cytokines should await the results of the currently ongoing studies.

Duration of Therapy

Most women treated with combination chemotherapy regimens whose disease responds experience only a partial response of their disease. A minority of the women have a complete response, i.e., complete disappearance of all signs and symptoms of disease. For those women whose disease responds to therapy, one might reasonably ask how long such toxic or potentially toxic therapy should continue. There are no good studies to define the answer to these questions, and many of the cooperative group trials have continued the therapy until the time of progression, sometimes in excess of 2 years. Such an approach seems contrary to the initial priority goals set out for the treatment of metastatic disease: comfort, function, and then longevity. An alternative approach might be to give a fixed number of chemotherapy cycles (e.g., four to six, or until a maximum response is achieved) and then allow the woman a "rest" period off all chemotherapy to enjoy the benefits of the response. Several investigators have noted that responses can be durable, especially the complete responses.[82,83] While not all women will be comfortable with such an approach, many women will be able to take advantage of the absence of treatment-related toxicities and the benefits of their response. Furthermore, when such rests are followed by the subsequent progression of the breast cancer, the women can return to the prior therapy or be switched to second-line combinations. As is true for response after adjuvant therapy, if the disease progression occurs after only a short rest, then the original regimen is not likely to have worked much longer and is unlikely to generate further response. In contrast, when there has been a fairly long rest period (e.g., >3 months), then there is a reasonable chance that the prior regimen will again generate some response, and it is further likely that such a patient could be an excellent candidate for new investigational agents. Such a philosophy has been advocated in small-cell lung cancer (SCLC), where second-line chemotherapy has been particularly unsuccessful when it follows immediately upon prior treatments, but has shown response to second-line treatment when there is a $\geq$90-day pause from the prior therapies.[84] Several investigators have advocated this clinical situation for new drug discovery in SCLC, and a similar philosophy would be very practical in breast cancer.

The Role of 5-Fluorouracil

5-Fluorouracil (5-FU) was originally included on a weekly basis in the five-drug regimen described by Cooper et al.[55] The various permutations of these regimens have used various doses and schedules of the 5-FU which range from weekly injections to one injection on day 1 and 8 of a 28-day cycle to once every 3 weeks.[49] Furthermore, studies by investigators from Arizona and the Southwest Oncology Group (SWOG) have suggested that CA is essentially equivalent to CAF[85]; however, in comparison trials, the response is marginally better with CAF than CA and the duration of response appears greater.[86] One might still question the role of 5-FU in CAF regimens specifically and in breast cancer in general. 5-FU has been studied as a single agent in breast cancer and has been shown to be an active agent.[49,53] 5-FU has also been studied extensively in colorectal cancers where investigations into the dose and schedule have identified certain ways to optimize its use.[87,88] For example, infusional therapy spread over several days is generally superior to intermittent bolus use, and multiple consecutive-day administration is superior to weekly administration.[87,88] These observations in gastrointestinal malignancies suggest that 5-FU has not been administered optimally for breast cancer. Therefore, before 5-FU is discarded from the combination regimens for breast cancer, further study seems urgently warranted. For example, the use of leucovorin (folinic acid) to modulate 5-FU in colorectal cancer has met with considerable success.[89] To take advantage of such favorable interactions, we at University of Maryland Cancer Center have completed a phase I study of CAF + leucovorin (CALF) as the pilot study for a randomized trial in metastatic visceral disease breast cancer in CALGB.[90]

Salvage Chemotherapy

A number of salvage chemotherapy regimens have been described and some are outlined in Table 5. In general, the salvage regimen of choice will likely depend on the woman's prior chemotherapy exposure history, the response to these therapies, and the duration of the treatment-free period as discussed above. The inconsistent results seen in most salvage regimens is due in part to imbalance in these very important prognostic factors. Furthermore, at this point in a woman's treatment, a careful reassessment of the goals of treatment, as in each instance of a change in therapeutic alternatives, is needed to balance the potential benefits of the second-line chemotherapy with its potential toxicities and their impact on the quality of survival. Sometimes the judicious use of irradiation to painful areas can have considerable palliative benefit. Some women will nevertheless benefit greatly from the application of such salvage regimens. Furthermore, the identification of new and highly active regimens in this setting will likely produce combinations worthy of testing as initial treatment combinations.

References

1. Silverberg E, Boring CC, Squires BA: Cancer Statistics, 1990. Ca-A Cancer J Clinicians 1990; 40:9-26.
2. Cutler S: Classification of extent of disease in breast cancer. Semin Oncol 1974; 1:91–96.
3. Fisher B, Slack N, Katrych D, et al: Ten-year follow-up results for patients with carcinoma of the breast in a cooperative group trial evaluating surgical adjuvant chemotherapy. Surg Gynecol Obstet 1975; 140:528–534.
4. Cutler S, Asire AJ, Taylor SG III: Classification of patients with disseminated cancer of the breast. Cancer 1969; 24:861-869.
5. Patterson AH, Zuck VP, Szafran O, et al: Influence and significance of certain prognostic factors on survival in breast cancer. Eur J Clin Oncol 1982; 18:937–943.
6. Tormey DC, Weinberg V, Leone LA, et al: A comparison of intermittent vs. continuous and of adriamycin vs. methotrexate 5-drug chemotherapy for advanced breast cancer. Am J Clin Oncol 1984; 7:231–239.
7. Aisner J, Weinberg V, Perloff M, et al: Chemotherapy v. chemoimmunotherapy (CAF v CAFVP v CMF, each + MER) for metastatic carcinoma of the breast: a CALGB study. J Clin Oncol 1987; 5:1523–1533.
8. Perry MC, Kardinal CG, Korzun AH, Ginsberg SJ, et al: Chemohormonal therapy in advanced carcinoma of the breast: Cancer and Leukemia Group B protocol 8081. J Clin Oncol 1987; 5:1534-1545.
9. Aisner J, Korzun A, Perloff M, Chiarieri D, et al: A randomized comparison of CAF, VATH, and VATH alternating with CMFVP for advanced breast cancer: a CALGB study. Proc Am Soc Clin Oncol 1988; 7:8 (abstract).
10. Hortobagyi GN, Smith TN, Legha SS, et al : Multivariate analysis of prognostic factors in metastatic breast cancer. J Clin Oncol 1983; 1:776.
11. Fey MF, Brunner KW, Sonntag RW: Prognostic factors in metastatic breast cancer. Cancer Clin Trials 1981; 4:237–247.
12. Chu FCH, Lin FJ, Kim JH, et al: Locally recurrent carcinoma of the breast. Cancer 1976; 37:2677–2681.
13. Schnipper LE, Come SE: Hypercalcemia in breast cancer. In: Harris JR, Hellman S, Henderson IC, Kinne DW (eds). Breast Diseases. J.B. Lippincott, Philadelphia, pp 552–538, 1987.
14. Stillman M, Foley K: Breast cancer and epidural spinal cord compression: diagnostic and therapeutic strategies. In: Harris JR, Hellman S, Henderson IC, Kinne DW (eds). Breast Diseases. J.B. Lippincott, Philadelphia, pp 488–497, 1987.
15. Byar DP, Sears ME, McGuire WL: Relationship between estrogen receptor values and clinical data in predicting the response to endocrine therapy for patients with advanced breast cancer. Eur J Cancer 1979; 15:299–310.
16. Paridaens R, Sylvester M, Ferrazi E, et al: Clinical significance of the quantitative assessment of estrogen receptors in advanced breast cancer. Cancer 1980; 46:2889–2895.
17. McGuire WL, Clark GM, Hubay CA, et al: Role of steroid hormone receptors as prognostic factors in primary breast cancer. NCI Monographs 1986; 1:19–33.
18. Stewart J, King R, Hayward J, et al: Estrogen and progesterone receptors: correlation of response rates, site and timing of receptor analysis. Breast Cancer Res Treat 1982; 2:243-250.
19. Osborne CK, Yochmowitz MG, Knight WA, et al: The value of estrogen and progesterone receptors in the treatment of breast cancer. Cancer 1980; 46:2884–2888.
20. Clarysse A: Hormone-induced tumor flare. Eur J Cancer 1985; 21:545.
21. Hall TC, Dedrick MM, Nevinny HB: Prognostic value of hormonally induced hypercalcemia in breast cancer. Cancer Chemother Rep 1963; 30:21–26.
22. Henderson IC: Endocrine therapy in metastatic breast cancer. In: Harris JR, Hellman

S, Henderson IC, Kinne DW (eds). Breast Diseases. J.B. Lippincott, Philadelphia, pp 398–428, 1987.

23. Ettinger DS, Allegra J, Bertino LR, et al: Megestrol acetate versus tamoxifen in advanced breast cancer: correlation of hormone receptors and response. Semin Oncol 1986; 13(Suppl 4):9-14.

24. Puga FJ, Welch JS, Bisel HF: Therapeutic oophorectomy in disseminated carcinoma of the breast. Arch Surg 1976; 111:880-887.

25. Ingle JN, Krook JE, Green SJ, et al: Randomized trial of bilateral oophorectomy versus tamoxifen in premenopausal women with metastatic breast cancer. J Clin Oncol 1986; 4:178–186.

26. Harvey HA, Lipton A, Max DT, et al: Medical castration produced by the GnRH analogue leuprolide to treat metastatic breast cancer. J Clin Oncol 1985; 3:1068–1072.

27. Mouridsen H, Palshof T, Patterson J, et al: Tamoxifen in advanced breast cancer. Cancer Treat Rev 1978; 5:131–141.

28. Belani CP, Pearl P, Whitley NO, Aisner J: Tamoxifen withdrawal response: a case report. Arch Int Med 1989; 149:449-450.

29. Caneta R, Florentine S, Hunter H, et al: Megestrol acetate. Cancer Treat Rev 1983; 10:141–157.

30. Johnson PA, Muss H, Bonomi P, et al: Megestrol acetate as primary therapy for advanced breast cancer. Semin Oncol 1988; (Suppl 1):34–37.

31. Pannuti F, Martoni A, DiMarco AR, et al: Prospective, randomized clinical trial of two different high dosages of medroxyprogesterone acetate in the treatment of metastatic breast cancer. Eur J Cancer 1979; 15:593–599.

32. Aisner J, Tcheckmedyian NS, Moody M, et al: High dose megestrol acetate for treatment of advanced breast cancer: dose and toxicities. Semin Hematol 1987; 24(Suppl 1):48–55.

33. Alexieva-Figusch J, Blankenstein MA, Hop WCJ, et al: Treatment of metastatic breast cancer patients with different dosages of megestrol acetate: dose relations, metabolic and endocrine effects. Eur J Cancer Clin Oncol 1984; 20:33–40.

34. Abrams JS, Cirrincione C, Aisner J, Berry D, et al: A phase III trial of megestrol acetate (MA) in metastatic breast cancer (MBC). Proc Am Soc Clin Oncol 1992; 11:A84 (abstract).

35. Santen RJ, Lipton A, Harvey H, et al: Use of aminoglutethimide and hydrocortisone as a "medical adrenalectomy" for treatment of breast carcinoma. Prog Clin Cancer 1982; 8:245-265.

36. Santen RJ, Worgul TJ, Samojlik E, et al: Randomized trial comparing surgical adrenalectomy with aminoglutethimide plus hydrocortisone in women with advanced breast cancer. N Engl J Med 1981; 305:545–551.

37. Brodie AMH: Aromatase inhibition and its pharmacologic implications. Biochem Pharmacol 1985; 34:3213–3219.

38. Willard EM, Carpenter JR: Low-dose aminoglutethimide is active in metastatic breast cancer. Proc Am Soc Clin Oncol 1991; 10:A96 (abstract).

39. Coombes RC, Goss P, Dowsett M, et al: 4-hydroxyandrostenedione in treatment of postmenopausal patients with advanced breast cancer. Lancet 1984; 2:1237–1239.

40. Raats JI, Falkson G, Falkson HC: A study of Fadrozole, a new aromatase inhibitor, in postmenopausal women with advanced metastatic breast cancer. J Clin Oncol 1992; 10:111–116.

41. Kennedy BJ: Hormonal therapies in breast cancer. Semin Oncol 1974; 1:119–130.

42. Cooperative Breast Cancer Group: Results of studies of the Cooperative Breast Cancer Group, 1961 to 1963. Cancer Chemother Rep 1961; 41:1–43.

43. Carter AC, Sedransk N, Kelley RM, et al: Diethylstilbestrol: recommended dosages for different categories of breast cancer patients. JAMA 1977; 237:2079–2085.

44. Bakker GH, Setyono-Han B, Portengen H, De Jong FH, et al: Treatment of breast cancer with different antiprogestins: preclinical and clinical studies. J Steroid Biochem Mol Biol 1990; 37:789–794.

45. Lee RL, Buzdar AU, Blumenschein GR, et al: Trioxifene mesylate in the treatment of advanced breast cancer. Cancer 1986; 57:40–43.
46. Fontana JA, Burrows-Mezu A, Clemmens DR, LeRoith D: Retinoid modulation of insulin-like growth factor-binding proteins and inhibition of breast carcinoma proliferation. Endocrinology 1991; 128:1115–1122.
47. Lippman ME, Dickson RB: Regulatory Mechanisms in Breast Cancer: Advances in Cellular and Molecular Biology of Breast Cancer. Kluwer Academic Publishers, Norwell, Massachusetts, 1991.
48. Carter SK: Integration chemotherapy into combined modality treatment of solid tumors. VII: Adenocarcinoma of the breast. Cancer Treat Rev 1976; 3:141–174.
49. Buzdar AU, Hortobagyi GN, Esparza LT, et al: Elliptinium acetate in metastatic breast cancer: a phase II study. Oncology 1990; 47:101–104.
50. Holmes FA, Walters RS, Theriault RL, et al: Phase II trial of taxol, an active drug in the treatment of metastatic breast cancer. J Natl Cancer Inst 1991; 83:1797–1805.
51. Taguchi T: Phase I and II clinical studies of CPT-11. Proceed Third Conference on DNA Topoisomerases in Therapy. October 15–18, 1990, New York, NY, p 33 (abstract).
52. Delozier T, Delgado FM, Fumoleau P, et al: Phase II trial with Navelbine (NVB) in advanced breast cancer (ABC). Breast Cancer Res Treat 1990; 16:149 (abstract).
53. Henderson IC: Chemotherapy for advanced disease. In: Harris JR, Hellman S, Henderson IC, Kinne DW (eds). Breast Diseases. J.B. Lippincott, Philadelphia, pp 428–479, 1987.
54. Greenspan EM: Combination chemotherapy for advanced mammary carcinoma: a twelve-year experience. Mt Sinai J Med (NY) 1972; 39:435–446.
55. Cooper R: Combination chemotherapy in hormone resistant breast cancer. Proc Am Assoc Cancer Res 1969; 190:15 (abstract).
56. Hart RD, Perloff M, Holland JF: One day VATH (vinblastine, adriamycin thio-tepa and halotestin) therapy for advanced breast cancer refractory to chemotherapy. Cancer 1981; 48:1522–1527.
57. Canellos GP, DeVita V, Gold GL, et al: Combination chemotherapy for advanced breast cancer: response and effect on survival. Ann Intern Med 1976; 84:389–392.
58. Carbone PP, Bauer M, Band P, et al: Chemotherapy of disseminated breast cancer. Cancer 1977; 39:2916–2922.
59. Henderson IC, Canellos GP: Cancer of the breast: the past decade. N Engl J Med 1980; 302:78–90.
60. Canellos GP, Pocock SJ, Taylor SG III, et al: Combination chemotherapy for metastatic breast carcinoma: a prospective comparison of multiple drug therapy with L-phenylalanine mustard. Cancer 1976; 38:1882–1886.
61. Brambilla C, DeLena M, Rossi A, et al: Response and survival in advanced breast cancer after two non-cross-resistant combinations. Br Med J 1976; 1:801–804.
62. Aisner J, Abrams JS, Tchekmedyian NS: Carcinoma of the breast. In: Rosenthal JC (ed). Neoplastic Diseases: Fundamentals of Clinical Oncology. Precept Press Inc., Chicago, pp 704–745, 1991.
63. Muss HB, White DR, Cooper R, et al: Combination chemotherapy in advanced breast cancer: a randomized trial comparing a three-vs. a five-drug program. Arch Int Med 1977; 137:1711–1714.
64. Bull J, Tormey D, Li SH, et al: A randomized comparative trial of adriamycin vs. methotrexate in combination chemotherapy. Cancer 1978; 41:1649–1657.
65. Muss H, White D, Richards F, et al: Adriamycin versus methotrexate in five-drug combination chemotherapy for advanced breast cancer. Cancer 1978; 42:2141–2148.
66. DeLena M, Brambilla C, Marabito A, et al: Adriamycin plus vincristine compared to and combined with cyclophosphamide, methotrexate, and 5-fluorouracil for advanced breast cancer. Cancer 1975; 35:1108–1112.
67. Morgan LR: Adriamycin and mitomycin-C in advanced breast cancer. In: Carter SK, Crooke ST (eds). Mitomycin-C. Academic Press, New York, 1979.

68. DeLena M, Jirillo A, Villa S, Volonterio A, et al: Preliminary results with adriamycin plus mitomycin combination in metastatic breast cancer. Proc Am Soc Clin Oncol/AACR 1981; 22:400 (abstract).
69. Denafrio JM, East DR, Troner MB, Vogel CL: Phase II study of mitomycin-C and vinblastine in women with advanced breast cancer refractory to standard cytotoxic therapy. Cancer Treat Rep 1978; 62:2113–2115.
70. Konits PH, Aisner J, Van Echo DA, et al: Mitomycin-C and vinblastine chemotherapy for advanced breast cancer. Cancer 1981; 48:1295–1298.
71. Shipp SK, Westrich MA, Muss HB, et al: Vincristine, doxorubicin and mitomycin-C in patients with metastatic breast cancer failing prior cyclophosphamide (C), methotrexate (M), and fluorouracil (F). Proc Am Soc Clin Oncol/AACR 1981; 22:381 (abstract).
72. Oster MW, Park Y: Vincristine, adriamycin and mitomycin (VAM) therapy for previously treated breast cancer. Cancer 1983; 51:203–205.
73. Friedman MA, Marcus FS, Cassidy MJ, et al: 5-Fluorouracil + oncovin + adriamycin + mitomycin-C (FOAM): an effective program for metastatic breast cancer, even for disease refractory to previous chemotherapy. Cancer 1983; 52:193–197.
74. Trump DL, Ettinger DS, Abeloff MD, et al: Doxorubicin, vincristine, and cisdiamminedichloroplatinum (II) therapy in patients with advanced breast cancer. Med Pediatr Oncol 1981; 9:1–8.
75. Mattson W, Arwidi A, Van Eyben F, et al: Phase II study of combined vincristine, adriamycin, cyclophosphamide, and methotrexate with citrovorum factor rescue in metastatic breast cancer. Cancer Treat Rep 1977; 61:527–529.
76. Longacre D, Donovan M, Paladine W, et al: Hexamethylmelamine, vincristine and methotrexate chemotherapy in advanced neoplasms. Cancer Treat Rep 1977; 61:919–922.
77. Hryniuk W, Bush H: The importance of dose intensity in chemotherapy of metastatic breast cancer. J Clin Oncol 1984; 2:1281–1288.
78. Frei E III, Canellos GP: Dose: a critical factor in cancer chemotherapy. Am J Med 1980; 69:585–594.
79. Budman D, Wood W, Henderson IC, et al: Initial findings of CALGB 8541: a dose and dose intensity trial of cyclophosphamide, doxorubicin, and 5-fluorouracil as adjuvant treatment of stage II, node +, female breast cancer. Proc Am Soc Clin Oncol 1992; 11:51 (abstract).
80. Hortobagyi GN, Buzdar AU, Bodey GP, et al: High-dose induction chemotherapy of metastatic breast cancer in a protected environment: a prospective randomized study. J Clin Oncol 1987; 5:178–184.
81. Peters WP, Shpall EJ, Jones RB, Ross M: High dose combination cyclophosphamide, cisplatin, and carmustine with bone marrow support as initial treatment of metastatic breast cancer. Proc Am Soc Clin Oncol 1990; 9:10 (abstract).
82. Legha SS, Buzdar AU, Smith TL, et al: Complete remissions in metastatic breast cancer treated with combination drug therapy. Ann Int Med 1979; 91:847–852.
83. Decker DA, Ahmann DL, Bisel HF, et al: Complete responders to chemotherapy in metastatic breast cancer. JAMA 1979; 24:2075-2079.
84. Aisner J: Strategies for the identification of new drugs in small cell lung cancer. Lung Cancer (in press).
85. Jones SE, Durie BGM, Salmon SE: Combination chemotherapy with adriamycin and cyclophosphamide for advanced breast cancer. Cancer 1975; 36:90–97.
86. Tranum B, McDonald B, Thigpen T, et al: Adriamycin combinations in advanced breast cancer. Cancer 1982; 49:835-839.
87. Petrelli N, Douglass HO Jr, Herrera L, et al: Fluorouracil with leucovorin in metastatic colorectal carcinoma: a prospective randomized phase III trial. J Clin Oncol 1989; 7:1419–1426.
88. Grage TB, Moss SE: Adjuvant chemotherapy in cancer of the colon and rectum: demonstration of effectiveness of prolonged 5-FU chemotherapy in a prospectively controlled trial. Surg Clin N Am 1981; 61:1321–1329.

89. Arbuck SG: 5-Fu/leucovorin: biochemical modulation that works? Oncology 1987; 1:61–67.
90. Parnes HL, Abrams JS, Tait N, et al: A phase I/II study of cyclophosphamide, doxorubicin, 5-fluorouracil and leucovorin for metastatic adenocarcinoma. J Natl Cancer Inst 1991; 83:1017-1020.

High-Dose Combination Alkylating Agent Therapy for Primary and Metastatic Breast Cancer:

A Brief Overview

William P. Peters

Introduction

The therapeutic approach to breast cancer has been undergoing a major and rapid evolution. Ten years ago, the use of adjuvant chemotherapy was controversial. Even 5 years ago, after the first overview analysis of adjuvant breast cancer therapy, the treatment with adjuvant chemotherapy of women with node-positive breast cancer over the age of 50 years was considered by some "experimental" and by others "contraindicated" even though the trends in the early curves were in favor of therapy but not statistically significant. Today, less than 5 years later, with additional trials and continued follow-up of the previously treated patients, adjuvant therapy for pre- and postmenopausal women with adjuvant therapy is considered state of the art, even for women with node-negative breast cancer. Similarly, the situation regarding dose-intensification is undergoing major evolution. Through the early part of this decade, metastatic breast cancer was considered an incurable disease and therapeutic decisions were based upon their palliative potential. However, with the demonstration that bone marrow transplant techniques could cure some cases of acute leukemia and lymphoma that were incurable by other techniques, the possibility of "curing" breast cancer was entertained as a strategic end in breast cancer using dose-intensification.

From: Wise L, Johnson H Jr (eds): *Breast Cancer: Controversies in Management*. Futura Publishing Company, Inc., Armonk, NY, © 1994.

Dose-Intensification in the Treatment of Breast Cancer

There has been increasing experimental and clinical evidence of the importance of dose-intensification in the treatment of breast cancer. Perhaps the strongest evidence to date comes from two randomized clinical trials in breast cancer: (1) a randomized trial of cyclophosphamide, methotrexate, and fluorouracil (CMF) in metastatic breast cancer by Tannock and his colleagues[1] and (2) a trial of three different doses of cyclophosphamide, doxorubicin, and fluorouracil (CAF) in primary breast cancer undertaken by the Cancer and Leukemia Group B (CALGB). In the first trial, patients with metastatic breast cancer were randomized to two doses of CMF for metastatic breast cancer. The results demonstrated an improved disease-free and overall survival for patients treated with the more intensive regimen, and further, an improved quality of life with the more intensive treatment. In primary disease, the use of more intensive therapy in a large, multicenter trial, CALGB 8541,[2] which has been reported at the recent ASCO national conference demonstrated convincingly that a more dose-intensive CAF was statistically superior to a lower dose CAF in both disease-free and overall survival in all patient subgroups analyzed. At the time of the initiation of this protocol, all the treatment arms were felt to represent ethical and effective treatment (i.e., not placebo) and even though the low-dose arm is modest by contemporary standards, it reflected reasonable therapy for breast cancer. While the intermediate-dose therapy was not statistically significantly different at the time of the initial analysis, the curves were in the appropriate position for indicating an intermediate effect; however, further follow-up is needed. Based on the results in other diseases, our group initiated in the beginning of the 1980s a series of sequential trials designed to evaluate the role, if any, of very high-dose therapy in breast cancer.[3-8] The philosophical underpinning of these studies was none other than to try to apply principles proven effective in other diseases to "cure" breast cancer. It was not known at the time whether this was possible, but the beginning philosophical position was to, in essence, pull out all the stops and go for broke. This approach was, as might be expected, criticized for its willingness to accept toxicity, of which there was plenty.

An initial clinical trial was undertaken to determine whether it was possible to combine multiple alkylating agents as escalated doses, ameliorating marrow suppression by using autologous bone marrow support. Preclinical data derived from the Southern Research Institute by Skipper, Schabel, and their colleagues, suggested that the use of combinations of alkylating agents might provide a unique opportunity since there was clear evidence of non-cross-resistance among selected agents, and in many cases, evidence of therapeutic synergy and even, in some cases, collateral sensitivity.

In an initial trial, patients with advanced, resistant breast cancer were treated with a high-dose combination of cyclophosphamide, cisplatin, and carmustine (CPA/cDDP/BCNU) with autologous bone marrow support in a phase I trial designed to establish the maximum tolerated dose and safety of this treatment. The trial identified a maximum transplant dose, limited by three novel side effects including veno-oclusive disease, resistant hypertension, and refractory thrombocytopenia. From a clinical point of view, the impressive fact about the trial was the unexpectedly high frequency of objective response. This was particularly evident in breast cancer where despite extensive previous treatment, all evaluable patients achieved at least an objective partial response, and nearly one-third had a clinical complete remission. While these responses were not durable, which was not unexpected given the advanced disease state and tumor volume, the trial did provide encouragement that application of high-dose therapy might show increased cytoreductive power in earlier disease or with smaller tumor volume.

A second phase II trial was undertaken to establish the activity of this regimen in metastatic breast cancer. Twenty-two women with measurable, metastatic breast cancer that was hormone receptor-negative and did not involve the brain or bone marrow and who had not received prior chemotherapy for metastatic disease were studied. Each received a single treatment with high-dose CPA/cDDP/BCNU and ABMS and no other therapy until relapse. Therapy-related mortality occurred in over 20% of patients. However, objective complete responses were seen in 54% of the treated patients. Importantly, 3/22 (14%) of these poor-prognosis patients have remained continuously disease-free at full performance status now for a minimum of 6 years with lead follow-up to beyond 9.5 years. While this is a small series, it is in contrast to previous efforts where the identification of patients remaining continuously disease-free for extended periods of time is essentially unknown. The high frequency of complete remissions and the fraction of patients with extended disease-free survival suggested that treatment at time of a lower tumor volume might result in a higher frequency of complete remissions and also a higher frequency of durable remissions.

We therefore instituted a trial in which patients with measurable, metastatic breast cancer were treated initially with an induction chemotherapy using an intensive doxorubicin-based regimen and followed this by high-dose consolidation using cyclophosphamide, cisplatin, and carmustine with ABMS. The results have shown an increase in the complete response frequency to 60% of all patients entered on study and 68% of all transplanted patients (5/45 patients were not able to go onto transplant either because of disease progression or refusal). The extended follow-up of these patients shows that 25% of the patients who achieved a complete remission remain continuously disease-free with minimum follow-up of 4 years.

These data suggest that tumor volume reduction may be important in improving the outcome after high-dose therapy. For this reason, we sought to evaluate high-dose therapy in patients with high-risk primary breast cancer. In a recently analyzed trial, we studied 102 patients with primary breast cancer that involved 10 or more axillary lymph nodes at the time of initial surgery. Patients were treated with four cycles of induction CAF and then planned high-dose CPA/cDDP/BCNU and ABMS. Eighty-five patients completed the treatment program and were eligible. Of these patients, 72% have remained event-free with a minimum follow-up of 16 months, a lead follow-up of over 5 years, and a median follow-up of 2.5 years. The program was associated with significant toxicity; the therapy-related mortality was 12%. There was also a high frequency of late toxicity, including pulmonary toxicity. Quality-of-life studies revealed, however, that patients 1 year or more post-transplant were functioning normally. These results, if confirmed in the ongoing, prospective randomized trials, have important implications for oncology practice. The extension of this type of therapeutic approach, perhaps coupled with more aggressive induction therapy, may prove useful in earlier breast cancer.

Conclusion

The use of high-dose therapy in breast cancer is in its infancy as a therapeutic modality in treatment. The data available from studies in both metastatic and primary breast cancer indicate, however, that this approach can result in a higher frequency of complete remission, which in some poor-prognosis patients has resulted in extended disease-free survival. The early results in high-risk primary disease are also encouraging and suggest that the treatment for breast cancer may not be as hopeless as some have suggested.

References

1. Tannock I, Boyd N, DeBoer G, et al: A randomized trial of two dose levels of cyclophosphamide, methotrexate, and fluorouracil chemotherapy for patients with metastatic breast cancer. J Clin Oncol 1988;6:1377–1387.
2. Budman DR, Wood W, Henderson IC, Korzun AH, et al: Initial findings of CALGB 8541: a dose and dose intensity trial of cyclophosphamide (C), doxorubicin (A), and 5-fluorouracil (F) as adjuvant treatment of stage II, node +, female breast cancer. Proc Am Soc Clin Oncol 1992;11:291.
3. Peters WP, Shpali EJ, Jones RB, Olsen G, et al: Critical factors in the design of high-dose combination chemotherapy regimens. In: Herzig TP (ed). Advances in Cancer Chemotherapy. Park Row, New York, pp 43–52, 1987.
4. Peters WP, Shpall EJ, Jones RB, Olsen GA, et al: High dose combination alkylating agents with bone marrow support as initial treatment for metastatic breast cancer. J Clin Oncol 1988;6:1368–1376.
5. Peters WP, Jones RB, Shpali EJ, Shogan J: Dose intensification using high-dose combination alkylating agents and autologous bone marrow support for the treatment of breast cancer. In: Dicke KA, Spitzer G, Jagannath S (eds). Autologous Bone Marrow Transplantation. Proceedings of the Fourth International Symposium. Univ. of Texas MD Anderson Cancer Center, Houston, pp 389–397, 1989.
6. Peters WP: Dose intensification using high-dose combination alkylating agents and autologous bone marrow support in the treatment of primary and metastatic breast cancer: a review of the Duke Bone Marrow Transplantation Program experience. In: Ragaz J, Ariel IM (eds). High-Risk Breast Cancer, Springer-Verlag, Berlin, pp 437–446, 1991.
7. Peters WP: High-dose chemotherapy and autologous bone marrow support for breast cancer. In: DeVita VT, Hellman S, Rosenberg SA (eds). Important Advances in Oncology. J.B. Lippincott Co, Philadelphia, pp 135–150, 1991.
8. Peters WP, Ross M, Vredenburgh JJ, Nadel S, et al: High-dose chemotherapy and autologous bone marrow support as consolidation after standard dose adjuvant therapy for high-risk primary breast cancer. J Clin Oncol, in press.

Section **VI**

Miscellaneous Topics

Editorial Commentary

Chapter 42

In this age of cost consciousness, we felt it would be worthwhile to compare the cost of conservative surgery versus mastectomy. We are, however, still of the "old school," and believe that cost should not play a role in choosing between these two forms of therapy. It is not uncommon that a side effect of progress is increased cost. Fortunately, until recently in the United States we have been able to deliver state-of-the-art medical therapy without regard for cost. As we move into the next century, however, we may have to prioritize and reassess how we can utilize our limited resources. This chapter raises some provocative ethical questions in this regard.

Chapters 43 and 44

Ten percent of the American population is African-American and statistics consistently show that African-American women have a worse outcome with breast cancer than white women. We feel that is important to point out that the factors influencing the differences in outcome are not easily identified. Further research is required to sort out the importance of socioeconomic versus biological factors.

Chapters 45 and 46

In two outstanding chapters, the role of immunology as a key for the evaluation of patients with breast cancer is discussed. Dr. Black advocates an expanded use for the immunological assessment of breast cancer patients and

From: Wise L, Johnson H Jr (eds): *Breast Cancer: Controversies in Management.* Futura Publishing Company, Inc., Armonk, NY, © 1994.

present arguments as to why an immunological evaluation of all breast cancer patients should be done routinely. In contrast, Drs. Wallack and Scoggin conclude from the available data that current immunology techniques provide no information that have demonstrably convincing prognostic value.

Chapter 47

Dr. Maguire cites a number of articles that indicate fewer body image problems with lumpectomy than with mastectomy. Some of these lumpectomy patients, however, experienced increased anxiety due to excessive fear of recurrence of their cancer (this anxiety may have been due to inadequate preoperative counseling). The foregoing seems to be the main evidence supporting Dr. Maguire's thesis that "breast conservation does not reduce psychological morbidity." In our own patients, we found (American Journal Psychiatry 1985; 34:142) that the lumpectomy patients had significantly less loss of feelings of attractiveness and femininity than the mastectomy patients. Additionally, lumpectomy patients rated their husbands' sexual behavior as having been enhanced after surgery whereas the mastectomy patients felt that their husbands' sexual behavior showed a decline. We also compared the two treatment groups with regard to the frequency of severe sexual dysfunction; this was almost three times as common in the mastectomy group as in the lumpectomy group.

Chapter 48

Dr. Mueller in a thoughtful study reemphasizes the fact that a decade or so ago the surgeon was the "captain" of the ship with regard to patients with breast cancer; nowadays, however, all the subspecialists, including the diagnostic radiologist (mammographer), the radiotherapist, the medical oncologist, the pathologist, the statistician, and to some degree, even the patient herself are fighting to be the "captain" of the ship, i.e., to be in charge, the net result being that no one is in charge.

Chapter 49

In this final chapter, Professor Forrest presents his views on breast cancer management, including prevention, screening, and treatment. He feels the approach for the future lies in multidisciplinary team management, where the surgeon may be the leader, but only if he devotes most, if not all, of his time to the management of breast disease.

42

The Cost of Breast Cancer Therapy:
Minimal Surgery Versus Mastectomy

Benjamin Pace, Eric Munoz,
Leslie Wise

Introduction

The art and science of surgery are applied for two principal indications: to save life or limb and to improve on the quality of life. Debate concerning the various surgical options for a given disease entity must, at the outset, take into consideration the success with which each option fulfills this charge. Breast cancer surgery is no different in this regard. Considerations of cost containment and appropriate use of hospital resources, though quite important, are of little value if the applied treatment does not deal with the disease process as well as improve on the quality of life of the patient.

Traditional radical mastectomy has slowly been replaced with modified radical mastectomy (MRM) and, more recently, with lumpectomy and axillary dissection plus radiation therapy (LAR). This approach is logical if one assumes that breast cancer is often a systemic disease from the start. Surgery, rather than chemotherapy and/or hormonal therapy, may be the *adjuvant* therapy, providing only local control of a widespread process. Regardless of the point of view, breast-conserving LAR has been convincingly shown to be *as effective* as MRM for the majority of patients with breast cancer.[1-3]

Both MRM and LAR have equally fulfilled their first charge, being associated with similar survival rates. Yet, what is the cost of these "equivalent" treatments? Unfortunately, we are forced to ask these questions. The rapid proliferation of medical technology during the past several decades has outstripped our

From: Wise L, Johnson H Jr (eds): *Breast Cancer: Controversies in Management.* Futura Publishing Company, Inc., Armonk, NY, © 1994.

485

ability as a nation to bankroll all available medical diagnostic and therapeutic interventions. Under these circumstances, priorities must be set. Until recently, a reticent physician population has been unwilling to establish these priorities, instead finding themselves the "victim" of government regulation. Physicians must confront this reality by questioning the cost-effectiveness of their common practices and determining *their* priorities.

In an attempt to further understand health care costs, a recent study by our group compared the cost of modified radical mastectomy alone versus lumpectomy with axillary dissection plus postoperative radiotherapy. It identified a significantly greater cost for breast-conserving surgery.[4] This study is reviewed for the benefit of the reader.[*]

Methods

Financial data were obtained for 79 of our patients with either stage I or stage II breast carcinoma treated during 1983/1984 at the Long Island Jewish Medical Center, an 805-bed voluntary teaching hospital in New York City. The studies were retrospective; financial data were computed for the total mean charges (hospital and physician) for the primary treatment for this disease. Treatment for lumpectomy patients consisted of lumpectomy, axillary dissection, and postoperative radiotherapy. Financial data for lumpectomy patients included hospital inpatient charges, surgeons' fees, and the cost of the standard 6-week course of the postoperative radiotherapy. The cost of radiotherapy included hospital outpatient charges and radiotherapist (physician) fees.

Patients treated by mastectomy had a standard modified radical mastectomy and did not receive any postoperative radiotherapy. Their financial charges were totaled to include hospital inpatient charges and surgeons' fees. No other physician charges, such as for anesthesiologists, consulting physicians, or chemotherapists, were included for either lumpectomy or mastectomy patients in this analysis.

Inpatient hospital charges for both therapies were computed by hospital service area, including room and board, laboratory (i.e., hematology, urinalysis, coagulation studies, blood chemistry, and microbiology), blood processing (i.e., blood and blood products), operating room/recovery room, central supply-pharmacy, diagnostic radiology, and other (pathology, estrogen receptors, respiratory therapy, etc.). Students' *t* test was used to compare statistical significance between the charges for lumpectomy and mastectomy.

Results

Seventy-nine patients were studied; 49 had lumpectomy and 30 had mastectomy. No patients in this series had complications or required reoperation. Mean length of stay (LOS) for lumpectomy patients was 7.9 ± 4.1 days, and for

---

[*]Portions reprinted by permission of the American Medical Association.

Table 1
Total Charges* for Lumpectomy and Mastectomy

	Mean ($\pm$ SEM) Charge per Patient, $	
	Lumpectomy (n = 49)	Mastectomy (n = 30)
Hospital inpatient	5741 $\pm$ 2805	7328 $\pm$ 3058
Surgeon	1943 $\pm$ 990	3016 $\pm$ 397
Hospital outpatient (radiotherapy)	5015 $\pm$ 81	–
Radiotherapist (physician)	2562 $\pm$ 123	–
Total*	$14,176 $\pm$ 4262[a]	$10,345 $\pm$ 3134[a]

*Sum of the mean for each individual service does not necessarily equal mean total charge per patient.
[a]Statistically significant at P <.01.
Reprinted by permission from Munoz E, Shamash F, Friedman M, Rosner G, Wise L: Lumpectomy vs. mastectomy: costs of breast preservation for cancer. Arch Surg 1986; 121:1298–1301.

mastectomy patients, 9.9 ± 4.5 days. Mean total physician charges per patient for lumpectomy included surgeon, 1943 ± 990, and radiotherapist, 2562 ± 123, for a total of $4505. Mean total physician charges for mastectomy included surgeon only, 3016 ± 397. Total physician charges per patient were 49.3% greater for lumpectomy than for mastectomy patients (P<.0001).

Hospital inpatient charges for lumpectomy were 5741 ± 2776 (mean total $\pm$ SEM per patient), and for mastectomy, 7328 ± 3007 (Table 1). Thus, hospital inpatient charges were 27.6% greater for mastectomy patients than for lumpectomy patients (P<.02). Each hospital service area demonstrated charges that were usually significantly greater for mastectomy than lumpectomy: room and board, 25.7% greater; laboratory 37.6% greater; diagnostic radiology, 37.6% greater; blood processing, 37.7% greater; operating room/recovery room, 28.5% greater; central supply-pharmacy, 27.8% greater; and other, 29.2% greater. Laboratory, diagnostic radiology, and blood processing demonstrated the greatest differences (expressed as percentages) between lumpectomy and mastectomy patients (Table 1). As noted, mean total hospital and physician charges were 37% greater (P<.01) for lumpectomy than for mastectomy patients ($14,176 vs. $10,345).

These results demonstrate that for the treatment of potentially curable breast cancer, the total charges for lumpectomy were 37% more expensive than those for mastectomy (P<.01). There was no significant difference in charges between stage I and stage II patients treated with either lumpectomy or mastectomy. Although hospital inpatient fees were significantly less (P<.02) for lumpectomy ($5741) than for mastectomy ($7328), mean total physician charges were significantly higher (P<.0001) for lumpectomy ($4505, surgeon plus radiotherapist) than for mastectomy ($3016, surgeon only). In addition, the substantial radiation therapy hospital outpatient charge for lumpectomy ($5015) makes total charges for this therapy higher than for mastectomy.

Discussion

Lumpectomy proved to be significantly more expensive than mastectomy, mainly due to the requirement for 6 weeks of costly postoperative radiotherapy. It seems clear that, purely from the standpoint of survival versus cost, MRM provides an equal survival rate while being 37% less expensive than LAR in the treatment of early breast cancer. With the present health care cost crisis, would it not be reasonable, then, to limit the option of women to just mastectomy?

The answer in the case of breast cancer surgery lies in the second charge of surgical therapy, the provision of an improvement in the quality of life. Despite the decrees of those who would enjoin breast-conserving therapy for *all* patients, many women are satisfied with the outcome of MRM without reconstruction. In our practice, this is especially true for the older patient. Indeed, across the country, about half the patients choose this option after lengthy discussion in which the choices are carefully weighed with physician, family, and friends. For these patients, MRM not only fulfills the charge of surgical therapy but also allows for the conservation of scarce health care resources.

In contrast, many other women (often in a younger age group) are quite concerned with body self-image. For them, mastectomy alone, while effectively treating the local disease, does not answer their needs in respect to quality of life. The addition of breast reconstruction to MRM, while beneficial for many, significantly alters the cost of MRM, resulting on average with a more expensive therapy than LAR. In addition, the results with postmastectomy reconstruction, in general, are less cosmetically acceptable than those after LAR. The balance of cost versus efficacy in MRM plus plastic surgical reconstruction versus LAR clearly favors LAR in those patients in whom body self-image is a significant factor.

Finally, the greatest loss in both human and economic terms is in those patients in whom body self-image is pivotal, yet a mastectomy alone is performed for whatever reason. The psychological impact may be great, resulting in a failure to fulfill the charge of surgical care. The patient's quality of life and productivity may be diminished, sometimes overtly, but often subtly. One cannot weigh the cost of this type of failure.

In summary, the increased cost of LAR versus MRM, as demonstrated, is an important factor that must be kept in mind by all breast surgeons. Yet, in treating breast cancer as in treating all other surgical diseases, the gold standard by which all therapies should be judged first is the efficacy with which it fulfills its charge in treating disease *as well as* in improving the quality of life for the patient. In dealing with breast cancer, therapy must be individualized. MRM *is* acceptable in patients with early breast cancer not focused on body self-image, who are afraid of recurring tumor or unwilling or unable to undergo weeks of radiation therapy. These patients should not be made to feel out of touch or old-fashioned for choosing a therapy which, while effective, conserves health care dollars. Conversely, it would be a mistake to move toward imposing MRM on patients quite concerned with body self-image (who understand and accept radiotherapy and the possible local recurrence associated with LAR) under the guise of saving society an added expense. As pointed out, the addition of breast reconstruction to MRM in these patients places the balance of cost savings in favor of LAR.

The greatest economic advantage to society is that of a *functional* member at peace with his/her disease and treatment. This balance can only be achieved by a lengthy discussion of the treatment options with each individual patient. The cost-effectiveness of these options vary from individual to individual, as noted. Therapy for breast cancer must be individualized, not legislated for society as a whole. In this manner, it is possible to reap the maximum benefit for the patient while simultaneously receiving the maximum return on the health care dollar.

References

1. Fisher B, Redmond C, Poisson R, Margolese R, et al: Eight-year results of a randomized clinical trial comparing total mastectomy and lumpectomy with or without irradiation in the treatment of breast cancer. N Engl J Med 1989; 320:822–828.
2. Veronesi U: Rationale and indications for limited surgery in breast cancer: current data. World J Surg 1987; 11:493–498.
3. Wise L, Mason AY, Ackerman L: Local excision and irradiation: an alternative method for the treatment of early mammary cancer. Ann Surg 1971; 174:392.
4. Munoz E, Shamash F, Friedman M, Rosner G, Wise L: Lumpectomy and mastectomy: costs of breast preservation for cancer. Arch Surg 1986; 121:1297–1301.

43

The Dubious Nature of Ethnicity as a Risk Factor in Breast Cancer

Vernon J. Henderson, Claude H. Organ, Jr., Maria Soler

Introduction and Background

Breast cancer is second only to lung cancer as a cause of cancer deaths in American women. Although white American women have a 30% higher incidence of developing breast cancer than African-Americans, the overall mortality rates are approximately equal in these populations.[1,2] Whites have a significantly higher long-term survival rate than blacks despite adjustments for age and tumor stage.[3,4] Blacks have larger, more undifferentiated tumors at presentation and a higher incidence of nodal metastases at presentation.[3,4] Estrogen and progesterone receptors—biological markers whose presence correlate directly with improved survival—are less frequent in black women than in whites.[5] Black women under the age of 40 have a higher incidence of breast cancer and a worse prognosis than age- and stage-matched whites.

When white American women are compared with native-born Japanese and Chinese women, the risk of breast cancer remains higher for whites, but the survival figures strongly favor Asian women.[6,7] These striking racial differences are reduced when comparing American-born Japanese and Chinese to white Americans, but the differences remain statistically significant.

Observed racial differences in breast cancer incidence and survival strongly imply that race may represent a significant factor in breast cancer risk and prognosis. This conclusion can be, and continues to be, drawn from a superficial analysis of international epidemiologic studies on breast cancer incidence and survival.[2,6–8] The dangers associated with drawing conclusions about the role of

From: Wise L, Johnson H Jr (eds): *Breast Cancer: Controversies in Management.* Futura Publishing Company, Inc., Armonk, NY, © 1994.

race in breast cancer epidemiology on the basis of incomplete data or insignificant analysis is demonstrated by several important epidemiologic reports. Differences in breast cancer incidence between native Oriental and American women are reduced after living for a single generation in a Westernized society.[9] This observation, and similar observations in other ethnic groups, provide a strong argument for the significance of an environmental contribution to breast cancer risk since this change could not occur so rapidly as a result of a fundamental genetic change in the transplanted population.[10] Several factors, not related to race, also appear to significantly impact on the risk and prognosis of breast cancer. As the list of important factors that account for the observed racial differences in breast cancer risk grows, the importance of race as an important isolated risk factor is greatly diminished. Race continues to be viewed as a significant predictor of breast cancer risk and survival in spite of our understanding of the multiplicity of breast cancer etiology and outcome.[11]

Epidemiology of Breast Cancer

Epidemiologic observations have fostered our understanding of the risks of developing breast cancer within a population. Female gender, increasing age, aspects of the menstrual history, family history, and personal history of breast cancer are increasingly well-documented factors that contribute to the risk of developing this disease. Of the additional factors that possibly contribute to breast cancer risk, socioeconomic status is one of the most influential. The exact manner in which this factor contributes to breast cancer risk is not fully understood. One possible explanation holds that women of higher socioeconomic status delay having children until later in life than women of lower socioeconomic status, thereby increasing their age at first pregnancy, a well-known factor that increases breast cancer risk. Race and socioeconomic status are directly related to breast cancer incidence in countries such as the United States, England, and South Africa where the population is diverse, racial discrimination is endemic, and segments of the population are forced to live in conditions of poverty despite great national wealth.[1,2,12–15]

Large-scale population mortality studies from England and Wales were among the first to document a definite correlation between breast cancer mortality and social class. Social class was determined by the husband's occupation in these population surveys. Women of high social class experienced a higher than expected mortality rate from breast cancer when compared with the expected overall mortality for their group. The converse was observed in women of lower social class.[16]

Mortality data from such studies has subsequently undergone more intensive scrutiny. Social class-associated mortality differences reflect an increased incidence of breast cancer in women of high social status, and a decreased incidence of breast cancer in women of lower social class. Since the mortality rates for breast cancer are virtually the same for both groups, the increased mortality witnessed in the early studies was a reflection of the increased incidence of breast cancer within the higher social class. The association of breast cancer risk and socioeconomic status has been observed in multiple international studies from Denmark, Scotland, Norway, Hong Kong, Australia, and Finland.[8,17,18]

Dietary fat intake, obesity, alcohol consumption, stress, and caffeine ingestion, all of which relate to socioeconomic status, are associated with an increased risk of developing breast cancer. Among this growing list of risk factors, which are of a distinct environmental nature, the white race is still considered a risk factor for breast cancer and the black race is still considered a risk factor which predicts poor prognosis for breast cancer survival.[11]

The importance of race among the growing list of factors determining breast cancer incidence and mortality remains unclear, but in light of our current understanding of nonracial factors that contribute to breast cancer risk and prognosis, the issue of race deserves reexamination. This review will examine the evidence supporting the influence of race on breast cancer risk and prognosis and interpret this influence in light of our current understanding of the pathogenesis of breast cancer.

Breast Cancer in Blacks: Effect of Race on Breast Cancer Incidence

Reliable information regarding the epidemiology of breast cancer in black women has become available only in the past few decades. Henschke,[19] in 1973, brought national attention to the increasing cancer mortality rates in the US black population. Mortality rates for a number of cancer sites (including breast cancer) were noted to be increasing at a significantly higher rate in blacks when compared to whites. Potential factors explaining this increased cancer mortality rate in the black population included differences in (1) reporting of mortality information, (2) age, (3) cure rate, and (4) environmental factors. Genetic differences were discounted as a possible explanation for the rising cancer mortality in blacks since the observed changes occurred over one generation, a time span too short for any substantial population genetic changes. Henschke called for a more thorough investigation of the racial differences in cancer incidence and mortality.

Since the report by Henschke, racial differences in cancer incidence and mortality have received more attention. Multiple epidemiologic studies have recently appeared that document several factors that affect the incidence and mortality of breast cancer in black women. Such studies have attempted to clarify the role of race in the epidemiology of breast cancer in blacks. These studies have examined factors that are race-related (but not genetically determined), which could potentially account for racial differences in breast cancer risk and survival. Several studies serve to focus our attention on the appropriate issues.

Devesa and Diamond[1] provided the first report demonstrating the association of socioeconomic variables such as education and income on the incidence of breast cancer in black women. Data from the 1969–1971 Third National Cancer

Survey (TNCS) were correlated with socioeconomic information on education and income obtained from the 1970 census. A direct correlation of breast cancer incidence with rising socioeconomic status was demonstrated for both blacks and whites. This correlation had previously been reported for US whites, but had not been previously examined in African-Americans. Adjustment of incidence data for level of education significantly reduced the incidence gap noted between white and black women. However, this difference remained statistically significant.

This report demonstrated that (1) the well-described pattern directly associating breast cancer incidence with increasing socioeconomic status was identical for black and white women, and (2) when information on breast cancer incidence was adjusted for socioeconomic factors such as income and education, the gap in incidence between whites and blacks was significantly reduced. Adjustments for socioeconomic status could not eliminate the black/white disparity in breast cancer incidence. However, this study was important because it convincingly demonstrated that factors other than race contributed significantly to the observed differences in breast cancer incidence between black and white women.

McWhorter and associates[13] examined data from the Cancer Surveillance, Epidemiology, and End Results Program (SEER), which included approximately 20,000 black patients with cancer involving various sites including the breast. This database, compiled over the period 1978–1982, was analyzed by adjusting the incidence data for socioeconomic factors such as poverty. This survey demonstrated that poverty accounted for most, if not all, of the observed racial differences in breast cancer incidence between blacks and whites. White women had been shown by this databank to have a 20% higher overall risk of developing breast cancer. This higher risk was virtually eliminated by adjusting the data for the incidence of poverty. This study concluded that the observed black/white differences in breast cancer incidence were largely a function of socioeconomic status and less a function of race.

The extent to which individual socioeconomic factors affect breast cancer incidence remains unclear; however, the growing list of factors that influence breast cancer risk continue to narrow the observed ethnic/racial differences in incidence described above. Furthermore, enumeration of factors affecting breast cancer incidence provides important clues to the pathogenesis of breast cancer.

Epidemiologic studies that identify such nongenetic, etiologic factors underscore the importance of environmental factors in breast cancer pathogenesis, and race emerges as a factor of secondary importance in breast cancer risk. Race, through its effect on socioeconomic variables, only indirectly influences breast cancer risk. Ample evidence exists to corroborate this effect. Black women of high socioeconomic status who have been able to overcome the effects of race in determining socioeconomic status have breast cancer rates that are as high as those experienced by whites of similar socioeconomic status.[20] Similarly, poor white women, who have overcome the effects of race in determining socioeconomic status, experience reduced breast cancer risks comparable to blacks who are matched for socioeconomic status.[1] Therefore, breast cancer incidence is significantly influenced by variables that are related to *socioeconomic status*. Highest *level of education* attained appears to have the most important influence on the breast cancer incidence in black females.

The association of breast cancer incidence with *age at first pregnancy* is well documented. Several studies have demonstrated that late age at first pregnancy is largely influenced by the socioeconomic variable of education, and is explained by the fact that women who seek higher education delay the time to their first pregnancy until later in life compared with women who do not seek higher education. Higher education directly determines socioeconomic status. Therefore, socioeconomic status, education, and later age at first pregnancy are linked. Black women who attain higher education and delay the time to their first pregnancy experience an increased incidence of breast cancer that is approximately equal to that of whites.[1]

Breast Cancer in Blacks: Effect of Race on Breast Cancer Survival

Dayal and associates[21] evaluated the effects of race and socioeconomic status on survival from breast cancer. Nine hundred and three patients (515 white and 388 black) treated at the Medical College of Virginia for pathologically confirmed breast cancer were reviewed. Survival results were correlated with socioeconomic status in a subset of 323 (117 white and 206 black) of these patients from Richmond, Virginia. Statistically significant correlations were found between race and socioeconomic status, race and survival, stage at diagnosis and survival, and socioeconomic status and survival *in a univariate analysis of these factors*. However, multivariate analysis revealed socioeconomic status as the only important independent variable that affected patient survival. Dayal concluded that the observed survival differences between black and white breast cancer patients are attributed to differences in socioeconomic status between these groups and not to inherent racial differences.

Bassett and Krieger[22] examined the effect of social class on the black/white differences in breast cancer survival. Survival data for 268 black patients and 1,293 white patients from northwestern Washington State were analyzed. These data were correlated with 1980 census block data as a measure of socioeconomic status. The forms of treatment offered, the first course of therapy given, and patient follow-up were similar for blacks and whites in this study. After adjustments of the data for social class, black and white survival differences, previously noted in each social stratum, disappeared. This study concluded that studies examining racial differences in survival were possibly incomplete and misleading if they neglected to consider jointly the role of social class on patient survival.

Cella and associates[14] examined the effect of socioeconomic status on initial performance status (IPS), a highly significant predictor of survival, in patients with various cancers including breast cancer. They found that income and education were independently predictive of survival. However, race was not an independent predictor of length of survival. Cella concluded that socioeconomic variables, because of their significance as prognostic variables, should be included in the data of all clinical trials to more accurately test the efficacy of therapeutic regimens in different patient subgroups.

Dansey and associates[15] compared breast cancer survival between South African whites and blacks and concluded that ethnic origin was not a significant independent variable that affected the prognosis for survival for women with breast cancer. Subsequent studies have described several potential factors that appear to influence the incidence and prognosis of breast cancer in black women. These include obesity,[2] nutritional status,[23] the attitudes and beliefs of patients,[24] and the medical profession.[25–27] The extent to which any one of these factors influence the observed differences in breast cancer risk and prognosis among blacks is dubious. In all of the studies cited above, any observed racial differences in outcome were reduced by consideration of socioeconomic factors. Such studies have served to discount the significance of race as an independent factor determining breast cancer risk and prognosis.

Clinical Studies that Promote Racial Mythology

Several large clinical surveys are frequently cited in the literature concerning black/white differences in breast cancer survival. The surveys conducted by the American College of Surgeons are frequently cited because they report large numbers of cases that include detailed classification of patients into risk groups based on clinical criteria alone. These studies have generally demonstrated reduced survival for black breast cancer patients at all stages of disease, and strongly imply that the black race is an important indicator of poor prognosis for patients with breast cancer. These studies will be reviewed to provide a background for further examination of the issue of race as a determinant of breast cancer risk and prognosis.

The second Annual National Cancer Survey conducted by the ACS in 1978 was devoted to the study of cancer of the breast.[3] Over 24,000 breast cancer cases were analyzed, which included 1,988 breast cancers in black women. This represented a sufficiently large cohort of cancers in black women to allow comparison of the treatment results with those observed in white patients. Black women had (1) a lower percentage of localized cancers, (2) a higher percentage of advanced cancers, (3) a higher percentage of large tumors, and (4) lower 5-year survival for breast cancer at all stages compared to white women. Clinical cure rates were similar for black and white women with small tumors and negative axillary lymph nodes, but the clinical cure rates were better for white women with larger tumors and negative nodes. The authors concluded that the reduced survival witnessed in blacks was attributable to the presence of more advanced cancers at presentation, and not to the presence of biologically more active tumors in blacks. These conclusions were reached despite clear evidence that blacks witnessed reduced survival rates for breast cancer at all stages of disease compared to whites.

The 1985 American College of Surgeons report included information from the 1982 National Cancer Survey.[4] Over 27,000 patients were analyzed in this study, including 2,296 black patients: (1) significantly more black patients presented with large and clinically advanced tumors, (2) black women had a significantly lower incidence of estrogen receptor-positive tumors compared to white women, and (3) blacks experienced significantly reduced overall survival rates when matched by stage with whites. Multivariate analysis of survival data revealed clinical stage of disease, race, age, and estrogen receptor status as independent variables that had a significant impact on length of survival. A number of epidemiologic variables were assessed in this study which revealed a statistically significant difference in black patients and included age at menopause, age at first pregnancy, average number of pregnancies, and mean delay between tumor discovery and diagnosis between black and white patients. The conclusions of this survey strongly implied that race represents an important independent risk factor in the incidence and, in particular, the prognosis for survival in breast cancer.

The two surveys cited above represent misleading studies which, despite their conduct and appropriate statistical methodology, lead to conclusions that reflect a superficial analysis of a complex topic. Both of these studies discount the importance of socioeconomic variables as important contributors to the observed racial differences in breast cancer risk and prognosis. The extent to which any one of these socioeconomic variables contributes to the overall risk of breast cancer incidence and prognosis remains in question. However, as demonstrated by Bassett[22] and Cella,[14] socioeconomic information such as education, income, and place of residence should be included in and adjusted for any analysis of breast cancer incidence and survival. If such factors are not considered, the conclusions drawn from such studies are likely to be misleading or incorrect.

A second major omission in the American College of Surgeons surveys cited is the lack of consideration for treatment variables in assessing the racial differences in breast cancer survival. McWhorter and Mayer[28] have demonstrated that significant differences emerge when the types of initial treatments offered black and white breast cancer patients are compared. Blacks are *offered* surgery, radiation therapy, and chemotherapy less frequently, and accept these suggested forms less frequently than white patients. Other surveys reveal significant differences in the *attitudes* of blacks and whites regarding the meaning and expected outcome of cancer diagnosis and treatment. Blacks who were surveyed regarding the meaning of a cancer diagnosis generally tend to view such a diagnosis as a death sentence, and that the form of therapy cannot alter that dismal outcome.[24] These factors may significantly affect the observed incidence of breast cancer reported in black women by affecting the reporting frequency. The potential effect of these negative attitudes on survival of black patients with breast cancer are more immediately obvious if blacks are unwilling to believe in or accept prescribed cancer therapies. The presence of such attitudes, which affect outcome in a negative fashion, should focus more sharply the educational commitment of our professional organizations.

Treatment-related data seldom appears in cancer surveys describing the survival of black breast cancer patients. A typical assumption is apparently made that all patients included in clinical surveys *receive the same levels of care;* and therefore, the effect of any treatment differences on clinical outcome is minimal. In light of what is known regarding the attitudes of blacks towards a cancer diagnosis and cancer therapy, this assumption is obviously not accurate. Multiple studies reveal that African-Americans have *limited access* to health care, and on entering the system are offered state-of-the-art therapies much less frequently than their white counterparts. Blacks receive kidney transplants less frequently than whites despite the fact that blacks make up a large percentage of those on the waiting list for kidney transplants.[25,26] Similar forces undoubtedly apply to cancer therapeutic regimens, which often involve complex treatment and follow up protocols, and are assumed to be too complex and demanding for poor black patients. These assumptions have been proven false by studies that offer blacks state-of-the-art cancer care.

Briele and associates[29] reported on the results of treatment of stage I through stage III breast cancer patients at Cook County Hospital in Chicago over the period 1973–1987. This study analyzed the treatment results of 526 black women diagnosed and treated at Cook County Hospital. Their treatment outcomes were compared with published survival figures from large-scale clinical studies such as the NSABP and Milan Cancer Institute study protocols. This study is significant because it addresses *treatment outcome* in a traditionally high-risk population of poor black women. It reports in detail treatment outcomes *based on* (1) forms of initial therapy, (2) adjuvant chemotherapy prescribed, (3) rates of completion of prescribed chemotherapy and radiotherapy, and (4) reasons for failures to complete prescribed therapy. This study demonstrated projected 5- and 10-year overall survival rates of 83.9% and 76.6%, respectively, for 272 *node-negative* women, and 58.1% and 35.2%, respectively, for 72 *node-positive* women. These rates compare quite favorably with the projected 5- and 10-year overall survival rates reported by the NSABP and the Milan Cancer Institute. This study demonstrates convincingly that breast cancer outcome in black patients is highly influenced by treatment, as it is in white patients, and that race and low socioeconomic status do not necessarily predict a poor outcome if patients are offered and accept conventional therapy. It is clear that poor black women *can be entered* into complex treatment protocols and *can successfully complete* such protocols with similar results obtained in stage-matched nonblack patients.

Studies such as this negate the significance of race as a risk factor for breast cancer survival by demonstrating that when given equal access to treatment and follow up, there are no racial differences in treatment outcome.

Tumor Biology and the Pathogenesis of Breast Cancer

Biological markers that serve as predictors of tumor behavior are important tools in cancer therapy and also provide important clues regarding the pathogenesis of breast cancer. Several predictors of the clinical behavior of breast cancers have been identified and include tumor size, axillary node status, steroid hormone receptors, histopathological tumor grade, cellular kinetics and DNA content, and oncogene expression.[30] These prognostic indicators predict with varying accuracy the time to relapse of breast cancer and the overall survival. Racial differences in these biological markers have received attention as potential clues to explaining the reduced survival of breast cancer witnessed in black patients in several studies. The significance of the observed racial differences in biological markers are subject to various interpretations. Some interpret racial differences in markers (such as tumor grade and estrogen receptor status) as evidence of biologically more aggressive tumors in black women. Such differences in tumor phenotypic expression are viewed as evidence of a *fundamental difference* in the nature of breast cancers that develop in black women compared with other ethnic groups. Other evidence suggests that observed racial differences in biological markers *represent epiphenomena* reflective of the advanced clinical stage at presentation of breast cancers in black women, which are the result of socioeconomic factors or patient attitudes. Conflicting reports from recognized centers that support either viewpoint have not served to resolve this issue. Some of the major points will be outlined below.

Several large studies have compared the incidence of large tumors and axillary lymph node metastasis in black and white patients. Nemoto,[3] in 1978, surveyed 1,988 black women with breast cancer and found that black women had larger tumors with more frequent axillary nodal metastases at presentation than white women. The reduced survival witnessed in black women was attributed to *late stage* of presentation. In a subsequent study, Natarajan[4] confirmed that black women had differences in tumor size and frequency of nodal metastases at presentation when compared with white women (statistically significant). The authors concluded that these differences were unlikely to be due to socioeconomic factors alone, and suggested that some inherent differences in the malignant behavior of breast cancers existed between black and white patients. Multiple studies have demonstrated that black women present with large tumors with a higher frequency of axillary nodal metastases. Most studies, however, attribute this observation to (1) delays in seeking treatment *after* breast masses have been discovered, or (2) lack of access to health care and utilization of early detection measures such as mammography and breast self-examination. Currently there is no information that could attribute these observed differences to race or some genetically determined difference between blacks and other ethnic groups. In fact, studies that document no differences in time to treatment and treatment received between blacks and whites show *no differences* in the outcome of black patients compared with white patients.[13,20–22,29]

Estrogen and progesterone receptor status have been demonstrated to have an independent effect on prognosis for breast cancer recurrence and overall survival and represent useful prognostic information regarding breast cancer clinical behavior. Estrogen receptor-positive patients are considered to have an improved disease-free survival when compared to estrogen receptor-negative patients at all stages of disease. This information may be helpful in patients who have early stage disease with negative axillary nodes. Although the overall prognosis for these patients (lymph node-negative) is good, those who are estrogen receptor-negative experience a worse prognosis but their long-term survival may improve with adjuvant chemotherapy. Positive progesterone receptor status appears to be helpful for patients with stage II disease and has been demonstrated to be as predictive as the number of positive axillary nodes in predicting disease recurrence. Steroid receptor status is also important in predicting response to endocrine therapy. Pegorano[31] has described the racial distribution of estrogen and progesterone receptor status in tumors in a large cohort of different ethnic groups in South Africans. He observed a significantly higher percentage of estrogen receptor-positive tumors in white South Africans compared to mixed race individuals, Asians, and blacks. Pegorano suggested that these differences represented inherent tumor biological differences and that race plays a strong role in racial differences of tumor behavior.

Mohla[5] and associates examined estrogen and progesterone receptor status in 146 black women treated at Howard University Hospital, and compared their results to reported rates of distribution of estrogen and progesterone receptors. Their patients *differed significantly* from reported norms established in white patients in three areas: (1) incidence of estrogen receptor-positive and -negative tumors, (2) incidence of poorly differentiated tumors, and (3) percentage of patients discovered with advanced disease. Black patients had (1) a *lower* incidence of estrogen receptor-positive tumors, (2) a *higher* incidence of estrogen receptor-negative tumors, (3) a higher incidence of poorly differentiated tumors, and (4) a higher percentage of patients discovered with advanced disease at presentation. Briele,[29] reporting on a series of 526 poor black patients, described estrogen- and progesterone-positive tumors with a frequency approximately equal to other large reported series of breast cancer patients.

Although differences in estrogen and progesterone receptor status have been noted by several investigators, there is presently no data to support a racial or genetic cause for these observations. Environmental factors such as estrogen and progesterone use in the form of oral contraceptives are known to affect the subsequent receptor status of female breast cancers.[32,33] The nature of these interactions is being worked out. Several of the proto-oncogene amplifications associated with the development of human breast cancer have been demonstrated to vitro using breast cancer cell lines exposed to exogenous steroid hormones.[32] Environmental factors (such as oral contraceptives) are likely to influence the steroid receptor status of individual breast cancers, and therefore the racial basis for differences in steroid receptor status is questionable.

Cell kinetic and DNA content studies have recently emerged as potentially important prognostic indicators of breast cancer clinical behavior. Cell kinetics, as determined by the percentage of cells in the DNA synthesis (S) phase of the cell cycle, is a measure of cellular proliferation. Thymidine-labeling index represents the proportion of cells in active DNA synthesis, and has been correlated with disease-free survival and overall survival.

Flow cytometry is used to assess the growth characteristics of tumors and determine their DNA index, the ratio of measured nuclear DNA content compared to the normal nuclear diploid DNA content, and percentage of cells in the DNA synthesis phase (%S phase). These parameters correlated with disease-free and overall survival. Currently the techniques of cell kinetics and flow cytometry have *not* demonstrated, in a large-scale clinical comparison of tumors of black and whites, any racial differences in flow cytometry or DNA content.

Molecular genetics has recently provided some interesting clues in identifying prognostic indicators for breast cancer behavior. Proto-oncogenes (normal cellular genes involved in normal cellular growth and differentiation) have been identified which undergo mutations to oncogenes and may play a role in the pathogenesis of some cancers. HER-2/Neu oncogene, also known as *c-erb* B-2 oncogene, has been shown to correlate with time to relapse and overall survival in women with breast cancer.[34,35] Although this area of research is undergoing intense investigation, no consistent pattern of association of HER-2/Neu with breast cancer prognosis has emerged. Amplification of this oncogene has generally been associated with larger, more advanced tumors, and its presence may simply reflect a tendency of more advanced tumors to express oncogene amplification. To date, this oncogene has not been correlated with breast cancers in black women.

The above techniques are described because they are currently being actively applied in prospective studies of the management of breast cancer as prognostic indicators of outcome and therapy response. An important outcome of this active area of research is an understanding of the fundamental cellular mechanisms responsible for the phenotypic expression of malignant behavior. Current theories suggest that a series of intracellular molecular events must occur in any given individual to result in malignant transformation. A number of proto-oncogenes have been linked to breast cancer development. Mechanisms by which these proto-oncogenes can escape their normal regulatory mechanisms and cause malignant transformation are currently being elucidated. Research in this area is likely to uncover many other environmental factors that could possibly account for the observed racial differences in breast cancer incidence and survival. It seems unlikely that a single genetic defect will be discovered that would account for all of these complex interactions.

Discussion

Debate continues over the role of race as an independent predictor of risk and prognosis in breast cancer. This issue is distorted by international epidemiologic studies that reveal large differences in the risk and survival of breast cancer patients in different countries. Such studies poignantly depict the dismal survival figures for African-American patients when compared to other racial and ethnic groups. Issues of race naturally result from examination of these studies because racial and ethnic differences are the most obvious differences between the populations studied. However, the strength of racial differences is weakened significantly when intra-national studies are performed and reveal a spectrum of risk and survival for breast cancer within countries that vary by social class. The intra-national spectrum is quite narrow in countries that are homogenous with respect to race/ethnicity and socioeconomic variables. However, the spectrum of breast cancer risk and survival is quite broad in countries, such as the United States, which are diverse in terms of race/ethnicity and socioeconomic variables.

The Japanese present the most favorable figures with respect to breast cancer incidence and survival. Japanese women have a lower overall risk of developing cancer of the breast, and their overall survival is better stage for stage than any other ethnic group in the world. The Japanese are a homogenous population with a high standard of living, and are among the most highly educated societies in the world. There are vast differences between the richest and poorest Japanese in terms of income; however, the number of Japanese who live in poverty is quite small. Access to health care is excellent in Japan, and the Japanese are quite well informed regarding health-related issues. A number of malignancies—gastric, pancreatic and liver—that predict a dismal prognosis in the United States have significantly better outcomes in the Japanese. Public awareness of these malignancies and widespread screening programs are largely responsible for these improvements. Such enlightened approaches to public health issues underscore the effectiveness and responsiveness of the Japanese people to their health needs.

When native-born Japanese women migrate to Western countries, significant changes in the risk and prognosis for breast cancer in the women of these families are noted within a single generation.[9] This represents too short a time period for purely genetic events through mutation and natural selection to impact on a population. Such a rapid change in the epidemiology of breast cancer could only occur as a result of environmental factors such as diet or environmental exposure. Factors other than race appear to explain the observed differences in breast cancer incidence and survival between Japanese women and other ethnic groups.

Epidemiologic studies in white women document a now familiar pattern of risk for breast cancer incidence and prognosis. Poor women experience a reduced risk of developing breast cancer compared to women of higher socioeconomic status. Their mortality rates are equal to or higher than the mortality rates experienced by women of higher social class. This pattern of risk and prognosis has been demonstrated in many ethnic groups, and verifies the strong association of breast cancer incidence and mortality with socioeconomic variables. Patterns of breast cancer incidence and mortality have been demonstrated in black patients in the United States and South Africa. These patients are generally of low socioecomomic status, and although the incidence of developing breast cancer is low in these patients, their mortality rates for breast cancer are equal to or higher than age- and stage-matched white women.

A number of clinical reports have appeared in the medical literature to explain the observed racial differences in breast cancer incidence and survival between blacks and whites. These reports have examined a number of factors to which the racial differences could be attributed. The conclusions reached by such studies relate directly to the number of nonracial factors that have been taken into account to examine these differences. Studies that did not take socioeconomic variables into account in their analysis generally conclude that race is an important independent factor that determined a woman's risk for developing breast cancer and affects the prognosis for survival after the diagnosis of breast cancer has been made. Studies that take into account the influence of multiple socioeconomic variables tend to discount the influence of race as an independent factor of importance in breast cancer risk and prognosis. Finally, the few studies that have accounted for both treatment variables and socioeconomic status in their analysis have totally discounted the influence of race as an important factor in breast cancer risk and prognosis.

Racial differences in breast cancer incidence and survival disappear when patients are matched by socioeconomic status, treatment received, age, and stage of disease. The list of factors that affect the risk and outcome of breast cancer patients continues to grow. As these factors are identified, they must be taken into consideration when designing and interpreting clinical trials. Identification of populations at risk for a poor outcome with breast cancer has been the focus of intense investigation in recent years, particularly with recognition of the important role that adjuvant chemotherapy may play in improving the results of breast cancer survival in early stage, node-negative patients. Large-scale epidemiologic studies have identified black breast cancer patients at high risk for a poor long-term survival. This identification has been based largely on incomplete analysis of large clinical surveys. The deficiencies of such surveys, which generally result from incomplete adjustment for known socioeconomic factors that affect prognosis, have been demonstrated. Unfortunately, black women have been identified as high-risk patients based on these misleading surveys, and many potential dangers exist in such false identification.

Cancer centers will be competing for ever-decreasing available research funds and limited patient resources to help fund their programs. These centers will increasingly equate their ability to compete for patients and research funds with the success of their cancer programs as measured by the treatment outcomes in their patients. If race is identified as a potentially negative predictor of patient outcome, it may well become a means of further exclusion of blacks and other minorities from quality health care in this country.[36] This phenomenon is presently operative in a number of organ transplantation centers around the United States, and the exact extent to which this form of institutional racism is operative is presently unknown.[25,36] In the absence of clear evidence of a genetically determined etiologic factor that is unique to the forms of breast cancer seen in blacks, and not present or operative in the etiology of breast cancer in whites, race cannot be considered an important independent risk factor in breast cancer incidence and survival.

References

1. Devesa SS, Diamond EL: Association of breast cancer and cervical cancer incidences with income and education among whites and blacks. *J Natl Cancer Inst* 1980; 65:515–528.
2. Ownby HE, Frederick J, Russo J, et al: Racial differences in breast cancer patients. *J Natl Cancer Inst* 1985; 75:55–60.
3. Nemoto T, Vana J, Bedwani RN, et al: Management and survival of female breast

cancer: results of a national survey by the American College of Surgeons. *Cancer* 1980; 45:2917–2924.

4. Natarajan N, Nemoto T, Mettlin C, et al: Race-related differences in breast cancer patients: results of the 1982 National Survey of Breast Cancer by the American College of Surgeons. *Cancer* 1985; 56:1704–1709.

5. Mohla S, Sampson CC, Khan T, et al: Estrogen and progesterone receptors in breast cancer in black Americans. *Cancer* 1982; 50:552–559.

6. Natarajan N, Nemoto D, Nemoto T, Mettlin C: Breast cancer survival among orientals and whites living in the United States. *J Surg Oncol* 1988; 39:206–209.

7. Young JL, Ries LG, Pollack ES: Cancer patient survival among ethnic groups in the United States. *J Natl Cancer Inst* 1984; 73:341–352.

8. Mandelblatt J, Andrews H, Kerner J, et al: Determinants of late stage diagnosis of breast and cervical cancer: the impact of age, race, social class, and hospital type. *Am J Public Health* 1991; 81:646–649.

9. Buell P: Changing incidence of breast cancer in Japanese-Americans. *J Nat'l Cancer Inst* 1973; 51:1479–1483.

10. Staszewski J, Haenszel WM: Cancer mortality among Polish-born in the United States. *J Nat'l Cancer Inst* 1965; 35:291–297.

11. Mesko TW, Dunlap JN, Sutherland CM: Conspectus: risk factors for breast cancer. *Compr Ther* 1990; 16:3–9.

12. Freeman HP, Wasfie TJ: Cancer of the breast in poor black women. *Cancer* 1989; 63:2562–2569.

13. McWhorter WP, Schatzkin AG, Horm JW, Brown CC: Contribution of socioeconomic status to black/white differences in cancer incidence. *Cancer* 1989; 63:982–987.

14. Cella DF, Orav EJ, Kornblith AB, et al: Socioeconomic status and cancer survival. *J Clin Oncol* 1991; 9:1500–1509.

15. Dansey RD, Hessel PA, Browde S, et al: Lack of a significant independent effect of race on survival in breast cancer. *Cancer* 1988; 61:1908–1912.

16. Logan WPD: Social variations in mortality. *Pub Health Reports* 1954; 69:1217–1223.

17. Lilienfeld AM: The epidemiology of breast cancer. *Cancer Res* 1963; 23:1503–1513.

18. Wynder EL, Bross IJ, Hirayama T: A study of the epidemiology of cancer of the breast. *Cancer* 1960; 13:559–601.

19. Henschke UK, Leffall LD Jr, Mason CH, et al: Alarming increase of the cancer mortality in the U.S. black population (1950–1967). *Cancer* 1973; 31:763–768.

20. Polednak AP: Cancer mortality in a higher-income black population in New York State: comparison with rates in the United States as a whole. *Cancer* 1990; 66:1654–1660.

21. Dayal HH, Power RN, Chiu C: Race and socio-economic status in survival from breast cancer. *J Chron Dis* 1982; 35:675–683.

22. Bassett MT, Krieger N: Social class and black-white differences in breast cancer survival. *Am J Public Health* 1986; 76:1400–1403.

23. Coates RJ, Clark WS, Eley JW, et al: Race, nutritional status, and survival from breast cancer. *J Natl Cancer Inst* 1990; 82:1684–1692.

24. Black Americans' attitudes toward cancer tests: highlights of a study, *CA* 1981; 31:21–219.

25. Sanfilippo FP, Vaughn WK, Peters TG, et al: Factors affecting the waiting time of cadaveric kidney transplant candidates in the United States. *JAMA* 1992; 267:247–252.

26. Council on Ethical and Judicial Affairs: Black-white disparities in health care. *JAMA* 1990; 263:2344–2346.

27. Belanger D, Moore M, Tannock I. How American oncologists treat breast cancer: an assessment of the influence of clinical trials. *J Clin Oncol* 1991; 9:7–16.

28. McWhorter WP, Mayer WJ: Black/white differences in type of initial breast cancer treatment and implications for survival. *Am J Public Health* 1987; 77:1515–1517.

29. Briele HA, Walker MJ, Wild L, et al: Results of treatment of stage I–III breast cancer in

black Americans: the Cook County Hospital exerience, 1973–1987. *Cancer* 1990; 65:1062–1071.
30. Sunderland MC, McGuire WL: Prognostic indicators in invasive breast cancer. *Surg Clin North Am* 1990; 70:989–1003.
31. Pegorano RJ, Karnan V, Nirmul D, et al: Estrogen and progesterone receptors in breast cancer among women of different racial groups. *Cancer Res* 1986; 46:2117–2120.
32. Olsson H, Borg A, Ferno M, et al: HER-2/Neu and INT2 proto-oncogene amplification in malignant breast tumors in relation to reproductive factors and exposure to exogenous hormones. *J Natl Cancer Inst* 1991; 83:1483–1487.
33. Read LD, Keith D Jr, Slamon DJ, Katzenellenbogen BS: Hormonal modulation of HER-2/Neu protooncogene messenger ribonucleic acid and p185 protein expression in human breast cancer cell lines. *Cancer Res* 1990; 50:3947–3951.
34. Slamon DJ, Clark GM, Wong SG, et al: Human breast cancer: correlation of relapse and survival with amplification of the HER-2/Neu oncogene. *Science* 1987; 235:177–182.
35. Moe RE, Moe KS, Porter P, et al: Expression of HER-2/Neu oncogene protein product and epidermal growth factor receptors in surgical specimens of human breast cancers. *Am J Surg* 1991; 161:580–583.
36. Osborne NG, Feit MD: The use of race in medical research. *JAMA* 1992; 267:275–279.

44

Racial Differences in Breast Cancer:

Fact or Fiction?

Benjamin W. Pace, Houston Johnson, Jr.

Introduction

Despite a significantly lower incidence of the disease, black Americans are dying of breast cancer at nearly the same rate as whites. While race has been implicated as an independent risk factor by some authors, others have dissected the problem from this seemingly superficial interpretation to those of racially oriented differences in environment, socioeconomic and nutritional status, stage, hormone receptor status, and treatment.

This chapter reviews the relevant literature on the controversial topic of racial differences in breast cancer. It concludes with the formulation of screening and treatment plans for the future based on the evidence provided.

Breast cancer is a leading cause of cancer deaths among women in the United States, second only to lung cancer.[1] Though it affects all racial and ethnic groups, it does so unequally, with the incidence and mortality statistics differing for each set. This fact is most striking in the black population where the incidence of breast cancer is significantly lower than that in whites, while the mortality to incidence ratio is significantly higher (38% blacks, 32% whites).[2] In addition, screening programs and new treatment modalities implemented over the past several decades have not only failed to alter the breast cancer death rate significantly for the population as a whole (26.3 per 100,000 1955–1957 vs. 27.2 per 100,000 1985–1987, not statistically significant), but have been associated

---

From: Wise L, Johnson H Jr (eds): *Breast Cancer: Controversies in Management.* Futura Publishing Company, Inc., Armonk, NY, © 1994.

with a 29% *increase* in the breast cancer death rate for blacks during that same period.[3]

The enormity of this health problem is placed in perspective when one notes that, in 1991, an estimated 15,000 new cases of *invasive* breast cancer were diagnosed among black women in the United States.[3] Apart from this relatively large number of new cases is the significantly lower survival rate among blacks, over both the short and the long term.[2,4-14] Bain et al. found the 3-year survival rate to be 71% among blacks compared to 83% among whites, while a 1984 report from the NCI (National Cancer Institute) identified a 5-year survival rate of 63% for blacks and 75% for whites.[4,5] Gloeckler et al., reviewing the 1983 SEER data (Surveillance, Epidemiology, and End Results Project, NCI, 1983 report covering data for 1973–1979), found a difference in survival for blacks and whites: 61% and 73%, respectively.[6] Similarly, McWhorter and Mayer calculated that, controlling for stage, there was at least a 10% decrease in relative survival for blacks.[12] These results are echoed in numerous other studies.[2-14]

Having acknowledged racial differences in incidence and mortality rates, authors vary widely as to their interpretation of these results. The heart of the controversy may be divided into three components: (1) Is race an *independent* factor linking genetics and breast cancer incidence, treatment response, and survival? (2) If not, what factors can be identified (i.e., socioeconomic, treatment differences) that may account for the observed racial disparity, and, most importantly, (3) how may these findings be translated into programs designed to successfully impact on this growing health care crisis?

Race As an Independent Factor

Numerous studies are available in which race has been analyzed as an independent factor, controlling for the stage of disease at presentation. This standardization may be important, as other authors have emphasized that blacks often present with the later stages of breast cancer at the time of diagnosis.[10,15-25] In a large series, Nemoto et al. reviewed the American College of Surgeons' data prior to 1972.[20] Controlling for stage, they found race to indeed be an independent variable affecting survival. Studies headed by Vernon, Sondik, and Young have come to similar conclusions.[7,14,26] In addition to stage, other authors have also controlled for various combinations of age, delays in treatment, type of surgery, histology, and socioeconomic status with comparable results. In one such study, Bassett and Kreiger, controlling for age, stage and histology, found the mortality rate among blacks to be 1.35 times that found in whites.[9]

While these studies all conclude that race has an independent effect on survival, they all fall short in controlling for some, but not all, of the possible determinants of breast cancer survival. Most do not entertain the effects of education, income, access to health care (both before and after diagnosis), nutritional status, hormone receptor status, and treatment differences in evaluating their data. The extent to which these shortcomings affect their results is unknown.

Social, Environmental, and Other Acquired Factors

What role do social and environmental factors play in determining the survival from breast cancer as it relates to race? In one of the most telling studies investigating health care, breast cancer, and race, the effects of a uniformly applied breast screening program and adequate access to health care were outlined. Shapiro et al. reviewed data from the Health Insurance Plan (HIP) of New York, a prepaid health care organization providing a full range of inpatient and outpatient services utilizing their own hospitals, clinics, and staff. In this highly standardized environment, 3,000 patients were randomized into a control group without a breast screening program while 3,000 patients were randomized into a study group offering routine breast screening exams and yearly mammography. Sixty-five percent of those who were offered screening participated. Nonwhite patients in the control group had a lower survival rate than did their white counterparts at 5-year follow-up, consistent with the data presented above. However, there were *no* racial differences noted in the group for which screening was made available.[13]

The importance of this study stems not only from these surprising results but also from the fact that many key factors potentially influencing survival from breast cancer were controlled. Socioeconomic status differences as they relate to access to and quality of treatment and follow-up care were eliminated. Even the potential additional effects of nutrition, to some degree controlled, as these patients were partially preselected in their ability, on their own or through the level of their employment, to have access to this type of health care plan. Based on the data, the authors appropriately concluded that "secondary prevention measures may offer the possibility of reducing or closing the gap in breast cancer survival rates between white and nonwhite women."

Shapiro et al. are not alone in determining that, when acquired social and environmental factors are adequately controlled, there appears to be no purely race-related genetic influences on breast cancer survival. Schatzkin et al. analyzed data on 529 black and 589 white patients in an attempt to identify differences in risk factors, concluding that "the risk profile for breast cancer in black women was similar to that in white women."[27] Sutherland et al., in an early study out of the Charity Hospital of Louisiana at New Orleans, looked at survival in an indigent population.[28] They found that only differences in tumor size and lymph node status accounted for the noted long-term survival advantage of white patients. In a similar but later analysis, Sutherland and Mather found that race had no influence when controlling for socioeconomic status.[29]

Dansey et al. pointed to the fact that TNM staging is flawed in that it arbitrarily lumps together close but dissimilar tumor, nodal, and metastatic indices into larger staging groups.[15] In patients with localized disease, they determined that disaggregating their patients according to TNM indices rather than TNM staging eliminated any effect of race on survival. Finally, reviews by Daly et al. and by Zippin and Petrakis failed to identify race as an independent variable in breast cancer survival.[11,30] Daly's report controlled for lymph node and hormone receptor status, while Zippin's analysis controlled for socioeconomic status and age.

These data appear to contradict those supporting race as an independent variable in survival from breast cancer. As mentioned previously, this may be explained by the lack of adequate control in the "race as an independent variable" group of the myriad of potential social and environmental variables that may influence survival. In this regard, it would appear from the studies noted above that the variable(s) affecting survival differ with each group studied, ranging from local tumor factors and access to health care to age and socioeconomic factors. Yet, the reality is that these are probably not independent elements. Age and local tumor factors may be influenced by nutrition and access to health care, all of which are modulated by more global socioeconomic factors.

Identifiable Factors Influencing Breast Cancer Survival in Blacks

If, as the literature would suggest, the potential exists that survival from breast cancer is partially or fully independent of race or other genetic predeterminants, then every attempt should be made to identify and ameliorate the negative social and environmental variables affecting survival. First, what are these variables and what is the evidence of their interaction with survival?

Several studies have indicated that breast cancer develops at an earlier age in blacks. In Feldman's study population, blacks developed breast cancer, on average, 8 years earlier than did whites.[31] Similarly, Bain et al. found a significant difference in age at presentation, but to a lesser degree (average age at diagnosis 55.0 ± 15.8 years for blacks and 58.9 ± 14.4 years for whites).[4] Muller and associates from South Africa indicated that the poorer prognosis of their younger black patients may well be explained by the fact that there was a significantly greater proportion of these patients who fell into the higher risk premenopausal subgroup ($P<0.0001$).[14] This theory is not universally accepted, however. Natarajan et al., for example, found that, in Hawaii, Orientals develop breast cancer at a younger age than Hawaiian whites, yet they enjoy a better long-term survival.[32]

It is important to bear in mind that, in the United States, breast cancer screening programs have been formulated on statistics available for the population as a whole. As such, ages chosen for initial and follow-up screening mammography were heavily weighted toward the more populous white community. This being true, the imposition of this age-dependent screening system on the black population, where breast neoplasms occur at an earlier age, should have resulted in the detection of larger and more advanced tumors in black patients. This is exactly the finding of numerous large series. The American College of Surgeons' data from 1982[18] are illustrated in Table 1. These results are similar to those of a study of the 1978 American College of Surgeons' data where, again, blacks were found to have fewer tumors of limited size and more favorable prognosis. In addition, in reviewing the 1978 data, Nemoto and associates identified racial differences not only by tumor size, but by the presence or absence of positive

Table 1
Race and Tumor Size at the Time of Diagnosis*

Tumor Size	% Black	% White
< 1 CM	6.5	10.1
1.1–2.0	27.6	35.2
2.1–3.0	25.9	26.8
3.1–5.0	24.0	18.9
> 5 CM	15.9	9.0

*Reprinted by permission, Natarajan et al.[18]

axillary lymph nodes within each size category. Blacks had a significantly higher incidence of positive lymph node involvement per given size than their white counterparts.[8] The study by Bain's group, among others, confirmed these results. They indicated that 48% of blacks and 58% of whites were axillary node-negative at the time of surgery, while 14% of blacks and only 9% of whites were found to have more than eight lymph nodes involved with tumor.[4]

It would appear from these reports that a readjustment of screening programs taking into account racial differences holds the potential to significantly reduce mortality. Tumors would be identified earlier and, as such, be smaller with less likelihood of axillary or distant metastases.

The effect of tumor histology and grade as a race-related survival factor appears to be more controversial. Several authors have identified ethnic differences in tumor histology in various world populations[33–35]; however, the American data favor the conclusion that tumor histology is not a factor.[4,18,22] Differences in tumor grade among the races in America does appear to have some validity, but this may be interrelated with age and/or hormonal status.[21,22]

The literature indicates that hormone receptor status clearly influences survival in the population in general[36–39] and contains many references to the fact that black patients more often fall into the less favorable hormone receptor-negative category.[8,11,18,19,21,24,25,40–47] Beverly et al. determined that, after adjustment was made for age, menopausal status, tumor size, and nodal or distant metastases, only 54% of black breast cancer patients were estrogen receptor-positive while 60% were progesterone receptor-positive. The corresponding figures in whites were 72% receptor-positive for both estrogen and progesterone.[42] In their South African patient group, Pegoraro et al. found that 49% of blacks, 41% of Asians, and 67% of whites were estrogen receptor-positive.[47] These trends were confirmed by many other investigators. In contradistinction, a few authors have found no race-related difference in some hormonal status subgroups,[18,22] and a small series reported by Johnson and Carstens even identified a higher degree of estrogen-receptor positivity in premenopausal black women when controlling for socioeconomic status.[48]

Indeed, hormone receptor status may be one more factor in which socioeconomic status influences race-related survival. Unfortunately, socioeconomic factors often weigh heavily in our society regarding access to, and quality of, screening, treatment, and follow-up care. In addition, education, malnutrition, alcoholism, drug dependency, and other factors affecting host resistance may all be socioeconomic modulators of race-related survival from breast cancer as from cancers of all types. Lackland et al. found that in South Carolina, 13% of blacks and 6% of whites did not know how to perform breast self-examination while 18% of blacks and 5% of whites had never heard of mammography.[49] Bassett and Krieger found that, controlling for socioeconomic status, the black/white breast cancer survival difference was only 1.1 times higher in blacks.[9] Dayal et al. found that controlling for age and stage resulted in a residual race-related survival difference that was completely eliminated when standardization of socioeconomic factors was included.[50] In addition, even solely among blacks, Freeman and Wasfie indicated that those considered to be in a low socioeconomic subgroup had significantly worse survival rates than those identified as belonging to a higher socioeconomic subgroup.[51]

Nutrition may be a significant modulator of survival in breast cancer. In numerous studies of breast cancer survival unrelated to race, patients with a greater relative body weight were found to have a poorer prognosis.[22,52–57] Patients from lower socioeconomic groups tend to have higher relative body weights and, in the studies headed by Donegan, Tartter, Boyd, and Wynder, this correlation of higher average relative body weight and a poorer prognosis for blacks held true.[52–54,58] Within the black population, Schatzkin et al. identified that obesity is not only a variable influencing survival but also a risk factor for the *development* of breast cancer.[27] Coates and associates, in a 1990 report, indicated that adjustment for nutritional status in advanced stage III disease explained approximately three-fourths of the increased mortality among blacks.[59] They comment that "within each stage classification, lower levels of serum albumin and hemoglobin and higher relative body weight were more common among blacks and were independently associated with poorer survival." Clearly, nutrition appears to influence race-related survival.

Once diagnosed with breast cancer, blacks may receive different treatment than other groups. Bain et al. discovered that a smaller proportion of black patients with advanced disease received surgery.[4] McWhorter and Mayer found this to be true even after adjusting for age, stage, and histology.[12] In addition, black patients in their study were found to have received less aggressive therapy on the whole with more black patients having received *no* cancer-directed therapy. Feldman et al. noted that, among those having undergone appropriate treatment, more black patients were left with functional disabilities.[31]

Strategies for the Future

Educational programs need to reach as much of the population as possible. Adding awareness of breast cancer, self-examination, and mammography to already existing junior and senior high school health classes may aid in this effort. Screening recommendations need to be refined so as to take into account race-related age differences in breast cancer. Specifically, the data would indicate that the age of first mammography for black Americans be adjusted downward by at least 5 years in order to capture greater numbers of black patients with early disease. Follow-up studies of the efficacy of such a move would be warranted to confirm that the intended end was indeed achieved.

Once diagnosed with breast cancer, consideration should be given in all patients as to socioeconomic factors affecting survival. Nutritional status should be investigated and counseling offered with the goal of reducing relative body weight, improving overall nutritional status, and eliminating, or at least controlling, comorbid factors such as alcohol and drug dependency.

Proper therapy should be instituted in each case without deviation from the accepted therapy because of race. Hormonal receptor status should be obtained in every case and the knowledge gained applied where appropriate.

Clearly, these goals are most difficult to achieve for the indigent patient. Care for the indigent patient is often rendered in the setting of public clinics where, more often than not, staff is extremely limited, resources scarce and time for providing individual attention lacking. However, by striving toward these goals in all settings, physicians may best be able to improve survival from breast cancer in black Americans while improving health care for all Americans.

Only by improving the standard of living of each of its members may society hope to improve the standard of living for society as a whole.

References

1. Boring CC, Squires TS, Heath CW Jr: Cancer statistics for African Americans. Ca-A Cancer J Clinicians 1992; 42(1):19–38.
2. Whitman S, Ansell D, Lacey L, Chen EH, et al: Patterns of breast and cervical cancer screening at three public health centers in an inner-city urban area. Am J Public Health 1991; 81(12):1651–1653.
3. Bal DG: Cancer in African Americans. CA-A Cancer J Clinicians 1992; 42(1):5–18.
4. Bain RP, Greenberg RS, Whitaker JP: Racial differences in survival of women with breast cancer. J Chronic Dis 1986; 39(8):631–642.
5. National Cancer Institute. Seer Program: Cancer Incidence and Mortality in the United States, 1973. DHHS Publ No. 85–1837, Washington, DC. US Government Printing Office, 1984.
6. Gloeckler RL, Pollack ES, Young JL Jr: Cancer patient survival: surveillance, epidemiology, and end results program, 1973–79. J Natl Cancer Inst 1983; 70:693–697.
7. Young JL Jr, Gloeckler RL, Pollack ES: Cancer patient survival among ethnic groups in the United States. J Natl Cancer Inst 1984; 73:341–342.
8. Nemoto T, Vana J, Natarajan N, et al: Observation on short-term and long-term surveys on breast cancer by the American College of Surgeons II: estrogen receptor assay in the US in 1977. Int Adv Surg Oncol 1981; 4:224–239.
9. Bassett MT, Krieger N: Social class and black-white differences in breast cancer survival. Am J Public Health 1986; 76(12):1400–1403.
10. National Cancer Institute: 1987 Annual Cancer Statistics Review Including Cancer Trends: 1950–1985. DHHS Publ No. (NIH)88-2789. Washington, DC, US Government Printing Office, 1988.
11. Daly MB, Clark GM, McGuire WL: Breast cancer prognosis in a mixed Caucasian-Hispanic population. J Natl Cancer Inst 1985; 74(4):753–757.
12. McWhorter WP, Mayer WJ: Black/white differences in type of initial breast cancer treatment and implications for survival. Am J Public Health 1987; 77(12):1515–1517.

13. Shapiro S, Venet W, Strax P, Venet L, et al: Prospects for eliminating racial differences in breast cancer survival rates. Am J Public Health 1982; 72(10):1142–1145.
14. Vernon SW, Tilley BC, Neale AV, Steinfeldt L: Ethnicity, survival, and delay in seeking treatment for symptoms of breast cancer. Cancer 1985; 55(7):1563–1571.
15. Dansey RD, Hessel PA, Browde S, Lange M, et al: Lack of a significant independent effect of race on survival in breast cancer. Cancer 1988; 61(9):1908–1912.
16. Le Marchand L, Kolonel LN, Nomura AM: Relationship of ethnicity and other prognostic factors to breast cancer survival patterns in Hawaii. J Natl Cancer Inst 1984; 73(6):1259–1265.
17. Mandelblatt J, Andrews H, Kerner J, Zauber A, et al: Determinants of late stage diagnosis of breast and cervical cancer: the impact of age, race, social class, and hospital type. Am J Public Health 1991; 81(5):646–649.
18. Natarajan N, Nemoto T, Mettlin C, Murphy GP: Race-related differences in breast cancer patients: results of the 1982 national survey of breast cancer by the American College of Surgeons. Cancer 1985; 56(7):1704–1709.
19. Muller AGS, Van Zyl JA, Joubert G: Analysis of prognostic factors in 568 patients treated for breast cancer by surgery. J Surg Oncol 1989; 42(2):126–131.
20. Nemoto T, Vana J, Bedwani RN, Baker HW, et al: Management and survival of female breast cancer. Cancer 1980; 45(12):2917-2924.
21. Mohla S, Sampson CC, Khan T, et al: Estrogen and progesterone receptors in breast cancer in black Americans: correlation of receptor data with tumor differentiation. Cancer 1982; 50:552-559.
22. Ownby HE, Frederick J, Russo J, Brooks SC, et al: Racial differences in breast cancer patients. J Natl Cancer Inst 1985; 75(1):55–60.
23. Wilson RE, Donegan WL, Mettlin C, Smart CR, et al: The 1982 National Survey of Carcinoma of the Breast in the United States by the American College of Surgeons. Surg Gynecol Obstet 1984; 159(4):309–318.
24. Winters Z, Mannell A, Esser JD: Breast cancer in black South Africans. S African J Surg 1988; 26:34–46.
25. Valanis B, Wirman J, Hertzberg VS: Social and biological factors in relation to survival among black vs. white women with breast cancer. Breast Cancer Res Treatment 1987; 9(2):135–143.
26. Sondik EJ, Young JL, Horm JW, et al: Annual Cancer Statistics Review. Washington, DC, US Government Printing Office, 1987.
27. Schatzkin A, Palmer JR, Rosenberg L, Helmrich SO, et al: Risk factors for breast cancer in black women. J Natl Cancer Inst 1987; 78(2):213–217.
28. Sutherland CM, Mather FJ: Long-term survival and prognostic factors in breast cancer patients with localized (no skin, muscle, or chest wall attachment) disease with and without positive lymph nodes. Cancer 1986; 57(3):622–629.
29. Sutherland CM, Mather FJ: Charity Hospital experience with long-term survival and prognostic factors in patients with breast cancer with localized or regional disease. Ann Surg 1988; 207(5):569–580.
30. Zippin C, Petrakis NL: Identification of high-risk groups in breast cancer. Cancer 1971; 42:1381–1387.
31. Feldman JG, Gardner B, Carter AC, Alfonso A, et al: Relationship of race to functional status among breast cancer patients after curative surgery. J Surg Oncol 1979; 11(4):333-339.
32. Natarajan N, Nemoto T, Mettlin C: Breast cancer survival among Orientals and whites living in the United States. J Surg Oncol 1988; 39(3):206–209.
33. Sacks M, Selzer G: Breast cancer in Israel: histopathologic types in the different population groups. Israel J Med Sci 1981; 17(9–10):882–887.
34. Stemmermann GN: The pathology of breast cancer in Japanese women compared to other ethnic groups: a review. Breast Cancer Res Treatment 1991; 18:S67-S72.
35. Stemmermann GN, Catts A, Fukunaga FH, Horie A, et al: Breast cancer in women of Japanese and Caucasian ancestry in Hawaii. Cancer 1985; 56(1):206–209.

36. Osborne CK, Yochmowitz MG, Knight WA, McGuire WL: The value of estrogen and progesterone receptors in the treatment of breast cancer. Cancer 1980; 46:2884–2888.
37. Leake RE, Laing L, McArdle C, Smith DC: Soluble and nuclear estrogen receptor status in human breast cancer in relation to prognosis. Br J Cancer 1981; 43:67–71.
38. Clark GM, McGuire WL, Hubay CA, Pearson OH, et al: Progesterone receptors as a prognostic factor in stage II breast cancer. N Engl J Med 1983; 309:1343–1347.
39. Mason BH, Holdaway IM, Mullins PR, Yee LH, et al: Progesterone and estrogen receptors as prognostic variables in breast cancer. Cancer Res 1983; 43:2985–2999.
40. Hulka B, Chambless LE, Wilkinson WE, Deubner D, et al: Hormonal and personal effects on estrogen receptors in breast cancer. Am J Epidemiol 1984; 119:692–704.
41. Mohla S, Enterline JP, Sampson CC, Kahn T, et al: Predominance of poorly differentiated tumors among black breast cancer patients: management and screening indication. In: Metlin C, Murphy G (eds). Progress in Clinical and Biological Research Issues in Cancer Screening and Communication. New York, 83:249-258, 1982.
42. Beverly LN, Flanders WD, Go RC, Soong SJ: A comparison of estrogen and progesterone receptors in black and white breast cancer patients. Am J Public Health 1987; 77(3):351–353.
43. Stanford JL, Greenberg RS: Breast cancer incidence in young women by estrogen receptor status and race. Am J Public Health 1989; 79(1):71–73.
44. Stanford JL, Szklo M, Boring CC, et al: A case control study of breast cancer stratified by estrogen receptor status. Am J Epidemiol 1987; 125:184–194.
45. Crowe JP Jr, Gordon NH, Hubay CA, Pearson OH, et al: The interaction of estrogen receptor and race in predicting prognosis for stage I breast cancer patients. Surgery 1986; 100:599–605.
46. Savage N, Levin J, De Moor NG, Lange M: Cystosolic oestrogen receptor content of breast cancer tissue in blacks and whites. S Afr Med J 1981; 59(18):623–624.
47. Pegoraro RJ, Nirmul D, Reinach SG, Jordan JP, et al: Breast cancer prognosis in three different racial groups in relation to steroid hormone receptor status. Breast Cancer Res Treatment 1986; 7(20):111–118.
48. Johnson H Jr, Carstens R: Interracial differences in sex-steroid receptor status of breast cancers. J Nat Med Assoc 1988; 80(4):397–400.
49. Lackland DT, Dunbar JB, Keil JE, Knapp RG, et al: Breast cancer screening in a biracial community: the Charleston tri-county experience. South Med J 1991; 84(7):862–866.
50. Dayal HH, Power RN, Chiu C: Race and socio-economic status in survival from breast cancer. J Chronic Dis 1982; 35(8):675-683.
51. Freeman HP, Wasfie TJ: Cancer of the breast in poor black women. Cancer 1989; 63(12):2562–2569.
52. Donegan WL, Hartz AJ, Rimm AA: The association of body weight with recurrent cancer of the breast. Cancer 1978, 41:1590-1594.
53. Tartter PI, Papatestas AE, Ioannovich J, et al: Cholesterol and obesity as prognostic factors in breast cancer. Cancer 1981; 47:2222–2227.
54. Boyd NF, Campbell JE, Germanson T, et al: Body weight and prognosis in breast cancer. JNCI 1981; 67:785–789.
55. Zumoff B, Gorzynski JG, Katz JL, et al: Nonobesity at the time of mastectomy is highly predictive of 10 years disease-free survival in women with breast cancer. Anticancer Res 1982; 2:59-62.
56. Herbert J, Augustine A, Barone J, et al: Weight, height, and index in the prognosis of breast cancer patients: early results of a prospective study. Am J Epidemiol 1988; 128:931–932.
57. Mohle-Boetani JC, Grosser S, Whittemore AS, et al: Body size, reproductive factors, and breast cancer survival. Prev Med 1988; 17:634–642.
58. Wynder EL, Cohen LA: A rationale for dietary intervention in the treatment of postmenopausal breast cancer patients. Nutr Cancer 1982; 3:195–199.
59. Coates RJ, Clark WS, Eley JW, Greenberg RS, et al: Race, nutritional status and survival from breast cancer. J Natl Cancer Inst 1990; 82(21):1684–1692.

45

Immunological Evaluation of Patients with Breast Cancer Has a Significant Role in their Management

Maurice M. Black, Reinhard E. Zachrau

Introduction

The verity of the title statement depends on the ability to demonstrate:
1. the existence of immunological responses to autologous breast cancer in an appreciable proportion of breast cancer patients;
2. the prognostic significance of such immunological responses;
3. therapeutic implications of immunological reactivity in terms of
   a. currently available treatment alternatives, and
   b. therapeutic benefits of augmentation of specific immunity in individual patients; and
4. prophylactic implications of induced immunity in control individuals.

Supported in part by Grant No. 5R01-CA25165 from the National Cancer Institute, U.S.D.H.H.S., a grant from the Cancer Research Institute, Inc., New York, NY, and contributions from the H-O Foundation, Inc., the Abner and Mildred Levine Family Foundation, the Meyer Steinberg Foundation, Inc., the Morris Morgenstern Foundation, Newmark Associates, the Irwin and Sylvia Schnurmacher Foundation, Inc., and from Benjamin G. Kerr, MD.

From: Wise L, Johnson H Jr (eds): *Breast Cancer: Controversies in Management*. Futura Publishing Company, Inc., Armonk, NY, © 1994.

Immunological Responses to Autologous Breast Cancer

It has long been known from studies of infectious diseases and experimental immunology that immunogens induce focalized aggregations and differentiation of cells of the lymphoreticulo-endothelial (LRE) system at the site of the immunogens and in the regional lymph nodes. So distinctive and well defined are such responses in tissues and lymph nodes that pathologists regularly exploit them to distinguish the type of immunity, i.e., immediate (antibody-mediated) and delayed (cell-mediated), and even for specific diagnosis, e.g., tuberculosis.

Accordingly, if breast cancer tissues were not associated with non-self-immunogens, there should be no evidence of immunological responses against the autologous cancer tissue, either in vivo or in vitro. On the other hand, if breast cancer tissue is associated with non-self-immunogenic changes, there should be representation of specific immunological responses in the host in the form of structural and analytical measurements.

Pathologists have long recognized the existence of pronounced lymphoid/plasma cell infiltrations in some cancers, e.g., medullary carcinoma of the breast and Steiner's "blue" cancer of the stomach.[1-3] However, it was and still is often overlooked that distinctive but more subtle LRE responses are commonly present in primary breast cancers and in their draining lymph nodes. In the breast, these responses are seen as perivenous infiltrations of lymphoid cells (PVI), associated with in situ and invasive breast cancer.[4-7] In the lymph nodes, distinctive responses are seen as sinus histiocytosis and paracortical hyperplasia.[8-10] Such responses are found in approximately one-third of invasive breast cancer patients but are rarely found in patients with normotypic breast lesions (~5%). More specifically, the cellular responses to the primary cancer and in the regional lymph nodes indicate that, in most instances, the immunological response is of a cell-mediated rather than an antibody-mediated type of hypersensitivity. The cell-mediated immunity (CMI) nature of the LRE responses to autologous breast cancer was specifically recognized as early as 1959 and has been repeatedly documented since then.[11-15]

CMI to autologous invasive breast cancer is also demonstrable by postoperative in vitro and in vivo tests. In vitro tests from a number of laboratories, including our own, have demonstrated CMI to autologous breast cancer tissue sections or extracts in approximately one-third of unselected postoperative patients with invasive breast cancer.[16-20] In 1970, Black and Leis reported that Rebuck's skin window (SW) procedure[21] could be used to visualize in vivo CMI responses to autologous breast cancer.[22-24] Originally (1970–1979), our SW tests utilized cryostat sections of fresh tissue, fixed in ether-alcohol, as targets. Subsequently, we found that the same results could be obtained when sections of paraffin-imbedded tissues were used as targets. The procedure is thus readily applicable to previously diagnosed individuals, since we have found antigenicity retained in tissues from paraffin blocks that were more than 10 years old.[25]

A detailed description of all the variations in type and extent of cellular responses to autologous breast cancer tissue is beyond the purpose of this presentation. However, it is pertinent to indicate that one can readily recognize cellular responses that are consistent with CMI and analogous to those in primary breast cancers and regional lymph nodes. In a series of 262 unselected patients with invasive breast cancer who were SW tested 1–24 months postoperatively (mpo), approximately one-third showed positive responses. Note that breast cancer patients who are responsive to autologous breast cancer are *not* simultaneously responsive to normotypic areas of cancerous breasts by *any* of the aforementioned indices; nor are patients with benign breast lesions responsive to autologous benign or homologous benign or malignant breast lesions as judged by LMT procedures.[26] Thus, structural and analytical observations indicate that an appreciable minority of patients with invasive breast cancer have a type of CMI which is *specifically directed against an antigenic determinant expressed by breast cancer cells.*

However, the demonstration of specific immunity against autologous invasive breast cancer does not, per se, prove that cancer-associated antigenicity and host immunity are developmentally or prognostically significant. It could be that the antigenic change associated with invasive cancer is an epiphenomenon that is unrelated to the development and behavior of breast cancer. It is, therefore, necessary to determine the relationship between mammary carcinogenesis and immunogenicity and the nature of the relationship, if any exists, between specific immunity and the clinical behavior of breast cancer.

Pathologists have long noted the presence of lymphoid cell aggregations at the site of *developing* carcinomas. For example, Couperus and Rucker emphasized the association of developing melanomas and "an inflammatory infiltrate of lymphocytes and plasma cells."[27] Black pointed out the analogy between such reactions to developing cancer foci and the lymphoid cellular aggregates that are associated with the rejection of homologous skin grafts.[13] In 1969, Black and Chabon called specific attention to the immunological implications of LRE responses associated with the *preinvasive* phase of mammary carcinogenesis.[4] They indicated that immunogenicity was expressed in precancerous mastopathy as well as in the more advanced phases of in-situ carcinoma (ISC) of the breast. Such observations were expanded in a series of studies that utilized in vitro and in vivo indices of CMI against autologous ISC. These studies clearly demonstrated that immunogenicity and specific CMI were more regularly associated with preinvasive than with invasive breast cancer.[13,15,28–30] It was also shown that the breast cancer-associated CMI is cross-reactive with determinants expressed by in situ and invasive breast cancers of different individuals and by the principal envelope glycoprotein of the RIII-murine mammary tumor virus, designated as gp55.[31–33] It should also be noted that Springer et al. have shown that the early phases of carcinogenesis are associated with the "unmasking" of T and Tn antigens, changes which have diagnostic and predictive significance.[34]

Considered in toto, diverse types of structural and analytical data indicate that specific immunogenicity and CMI are associated with breast cancer. However, an association does not, per se, demand a prognostic relationship. In fact, if CMI against autologous breast cancer was universally demonstrable in all breast cancer patients, it would indicate that such reactivity is not prognostically significant. The prognostic significance of specific CMI can only be assessed by relating it to the behavior of breast cancers in individual patients over defined postoperative intervals.

Prognostic Significance of CMI to Autologous Breast Cancer

Metastatic Progression

Starting in the early 1950s, Black and associates initiated a series of studies that repeatedly demonstrated that the postoperative survival of breast cancer patients correlated more closely with the morphological characteristics of the cancer cell nuclei and the tumor-retarding responses by the host than with the type of primary therapy.[7,35,36] As described by Black and Speer,[37] the intrinsic aggressive potential of the cancer was inversely correlated with the degree of nuclear differentiation, designated as nuclear grade (NG). Studies of breast cancer patients from diverse geographical areas, under "blinded" conditions, demonstrated that NG is so powerful a prognostic variable that, when considered *alone*, it is capable of identifying subgroups of patients who are destined to have significantly different subsequent survivals. The mean 5-year postoperative survival rates according to NG were: 44% for cancers with poorly differentiated nuclei (NG I), 64% for those with moderately differentiated nuclei (NG II), and 88% for those with highly differentiated nuclei (NG III). It should be emphasized that these NG/survival relationships were derived from unselected breast cancer patients, without regard to tumor size, stage, and histologic type, patient age, immunological status, and type of treatment. In fact, the prognostic significance of the NG is *not dependent on curability*, since the relationship between NG and 5-year survival is maintained in patients who subsequently died of breast cancer.[38] Since NG is the microscopic correlate of DNA content and chromosomal characteristics, it is not surprising that analytical evaluations of DNA content and synthesis, such as by flow cytometry, show a correlation with NG.[39] Variations in the intrinsic aggressive potential of breast cancers have also been reported to correlate with the relative frequency in unmasking of the cryptic blood group substances T and Tn. Thus, Springer et al. indicate that a relative predominance of the Tn compared to the T antigen is more regularly associated with anaplastic than with well-differentiated breast cancer cells.[34] The point we would emphasize is the reality of the existence of variations in the intrinsic aggressive potential between individual breast cancers and of the recognizable correlates of such properties.

In addition to the prognostic influence of the intrinsic characteristics of a cancer, there are variations in survival that are associated with the presence or absence of CMI against a cancer, as evidenced by LRE responses.[7] Such intra-NG prognostic distinctions have been demonstrated in studies from geographically diverse populations. In each NG series, the survivals among LRE-positive patients were superior to those among LRE-negative patients. The correlation between CMI against NG-characterized breast cancer and subsequent metasta-

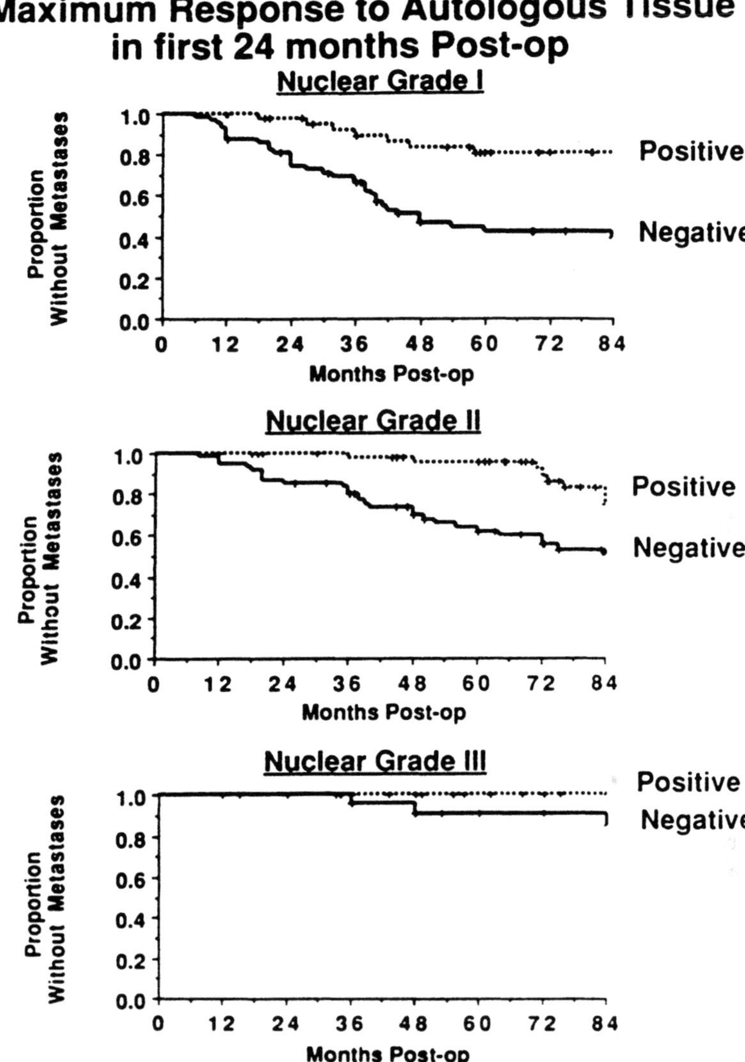

Figure 1: *Kaplan-Meier curves, showing proportions of patients with invasive breast cancer clinically free of recurrent disease at increasing postoperative intervals, in relation to nuclear grade (NG) and maximal skin window (SW) reactivity against autologous carcinoma, tested 1–24 months postoperatively. Patients were categorized as to the NG of their cancers, from NG I (poorly) to NG III (highly differentiated), at the time of diagnosis. Patient numbers by category are: NG I: SW-positive, 43, and SW-negative, 63: NG II: SW-positive, 54, and SW-negative, 62;NG III: SW-positive, 32, and SW-negative, 25. Reproduced with permission by the publisher.[33]*

sis-free survival is similarly evident when CMI is evaluated postoperatively by SW tests. The existence of distinctive survival characteristics according to NG and SW reactivity was reported in 1988 and 1989.[25,33] These studies demon-

Table 1

Survival Characteristics Among Breast Cancer Patients in Relation to Nuclear Differentiation of and Skin Window Reactivity Against Autologous Breast Cancer (Maximal Reactivity per Patient, 1–24 Months Postoperatively)

Nuclear Differentiation of the Cancer	Intensity of Skin Window Reactivity against Autologous Breast Cancer			
	1	2	3	Total
Low	39/19 (1.89)[a,b,c]	5/6 (0.83)	7/24 (0.29)[b,d]	48/49 (0.98)[e]
Intermediate	22/36 (0.61)[c,f]	3/16 (0.19)	1/31 (0.03)[d,f]	26/83 (0.31)[e,g]
High	3/18 (0.17)	0/7	0/21	3/46 (0.07)[g]
Total	61/73 (0.84)[h]	8/29 (0.28)	8/76 (0.11)[h]	77/178 (0.43)

[a]Numbers of patients with systemic metastases within 60 months/numbers of patients without clinical evidence of recurrent disease for ≥60 months postoperatively (ratios).
[b,e,h]$P < 0.0005$.
[c]$P < 0.01$.
[d]$P = 0.053$.
[f]$P < 0.001$.
[g]$P < 0.02$.

strated that positive SW reactivity against autologous breast cancer (1-24 mpo) is associated with significantly ($P<0.0001$) superior metastasis-free survivals among patients with NG I and NG II cancers compared to those among matched patients without such SW reactivity (Fig. 1). Among patients with NG III cancers, the survivals are intrinsically so favorable that SW reactivity, while still advantageous, has only little room for improvement.

The prognostic significance of SW reactivity against NG-characterized autologous breast cancer is further documented in Table 1. The ratio of patients with metastases <60 mpo to those without metastases ≥60 mpo is clearly influenced by both NG *and* specific SW reactivity. These data, as well as the previously cited observations, leave no doubt that the clinical behavior of breast cancer reflects intrinsic features of host as well as cancer. Moreover, as mentioned above, *the observed variations in clinical behavior are not dependent on cure.*

Second Primary Breast Cancers

If SW reactivity to autologous breast cancer reflects a CMI response that impedes metastatic progression, and if the immunogens expressed in different breast cancers are similar to one another and are most regularly associated with the in situ phase, it would be expected that SW reactivity to autologous breast cancer would impede the in situ-to-invasive progression of subsequent de novo breast cancers. It is noteworthy in this context that we have indeed found SW reactivity against autologous breast cancer to be inversely correlated with the proximate development of subsequent *invasive* primary breast cancers.[25]

Twenty-three of our patients who had been tested for SW reactivity against their autologous first breast cancers and/or gp55 1 to 24 mpo developed invasive second primary breast cancers. Thirteen of these patients had positive responses during the 1–24 months postoperative interval. In *none* of these 13 patients did the invasive second primary breast cancer develop *within 30 months* and in only *one within 60 months* after the first breast cancer. In contrast, among the 10 patients who lacked such reactivity, the second invasive breast cancers developed within 30 mpo in three and within 60 mpo in eight patients (P<0.005 for the 60 months interval).

It is important to note that the retarding influence of specific CMI is observable over a wide range of postoperative intervals, i.e., 2 months to more than 10 years. Among the 12 patients who developed a second primary invasive breast cancer within 30 months of a SW test against autologous breast cancer and/or gp55, *none* had a positive SW response in a total of 32 tests. Among 15 patients who developed a second primary invasive breast cancer within 60 months of SW testing, five (33%) had at least one positive response, and a total of 9 of 69 such tests (13%) were positive. These data suggest that specific CMI retards the in situ-to-invasive cancer progression. This interpretation is supported by the contrasting relationship between SW reactivity and the proximate development of second primary *in-situ breast cancers* (Table 2). These data indicate that the *in situ-to-invasive cancer progression is a nonobligate, immunologically impeded event.* This interpretation is further supported by our observations that in five of the six in-situ breast cancers that developed within 30 months of a positive SW response, there was an associated intense LRE response and a "self-healing" type of necrosis, as exemplified in Figure 2.

The foregoing observations on the existence and prognostic significance of breast cancer-associated cell-mediated immunity are made all the more specific by the lack of analogous findings regarding antibody-mediated immunity. Xenogenic antibodies against gp55 do react with an appreciable proportion of breast cancer tissues.[40-42] However, unlike CMI, these antibodies are *less* regularly reactive with in-situ than with invasive cancer foci. Moreover, the antibody-reactive determinant is associated with the protein moiety of gp55, while the CMI determinant is associated with the carbohydrate moiety (unpublished observations). In addition, we found no correlation upon

---

Table 2
Relative Frequency of Positive Skin Window Reactivity (SW — 3) Against Autologous First Breast Cancer and/or gp55, Among Patients in Whom a De Novo Breast Cancer was Diagnosed Within 30 Months After Skin Window Testing, by Stage of the Second Cancer (Maximal Response per Patient During the 30 Months Interval)

Type of Second Primary Breast Cancer	Patients with SW — 3/Total Tested
Invasive	0/12[a]
In situ	6/7 (86%)[a]

[a]P < 0.001.

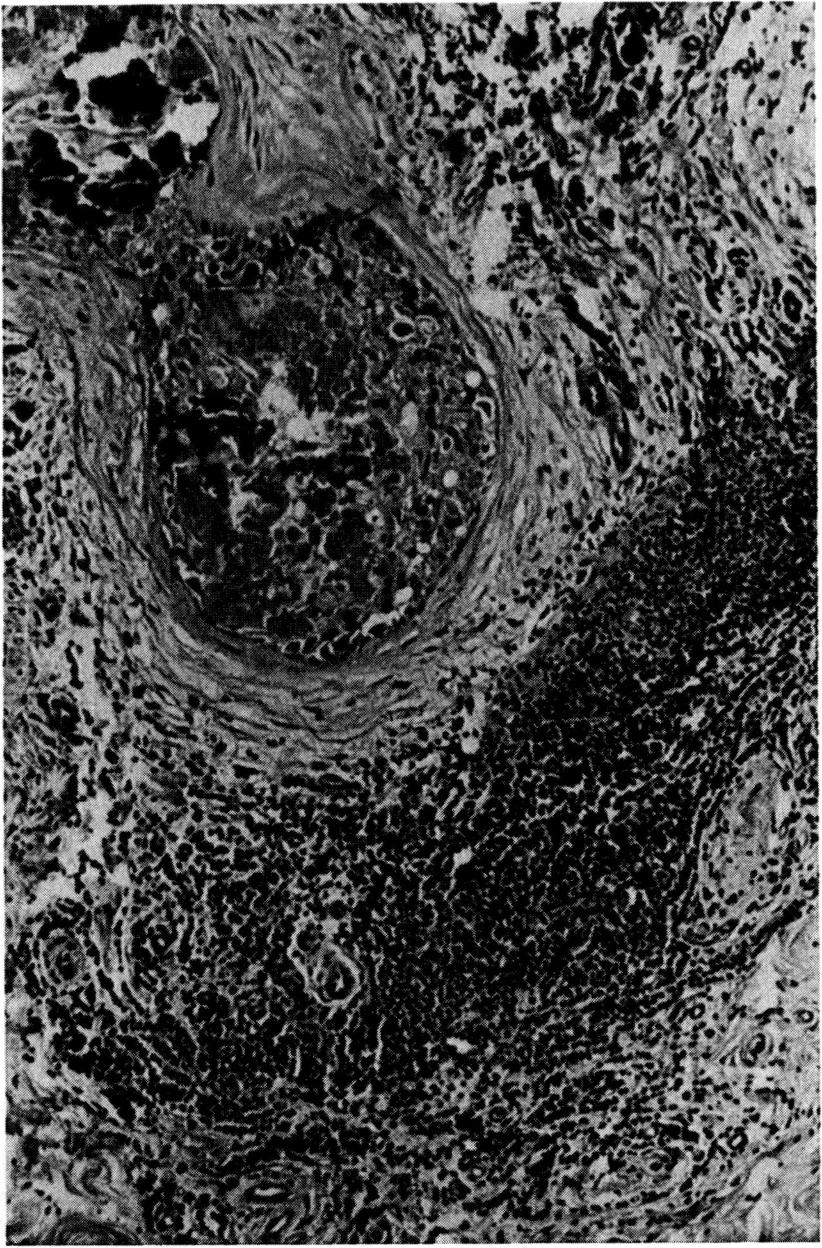

Figure 2: *Ipsilateral second primary in situ breast carcinoma, diagnosed 72 months after lumpectomy-treated invasive breast cancer, of a patient (code no. 86-0770) with positive skin window reactivity (SW-3) against gp55, 24 months prior to this second lesion. Note the intense lymphoreticulo-endothelial response to and the cytonecrotic changes of the cancer cells. Reproduced with permission by the publisher.[70]*

testing the same target tissues for CMI and antibody determinants, nor was the occasional presence of anti-gp55 antibodies in the sera of some breast cancer patients related to CMI against gp55 or to clinical behavior. Furthermore, immunohistochemical studies did not demonstrate binding of IgG, IgA, or IgE to autologous breast cancer. It is, therefore, highly unlikely that antibody-mediated immunity plays a role in the biological behavior of breast cancer. This is not to say that breast cancer cells might not be antigenically different from normotypic breast parenchymal cells, as judged by xenogenic responses. In fact, it would be surprising if they were not, since they are clearly different by so coarse a discriminant as microscopic examination. However, such antigenic markers are apparently *not immunogenic in the host of origin*. There is neither a priori nor empirical evidence that xenogenic antibodies exert any retarding influence on the development and/or metastatic progression of breast cancer.

Therapeutic Implications

The prognostically significant variables of both tumor and host provide the basis of intra-stage prognostic heterogeneity and should be considered in the selection of currently available therapeutic alternatives. Even more importantly, an appreciation of the clinical significance of tumor-associated antigenicity and specific immunity of the host may point the way toward the immunological control and prevention of breast cancer. The prognostically significant features with therapeutic implications include:

1. Breast cancer is characteristically immunogenic in its in-situ phase.

2. The in-situ carcinoma-associated immunogen activates the LRE system and provokes a CMI type of response.

3. The immunogenic CMI determinants, expressed by breast cancers in different stages and in different individuals, appear similar to one another and similar to a CMI determinant expressed by gp55.

4. The ISC-associated, gp55-like CMI *determinant* is "lost" in approximately one-fourth to one-third of invasive breast cancers.

5. *Reactivity* against the ISC-associated, gp55-like CMI determinant may vary in individual patients.

6. The metastatic progression of invasive breast cancer correlates inversely with the degree of nuclear differentiation of the cancer cells and with the proximate host CMI against the autologous cancer.

7. The development of subsequent invasive primary breast cancer is impeded by CMI against the autologous first breast cancer and/or against gp55.

In short, nuclear differentiation, specific antigenicity, and a specific type of host CMI constitute a clinically significant system that yields insight into the risk of metastatic progression of invasive breast cancer and the risk of development of a subsequent invasive primary breast cancer. This prognostic system differs from the TNM system, which is based on cancer size and stage but ignores the heterogeneities of tumor and host and the clinical reality that, *in the majority of breast cancer patients, dissemination has already occurred at the time of diagnosis.*[43]

The TNM staging system is a residue of the classic presumption that breast cancer is a homogenous entity, which undergoes a stepwise progression that is linearly dependent on time. It is this presumption that formed the basis of radical mastectomy and blamed the patient for not being cured.[44] The TNM system is impervious to the risk of second primary breast cancers and provides no conceptual guide to selection of the most appropriate of the currently available alternative types of primary and adjuvant therapy. Most distressingly, its general use obscures the need for and the potential development of new approaches to treatment and prevention. In contrast, a recognition of the diverse permutations of tumor and host that may occur in individual patients provides a rational basis for the selective use of currently available therapeutic alternatives and the exploitation of the therapeutic and prophylactic potential of immunological manipulation.

Currently Available Therapeutic Alternatives

Experience has demonstrated that, after surgical removal of the primary lesion, there remains a continued risk of systemic recurrences over extended postoperative intervals. This risk is *not* significantly reduced by increasing the extent of the primary surgical procedure, nor is it increased by the incomplete eradication of the local lesion. Since the aim of therapy should be to obtain maximal control of a disease with minimal attendant morbidity, it appears reasonable to utilize the least disfiguring procedure, i.e., lumpectomy, wherever this is consistent with the size of the tumor relative to the size of the breast. While the post-lumpectomy use of radiation therapy tends to reduce local recurrences, it has no demonstrable benefit on survival[45] and carries the intrinsic risk of regional tissue damage, leukemia, and a reduction in prolonged survival.[46] It remains to be shown that the routine use of post-lumpectomy adjuvant radiation therapy results in a net reduction in morbidity and mortality in all or in any particular subset of NG- and CMI-characterized patients.

The unsatisfactory control of breast cancer mortality by mastectomy led to the use of adjuvant cytotoxic chemotherapy. However, after more than a decade of observations, meta-analyses, and consensus meetings, it appears that the adjuvant use of CMF improves the overall survival to only a limited degree.[47] It is distressing that the extensive national and international clinical trials of adjuvant chemotherapy have made no attempt to relate their findings to intra-stage heterogeneity in terms of NG and specific immunity, despite the fact that such chemotherapeutic agents affect the replication and function of the DNA in *both* the cancer cells and the lymphoid cells. The conceptual and practical need for such studies has been repeatedly emphasized by this laboratory since 1959.[11,48] As shown in Table 3, among our stage II patients with NG I and NG II

Table 3

Postoperative Survival Characteristics Among Lymph Node-Positive Patients with Poorly or Moderately Differentiated Nuclear Grade Breast Cancers; Relationship to Skin Window (SW) Reactivity Against Autologous Cancer, 1–24 Months Postoperatively (mpo), and to Adjuvant CMF Therapy

	Adjuvant Therapy	
Skin Window Reactivity	*None*	*CMF*
	Number with SW − 3/Total Number Tested[a]	
All patients	12/85 (14%)	3/29 (10%)
	No. with MET <60 mpo/No. NED ≥60 mpo[b]	
SW − 3	2/10 [0.20][c,d]	0/3[e]
SW<3	38/30 [1.27][d]	13/9 [1.44][e]
Total	40/40 [1.00]	13/12 [1.08]

[a]Maximal reactivity/patient, 1–24 mpo.
[b]MET = systemic metastasis; NED = without clinical evidence of recurrent disease.
[c]Numbers in brackets are ratios.
[d]$P < 0.05$.
[e]Not significant.

cancers who were treated with adjuvant CMF, their survival was *not* improved over that expected according to NG and CMI.

Our data provide no support for adjuvant cytotoxic chemotherapy of breast cancers with well-differentiated nuclei, in patients having demonstrable CMI against their cancers, since there is little room for therapeutic benefit. In contrast, therapeutic assistance in the form of adjuvant therapy, including immune augmentation, would be indicated for breast cancers with poorly differentiated nuclei, in patients lacking CMI against their cancers. Although some attention has been given, of late, to the NG-related effects of adjuvant chemotherapy, there has not yet been a critical examination of the influence of cytotoxic adjuvant chemotherapy on the development of metastases and second breast cancers in patients characterized as to the NG of and the specific host CMI against the first breast cancer.

Immunological Manipulations

Amplification of Self-Selecting Populations of Prognostically Significant LRE Cells

In 1973, Black suggested that lymphoid cells collected from patients having SW reactivity to autologous breast cancer might be therapeutically beneficial if they were returned to the donor at the time of subsequently reduced SW reactivity or recurrence.[49] More recently, Rosenberg and associates[50-52] and others[53,54] have used lymphokines for the in vitro amplification of populations of lymphoid cells from the peripheral blood of patients with advanced cancer, to generate so-called lymphokine-activated killer cells (LAK). Lymphoid cells for amplification have also been derived from within advanced cancers or metastatic foci, so-called tumor-infiltrating lymphocytes (TIL). Both types of amplified cell populations have been used, with and without concomitant injections of inter-leukin-2, to treat patients with a variety of cancers. Such ingenious procedures have resulted in some striking benefits. However, such benefits have been limited to particular types of cancer, and the beneficial results have been sporadic. The lack of benefit in most patients may be related to our observations that *prognostically favorable, specifically reactive cells are uncommon* in lymph nodes, peripheral blood and cancer foci of patients with metastatic lesions. Accordingly, we would *not* expect that LAK or TIL, derived from such sources, would commonly express prognostically favorable anti-tumor CMI. On the other hand, our data suggest that it would be more productive *to isolate and amplify populations of lymphoid cells derived from positive SW tests against autologous breast cancer. This procedure would provide cells that have demonstrated an ability to focalize in a prognostically favorable fashion in response to the autologous cancer.* It would be of great interest to determine whether stored populations of such cells could restore prognostically favorable specific SW reactivity and impede the develop-ment of metastases in the donor.

Expanded populations of SW-derived, prognostically significant LRE cells should also be of value in the evaluation and potential use of transfer factor (TF). In 1949, Lawrence demonstrated the cellular transfer of cutaneous hypersensi-tivity in man[55] and, in 1955, showed that transfer of delayed hypersensitivity could be accomplished by use of soluble extracts of leukocytes, the active component of which was designated as TF.[56] As indicated in a recent extensive review by Fudenberg and Fudenberg, the subsequent history of TF included its use in diverse types of immunodeficiencies, infectious diseases, and cancer.[57] Although an initial soaring optimism was replaced by almost total oblivion, there remain therapeutic possibilities worthy of further examination. However, clini-cal evaluation requires, as a minimum, the demonstration that the donor cells possess the CMI in question and that the transfer procedure does in fact induce the desired specific immunity in the recipient. In short, to be effective, TF has to induce a demonstrable negative-to-positive change in specific CMI in the recipient. This caveat was previously emphasized by Black and Zachrau.[58] The point we would make at *this* time is that expanded populations of cells, derived from positive SW tests against autologous breast cancer, should provide a unique source for testing the ability of cellular extracts to restore prognostically significant immunity in autologous hosts. Similar benefits should extend to homologous hosts and control individuals, since TF is non-antigenic and, by definition, has the ability to impart *specific* CMI from sensitized to "naive" individuals. Accordingly, TF derived from sensitized cells should be able to impart anti-breast cancer CMI to control subjects.

In a 1973 report on human breast cancer as a model for cancer immunology, Black indicated that "in theory at least, transfer factor derived from the leukocytes of patients having high levels of cellular hypersensitivity against breast cancer should possess therapeutic potential in breast cancer patients and be a safe means of imparting heightened resistance to control populations. The most appropriate donors would be patients with in situ or microinvasive breast cancers who exhibit well-defined LRE and skin window reactivity against their autologous cancers. The transfer of cellular hypersensitivity from such patients to cancer-free individuals could then be monitored by the skin window technique and various in vitro techniques."[49] Our subsequent observations on the prognostic and prophylactic significance of SW reactivity to autologous breast cancer and/or gp55 makes this early suggestion all the more attractive. Moreover, the current ability to amplify populations of LRE cells with commercially available lymphokines should make such a study all the more feasible.

Note, however, that specifically reactive cells should not impede the metastatic progression of those autologous or homologous breast cancer cells that have "lost" the ISC-associated, gp55-like antigen determinant. The possibility of change in antigen expression should be considered in the evaluation of putative immunotherapeutic procedures, since the failure to do so compromises the validity of such evaluation.

Immune Augmentation

Procedures that favor the maintenance or restoration of specific CMI in breast cancer patients should reduce the risk of metastatic progression and the

Table 4

Maximal Skin Window (SW) Reactivity of Breast Cancer (BCa) Patients Against Autologous Carcinoma, 1–12 Months Before and 1–12 Months After Adjuvant Therapy with Vitamin A and/or Vitamin E, at Diverse Postoperative Intervals, Ranging from 3 to 120 Months

	Post-Therapy		
Pre-Therapy	SW − 3[a]	SW < 3[b]	Total
	Patients with In Situ BCa		
SW − 3	2	1	3 (33)[c,e]
SW < 3	3 [50][d]	3	6 [100]
Total	5 (56)[e]	4	9 (100)
	Patients with Invasive BCa		
SW − 3	5	6	11 (21)[f]
SW < 3	23 [56]	18	41 [100]
Total	28 (54)[f]	24	52 (100)

[a]SW − 3 = positive reactivity.
[b]SW < 3 = negative or intermediate reactivity.
[c]Numbers in parentheses, percentages relative to total in parentheses.
[d]Numbers in brackets, percentages relative to bracketed total.
[e]Not significant.
[f]P < 0.002.

Table 5
Maximal Skin Window (SW) Reactivity of Breast Cancer (BCa) Patients Against RIII-MuMTV gp55, 1–12 Months Before and 1–12 Months After Adjuvant Therapy with Vitamin A and/or Vitamin E, at Diverse Postoperative Intervals, Ranging from 3 to 120 Months

| Pre-Therapy | Post-Therapy | | |
	SW − 3[a]	SW < 3[b]	Total
	Patients with In Situ BCa		
SW − 3	3	2	5 (38)[c,e]
SW < 3	4 [50][d]	4	8 [100]
Total	7 (54)[e]	6	13 (100)
	Patients with Invasive BCa		
SW − 3	17	4	21 (36)[f]
SW < 3	26 [70]	11	37 [100]
Total	43 (74)[f]	15	58 (100)

[a]SW − 3 = positive reactivity.
[b]SW < 3 = negative or intermediate reactivity.
[c]Numbers in parentheses, percentages relative to total in parentheses.
[d]Numbers in brackets, percentages relative to bracketed total.
[e]Not significant.
[f]P < 0.0001.

development of second primary invasive breast cancers. While the literature is replete with reports of agents and procedures that were initially thought to possess immunologically mediated therapeutic effects against different types of cancer, almost all such promises were followed by disappointment. Such results could well have been expected since the "immunotherapeutic" procedures were neither chosen nor evaluated on the basis of their ability to transfer or induce prognostically favorable specific immunity. In the absence of such data, it is difficult to know whether a lack of clinical benefit reflects lack of stimulation of specific immunity, lack of target antigenicity, or whether the clinical behavior is indeed unaffected by treatment-induced specific immunity.[59]

Since we observed that spontaneously occurring postoperative specific SW reactivity is prognostically significant, it was of interest to determine whether such reactivity could be augmented iatrogenically. Prompted by reports of an immunoadjuvant influence of retinoids and alpha-tocopherol,[60–63] we initiated a study of the adjuvant influence of these agents on SW reactivity against autologous breast cancer and gp55. We found that retinol in the form of 200–300 K units of vitamin A (VA) per day and alpha-tocopherol in the form of 1,200–1,600 units of vitamin E (VE) per day, singly or in combination, for 1 to 2 months, increased SW reactivity against autologous breast cancer and/or gp55.[64,65] As shown in Tables 4 and 5 and exemplified in Figure 3, such treatments were capable of inducing negative-to-positive changes in SW reactivity against autologous breast cancer and against gp55. These effects were demonstrable over a wide range of postoperative intervals.

The observed increase in specific SW reactivity, associated with the adjuvant

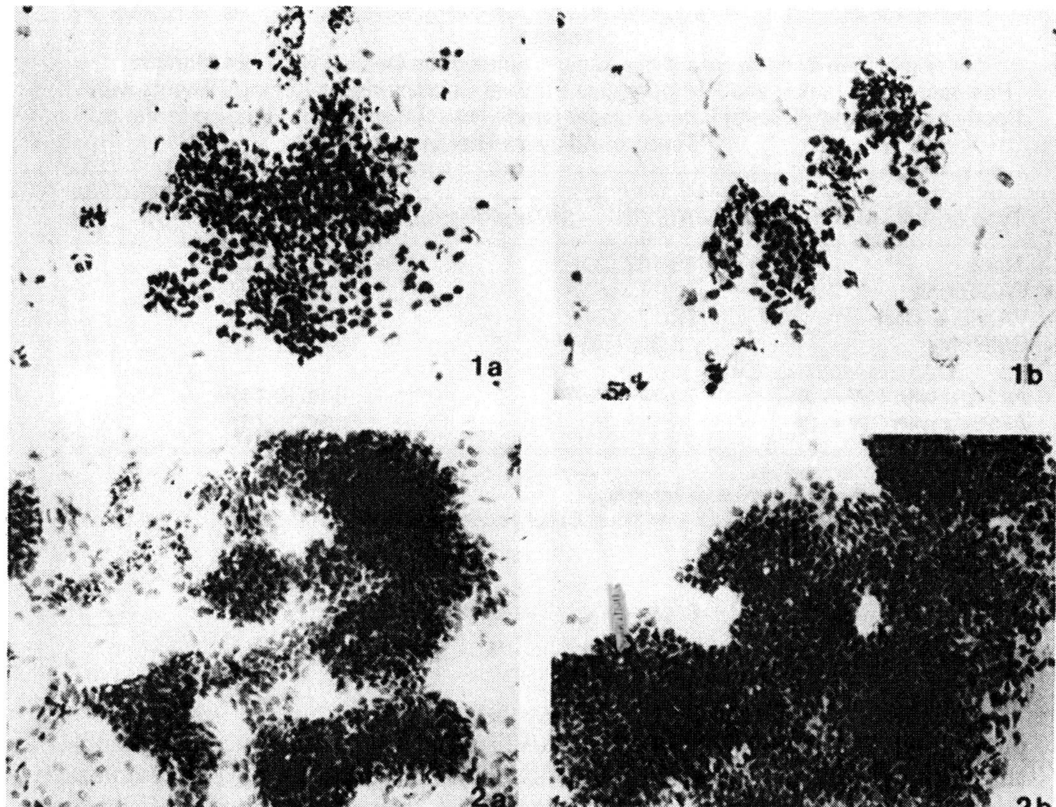

Figure 3: *Vitamin therapy-associated negative-to-positive changes in skin window reactivity. Simultaneous tests of a patient (code no. 80-3086) against gp55 and autologous in situ breast cancer before (1a, 1b) and after (2a, 2b) 25 days of treatment with 1,200 IU vitamin E per diem. Such negative-to-positive changes in prognostically significant immune reactivity should be demonstrable with any effective immunotherapeutic procedure. Reproduced with permission by the publisher.[70]*

VA/VE treatment of breast cancer patients, made it pertinent to determine whether treatment-associated reactivity against NG-characterized autologous breast cancer bears a similar relationship to survival as spontaneous reactivity. In Figure 1 and in Table 1, we demonstrated that the postoperative survival characteristics of NG-classified breast cancer patients correlate with SW reactivity against the autologous cancer. Such a relationship was also observed among patients who received adjuvant CMF therapy (Table 3). We now demonstrate that the VA/VE-associated increase in specific CMI is accompanied by a reduction in the relative frequency of early metastases.

As shown in Table 6, among different subgroups of patients with NG I and NG II breast cancers, the ratios of those with systemic metastases within 60 mpo to those who remained clinically free of recurrent disease for ≥60 mpo varied with the proportion of positive SW responses to autologous breast cancer. More

Table 6
Maximal Skin Window Reactivity Against Autologous Carcinoma, 1–24 Months
Postoperatively (mpo), and Postoperative Survival Characteristics Among Patients with
Poorly or Moderately Differentiated Nuclear Grade Breast Cancers, in Relation to Various
Types of Adjuvant Therapy

Type of Adjuvant Therapy	No. SW − 3[a]/Total Tested	No. with MET <60 mpo/No. NED ≥60 mpo[c]
None	46/162 (28)[d,e]	49/95 [0.52][f,g]
VA/VE only	11/17 (65)[d]	1/13 [0.08][f]
VA/VE + CMF	12/17 (71)[h]	3/8 [0.38][i]
CMF only	3/30 (10)[e,h]	13/13 [1.00][g,i]
All Pat's with SW − 3[a]	72/72 (100)	8/56 [0.14][k]
All Pat's with SW < 3[b]	0.162 (0)	63/80 [0.79][k]

[a]SW − 3 = positive reactivity.
[b]SW < 3 = negative or intermediate reactivity.
[c]MET = systemic metastasis; NED = without clinical evidence of recurrent disease.
[d]$P < 0.01$.
[e]$P = 0.061$.
[f]$P = 0.082$.
[g,i]ns.
[h,k]$P < 0.0001$.

particularly, the survival ratio in the VA/VE-treated series fits a linear relationship between SW reactivity and survival as defined in NG I and NG II breast cancer patients who did not receive adjuvant therapy ($r = 0.88$). In short, adjuvant therapy with VA/VE is clinically beneficial in accord with the degree of immune augmentation. These observations parallel those of Eccles et al. on the influence of a retinol derivative on the progression of experimental tumors having varying antigenicity.[66,67] They, too, found a treatment-associated retardation of tumor growth and metastases that appeared to be immunologically mediated rather than to result from a direct effect of retinol on the cancer cells.

Since the precursor-to-invasive progression of breast cancer is impeded by spontaneous proximate specific CMI, it should follow that procedures that augment ambient CMI against ISC-associated immunogens should impede the subsequent development of invasive breast carcinomas. Accordingly, the increase in SW reactivity against autologous breast cancer and/or gp55, associated with adjuvant VA/VE treatment, should be accompanied by a reduction in risk of subsequent de novo *invasive* breast cancers. In our patients who developed second primary breast cancers and did not receive VA/VE therapy, 22 of 28 (79%) of these second cancers were invasive. In contrast, among six patients who developed second primary breast cancers subsequent to VA/VE therapy, only two were invasive. These data are consistent with what should be obtained if there is indeed a treatment-related reduction in the precursor-to-invasive cancer progression. An extended study of this provocative possibility is certainly warranted.

Considered singly and in aggregate, data derived from diverse populations and over extended time periods demonstrate that the immunological evaluation of patients with breast cancer is prognostically important and warrants consideration in the choice of currently available primary and adjuvant therapeutic alternatives.

Immunization

The demonstration that the precursor phase of mammary carcinogenesis is characteristically immunogenic and associated with the expression of a CMI determinant that is similar in different breast cancers should have immunoprophylactic implications.[28,29,68-70] Such an expectation also follows from the observed inverse relationship between SW reactivity against autologous breast cancer and/or gp55 and the proximate development of subsequent invasive breast cancers. *Accordingly, it would be expected that the immunization of control individuals against the ISC-associated immunogen should prevent the development of first invasive breast cancers.*

Our observations suggest that gp55, or its isolated carbohydrate component, might be used as the immunogen in control individuals. However, we would emphasize that, before any clinical trial of immunoprophylaxis is undertaken, it should be demonstrated that the putative immunizing procedure can indeed induce CMI against gp55 and/or representative in-situ breast cancer tissues. *If this preliminary end-point can be attained, there would be ample justification for undertaking a clinical trial of the prophylactic effect of such immunization.*

More than three decades ago, it was evident that ". . . many, if not most, of our best survival rates represent bodily control of so-called autonomous malignant tumors, a control accomplished without the use of marrow toxic chemicals . . . , or the loss of goodly portions of our anatomy . . ."[36] The ensuing years have provided support for the validity and clinical importance of this appraisal. We submit that the exploitation of measurable immunological variables of tumor and host in breast cancer patients offers a high probability of reducing morbidity and mortality from the disease. Even more importantly, such procedures offer the potential for preventing the disease by immunoprophylactic manipulation.

Summary and Conclusions

1. The postoperative survival of breast cancer patients is significantly related to the nuclear differentiation of the cancer cells and the CMI against autologous breast cancer. The former can be evaluated microscopically, while the latter can be evaluated by a SW procedure. Although these parameters vary independently of one another, each exerts a highly significant influence on subsequent survival.

2. The immunogenicity that provokes prognostically significant CMI becomes manifest in the precursor phase of mammary carcinogenesis and reflects

a CMI determinant that is similar to a CMI determinant expressed in the gp55 component of the RIII-MuMTV. This determinant is expressed in most preinvasive breast cancers and in approximately 50–70% of invasive breast cancers.

3. Measurements of SW reactivity against NG-characterized autologous breast cancer provide a prognostic classification system that is pertinent to the selection of currently available primary and adjuvant therapies. More importantly, they provide a guide to the development of immunotherapeutic procedures.

4. The shared nature of the in situ carcinoma-associated immunogen and the negative correlation between specific CMI and the in situ-to-invasive cancer progression are consistent with the development of immunoprophylaxis.

5. The adjuvant use of high-dose retinol and/or alpha-tocopherol augments SW reactivity to autologous breast cancer and/or gp55. Such effects appear intrinsically and prototypically significant in regard to both immunotherapy and immunoprophylaxis.

In essence, immunological evaluation of patients with breast cancer does, indeed, have a significant role in their management by currently available procedures and an even more important role in the ultimate development of immunotherapy and immunoprophylaxis.

References

1. MacCarty WC, Mable AE: Relation of differentiation and lymphocytic infiltration to post-operative survival in gastric carcinoma. J Lab Clin Med 1921; 6:473–489.
2. Steiner PE, Maimon SN, Palmer WL, Kirzner JB: Gastric cancer: morphologic factors in five year survival after gastrectomy. Am J Pathol 1948; 24:947–961.
3. Moore OS, Foote FW Jr: The relatively favorable prognosis of medullary carcinoma of the breast. Cancer 1949; 2:635–642.
4. Hamlin IME: Possible host resistance in carcinoma of the breast: a histologic study. Br J Cancer 1968; 22:383–401.
5. Black MM, Chabon AB: In situ carcinoma of the breast. Pathol Annu 1969; 4:185–210.
6. Black MM, Chabon AB: Incipient carcinoma of the breast: structural characteristics and host reactivity. In: Severi L (ed). Immunity and Tolerance in Oncogenesis. Division of Cancer Research, Perugia, Italy, pp 923–936, 1970.
7. Black MM, Barclay THC, Hankey BF: Prognosis in breast cancer utilizing histologic characteristics of the primary tumor. Cancer 1975; 36:2048–2055.
8. Black MM, Speer FD: Sinus histiocytosis of lymph nodes in cancer. Surg Gynecol Obstet 1958; 106:163–175.
9. Black MM, Speer FD: Lymph node reactivity in cancer patients. Surg Gynecol Obstet 1960; 110:477–487.
10. Anastassiades OT, Pryce DM: Immunological significance of the morphological changes in lymph nodes draining breast cancer. Br J Cancer 1966; 20:239–249.
11. Black MM, Speer FD: Immunology of cancer. Surg Gynecol Obstet 1959; 109:105–116.
12. Black MM, Asire AJ: Palpable axillary lymph nodes in cancer of the breast: structural and biological considerations. Cancer 1969; 23:251–259.
13. Black MM: Immunology of breast cancer: clinical implications. In: Ariel I (ed). Progress in Clinical Cancer, Volume 6. Grune & Stratton, New York, pp 115–138, 1975.

14. Hirschl S, Black MM, Kwon S: Ultrastructural characteristics of sinus histiocytosis in lymph nodes during various stages of breast cancer. Cancer 1976; 38:807–817.
15. Black MM: Immunopathology of breast cancer. Pathobiol Annu 1977; 7:213–230.
16. Black MM, Leis HP Jr, Shore B, Zachrau RE: Cellular hypersensitivity to breast cancer: assessment by a leukocyte migration procedure. Cancer 1974; 33:952–958.
17. Rieche K, Arndt A, Pasternak G: Cellular immunity in mammary cancer patients as measured by the leukocyte migration test (LMT): a follow-up study. Int J Cancer 1976; 17:212–218.
18. Akiyoshi T, Nakamura Y, Kawaguchi M, Tsuji H: Cellular hypersensitivity to autologous tumor extracts in patients with breast carcinoma. Jpn J Surg 1978; 8:236–241.
19. Cannon GB, Dean JH, Herberman RB, Keels M, et al: Lymphoproliferative responses to autologous tumor extracts as prognostic indicators in patients with resected breast cancer. Int J Cancer 1981; 27:131–138.
20. Inamoto T, Ohgaki K, Hikasa Y, Kodama H: Specific antitumor immunity in pre- and postoperative state and 5-year survival of breast cancer patients. Nippon Geka Hokan 1984; 53:345–353.
21. Rebuck JW: Cytology of acute inflammation in man by two original technical procedures with particular reference to the role of lymphocytes. Doctoral thesis, University of Minnesota, 1947.
22. Black MM, Leis HP Jr: Human breast carcinoma: III. Cellular responses to autologous breast cancer: skin window procedure. NY State J Med 1970; 70:2583–2589.
23. Black MM, Leis HP Jr: Cellular responses to autologous breast cancer tissue: correlation with stage and lymphoreticuloendothelial reactivity. Cancer 1971; 28:263–273.
24. Black MM, Leis HP Jr: Cellular responses to autologous breast cancer tissue: sequential observations. Cancer 1973; 32:384–389.
25. Black MM, Zachrau RE, Hankey BF, Wesley M: Skin window reactivity to autologous breast cancer: an index of prognostically significant cell-mediated immunity. Cancer 1988; 62:72–83.
26. Black MM, Zachrau RE: Antitumor immunity in breast cancer patients: biological and therapeutic implications. J Reprod Med 1979; 23:21–32.
27. Couperus M, Rucker RC: Histopathological diagnosis of malignant melanoma. AMA Arch Dermat Syph 1954; 70:199–216.
28. Black MM: Cellular and biologic manifestations of immunogenicity in precancerous mastopathy. Natl Cancer Inst Monogr 1972; 35:73–82.
29. Black MM: Structural, antigenic and biological characteristics of precancerous mastopathy. Cancer Res 1976; 36:2596–2604.
30. Black MM, Kwon CS: Precancerous mastopathy: structural and biological considerations. Pathol Res Pract 1980; 166:491–514.
31. Black MM, Zachrau RE, Shore B, Dion AS, et al: Cellular immunity to autologous breast cancer and RIII-murine mammary tumor virus preparations. Cancer Res 1978; 38:2068–2076.
32. Zachrau RE, Black MM, Dion AS, Shore B, et al: Specificity of the simultaneous cell-mediated immune reactivity to RIII-murine mammary tumor virus glycoprotein 55 and human breast cancer tissues. Cancer Res 1978; 38:3414–3420.
33. Black MM, Zachrau RE, Ashikari RH, Hankey BF: Prognostic significance of cellular immunity to autologous breast carcinoma and glycoprotein 55. Arch Surg 1989; 124:202–206.
34. Springer GF, Desai PR, Wise W, Carlstedt SC, et al: Pancarcinoma T and Tn epitopes: autoimmunogens and diagnostic markers that reveal incipient carcinoma and help establish prognosis. In: Herberman RB, Mercer DW (eds). Immunodiagnosis of Cancer, Second Edition. Marcel Dekker, New York, pp 587–612, 1990.
35. Black MM, Speer FD, Opler SR: Structural representations of the tumor-host relation-

ships in mammary carcinoma: biologic and prognostic significance. Am J Clin Pathol 1956; 26:250–265.

36. Black MM, Speer FD, Opler SR: Some components of biologic predeterminism in cancer. Surg Gynecol Obstet 1956; 102:223–230.

37. Black MM, Speer FD: Nuclear structure in cancer tissues. Surg Gynecol Obstet 1957; 105:97–102.

38. Black MM, Kwon CS: Prognostic factors. In: Gallager HS, Leis HP Jr, Snyderman RK, et al. (eds). The Breast. CV Mosby, St. Louis, pp 297–319, 1978.

39. Moran RE, Black MM, Alpert L, Straus MJ: Correlation of cell-cycle kinetics, hormone receptors, histopathology and nodal status in human breast cancer. Cancer 1984; 54:1586–1590.

40. Mesa-Tejada R, Keydar I, Ramanarayanan M, Ohno T, et al: Detection in human breast carcinoma of an antigen immunologically related to a group-specific antigen of mouse mammary tumor virus. Proc Natl Acad Sci USA 1978; 75:1529–1533.

41. Mesa-Tejada R, Branwood AM, Keydar I, Fenoglio CM, et al: Increased incidence of immunohistochemically detectable mouse mammary tumor virus-related antigen in breast carcinoma tissues of patients with a family history of this disease. Proc Am Assoc Cancer Res Am Soc Clin Oncol 1979; 20:276.

42. Keydar I, Selzer G, Chaitchik S, Hareuveni M, et al: A viral antigen as a marker for the prognosis of human breast cancer. Eur J Cancer Clin Oncol 1982; 18:1321–1328.

43. Black MM, Speer FD: Biological variability of breast cancer in relation to diagnosis and therapy. NY State J Med 1953; 53:1560–1563.

44. Black MM, Zachrau RE: The use and abuse of therapeutic modalities in breast cancer. Prev Med 1990; 19:723–729.

45. Fisher B, Bauer M, Margolese R, Poisson R, et al: Five-year results of a randomized clinical trial comparing total mastectomy and segmental mastectomy with or without radiation in the treatment of breast cancer. N Engl J Med 1985; 312:665–673.

46. Cuzick J, Stewart H, Peto R, Baum M, et al: Overview of randomized trials of postoperative adjuvant radiotherapy in breast cancer. Cancer Treatment Rep 1987; 71:15–29.

47. US General Accounting Office/Program Evaluation and Methodology Division: Report to the Chairman, Subcommittee on Health and the Environment, Committee on Energy and Commerce, House of Representatives. GAO/PEMD 1989; 89–9:2–52.

48. Black MM, Hankey BF, Barclay THC: Intrastage prognostic heterogeneity: implications for adjuvant chemotherapy of breast cancer. J Natl Cancer Inst 1982; 68:445–447.

49. Black MM: Human breast cancer: a model for cancer immunology. Israel J Med Sci 1973; 9:284–299.

50. Rosenberg SA, Lotze MT, Muul LM, Chang AE, et al: A progress report on the treatment of 157 patients with advanced cancer using lymphokine-activated killer cells and interleukin-2 or high-dose interleukin-2 alone. N Engl J Med 1987; 316:889–897.

51. Rosenberg SA, Packard BS, Aebersold PM, Solomon D, et al: Use of tumor-infiltrating lymphocytes and interleukin-2 in the immunotherapy of patients with metastatic melanoma: a preliminary report. N Engl J Med 1988; 319:1676–1680.

52. Topalian SL, Solomon D, Avis FP, Chang AE, et al: Immunotherapy of patients with advanced cancer using tumor-infiltrating lymphocytes and recombinant interleukin-2: A pilot study. J Clin Oncol 1988; 6:839–853.

53. Kradin RL, Boyle LA, Preffer FI, Callahan RJ, et al: Tumor-derived interleukin-2 dependent lymphocytes in adoptive immunotherapy of lung cancer. Cancer Immunol Immunother 1987; 24:76–85.

54. Kradin RL, Kurnick JT, Lazarus DS, Preffer FI, et al: Tumor-infiltrating lymphocytes and interleukin-2 treatment of advanced cancer. Lancet 1989; i(#8638):577–580.

55. Lawrence HS: The cellular transfer of cutaneous hypersensitivity to tuberculin in man. Proc Soc Exp Biol Med 1949; 71:516–22.

56. Lawrence HS: The transfer in humans of delayed skin sensitivity to streptococcal M

  substance and to tuberculin with disrupted leukocytes. J Clin Invest 1955; 34:219–30.
57. Fudenberg HH, Fudenberg HH: Transfer factor: past, present and future. Annu Rev Pharmacol Toxicol 1989; 29:475–516.
58. Black MM, Zachrau RE: Immunotherapy of breast cancer? In: Gallager HS, Leis HP Jr, Snyderman RK, et al. (eds). The Breast. CV Mosby, St. Louis, pp 393–408, 1978.
59. Black MM, Zachrau RE: Immune mechanisms: prognostic therapeutic and preventive significance. In: Ariel IM, Cleary JB (eds). Breast Cancer: Diagnosis and Treatment. McGraw-Hill, NY, pp 128–142, 1986.
60. Cohen BE, Gill F, Cullen PR, Morris PJ: Reversal of postoperative immunosuppression in man by vitamin A. Surg Gynecol Obstet 1979; 149:658–662.
61. Patek P, Collin JL, Yogeeswaran G, Dennert G: Antitumor potential of retinoic acid: Stimulation of immune-mediated effectors. Int J Cancer 1979; 24:624–628.
62. Beisel WR: Single nutrients and immunity. Am J Clin Nutr 1982; 35(Suppl):417–468.
63. Bellag W: Vitamin A and retinoids: from nutrition to pharmacotherapy in dermatology and oncology. Lancet 1983; i(#8329):860–863.
64. Black MM, Zachrau RE, Dion AS, Katz M: Stimulation of prognostically favorable cell-mediated immunity of breast cancer patients by high dose vitamin A and vitamin E. In: Prasad KN (ed). Vitamins, Nutrition and Cancer. S. Karger, Basel, pp 134–146, 1984.
65. Black MM, Zachrau RE, Katz MF: Adjuvant immunotherapy of breast cancer: prototypic observations with alpha-tocopherol and retinol. In: Prasad KN, Meyskens FL Jr (eds). Nutrients and Cancer Prevention. Humana Press, Clifton, New Jersey, pp 319–328, 1990.
66. Eccles SA, Barnett SC, Alexander P: Inhibition of growth and spontaneous metastasis of syngeneic transplantable tumours by an aromatic retinoic acid analogue. 1. Relationship between tumour immunogenicity and responsiveness. Cancer Immunol Immunother 1985; 19:109–114.
67. Eccles SA, Parvies HP, Barnett SC, Alexander P: Inhibition of growth and metastasis of syngeneic transplantable tumours by an aromatic retinoic acid analogue. 2. T cell dependence of retinoid effects in vivo. Cancer Immunol Immunother 1985; 19:115–120.
68. Black MM, Zachrau RE: Immunoprophylaxis of breast cancer: a conceptual appraisal. In: Paterson AHG, Lees AW (eds). Reviews on Endocrine-Related Cancer; Fundamental Problems in Breast Cancer. ICI Pharma, Mississauga, Ontario, pp 137–143, 1984.
69. Black MM, Zachrau RE: Stepwise mammary carcinogenesis: immunological considerations. In: Zander J, Baltzer J (eds). Advances in Early Detection and Treatment of Breast Cancer. Springer, Berlin-Heidelberg, pp 64–72, 1985.
70. Black MM, Zachrau RE: In situ carcinoma-associated immunogenicity: therapeutic and prophylactic implications in breast cancer patients. In: Klein G, Vande Woude G (eds). Advances in Cancer Research Vol 56. Academic Press, NY, in press.

46

Immunological Evaluation of Patients with Breast Cancer Has No Significant Role in Their Management

Marc M. Wallack, Stephen D. Scoggin

Cancer was the leading cause of death for women ages 35 to 74 in the United States in 1987 and was responsible for 476,927 reported deaths. Since 1950, breast carcinoma has been the leading cause of cancer deaths, only recently being overtaken by lung cancer. Survival improved significantly from 1960 to 1990. White patients diagnosed with breast carcinoma between 1981 and 1986 had a 78% chance of surviving 5 years compared to 75% if diagnosed between 1974 and 1980; however, a black patient's survival odds have remained unchanged at 63–64% since 1975. While the 3% improvement for white patients is statistically significant (P<.05), it is unclear whether or not this reflects more widespread screening and earlier diagnosis or actual improvement of the odds of surviving breast cancer. Though we have learned a great deal about the nature of this disease, the death rate has remained relatively constant at about 28 per 100,000 women and there will be approximately 175,000 new cases in the US this year. Questions regarding optimal surgical therapy have in large part been answered and of course surgery is the mainstay of therapy, but it is clear it is not as simple as removing the disease from the patient; adjuvant therapy is also an important part of treatment of a systemic disease. There are still questions to be answered concerning adjuvant therapy, but the modalities of radiation, chemotherapy, and hormal therapy are at present being employed with proven usefulness and have been practically optimized. Diagnosis relies on patient detection, physical examination, mammographic screening, and biopsy and, in truth, has become very good, yet women are still dying of breast cancer. With the

From: Wise L, Johnson H Jr (eds): *Breast Cancer: Controversies in Management*. Futura Publishing Company, Inc., Armonk, NY, © 1994.

explosion of knowledge in immunology in recent years, many heads have turned to this field for answers to basic questions concerning tumor behavior, the relationship of breast cancer to the immune system, and for immunodiagnostics and immunotherapeutics. With the elucidation of the basic mechanisms and components of the immune system, the development of hybridoma technology, and the characterization and production of many biological response modifiers, much excitement has been generated concerning the possibility of the application of this knowledge to the management of the breast cancer; however, to date it has failed to find a practical application. In fact, the National Institutes of Health (NIH) Consensus Conference on the Treatment of Early Stage Breast Cancer did not mention immunology in its report when it convened in June 1990. Nonetheless, it is an active area of research and practical use is on the horizon though that horizon is a little farther away than initially believed for breast cancer.

A long-held premise has been that of immunosurveillance. It stands to reason that cancer cells are not normal cells and it has been thought that in those with an intact immune system, any cell transformed to a neoplastic one would be recognized as foreign and thus eliminated. This concept was first put forth by Paul Ehrlich who envisioned a "positive mechanism" capable of eliminating "aberrant cells" providing protection from neoplastic cells. The idea that the development of a tumor was a result of a defect in immunosurveillance or, in other words, an immunodeficiency is perfectly logical and there is ample evidence to support such a position. Malignant tumors peak in childhood and old age when the argument can be made that the immune system is not fully functional. The incidence of malignancy in transplant patients taking immunosuppressive drugs is higher though restricted to a few types of tumors. The experience with acquired immunodeficiency from HIV virus infection is often cited as an example; however, it can also be used to argue against the concept as these patients do not have an increase in the most common tumors, i.e., breast, colon, and lung. Tumors removed at surgery are frequently characterized by a marked mononuclear infiltrate unrelated to tumor necrosis, and in fact, tumor infiltrating lymphocytes plus interleukin-2 have recently been shown to mediate regression of metastatic melanoma. In the case of breast cancer, approximately 80% of patients with in-situ carcinoma have lymphoid cellular responses in the region of the tumor and associated sinus histiocytosis of regional lymph nodes. These findings are associated with a more favorable prognosis. In addition, there is an inverse correlation between peripheral lymphocyte count and chance of recurrence.

The above observations support the idea that immunocompetence is an important variable in the tumor-"host" relationship, and tests for immunocompetence (Table 1)[1] would identify patients at risk for development of a tumor and those at risk for recurrence and provide an index of prognosis. One must remember, however, that in order to mount an immune response, an immunogen must be recognized. Breast carcinoma is decreasingly immunogenic with increasing stage[2,3] and immunological responsiveness is more a function of the antigenicity of the tumor than of the general immunocompetence of the patient. To be sure, as tumor burden increases and metastasis occurs, the ability to mount an immune response to a neoantigen decreases; however, the majority of

Table 1
Tests for Immunocompetence

Immune Cells	Detection or Enumeration	Function
T Cells	FCM[1] with MAbs[2] for CD2, 3, or 5	Lymphocyte proliferation to mitogens or antigens, DHS[3] skin test
T Cell Subsets	FCM with MAbs for CD4 (helper inducer) and CD8 (suppressor cytotoxic)	Functional assays for help, suppression cytotoxicity
B Cells	FCM with MAbs for CD19, 20, anti-H and Anti-L Chains	Serum immunoglobulins or subclasses, antibodies especially postimmunization
NK Cells	FCM with MAbs for CD16 or 56	K562 cellular cytotoxicity, ADCC
Complement	Immunochemical component detection	CH_{50} or specific hemolytic assay for components
Neutrophils	Morphologic or histochemical features by cell counter	Biochemical and microbicidal
Monocyte–Macrophages	Morphologic histochemical or features MAb to CD14	Biochemical and microbicidal

[1]FCM = flow cytometry.
[2]MAbs = monoclonal antibodies.
[3]DHS = delayed hypersensitivity.
Borrowed from Stites DP: Laboratory evaluation of immune competence. In: Stites DP, Terr Al (eds). Basic and Clinical Immunology, 7th ed. Appleton & Lang, Norwalk, CT, 1991.

breast cancer patients remain reasonably immunocompetent. They display few consistent abnormalities in immune function as evidenced by mixed lymphocyte cultures, delayed hypersensitivity, absolute numbers of lymphocytes, T and B cell numbers or ratios, the blastogenic response to mitogens, or immunoglobulin levels.[5] The evidence indicates that general immunocompetence does not correlate with prognosis. In fact, some investigators have reported the converse to be true,[6,10] a possible mechanism being the reduction of T-suppressor cells.

Indications for testing for immune competence are listed in Table 2. In the context of breast cancer, the indications at present are for research or monitoring neutropenia induced by cytotoxic chemotherapeutic agents, which is assessed simply by a white blood cell count. Evaluation for immunocompetence otherwise does not play a significant role in management.

This is not to argue that an intact immune system or immune recognition of breast cancer is not an important natural defense. But an intact immune system does little against a nonimmunogenic tumor. Immunologically mediated tumor retardation depends on both retention of the specific antigenicity of the cancer cells and the specific cell-mediated immunity of the host, and these can vary independently.[7] As mentioned previously, immunogenicity of breast carcinoma is inversely proportional to stage. The concept of heterogeneity of breast carcinoma and that antigen expression is a dynamic, changing process as the tumor develops, and that those changes that favor tumor growth are selected for is an important

---

Table 2
Indications for Testing Immunocompetence

Clinical diagnosis, therapeutic monitoring, or prognosis of[1]:
1. Congenital and acquired immunodeficiency diseases.
2. Immune reconstitution following bone marrow or other lymphoid tissue grafts.
3. Immunosuppression induced by drugs, radiation or other means for transplant rejection or cancer treatment.
4. Autoimmune disorders, as a possible adjunct to diagnosis (rarely useful).
5. Immunization, to monitor efficacy or immune status.
6. Clinical or basic research.

---

[1]Tests must be interpreted in the clinical context, particularly in conjunction with a thorough history and physical examination.
Borrowed from Stites DP: Laboratory evaluation of immune competence. In: Stites DP, Terr AI (eds). *Basic and Clinical Immunology*, 7th ed. Appleton & Lang, Norwalk, CT, 1991.

one as it is in large part responsible for the changing relationship seen between tumor and immune system as a tumor progresses. Antigenic modulation is one of many proposed mechanisms of "immunological escape" (Fig. 1) that tips the balance in favor of tumor growth, but seems to be one of the most important ones in breast cancer. Heterogeneity occurs to such an extent that cells from different portions of a single cancer in a single host may have markedly different potentials for hematogenous or lymphatic spread, organ-specific lodgement and growth, hormonal receptor content, hormonal sensitivity and response, chemotherapy response, production of angiogenic compounds, and many other features of cancer cell behavior and histologic appearance.[20] Monoclonal antibody studies of breast carcinoma antigens have all demonstrated marked heterogeneity and, in general, there is a decrease in the expression of any given antigen as tumors metastasize. Metastatic deposits likely begin as clonal expansions, but as they progress, substantial heterogeneity develops as well as it does in the primary tumor. Another mechanism of immune escape is loss of major histocompatibility complex (MHC) antigens. CD4 T cells (helper) recognize antigens in the context of class II molecules and CD8 T cells (cytotoxic and suppressor) in association with MHC class I molecules; however, studies have failed to correlate survival with expression of these antigens.[13] The study of the location of milk fat globule membrane provides a good model of antigenic modulation. Milk fat globule membrane is derived from the apical membrane of epithelial cells. Localization has been assessed using post-fixation immunoelectron microscopy. In normal and benign breast tissue as well as in well-differentiated tumors, localization is in relation to the apical membranes. Moderately differentiated carcinomas showed a combined picture of cell membrane, vesicular, and intracytoplasmic localization which is a feature of lobular carcinoma. Poorly differentiated carcinomas label throughout the cytoplasm with no cell membrane localization. Heterogeneity of labeling in the same sample is common. Apparently, breast carcinomas acquire a defect in intracellular transport of milk fat globulin, resulting in failure of expression at the cell surface and accumulation of vesicles within the cytoplasm, the

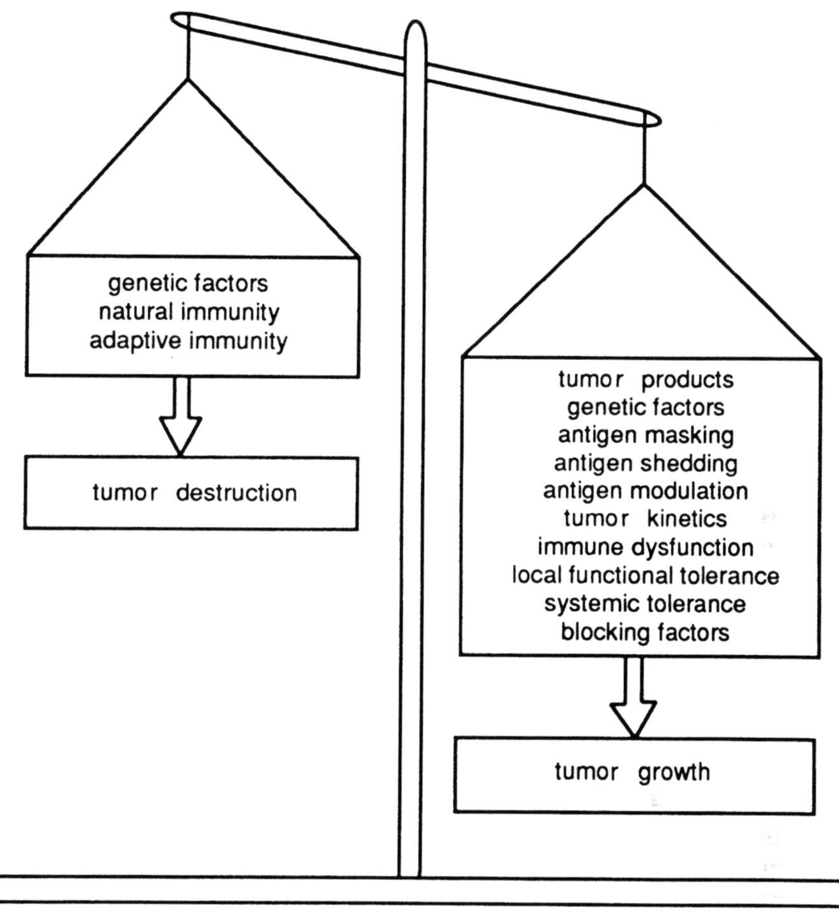

Figure 1: *Immunological escape (Borrowed from Dawson M, Moore M: Tumor immunology. In: Roitt IM, Brostoff J, Male DK (eds). Immunology, 2nd ed. CV Mosby, Cower Medical Publishing 1989.)*

extent of this correlating with the change in differentiation.[12] This progressive loss of antigen expression correlates with the finding that many times lymphoreticuloendothelial responses to in-situ carcinoma will be absent in areas of invasive carcinoma. This is supported by direct measurements of cell-mediated immunity from the same breast.[2]

As stated earlier, a cellular-immune response to autologous tumor is associated with a longer disease-free interval, a decreased chance of recurrence and longer survival.[2,3,6,7,10,11,17,19] These responses are not found against autologous normal breast and reactivity measured by the leukocyte migration inhibition and the skin window procedure is greatest for stage TIS > stage I > stage II.[2] Positive responses are uncommon among patients who develop metastases. The determinant that elicits a cellular response in the skin window procedure developed by Black[17] is similar to that of glycoprotein 55 (gp55), an envelope protein of the RIII murine mammary tumor virus. The frequency of response to the antigen is more commonly seen than with autologous tumor in patients with invasive cancer, further affirming the loss of this determinant in these tumors. In nuclear grades I and II tumors, a positive skin window test portends a better prognosis, however, it has no predictive value for nuclear grade III tumors which have a good prognosis independent of response. Nuclear grading itself has not yet come into widespread use; however, testing patients against autologous tumor or gp55 may prove useful in the future but at present does not play a significant role in patient management.

Agents that enhance the immunogenicity of a tumor and/or enhance recognition of antigens logically would enhance immunologically mediated tumor control. Nonspecific immunotherapy has generally been a failure as a therapeutic modality. Recent results from the National Surgical Adjuvant Breast and Bowel Project B-10 failed to demonstrate benefit from *C. parvum* administration in prolonging the disease-free survival[32] and this is in keeping with the failure of other nonspecific immunostimulating agents to find a role in therapy.[5] The phenomenon of virus augmentation of responses to tumor antigens that alone are weakly immunogenic has been described in many virus tumor cell combinations and is a promising approach to active immunotherapy. Melanoma cells lysed with vaccinia virus termed *vaccinia melanoma oncolysate* have shown promising initial results in the treatment of melanoma[31] and a phase III clinical trial is currently under way to assess the value of this modality. It is our practice to routinely evaluate these patients' immune status as immunocompetence correlates with response and prognosis in melanoma. Serological studies are also performed to monitor the development of antimelanoma antibodies in this trial. Although breast cancer has not been treated with oncolysates, vesicular stomatitis virus-infected breast tumor line extracts have been shown to elicit positive skin tests in a greater proportion of breast cancer patients than extracts prepared from uninfected cells.[4,5] Black has also reported the development of reactivity to autologous tumor and gp55 with the administration of tocopherol and retinol.[11]

Passive specific immunotherapy with monoclonal antibody has been a hope since the advent of hybridoma technology in 1975; however, the lack of progress in bringing it to useful fruition has been frustrating for most investigators. More than 20 antibodies have been identified as differentially reactive with breast cancer and probably as many as several hundred could be developed. The hopes that monoclonal antibody to breast tumor antigens could result in direct cytotoxicity, antibody-dependent cellular cytotoxicity, or complement-mediated cytotoxicity have not been realized as yet. Monoclonal antibody conjugated to toxins or radionuclides is an area of investigation. The trouble with this therapy is severalfold. First is the vast amount of antigenic heterogeneity that has been observed in most tumor masses using monoclonal antibody which impedes binding to all cells of the tumor for effective killing. Secondly, monoclonal antibodies do not internalize in carcinoma as they do in many monoclonal antibody-lymphocyte cell surface antigen complexes. Delivery of an effectively killing radionuclide to a tumor would obviate the need for binding to every cell or internalization. If these two modalities prove effective in the future, then immunological evaluation of breast tumors would be important to determine the most appropriate monoclonal antibody for delivery, but at present, immunological evaluation of tumor plays no significant role.

Monoclonal antibody conjugated with radionuclides has also been used for localization purposes and its use has even been reported for radioimmunoguided surgery using a hand-held gamma counter at surgery.[16] Monoclonal antibody has been used to evaluate the presence of serum antigens and antibodies associated with breast carcinomas, but as yet has not had an impact for diagnostic or prognostic purposes, and evaluation for the presence of circulating antigen or antibody has not found a role in the management of breast cancer. In addition, the presence of antigen/antibody complexes does not have diagnostic or prognostic significance.[9]

The modalities outlined have prognostic capabilities, however, at present do not meet the criteria set out for a useful prognostic factor outlined by the NIH Consensus Conference. These are:

- It has significant and independent predictive value that has been validated by clinical testing.
- Its determination must be feasible, reproducible, and widely available with quality control.
- It must be readily interpretable by the clinician and have therapeutic implications.[24]

Nuclear grade is a well-documented prognostic factor that is not widely used as is determination of S-phase fraction by flow cytometry. S-phase fraction determination is an independent prognostic factor and its clinical value is still being defined. It is recommended that determination of nuclear grade become routine.

Prognostic factors are of primary importance, of course, for determining therapy. Currently, the accepted, most widely applicable and reliable prognostic features are tumor size and nodal and receptor status. Trials are under way to evaluate adjuvant therapy in node-negative patients and, if all patients are eventually treated regardless of nodal status, this will eliminate the need for node dissection except for progressive axillary disease. The need for precise and reliable prognostic indicators is critical, particularly in patients without node metastasis to determine which are at high risk for recurrence, and those that are not can be spared adjuvant therapy. Immunologic evaluation may be able to fill that role but, at present, it does not.

In summary, at present, immunological evaluation for immunocompetence, tumor evaluation, diagnostic, therapeutic, or prognostic purposes does not play a significant role in the management of the breast cancer patient. A great deal of work is being done in this field and knowledge is increasing at an astonishing rate, and may well make a chapter with this title of historical interest only in the near future.

References

1. Stites DP: Laboratory evaluation of immune competence. In: Stites DP, Terr AI (eds). Basic and Clinical Immunology, 7th ed. Appleton & Lang, Norwalk, CT, 1991.
2. Black MM, Zachrau RE: Stepwise mammary carcinogenesis: immunological considerations. In: Zander J, Baltzer S. (eds). Early Breast Cancer Histopathology, Diagnosis, and Treatment. Springer-Verlag, NY, 1985.
3. Black MM, Zachrau RE: Immune mechanisms: prognostic, therapeutic, and preventive significance. In: Ariel IM, Cleary JB (eds). Breast Cancer Diagnosis and Treatment. McGraw-Hill, NY 1987.
4. Wallack MK, Bash JA: Immunology and immunotherapy of mammary tumors. In: Donegan WL, Spratt JS (eds). Cancer of the Breast, 3rd ed. WB Saunders, Philadelphia, 1988.
5. Smally RV, Oldham RK: Newer methods of cancer screening and treatment with biologics. In: Grundfest-Bromatowski S, Esselstyn CB Jr (eds). Controversies in Breast Disease: Diagnosis and Management. Marcel Dekker, Inc, NY, 1988.
6. Cannon CB Pomerantz R: Cell-mediated immune responses prognostic indications of survival from breast cancer. Int J Cancer 1989; 44:995–999.
7. Black MM, et al: Prognostic significance of cellular immunity to autologous breast carcinoma and glycoprotein 55. Arch Surg 1989; 124:202–206.
8. Schlom J: Future prospects in breast cancer research and management. In: Lippman ME, et al (eds). Diagnosis and Management of Breast Cancer. WB Saunders Company, Philadelphia, 1988.
9. Herberman RB, et al: Report on international comparative evaluations of possible value of assays for immune complexes for diagnosis of human breast cancer. Int J Cancer 1981; 27:569–576.
10. Cannon CB, et al: Lymphoproliferative responses to autologous tumor extracts as prognostic indicators in patients with resected breast cancer. Int J Cancer 1981; 27:131–138.
11. Black, MM, Zachrau RE: Prognostically significant skin window reactivity to breast cancer: influence of adjuvant therapy with retinol and tocopherol. Cancer Invest 1990; 8(2):277–278.
12. Coccoran D, Walker R: Ultrastructural localization of milk fat globule membrane antigens in human breast carcinomas. J Pathol 1990; 161:161–166.
13. Winizer HO, et al: Lacking prognostic significance of B2 microglobulin, MHC class I and class II antigen expression in breast carcinomas. Br J Cancer 1990; 62:289–295.
14. Blamey R: Does biological understanding influence surgical practice? Br J Cancer 1989; 60:271–274.
15. Walker RA, et al: An evaluation of immunoreactivity of c-erb B2 protein as a marker of poor short-term prognosis in breast cancer. Br J Cancer 1989; 60:426–429.
16. Martin EW, et al: Radioimmunoguided surgery using monoclonal antibody. Am J Surg 1988, 156:386–392.
17. Black MM, et al: Skin window reactivity to autologous breast cancer: an index of prognostically significant cell mediated immunity. Cancer 1991; 62:72–83.
18. Boring CC, Squires TS, Tong T: Cancer statistics, 1991. Ca - Cancer J Clinicians 1991; 41:19–36.
19. Black MM, et al: Cellular hypersensitivity to breast cancer: assessment by a leukocyte migration procedure. Cancer 1974; 33:952–958.
20. Cady B: New diagnostic, staging and therapeutic aspects of early breast cancer. Cancer 1990; 65:634–647.
21. Rush BJ Jr: Breast. In: Schwartz S, et al (eds). Principles of Surgery, 5th ed. McGraw Hill, NY, 1989.
22. Aust JB: Editorial comment. Am J Surg 1988; 156:392.
23. Clark GM, McGuire WL: Steroid receptors and other prognostic factors in primary

breast cancer. Semin Oncol 1988; 15 (Suppl 1):20–25.
24. NIH Consensus Conference: Treatment of early stage breast cancers. JAMA 1991; 265:391–395.
25. Fisher B, Costantino J, Redmond C, et al: Eight-year results of a randomized trial comparing total mastectomy and lumpectomy with or without radiation in the treatment of breast cancer. N Engl J Med 1989; 320:822–828.
26. Dawson M, Moore M: Tumor immunology. In: Roitt IM, Brostoff J, et al (eds). Immunology, 2nd ed. CV Mosby, Cower Medical Publishing, St. Louis, 1989.
27. Rosenberg SA, et al: Gene transfer into humans: immunotherapy of patients with advanced melanoma, using tumor-infiltrating lymphocytes modified by retroviral gene transduction. N Engl J Med 1990; 323:570–578.
28. Rosenberg SA, Spiess P, Lafreniere R, et al: A new approach to the adoptive immunotherapy of cancer with tumor infiltrating lymphocytes. Science 1986; 233:1318–1321.
29. Rosenberg SA, Packard BS, Aebersold PM, Solomon D, et al: Use of tumor-infiltrating lymphocytes and interleukin-2 in the immunotherapy of patients with metastatic melanoma: a preliminary report. N Engl J Med 1988; 319:1676–1680.
30. Mastrangelo MJ, Berd D, Maguire HC Jr, et al: Current conditions and prognosis of tumor immunotherapy: a second opinion. Cancer Treatment Rep 1984; 68:207.
31. Wallack MK, et al: Positive relationship of clinical and serologic responses to vaccinia melanoma oncolysate. Arch Surg 1987; 122:1460–1463.
32. Fisher B, Brown A, Wolmark N, Fisher ER, et al: Evaluation of the worth of corynebacterium parvum in conjuction with chemotherapy as adjuvant treatment for primary breast cancer: eight-year results from the National Surgical Adjuvant Breast and Bowel Project B-10. Cancer 1990; 66:220–227.

47

Breast Conservation Does Not Reduce Psychological Morbidity

Peter Maguire

Introduction

More and more surgeons are choosing breast conservation procedures as an alternative to mastectomy in the treatment of early breast cancer. They are doing this on the assumption that breast conservation lessens psychological morbidity because body image problems are reduced compared to patients undergoing mastectomy. Unfortunately, recent studies have shown that this assumption is incorrect. These studies will be reviewed and the implications for patient management discussed.

The Effect of Mastectomy

Controlled studies in the late 1970s using standardized questionnaires[1] or standardized psychiatric interviews[2] found that up to a quarter of women undergoing a mastectomy for early breast cancer developed an anxiety state and/or depressive illness within the first year of treatment. This morbidity was significantly greater than that found in women treated for benign breast disease. The use of adjuvant chemotherapy further increases the risk of affective disorders especially when chemotherapy is continued for a year.[3] Later studies have confirmed that the morbidity associated with mastectomy remains high.[4]

The risk of anxiety and depression is related to an inability to adapt to the loss of a breast and consequent problems such as increasing self-consciousness, a reluctance to look at the chest wall, and a heightened sense of vulnerability because the woman no longer feels whole.[5] Patients with body image problems

From: Wise L, Johnson H Jr (eds): *Breast Cancer: Controversies in Management*. Futura Publishing Company, Inc., Armonk, NY, © 1994.

are nine times more likely to develop sexual problems than those without. Up to a third of patients who had a satisfactory sexual relationship before surgery develop sexual difficulties.[2]

Complications such as pain and lymphoedema in the arm caused by surgery also provoke anxiety and depression,[5] because they hinder physical recovery and remind the patient that she has had a cancer removed. This association between mastectomy, anxiety, depression, body image problems and sexual difficulties has prompted surgeons to adopt breast-conserving procedures in the hope that this would reduce morbidity.

The Effect of Breast-Conservation

Sanger and Reznikoff[6] compared 20 women who had undergone a modified radical mastectomy with 20 women who had had breast conservation plus radiotherapy. They found fewer body image problems in the breast-conserved group but no difference in overall psychological adjustment scores. They commented that both groups appeared reasonably well-adjusted. However, this conclusion was of dubious value because the cooperating physicians refused to refer any women deemed to be having psychological difficulties as a result of diagnosis and treatment.

In an even smaller study of 11 patients who underwent breast conservation and 11 patients who underwent mastectomy, similar findings emerged.[7] Women undergoing mastectomy showed greater body image problems and sexual difficulties.

De Haes, van Oostram, and Welvaart[8] used the Rotterdam symptom checklist to assess patients 11 and 18 months after randomization to breast conservation plus radiotherapy or modified radical mastectomy. Of the 41 who were eligible, 34 (83%) patients (17 in each group) completed both assessments. While the body image of women was more severely impaired after mastectomy regardless of age, there were no differences in overall psychological effects.

The first study to examine the relationship between type of surgery and psychiatric morbidity was reported in 1986 by Fallowfield and colleagues.[9] Their sample included 101 women who agreed to take part in a randomized trial of breast conservation plus radiotherapy versus a modified radical mastectomy. None of the women had strong preference for either treatment. They were interviewed at home an average of 16 (range 4 to 32) months after surgery by trained interviewers using standardized psychiatric interviews. Against the study's main hypothesis, women undergoing breast conservation had a higher incidence of anxiety and depression (38%) than those undergoing mastectomy (32%). But there were fewer body image problems in the breast-conserved group. Interviews with the women suggested some important reasons why breast conservation failed to reduce morbidity. They were more afraid that some cancer remained, were more worried about recurrence, and interpreted having radiotherapy as meaning that they had a worse prognosis. So the benefits of reducing body image problems appeared to be offset by greater fears about their cancer.

Importantly, a large prospective though not randomized study carried out in Quebec[4] has confirmed these findings. Of 235 eligible women, 227 (96%) patients were seen 3 months after surgery and 205 (87%) were seen again approximately 18 months later. They measured psychiatric morbidity using a psychiatric symptoms index and calculated the proportion of high scorers in each group. Thirty-one (38.8%) of those 80 women who had undergone breast conservation were deemed to have high scores 3 months after surgery compared with 37 (25%) of those 147 subjects undergoing mastectomy. At 18 months, the proportion of high scorers (35%) in the breast-conserved (74) and mastectomy groups (131) was identical.

In a further prospective study,[10] 269 women diagnosed as having breast cancer were followed up for 1 year; there was no significant difference in psychiatric morbidity between the breast-conserved (anxiety 27%, depression 19%) and mastectomy groups (anxiety 28%, depression 21%). Sexual dysfunction was also high in both groups.

Thus, it has to be concluded that while breast conservation reduces body image problems, the benefits are offset by fears about disease and other treatments such as radiotherapy. Consequently, those involved in the management of women with early breast cancer must seek to reduce this psychological morbidity.

The Role of Choice

Morris and Royale[11] examined the effects of surgeons offering patients a choice of surgery. Patients were interviewed before surgery and every 2 and 3 months thereafter for 1 year and self-rating scales were administered. Before surgery, patients who had no choice were found to be more anxious and more depressed. Their spouses were also more adversely affected. In those offered a choice, there was no difference in psychological morbidity between those offered wide local excision or mastectomy. Two to 3 months after surgery, clinical anxiety and depression were significantly more evident in patients who had not been given a choice.

Patients who had no choice also had a greater fear of recurrence and were less interested in their normal hobbies and social activities. They felt they were less able to work at the same level as before and were less positive about the future.[12] In the group offered a choice, the only difference between the breast-conservation group and the mastectomy group was the former group's greater fear of recurrence.

Wolberg et al.[13] used a battery of self-report scales to assess women 4 months, 8 months, and 16 months after surgery for breast cancer or benign breast disease. They used the Psychological Adjustment to Illness Scale to measure psychological, social, and sexual changes. Adjustment problems were significantly greater in patients with cancer compared to those with benign disease. While there was an improvement in adjustment scores over time, there were still considerable residual problems 18 months after surgery. There were few differences between the mastectomy and the breast-conservation groups, but those who elected breast conservation reported more vigor and better sexual adjustment at follow-up compared to the mastectomy group. The authors concluded that the absence of major differences between the breast-conservation and the mastectomy groups in psychological morbidity was due to the fact that they had been completely informed and responsible for the choice of surgery.

Fallowfield et al.[10] have also been examining the effect of choice on psychological outcome. They have compared the patients of surgeons who offer choice with those whose surgeons prefer mastectomy or breast conservation. Patients who were given a choice or who realized they would have been given a choice had it been technically possible fared better psychologically than patients who were not given a choice. Hence, one important way of reducing psychological morbidity is to thoroughly discuss surgical options with patients with breast cancer when these are possible or explain why a choice is not viable. The psychological effects on women who develop a recurrence but were offered a surgical choice remain to be determined.

Patients who perceive that the information they were given about diagnosis and treatment was inadequate are more likely to become anxious or depressed.[9] Being told the diagnosis in the absence of a close friend or family member also increases the psychological morbidity. Hence, it is worth asking the patient if she would like to have someone present and if she has any questions about her diagnosis and treatment options.

Monitoring of Progress

Whatever preventive measures are taken, it is likely that a proportion of women will develop psychological morbidity. So, the question is how best to detect and help them.

Role of Specialist Nurses

When specialist nurses are employed and trained in interviewing and psychological assessment skills,[14] they recognize over 90% of those patients with breast cancer who develop problems that warrant psychological intervention. In contrast, less than 20% of those followed up routinely who are similarly affected and need help are detected. Importantly, psychiatric referral by the specialist nurse followed by treatment of her patients led to a three- to fourfold reduction in psychological morbidity compared to the control arm.

The monitoring was carried out through regular two monthly home visits. This distressed some women because it reminded them of their cancer and/or surgery. A limited intervention approach[15] was developed where specialist nurses restricted their visits to one home visit within 6 weeks of surgery and a controlled trial conducted to compare its efficacy with that of the original full intervention by specialist nurses. The limited intervention proved to be as effective as the full intervention. This approach now forms the basis of routine monitoring of patients undergoing treatment for breast cancer in our health district. Those found to have problems are referred to a psychiatric backup team or to their general practitioner.

A key question is to what extent surgeons and nurses involved in breast cancer care who do not have such specialist nurses can acquire and apply the relevant monitoring skills.

Monitoring Skills

Initial Assessment

When the patient first presents, there are key questions that should be asked which will inform the patient immediately that you are interested in her psychological well-being and prompt her to disclose any current concerns. Thus, when taking a history of the breast lump and associated symptoms, it is worth asking her when she discovered the lump, what she thought it might be, and how she felt about it. This will reveal how aware she is that it could be serious. The extent of any worry can then be explored. If she proves to be very worried, the basis of this can be established by asking "what is it that makes you so worried?" This may reveal that she has a strong family history of breast cancer and that other relatives have died from it.

Monitoring after Surgery

General questions that indicate an interest in how the woman has been affected by her surgery or other treatments are also effective in promoting disclosure, for example: "how have you been getting on since your operation?" More directive questions such as "how have you felt about losing a breast?" will make the woman feel that it is legitimate for her to disclose any adverse psychological reactions such as anxiety, depression, body image problems, or sexual difficulties. Concerns about her prognosis can also be elicited by asking "how do you see things working out in the future?" Women who are plagued by worry about their prognosis will then usually reveal this. In a small but important proportion of women, it will become clear that they have become persistently anxious or depressed to the extent that they can no longer distract themselves out of it. They will usually have other signs and symptoms of anxiety and depression such as initial insomnia, repeated waking or early morning waking, loss of energy, impaired concentration, and irritability. If this persistent mood change also represents a significant change from how the woman feels normally, the need for psychiatric help should be considered. Most patients so affected respond well to appropriate anxiety management training or antidepressant medication.

Women who find it hard to look at their chest wall because they are upset by it or are dissatisfied with the external breast prosthesis should be offered help for their body image problems. This may involve counseling, graded exposure to looking after relaxation, cognitive therapy, or breast reconstruction. Women with sexual difficulties often respond to the Masters and Johnson conjoint approach providing the partner will agree to be involved.

Conclusion

Regardless of the type of breast surgery used and the extent to which treatment options are offered, a proportion of women develop psychological morbidity as a result of the diagnosis and treatment of early breast cancer. It is, therefore, important to monitor their progress and detect those who need psychological help so that they can make a full emotional recovery.

References

1. Morris T, Greer HS, White P: Psychological and social adjustment to mastectomy. Cancer 1977; 40:2381–2387.
2. Maguire GP, Lee EG, Bevington DJ, Kuchemann CS, et al: Psychiatric problems in the year after mastectomy. Br Med J 1978; 279:963–965.
3. Hughson AVM, Cooper AF, McArdle CS, Smith DC: Psychological impact of adjuvant chemotherapy in the first two years after mastectomy. Br Med J 1986; 293:1268–1271.
4. Maunsell E, Brissen J, Deschenes L: Psychological distress after initial treatment for breast cancer: a comparison of partial and total mastectomy. J Clin Epidemiol 1989; 42:765–771.
5. Maguire P: Psychiatric morbidity associated with mastectomy. In: Baum M, Kay R, Scheurten H (eds). Clinical Trials in Early Breast Cancer. Birkhauser Verlag, Basel, pp 373–380, 1982.
6. Sanger CK, Reznikoff M: A comparison of breast-saving procedures with the modified radical mastectomy. Cancer 1981; 48:2341–2346.
7. Beckman J, Johanson L, Richards C, Blichert-Toff M: Psychological reactions in younger women operated on for breast cancer. Danish Med Bull 1983; 30:10–12.
8. de Haes JCJM, Van Oostrom MA, Welvaart K. The effect of radical and conserving surgery on the quality of life of early breast cancer patients. Euro J Surg Oncol 1986;.
9. Fallowfield LJ, Baum M, Maguire GP: Effects of breast conservation on psychological morbidity associated with diagnosis and treatment of early breast cancer. Br Med J 1986; 293:1331–1334.
10. Fallowfield LJ, Hall A, Maguire GP, Baum M: Psychological outcomes of different treatment policies in women with early breast cancer outside a clinical trial. Br Med J 1990; 301:275–380.
11. Morris J, Royle GT: Offering patients a choice of surgery for early breast cancer: a reduction in anxiety and depression in patients and their husbands. Social Sci Med 1988; 6:583–585.

12. Morris J, Ingham R: Choice of surgery for early breast cancer: psychosocial considerations. Social Sci Med 1988; 27:1257–1262.
13. Wolberg WH, Romsaas EP, Tanner MA, Malec JF: Psychosexual adaptation to breast cancer surgery. Cancer 1989; 63:1645–1655.
14. Maguire GP, Tait A, Brooke M, Thomas C, Sellwood R: The effect of counselling on the psychiatric morbidity associated with mastectomy. Br Med J 1980; 281:1454–1456.
15. Wilkinson S, Maguire P, Tait A: Life after breast cancer. Nursing Times 1986; 84:34–37.

Breast Cancer:

Is Anyone in Charge?

C. Barber Mueller

Introduction

This chapter presents a clinical impression of the breast cancer world of 1993. As with any small personal sample of the world, it may not be applicable everywhere, but for me, reflecting on 50 years of change, it attempts to describe what exists today. Surgeons are no longer the focal point in the treatment of breast cancer, the only player in the game. Others have become important and everyone seems to have a piece of the action in decision-making regarding diagnosis and therapy.

Diagnostic Radiologists

The driving force in early diagnosis has become the radiologist. A large effort now recruits women for screening mammography, and improved radiography is an important force. When the mammographer stands alone as an independent agent serving a self-referred population, he assumes the role of a primary care physician without relationship to surgeons, pathologists, and/or oncologists and rarely has he put a system in place for discharging the obligations that are associated with that role under case law. He directs therapy by the nature of his report without actually participating in subsequent management and fulfilling the role of the primary care physician.[1] The clinical studies on the efficacy of mammography are praiseworthy since outcomes are not measured in cancers discovered but in patient survival and deaths due to breast cancer. Of several major studies, those most usually referred to are the controlled trials

Table 1
Results of HIP and Swedish Studies on Efficacy of Mammographic Screening

	A *Health Insurance Plan of New York Study:* *10-year mortality data*			**B** *Swedish National Board of Health and* *Welfare Study: 7-year mortality data*	
	No.	*%*		*No.*	*%*
No. of women screened*	31,888	100	No. of women screened	78,085	100
Death from breast cancer			Deaths from breast cancer		
Screened	146	0.458	Screened	87	0.111
Control	192	0.602	Control*	125	0.160
Reduction in death from breast cancer	46 (24% rel- ative)	0.144 (abso- lute)	Reduction in deaths from breast cancer	38 (30% rel- ative)	0.049 (abso- lute)
Death from all causes			Deaths from all causes		
Screened	2,235	7.009	Screened	4,846	6.206
Control	2,116	6.636	Control*	4,787	6.131
Increase in death from all causes	119 (6% rela- tive)	0.373 (abso- lute)	Increase in deaths from all causes	59 (1% rela- tive)	0.076 (abso- lute)

*Includes women who were offered screening but refused.

*Adjusted for different number in control group.

From Wright CJ: Breast cancer screening. Surgery 1986; 100:595–596.

from Sweden and New York City (HIP Study).[2-5] Both trials show equal overall (total) mortality rates between the screened and the control groups. They show a reduction in breast cancer mortality in the screened group with an equal increase in deaths due to other causes. There are enough deaths *due to breast cancer* in both groups to make the difference statistically significant. The *total number of deaths* in the two groups is such that the small difference in mortality is not statistically significant (Table 1A and 1B).

The crucial issue here is "cause of death," something not always easy to determine, for guidelines are generally not precisely defined and blinded observers are not required. Neither the Swedish nor the New York Study addresses the issue of the increase in mortality due to other causes in the screened group.[6]

In looking at deaths due to breast cancer, the most statistically significant difference between screened and control groups occurred in the group of women between 50 and 60 years of age and this has led to recommendations of the American Cancer Society, which advocates screening women between 40–50 and 50–60. Cost effectiveness is difficult to assess for cost is generated not only by the cost of the x-ray examination but by unnecessary operations, anguish, fear, and apprehension of women who have benign disease. As in any comparative trial, survival benefits are unable to be seen in any individual patient, for although groups may be different, it is impossible to identify which woman was benefitted. False-positive rates are probably in the 60–80% range and false-negative rates in the 15–20% range. At times, the benign-to-malignant operative rates are as high as 12:1 or 16:1.[7] The Scottish experience, which established breast cancer clinics containing mammographers, surgeons, pathologists, cytologists, and oncologists in one setting, has reduced that figure to below 1:1 by the use of extensive preoperative diagnostic efforts such as needle biopsy, cytology, and stereotactic cytology and histology.

Mammography was originally established as a screening activity in asymptomatic women and had no role in the diagnosis of breast masses that are palpable.[8] However, publicity pushes practitioners into radiological and ultrasonic examination of all breast masses rather than directing the patient who has one toward the surgeon and pathologist. Mammographers generally use the criteria of Wolfe,[9] who uses pathological terms to describe radiological pictures and thus carries overtones that are unwarranted. Kopans[10] proposes a two-step affair that acknowledges a difference between screening mammograms and diagnostic mammograms. The diagnostic mammograms are associated with x-ray control, needle biopsy, cytology, and if necessary, histology, so they actually become more than just mammograms, but a complex regimen that leads to a pathological diagnosis.

Pathologists

The pathologist holds the key position in diagnosis for only he makes the diagnosis of breast cancer; all others have only presumptive diagnoses. There are two basic pathological techniques: cytology and histology, the latter seen with core/punch biopsy or an operative specimen.

When cytology is unequivocally positive, it may be considered correct. When it is negative, it generally does not count. When doubtful, it usually pushes the patient to the operating room. There are too few studies that report on false-positive and true-positive values because the positive predictor value of cytology depends not only on the skill of the cytologist, but also on the skill of the individual who inserts the needle. Cytology is generally reported as a description of the microscopic appearance and not in the five-grade fashion utilized for Pap smears. Such a grading system has not generally been adapted for breast reporting but might well be of benefit.

Histology with paraffin section is the gold standard and an invasion of the basement membrane of the duct or gland is the ultimate criterion of cancer. In 1971, Gallagher and Martin[11] introduced the concept of minimal cancer which included intraductal carcinoma, lobular carcinoma in situ, and invasive cancer less than 1 cm in size. Mammography is now bringing smaller, newer (?), earlier (?) lesions. There is more intraductal carcinoma, more in-situ carcinoma, and

Table 2
Results of Review of Minimal Cancers Detected by BCDDP

Cases Interpreted as Benign on Review

| | | No. of Cases by Project Diagnosis | |
Review Diagnosis	Total No. of Cases (%)	In-Situ Carcinoma	Infiltrating Carcinoma, <1 cm
Atypical ductal hyperplasia	47 (71)	42	5
Atypical lobular hyperplasia	7 (11)	6	1
Atypical ductal and lobular hyperplasia	3 (4)	3	0
Other benign	9 (14)	5	4
Total	66 (100)	56	10

From Beahrs O, Shapiro S, Smart C: Report on the working group to review the NCI-ACS Breast Cancer Demonstration Project. J Natl Cancer Inst. 1979; 62:640–664.

carcinoma with microinvasion. It is not known if all of these are lethal lesions even though some of the microinvasive lesions have axillary metastases.

Beahrs[12] conducted a review of the minimal cancers found in the Breast Cancer Demonstration Project. Four expert pathologists found a false-positive misdiagnosis in 13% of the minimal cancers (Table 2).

If the pathologist defines a lesion as cancer, it will get into the registry and if the lesion is not ultimately lethal, the cure rate will be improved. If there is an undercall—a false-negative—and carcinoma is missed, the true cancer will sooner or later be recorded. Thus all errors will be false-positives, errors that will increase the incidence of cancer and improve the cure.

All pathologists are not equal. Ackerman,[13] when conducting a course that presented 100 slides to pathologists, found an approximate 10% variability in diagnostic reading. These were not all standard "garden variety" specimens but represented some of the more difficult interpretations. A study by Linders[14] reported the uniformity of pathological diagnosis and found a 5% variability in both directions. There is no way to control this or even measure it well. The early NSABP studies provided control by using one man, Edward Fisher, to read all sections. At least this created uniformity. Neilson,[15] in an autopsy study of 83 women, made multiple sections of each breast and found that 25% had pathological features that could be diagnosed as cancer or precancer.

Lobular carcinoma in situ used to be considered a malignant lesion. It is now classified with the malignancies, but three decades have provided an opportunity to see the outcomes of unoperated women.[16,17] This lesion is different from the standard breast cancer; it is a marker of forthcoming cancer.

Ductal carcinoma in situ, or intraductal carcinoma, is now called cancer and it is put into the registry as such. Its long-term outcomes have yet to be defined.

It appears to be a marker similar to that of lobular carcinoma in situ, but the subsequent appearance of invasive carcinoma is probably three times greater than that of lobular carcinoma in situ.[18]

When lumpectomy follows needle-localized biopsy of nonpalpable lesions, the pathologist's role becomes crucial. It is he who defines the cell and histologic type, i.e., calls it cancer—he looks at the margins, may propose re-excision, and has a central role in classification. In nonpalpable mammographically positive lesions, the surgeon assumes the role of a technician required to excise what the mammographer calls and to excise it as the pathologist demands.

Therapeutic Radiologists

In the days of radical mastectomy, it was customary to irradiate wound, axilla, parasternal, and supraclavicular areas in the postoperative period. This was almost always done in women with positive lymph nodes. Today, radiotherapy is recommended after lumpectomy and breast-conservation surgery. NSABP B-06[19] showed that survival following lumpectomy was no different than that following simple mastectomy and that x-ray treatment did not affect survival. Local recurrence with and without x-ray treatment was studied. In the node-negative untreated group, the local recurrences were reported as 38% and in the x-ray-treated group, 20%. In the node-positive untreated group, the local recurrence was reported as 43% and in the x-ray-treated group, 7%. Local recurrences, when reported by NSABP, are reported only if they are the *first* appearance of recurrent disease, and the rates in women treated by lumpectomy are generally higher than those reported in other series that report local recurrences after more extensive operative procedures. This probably represents inadequate excision of the primary tumor. A British study[20] also confirms that x-ray treatment delays the appearance of local recurrence but suggests that perhaps the ultimate incidence is not changed, the recurrence is merely delayed in time.

Measuring the degree of benefit in a group against the degree of harm to an individual is never easy. The radiotherapy recommendations propose that everyone be treated and that the improvement, i.e., the reduction in local recurrence, is approximately 20% to 30%. At the time of these initial reports, mastectomy was proposed as the treatment for recurrent disease and this would give a 25% reduction in mastectomies. More recently, re-excision of the area has become accepted and this helps to reduce mastectomy rates.

Oncologists

Oncology in general and surgical oncology in specific has become a specialty in its own right. Initially the oncologist confined his role to the treatment of primary hematologic malignancies and established metastatic disease in solid tumors. From the early days of cytoxan and 5FU, objective responses seen in approximately 30% of patients were accompanied by a subjective improvement in 75% to 80%. This was followed by L-PAM, methotrexate, and many other antineoplastic agents with varying degrees of toxicity, most of which have many side effects. When used for "salvage" in an individual patient, the illness incurred by the drug may be balanced against the benefit seen in relief of symptoms. The most remarkable drug, however, has been tamoxifen,[21-23] which frequently provides dramatic improvement in metastatic disease with minimal side effects.

The concept of treating micrometastases, i.e., breast cancer that is not visible, means that toxic drugs will be given following mastectomy to women who are clinically well. The subgroup of premenopausal, node-positive women has been found in clinical trials to have received some benefit with adjuvant cytotoxic therapy, benefits seen in 6% to 9% of the women by a delay in death of perhaps 14–18 months.[24] It has even been proposed for node-negative patients since some clinical trials reported an extension of the disease-free interval without a change in survival.[25] The US General Accounting Office attempted to identify the survival benefit achieved during a decade of treatment of premenopausal node-positive patients.[26] Their report showed that there was no improvement in 3-, 5-, or 7-year survival by the use of adjuvant chemotherapy in stage II premenopausal women. Despite minimal benefits, if any, there is a general thrust to administer adjuvant chemotherapy to every premenopausal stage II woman, with an additional thrust to do so for the stage I (node-negative) premenopausal group. The use of tamoxifen as an adjuvant to surgery poses fewer ethical issues since the side effects of tamoxifen therapy are relatively minimal when compared to those seen with cytotoxic chemotherapy. An unresolved issue is the use of conjugated estrogens—premarin—in postmenopausal women who are also candidates for tamoxifen therapy. The statistical/clinical evidence for benefit in stage II premenopausal women is marginal, at best, but an aggressive drive to treat all such women is held by many oncologists.

Statisticians

Statisticians have a major role in the scientific design and statistical significance of clinical trials, which having achieved a degree of emotional and political importance, are then converted to standard management. The gold standard of clinical trials includes the following:

1. Patient assignment is "really" randomized.
2. All clinically relevant outcomes are reported.
3. Patient group is similar to the "real" (outside) world.
4. Both clinical and statistical significance are considered.
5. The therapeutic maneuver is feasible and acceptable.
6. All patients entered into the study are accounted for at conclusion.

These standards are difficult to achieve, but certainly better than no defined standards at all. Patients in clinical trials are "subjects" and ethical considerations that play upon subjects in an experiment are different from ethical considerations that play upon patients in a patient/doctor relationship. In clinical trials, benefits are never seen in individual patients; they may be seen only in a group. Statistical manipulation of group data occurs without necessarily having clinical thoughtfulness, e.g., when reduction in mortality is reported it is a relative number rather than the actual difference between two groups. A concept about ethical issues has arisen that holds that it is unethical to withhold these benefits, thus creating justification for making well women ill. The ethical base for this position has never been satisfactorily established or documented. Statisticians do not see patients, they see numbers and deal with illness and benefits in the aggregate, but statistical pronouncements have considerable influence in determining general policy and individual choices.

Surgeons

Once the keystone of the system, surgeons are no longer in that position. Operations on the breast are essential but less central to the entire effort, and surgeons have less control than formerly over the subsequent radiological, therapeutic, or adjuvant therapy. There are some current efforts to provide preoperative chemotherapy and render operable some patients who would not have been so considered. The Edinburgh group has reported on 47 women with large local biopsy-proven breast cancer, given cytotoxic chemotherapy for 3 preoperative months. Thirteen had a complete clinical remission and eight had no histologic evidence of carcinoma in the resected specimen.[27] The follow-up was short and the numbers too few to determine any effect on survival. A preoperative chemotherapy treatment study is now in the clinical trial stage. If this becomes a popular sequence, surgeons will more and more become technicians since it will be the oncologist who first sees the patient and makes decisions about chemical and surgical care. Dr. Bernard Fisher has proposed a new paradigm for breast cancer, suggesting that surgeons are no longer central to the issue and that chemical treatments will change the role, the timing, and the type of resection.[28]

The Woman—The Patient

The "greening of America" has been a strong movement that includes a woman's control over her own body. Publicity from the American Cancer Society and the feminist movement in general have created the idea that cure is a right and that cure is just around the corner.[29] Breast Cancer Detection Clinics have strong political support and have begun to drive the system by setting into motion a chain of events that has some scientific support, some statistical support, plenty of emotion, and a feeling that this is a part of the human rights of today. All of these factors play a role. The woman must be consulted and informed, her wishes taken into account, and supposedly she is in charge.

However, the multiple ideas, conflicting claims, uncertain values, when mixed with visions of alopecia and illness due to chemotherapy, can hardly provide any woman with a clear idea of the correct course—if there is one. In the personal emotional turmoil of a recent diagnosis of carcinoma of the breast, few women are truly capable of giving "informed" consent to any therapeutic course.

Conclusion

The breast cancer movement is now so divided and fragmented that it is not easy to see a central theme that may provide a comprehensive view of the disease, its treatment, and patient management. At present, this author believes that no one is in charge.

References

1. Spratt JS, Spratt SW: Legal perspectives on mammography and self-referral. Cancer 1992; 69:599–600.
2. Shapiro S, Venet W, Strax P, et al: Ten to fourteen year effect of breast cancer on screening on mortality. J Natl Cancer Inst 1982; 69:349–355.
3. Tabar L, Fagerberg CJG, Gad A, et al: Reduction in mortality from breast cancer after mass screening with mammography. Lancet 1985; I:829–832.
4. Tabar L, Dean P: The control of breast cancer through mammography screening: what is the evidence? Radiol Clin NA 1987; 25:993–1004.
5. Schmidt JG: The epidemiology of mass breast cancer screening: a plea for a valid measure of benefit. J Clin Epidemiol 1990; 43:215–225.
6. Wright CJ: Breast cancer screening: a different look at the evidence. Surgery 1986; 100:594–598.
7. Walt AJ: Screening and breast cancer: a surgical perspective. Am Coll Surg Bull 1990; 75:6–10.
8. Young JD, Sadowsky NL, Young JW: Mammography of women with suspicious breast lumps. Arch Surg 1986; 121:807–809.
9. Roebuch EJ: The importance of mammographic parenchymal patterns. Br J Radiol 1982; 55:387–398.
10. Kopans DB: The breast imaging report. Breast disease update. Am Coll Radiol 1989; 14:1–11.
11. Gallagher HS, Martin JE: An orientation to the concept of minimal breast cancer. Cancer 1971; 28:1505–1510.
12. Beahrs O, Shapiro S, Smart C: Report on the working group to review the NCI-ACS Breast Cancer Demonstration Project. J Natl Cancer Inst 1979; 62:640–664.
13. Ackerman L: Personal communication.
14. Linden S, Cline JW, Wood DA, et al: Validity of pathological diagnosis of breast cancer. JAMA 1960; 173:143–146.
15. Nielson M, Jensen G, Anderson J: Precancerous and cancerous breast lesions during lifetime and at autopsy: a study of 83 women. Cancer 1984; 54:612–615.
16. Anderson JA: Lobular carcinoma in situ: a long-term follow up in 52 cases. Acta Pathol Mic Scan 1974; 82:519–525.
17. Hutter RVP, Foote FW Jr: Lobular carcinoma in-situ long-term follow up. Cancer 1969; 24:1081–1087.
18. Millis RR, Thynne GSJ: In-situ intraductal carcinoma of the breast: a long-term follow-up study. Br J Surg 1975; 62:957–961.

19. Fisher B, Redmond C, Poisson R, et al: Eight-year results of a randomized clinical trial comparing total mastectomy and lumpectomy with or without irradiation in the treatment of breast cancer. NEJM 1989; 320:822–828.
20. Tough ICK: The significance of recurrence in breast cancer. Br J Surg 1966; 53:897–905.
21. Allan SG, Rodger A, Smyth JF, et al: Tamoxifen as a primary treatment of breast cancer in elderly or frail patients. Br J Med 1985; 290:358–360.
22. Brinkley DM, Dossett JA, McPherson K, et al: Controlled trial of tamoxifen as single adjuvant agent in management of early breast cancer. Lancet 1985; I:836–839.
23. Davidson NE: Tamoxifen: panacea or pandora's box? NEJM 1992, 326:885–887.
24. Early Breast Cancer Trialists Collaborative Group: Systemic treatment of early breast cancer by hormonal, cytotoxic or immune therapy. Lancet 1992; 339:71–85.
25. Mueller CB: The disease-free interval in breast cancer trials: scientific or spurious? Surgery 1991; 110:629–635.
26. Breast cancer patients' survival, GAO/PEMD, 89–9 - pp 1–51 US General Accounting Office, Washington, DC 1989.
27. Anderson EDC, Forrest APM, Hawkins RA, et al: Primary systemic therapy for operable breast cancer. Br J Cancer 1991; 63:561–566.
28. Fisher B: Surgery for breast cancer in the era of molecular biology. Presented at Clinical Congress American College of Surgeons, Chicago 1991.
29. Patterson JT: The dread disease: cancer and modern American culture. Harvard University Press, Cambridge, 1987.

New Horizons in the Management of Breast Cancer

A. P. M. Forrest

Reflections on the Past

Before taking stock of the present or looking towards the future, one must consider the implications of the past: the era of radical surgery, epitomized by the radical operations of William Stewart Halsted and Willy Meyer. But the first planned radical operation combining mastectomy with extirpation of the axillary lymph nodes was performed not in the US but in Glasgow, Scotland, some 30 years before Halsted's classic paper. The surgeon was Joseph Lister, the patient his sister, Isabella Pim, whose breast cancer had been considered by James Paget in London and James Syme in Edinburgh to be too advanced for operation, and who consulted her brother as a last resort. Lister could see "no insuperable anatomical difficulty" to performing an operation, and having "rehearsed the procedure on the dead body," carried it out in the dining room of his residence in June 1867. Before doing so, he sought the advice of Syme, who considered Lister's carbolic acid treatment as "doubtless depriving the intended operation of danger." But it was then only 2 months since Lister had used carbolic as an antiseptic dressing for a surgical, as opposed to traumatic, wound. It was, as he wrote to his father, "a formidable procedure." His sister recovered rapidly, but died 3 years later from "a tumour of the liver."[1]

The Lister operation spread throughout Europe; and it was following a tour of European centers that Halsted perfected his operation on anatomical principles to prevent the high local relapse rates which he had observed during his visit. For, as is clear from the illustrations in his paper, many of his cases were of advanced disease. But he also accepted fallaciously that cure could be assumed

From: Wise L, Johnson H Jr (eds): *Breast Cancer: Controversies in Management*. Futura Publishing Company, Inc., Armonk, NY, © 1994.

"if 3 years had passed without detecting either local recurrence or symptoms of internal disease."[2]

Several theoretical beliefs, based on the postmortem studies of Virchow and Sampson Handley, supported his view; breast cancer became established as being primarily a locoregional disease. Spreading by "permeation" of the lymphatics to the regional lymph nodes, the disease was believed to be contained within these boundaries until such time as further dissemination with the formation of "secondary" deposits of tumor occurred. This was regarded as a late phenomenon so that the eradication of all cancer cells within the regional lymphatic boundaries gave the best opportunity for cure, even when regional lymph nodes were involved. It was for this reason that surgery was extended to include excision of the internal mammary and supraclavicular nodes and that postoperative radical radiotherapy was added. But, as is now clear from the results of controlled randomized trials, such extensions of local therapy did not improve survival.[3-5]

During the radical era, sparse attention was paid to the early spread of invasive breast cancer by embolization of lymphatic and vascular channels, which is now recognized as the primary cause of metastases and death. Only a few pioneers, such as Geoffrey Keynes in St. Bartholemew's Hospital, regarded radical surgical treatment as being not only mutilating but illogical, and feared that "the invaders were bound to gain the upper hand in the end."[6] But proof awaited the demonstration, from long-term follow-up studies such as those described by Mueller in this volume, demonstrating that once invasive breast cancer is established as clinically evident disease, cure, in statistical terms (the survival rate of breast cancer patients becoming parallel to that of the normal age-matched population), has not been demonstrated.[7-13] Breast cancer is a disease which, although it disseminates early, may take many years to recur. Even 30 years from the time of diagnosis, patients with invasive breast cancer who are treated only by local surgery and radiotherapy continue to show excess mortality from metastatic disease.

It is this variability of the natural history of breast cancer in the individual patient which makes management so complex and demands that we understand better the underlying biology of the tumor if therapy is to become logical.

Eradication of a Disease

To eradicate a disease there requires to be an effective method of prevention. In turn, this requires that its cause is fully understood. The cause of breast cancer is still obscure. Even if not preventable, a disease can be controlled if effective treatment is available. This already has been achieved, for example, for childhood leukemia and testicular cancer but not yet for breast cancer. Although advances in treatment are at hand, they do not guarantee cure, but only have the potential to prolong life. Because of our continued failure to eradicate or control the disease, resources are being allocated to programs of early diagnosis by mammographic screening of normal women. One of the principles to justify screening is that the treatment of the disease during its preclinical detectable phase (when discovered by screening) compared to its treatment when it is symptomatic prolongs life.[14] Evidence that mammographic screening increases the survival of women with breast cancer was reported by Feig and is now indisputable.[15,16]

The first study to demonstrate a reduction in mortality of breast cancer from screening normal women was the HIP randomized trial in New York.[17] In that trial, mammography and physical examination were offered annually on four occasions. With improvements in the quality of mammography, physical examination is no longer regarded as necessary for the initial screen, which in the Swedish Two-Counties Trial was by single oblique-view mammography.[18] Follow-up over an average of 11 years has now been reported, indicating that compared to the nonscreened control group, women offered screening have a 40% reduction in mortality from breast cancer.[19–21] In the Swedish trial, 90% of women attended. Smaller gains have been reported in other controlled trials and comparative studies in which compliance has been less, but overall there is no doubt of the benefit.[15,16] This is why, in the UK and other European countries, nationally funded programs of screening by mammography have been introduced.

The success of screening depends not only on women complying but also on the quality of screening which must be of the highest order. This applies not only to the basic mammographic screen, but also to the assessment of mammographic abnormalities, the performance of biopsies, and the histopathological interpretation and treatment of screen-detected lesions. In the UK this is being achieved by the development of multidisciplinary teams within the screening service and by a system of quality assurance, centrally controlled, which impinges on all its aspects.[22] Similar safeguards are noticeably absent in the United States, resulting in biopsy rates that would be unacceptable in the European programs.

It is likely that screening will continue to be promoted until such time as the cause of breast cancer is known or effective treatment developed. But screening is third best and its promotion is justified only if cost is minimized, so that resources that otherwise would be applied to fundamental research can be conserved.

Diagnosis of Breast Cancer

A big step forward has been made by the ability to make a firm diagnosis of breast cancer without surgical intervention. For a palpable tumor, it is straightforward, and based on the findings of physical examination, mammography, and fine-needle aspiration cytology, and if the cytology is equivocal, TRU-cut needle biopsy. Similar diagnostic accuracy is now being achieved for the nonpalpable cancer detected by mammography, although this requires ultrasonic or radiological guidance of the aspirating needle.

The value of making a preoperative diagnosis is not in doubt. It allows appropriate investigations to be arranged, treatment to be planned with knowledge of diagnosis, and the counseling of the patient. In the Edinburgh breast service, counseling is the responsibility of a trained breast care nurse, who is available to a woman from the time of diagnosis.

But if treatment is to be rationalized, we need to know more than the cytological diagnosis and have an index of the likely behavior of the disease. Current reliance on size, axillary node status, and tumor grade to indicate its aggressiveness and give a guide to the extent of local and systemic treatment will hopefully be replaced by biological indices. For it is the inherent biological behavior of the tumor that must be taken into account. Much information has already come from studies of the expression of oncogenes (c-*myc* and *erb*-B2), of receptors for growth factors (e.g., estrogen and epidermal growth) and of secreted protein products (e.g., cathepsin-D), which have been assayed on fresh and archival tumor tissue[23]; and with the development of specific immunocyto-chemical stains, it should be possible to apply such indices to cellular aspirates by flow cytometry. The availability of an immunohistochemical assay for estrogen receptor, which can be performed on cellular aspirates, has been shown to be of value for the selection of tamoxifen therapy in elderly women.[24,25]

Treatment

The management of breast cancer increasingly emphasizes systemic rather than local therapy.

But not surprisingly, a surgeon's concern is primarily with the need to ensure local control of the disease. But he should now be asking himself not "how radical" but "how conservative" can his surgery safely be. It is almost 60 years since Geoffrey Keynes first explored the use of radical radiation therapy (later combined with local excision of the tumor) for the treatment of localized breast cancer.[26] There is now no shortage of evidence that, in suitable cases, the results of local excision followed by radical radiotherapy equal those of regimes of therapy based on mastectomy.[27,28] It is also now accepted that relapse of the disease within the breast does not imperil ultimate outcome, provided this is treated promptly. Yet surgeons are obsessed with the need for perfection, paying more attention to a small risk of relapse affecting a few women, rather than freedom from relapse in the majority, for whom perfection is freedom of disease without loss of the breast.

The question of "how conservative" is particularly important for women whose cancers are detected through screening. Knowledge that treatment can be successful without loss of the breast will encourage them to attend. In the county of Gavleborg in Sweden, local excision alone is now practiced for all invasive tumors under 2 cm in diameter.[29] Controlled trials are under way to test the safety of this approach.[30]

The local management of ductal carcinoma in situ (DCIS), which accounts for almost 20% of screen-detected lesions, poses greater difficulty. By definition, this is the one form of breast cancer for which cure can be guaranteed by mastectomy and it is tempting to advise this approach. But increasingly local excision is being accepted as adequate treatment. Careful histopathological studies suggest that the size of the lesion is critical and, in Europe, local excision is now the preferred surgical treatment provided extensive calcifications are not present on the mammogram and that excision margins are clear.[31,32] The roles of radiotherapy and tamoxifen are under study in a UK National Trial in which women with DCIS are randomly allocated for excision alone or excision plus radical radiotherapy, both arms being further randomized to receive tamoxifen or not.[33]

Lobular carcinoma in situ is not cancer; it is a marker of increased risk. It is a histopathological diagnosis, there being no mammographic signs for this condition, and therefore it is a chance finding in a biopsy specimen.[34] Provided excision margins are free of change, no further treatment is required.

Systemic Therapy

It is clear that gains in survival for women with invasive breast cancer have followed the introduction of adjuvant systemic therapy. But although highly significant in statistical terms, they are, in real terms, modest.[35] Yet, as recently advised, the surgeon should now be seeking indications *not* to give systemic treatment rather than considering indications to give it.[36] It should be appreciated that systemic adjuvant therapy gives equal reduction in the annual odds of death in node-negative and node-positive disease. Because of its worse prognosis, absolute gains are greater in node-positive patients, but significant benefit is still achieved in those without nodal involvement. But before administering chemotherapy with its attendant morbidity, one wishes to know which node-negative patients have the more aggressive disease—a strong argument for the availability of a precise method to select patients for appropriate therapy.

One way to improve selectivity of suitable therapy that is under study is to reverse the orthodox approach of local therapy followed by adjuvant systemic therapy and to give the systemic therapy first, reserving local therapy for the management of residual local disease. By removing the primary tumor as the first step in orthodox management, one loses the only immediate indicator of the effectiveness of treatment. By leaving the primary tumor in situ, not only does its behavior enable one to assess the effectiveness of the systemic treatment, but one also exploits the potential effect of systemic treatment on the local disease. As a result of the reduction in size of the primary tumor, this may be amenable to control by more conservative means than would otherwise have been used. There is now good evidence from a Milan study that primary chemotherapy renders three-quarters of large but operable tumors (over 2 cm) suitable for breast-conserving therapy.[37] This study does not indicate that primary chemotherapy increases cure; but this information should come from the large NSABP trial B-18, in which, in women with operable disease, preoperative chemotherapy is being compared with the same chemotherapy given postoperatively.[38]

In the UK, studies in patients with large operable tumors initially concentrated on using the primary tumor as an indicator of appropriate systemic

Table 1
Regressions of Large Tumors Achieved by Antiestrogen and Chemotherapy*

Treatment	Number of Patients	Significant Regression (Complete)	No Change	Progression
Antiestrogen Therapy				
ER <20 f moles/mg	15	0	5	10
ER ≥20 f moles/mg	46	24	16	6
Chemotherapy				
primary (ER <20 f moles/mg)	27	23 (8)	4	0
following failed antiestrogens	20	11 (5)	9	0

*From: Br J Cancer 1991 (with permission).

therapy.[39-41] In the study that we reported, 88 patients with operable tumors of greater than 4 cm were treated initially with antiestrogens, reserving chemotherapy for nonresponding disease,[40] a policy that we altered knowing that tumors with estrogen-receptor concentration of less than 20 f.moles per mg cytosol protein failed to significantly regress with antiestrogen therapy.[42]

In all, 61 patients received antiestrogens, to which 24 responded, 21 remained static over a 3-month period, and 16 progressed. Forty-seven (27 as a primary mode of therapy and 20 following failed antiestrogens) of the 88 patients received chemotherapy, 34 (72%) with significant regression of their tumor.[43] Mastectomy was carried out 3 to 6 months after the start of primary systemic treatment in 82 patients and wide local excision in six. Complete clinical regression did not occur in any of those responding to antiestrogens (because the rate of response is slow) but was observed in 13 of those receiving chemotherapy, eight of whom had no histopathological evidence of tumor in the mastectomy specimen (Table 1). This regime of selective primary systemic therapy is now being studied in a controlled randomized trial, in which control patients receive orthodox treatment by mastectomy followed by adjuvant tamoxifen therapy.

While studies of primary systemic therapy are still in their infancy, there seems little doubt that the convergence of systemic and local therapy points the way to the future management of the disease, allowing not only curability but also the impact that systemic treatment may have on the requirements for local control and the extent of local surgery and radiation.

New Methods of Treatment

As indicated above, the gains made with the types of systemic therapy now available are modest. The development of more effective treatment is a necessary step towards better management. Intensification of chemotherapy regimes by escalating the dose of drugs and by measures to reduce toxicity are now being applied to locally advanced disease, not only to help control the local disease but to eliminate micrometastatic disease. Such measures include the administration of colony-stimulating factors (G-CSF and GM-CSF) and autologous bone marrow transplants. Attempts to increase the sensitivity of the target malignant cells by their recruitment into the synthetic phase of the cell cycle have not been accepted as being of clinical benefit.[44] Targeted chemotherapy, by encapsulation within liposomal membranes, by attachment to a chemical substrate (ligand) which binds to a specific cell receptor, or by attachment to an antibody to a specific cell constituent, is opening the way to more selective therapy—methods that also can be used to carry destructive radioisotopes into the tumor cell.[15] The introduction of foreign genes (e.g., that for tumor-necrosing factor) into lymphocytes harvested from the tumor (tumor-infiltrating lymphocytes, TIL-cells) is opening the way to gene therapy.[45] Aggressive therapy of this type can be associated with serious morbidity, which makes the correct selection of patients for such methods of treatment even more critical.

Advances are also being made in the development of more potent antiestrogens, such as gonadotrophin-releasing hormone agonists and antagonists to effect ablation of ovarian function in the young woman, and the aromatase inhibitors to inhibit the peripheral synthesis of estrogens in those who are postmenopausal.

The Elderly: A Special Case

At the present time, one-third of all breast cancers are diagnosed in women of 70 years of age or more; moreover, the incidence in elderly women would appear to be sharply increasing.[46] Elderly women have atrophic fatty breasts, which are lucent on a mammogram and therefore would be expected to be particularly suitable for screening, but their response to an invitation to be screened is poor, and most are referred with symptomatic disease.[47] The belief that the elderly present with breast cancer which is at a more advanced symptomatic stage is not borne out by fact. Nor is there support for the view that their disease runs a more favorable course.[48] In fact, there is evidence, first suggested by Mueller from the Syracuse Registry and recently confirmed from population studies, that the reverse is the case.[9,49–51] Effective and appropriate treatment is therefore still indicated, and there is no justification for modifying management on the grounds of chronological age alone. For example, it is reported both from the US and the UK that simple excision of the tumor as sole treatment gives unacceptable local relapse rates.[52–54]

The view that elderly women are liable to receive less than appropriate therapy has been supported by a study from seven US hospitals.[55] Local therapy, even when co-morbidity is taken into account, was less radical than would have been the case in younger patients. There is, however, one difference in the tumors of elderly women that should be taken into account. They are more likely to be rich in estrogen receptors, and therefore respond better to antiestrogen therapy.[56] The meta-analysis of adjuvant trials reported by the Early Breast Cancer Trialists Co-operative Group has shown that tamoxifen provides benefit in elderly women.[35] No such evidence is available for chemotherapy, but the numbers of elderly patients included in trials of adjuvant chemotherapy are small—another indication of how age can modify treatment policy. Nevertheless, the responsiveness of tumors to tamoxifen in these elderly patients suggests that all should be given tamoxifen as part of their primary treatment.

It was recognition of the value of tamoxifen, coupled with the knowledge that its administration as primary systemic therapy for primary breast cancer in infirm elderly patients led to objective regression of 50% of tumors, with disease stabilization in another 20%, which promoted interest in the use of tamoxifen alone in fit patients.[47] But it is now clear that the assessment of response can take many months; additionally, long-term studies indicate that control of the disease for 5 years or more can be expected only in 30%.[57] It is those with complete remission of their primary tumor who benefit best. Two controlled trials comparing tamoxifen alone with tamoxifen plus surgical removal of the tumor have given controversial results.[58,59] More informative is the trial recently reported by Baum and colleagues which addressed the question of whether tamoxifen alone provided equal control to tamoxifen plus "optimal" surgery.[60] The answer is negative; a recent report indicates that relapse rates in those treated by tamoxifen alone were significantly higher than those in which tamoxifen was combined with surgery.[61] Primary tamoxifen therapy should therefore be used solely for those who are unsuitable for surgery and then, as we have shown, only if estrogen receptor is present in more than 20% of the cells in the tumor.[25,62]

But, what is "optimal surgery?" In the CRC trial referred to above, it was left to the participating surgeons to decide; most elected for local excision of the tumor alone, which, as indicated above, is not optimal when performed in the absence of tamoxifen (but may still be in its presence). Trials currently being conducted under the auspices of the European Organization for Research and Treatment of Cancer which are comparing mastectomy with local excision and tamoxifen will help answer this question.[47]

Considering that older women dislike radiotherapy because of its need for frequent attendance, mastectomy with dissection of the axilla would appear to remain the standard optimal local treatment, But one must remember that older women may still wish to consider restoration of their breast, provided this can be done simply at the time of mastectomy. The insertion of a subpectoral sialastic prosthesis readily allows this.

Prevention

As indicated, the primary prevention of any disease, including breast cancer, rests upon determining its cause and then removing this. Of the factors that put a woman at risk from breast cancer, age and country of origin are the most relevant, indicating that exposure to an environmental factor is likely to be the causal agent. Breast cancer is a disease of western civilization; those who migrate to the west from low-risk countries take on the western incidence of the disease.[63]

The development of malignancy is a multistage process. Although the predominant cause of breast cancer is unknown, there is no doubt that female sex hormones influence every stage of the development of the disease. Functioning ovaries are necessary for its initiation. Oophorectomy before the age of 40 years reduces the incidence of the disease by half; prolonging the period of reproductive life increases risk.[64,65]

Estrogen is an essential promoting agent for the early stages of carcinogenesis. It also modifies the growth of established disease. It is such information that has led to the suggestion that the development of the disease might be impeded by the continuous administration of antiestrogens.[66] But concern about the potential risks of long-term antiestrogen therapy has been expressed, particularly regarding vascular disease and osteoporosis. These concerns have not been confirmed. Studies of long-term tamoxifen therapy in patients with breast cancer included in adjuvant trials and in a group of normal women have shown that tamoxifen, although acting as an estrogen-antagonist on the breast may act as an estrogen-agonist at other sites, e.g., liver and bone. Following the administration of tamoxifen, profiles of lipoproteins and clotting factors are altered favorably regarding their influence on cardiac and thrombotic disease while bone demineralization does not occur.[67,68]

Confirmation of a potentially beneficial effect from long-term tamoxifen on cardiac disease has come from the Scottish tamoxifen trial, in which the numbers of women suffering fatal myocardial infarction in those taking tamoxifen for 5 years was significantly less than in their control partners.[69] A report from Stockholm that the incidence of endometrial cancer is increased in women taking tamoxifen has not been substantiated in other studies, but this is a potential risk that must be kept under review.[70]

Large adjuvant studies have offered the opportunity to compare the incidence of contralateral breast tumors in those taking tamoxifen with untreated controls. As was first pointed out by Cuzick and Baum,[71] this is significantly reduced. A recent review indicates that the incidence is approximately halved; but before regarding this as demonstrating prevention rather than suppression of growth, one must be certain that these contralateral tumors were not present at the time of primary treatment or that they do not represent metastases.[68] Trials of tamoxifen therapy in normal women believed to be at risk from breast cancer are now under way in the US and the UK.

The administration of tamoxifen is not the only method by which estrogen action can be inhibited. Gonadotrophin-releasing hormone analogues which, by desensitizing the pituitary to normal pulsatile stimulation by the natural hormone, inhibit gonadotrophin production have been proposed as a method of suppressing ovarian function in young women.[72] By inhibiting both estrogen and progesterone secretion by the ovaries, Pike and colleagues suggest that not only will this prove to be an effective contraceptive but that it will exert a preventative effect on the development of both ovarian and breast cancer. They consider that the evidence that estrogen *alone* increases breast cancer risk is sparse and that it is the combination of estrogen and progesterone that occurs during the luteal phase of the menstrual cycle which is the promoting agent.

Evidence supporting their view comes from studies of cell turnover in the human breast, which indicate that maximal proliferative activity occurs during the luteal phase.[73] This concept allows the administration of a small dose of estrogen to maintain well-being during the period of "medical castration." A small feasibility study, in which gonadotrophin-releasing hormone analogues are combined with 0.625 mg of equine estradiol daily, has been started. To prevent the risk of endometrial proliferation, which is induced by estrogen alone, progesterone is being administered for a few days each 3 months.[74]

A third method of reducing estrogen secretion which is under study is by dietary intervention. The Womens' Health Trial Study Group in the US reported recently that reduction of fat intake from 40% to 20% of total calories led to a significant fall in plasma estrogens.[75] The implications of this finding are under consideration.

An essential requirement for studies of chemoprevention is the definition of those women at increased risk from breast cancer. Combinations of risk factors that can readily be obtained on enquiry—for example, family and reproductive history—do allow some measure of risk allocation but discrimination is not good. Three-quarters of all breast cancers arise in women without such factors.

The transformation of normal breast epithelium through hyperplasia to malignancy was described by Page in Chapter 18. Although currently regarded as pathological events defined by histological criteria, genetic and other biological markers are under study and are bound to be defined. Studies of fine-needle aspirates from normal breasts and of epithelial cells derived from nipple aspirates are in progress in normal women and may have great potential in determining whether changes in phenotype leading to malignancy have occurred.[76]

Conclusions

In this final review, I have not considered the management of advanced or metastatic disease which has been well documented in other chapters of this book. I have considered only "early" presymptomatic and symptomatic disease. It must be clear that the future management of early breast cancer does not lie in better surgery or more intense radiotherapy, which are but means of controlling the local manifestations of the disease. Local therapy is curative only when the cancer is truly localized to the breast.

Advances in the techniques of early diagnosis may result in a larger proportion of such tumors being recognized, which then can be cured by conservative local surgery; but for established symptomatic invasive disease, it is systemic treatment that determines outcome and must play the leading role.

This implies that as time goes on, surgeons will become less involved with decisions regarding management, unless they are prepared to cooperate closely with those in other fields. In Edinburgh and other specialized centers in the UK, breast cancer management is increasingly in the hands of a multidisciplinary team of which the surgeon is an active member and, in many instances, the leader. This is the approach for the future, for it is the only way to ensure that the best advice for the total care of women with this complex disease can be given within one clinical environment. But a surgical member of such a team must be prepared to devote most of his time to breast disease, as other surgeons must be prepared to reduce or relinquish practice in this area.

References

1. Forrest APM: Lister oration: breast cancer—121 years on. J Royal Coll Surg Edinb 1989; 34:239–248.
2. Halsted WS: The results of radical operations for the cure of carcinoma of the breast. Ann Surg 1970; 46:1–19.
3. Lecour J, Monique L, Caceres E, et al: Radical mastectomy versus radical mastectomy plus internal mammary dissection: ten-year results of an international co-operative trial in breast cancer. Cancer 1983; 51:1941–1943.
4. Cuzick J, Stewart HJS, Peto R, et al: Overview of randomised trials of post-operative adjuvant radiotherapy in breast cancer. Cancer Treat Rep 1987; 71:15–29.
5. Cuzick J, Stewart HJS, Peto R, et al: Overview of randomised trials comparing radical mastectomy without radiotherapy against simple mastectomy with radiotherapy in breast cancer. Cancer Treat Rep 1987; 71:7–14.
6. Keynes G: Gates of Memory. Oxford University Press, 1981.
7. Easson EC, Russell MJ: The Curability of Cancer in Various Sites. Pitman, London, 1968.
8. Adair F, Berg J, Houbert L, Robbins GF: Long-term follow-up of breast cancer patients: the thirty-year report. Cancer 1974; 33:1145–1150.
9. Mueller C, Ames F, Anderson GD: Breast cancer in 3558 women: age as a significant determinant in the role of dying and causes of death. Surgery 1978; 83:123–132.
10. Langlands AO, Pocock SJ, Kerr JR, Gore SM: Long-term survival of patients with breast cancer: a study of the curability of the disease. Br Med J 1979; 2:1247–1251.
11. Brinkley D, Haybittle JL: Long-term survival of women with breast cancer. Lancet 1984; 1:1118.
12. Le MG, Hill C, Rezvani A, Sarrazin D, et al: Long-term survival of women with breast cancer. Lancet 1984; 2:922.
13. Rutqvist LE, Wallgren A: Long-term survival of 458 young breast cancer patients. Cancer 1985; 55:658–665.
14. Wilson JMG, Jungner G: Principle and Practice of Screening for Disease. World Health Organization Public Health Paper, 1968.
15. Forrest APM: Breast cancer: the decision to screen. Fourth HM Queen Mother Fellowship. Nuffield Provincial Hospital Trust, London, 1990.
16. Forrest APM: Breast cancer: the decision to screen. J Pub Health Med 1991; 13:2–12.
17. Shapiro S, Venet W, Strax P, Venet L: Periodic Screening for Breast Cancer: The Health Insurance Plan Project and its Sequelae 1963–1986. The John Hopkins University Press, Baltimore and London, 1988.
18. Tabar L, Fagerberg CJG, Gad A, Baldetorp L, et al: Reduction in mortality from breast cancer after mass screening with mammography: randomised trial from the Breast Cancer Screening Working Group of the Swedish National Board of Health and Welfare. Lancet 1985;1:829–832.
19. Day NE: Screening for breast cancer. Br Med Bull 1991; 47(2):400–415.
20. Duffy SW, Tabar L, Fagerberg G, Gad A, et al: Breast screening, prognostic factors and survival: results from the Swedish two-county study. Br J Cancer 1991; 64:1133–1138.
21. Tabar L, Fagerberg G, Day NE, Duffy SW, et al: Breast cancer treatment and natural history: new insights from results of screening. Lancet 1992; 339:412–414.

22. Department of Health Advisory Committee: Breast cancer screening 1991: evidence and experience since the Forrest Report. NHSBSP Publications, Sheffield, 1991.
23. McGuire WL, Tandon AK, Allred DC, et al: How to use prognostic factors in axillary node-negative breast cancer patients. J Nat Canc Inst 1990; 82:1006–1015.
24. Greene GL, Jensen EV: Monoclonal antibodies as probes for estrogen receptor detection and characterization. J Steroid Biochem 1982; 16:353–359.
25. Gaskell DJ, Hawkins RA, Sangster K, Chetty U, et al: Relationship between immunocytochemical estimation of oestrogen receptors in elderly patients with breast cancer and response to tamoxifen. Lancet 1989; 1:1044–1045.
26. Keynes G: Radium treatment of primary carcinoma of the breast. Lancet 1928; ii:108–111.
27. Veronesi U, Banfi A, Salvadori B, Luini A, et al: Breast conservation is the treatment of choice in small breast cancer: long-term results of a randomised trial. Europ J Cancer 1990; 26:668–670.
28. Fisher B, Redmond C, Poisson R, Margolese R, et al: Eight-year results of a randomized trial comparing total mastectomy and lumpectomy with or without radiation in the treatment of breast cancer. N Engl J Med 1989; 320:822–828.
29. Lundgren B: Screening for breast cancer: a view from the front line. Biomed Pharmacother 1988; 42:443–446.
30. The Uppsala-Orebro Breast Cancer Study Group: Sector resection with or without postoperative radiotherapy for stage I breast cancer. J Nat Canc Inst 1990; 82:277–282.
31. Lagios MD, Margolin FR, Westdahl MD, Marye R: Mammographically detected duct carcinoma in situ. Cancer 1989; 63:618–624.
32. Holland R, Hendriks JLCL, Verbeek ALM, et al: Extent, distribution and mammographic histological correlations of breast ductal carcinoma in situ. Lancet 1990; i:519–522.
33. UK Co-ordinating Committee for Cancer Research: Protocol of the UK randomised trial for the management of screen-detected ductal carcinoma in situ (DCIS) of the breast. NHS Breast Screening Programme. Breast Screening Publications, Oxford, 1989.
34. Page DL, Japaze H: Non-Infiltrating (In Situ) Carcinoma in the Breast. In: Bland KI, Copeland EM (eds). WB Saunders, Philadelphia, p 185, 1991.
35. Early Breast Cancer Trialists' Collaborative Group: Systemic treatment of early breast cancer by hormonal cytotoxic or immune therapy: 133 randomised trials involving 31,000 recurrences and 24,000 deaths among 75,000 women. Lancet 1992; 339:71–85.
36. Glick JH: Meeting highlights: adjuvant therapy for breast cancer. J Natl Cancer Inst 1988; 80:474–475.
37. Bonadonna G, Veronesi U, Brambilla C, et al: Primary chemotherapy to avoid mastectomy in tumours with diameters of three centimetres or more. J Natl Cancer Inst 1990; 82:1539-1545.
38. Fisher B: A biological perspective of breast cancer: contributions of the National Surgical Adjuvant Breast and Bowel Project clinical trials. CA 1991; 41:97–111.
39. Thomlinson RH: Measurement and management of carcinoma of the breast. Clin Radiol 1982; 33:481–493.
40. Forrest APM, Levack PA, Chetty U, Miller WR, et al: A human tumour model. Lancet 1986; 2:840–842.
41. Mansi JL, Smith IE, Walsh G: Primary medical therapy for operable breast cancer. Eur J Cancer 1989; 25:1623–1627.
42. Anderson EDC, Forrest APM, Levack PA, Chetty U, et al: Response to endocrine manipulation and oestrogen receptor concentration in large operable breast cancer. Br J Cancer 1989; 60:223.
43. Anderson EDC, Forrest APM, Hawkins RA, Anderson TJ, et al: Primary systemic therapy for operable breast cancer. Br J Cancer 1991; 63:561–566.
44. Lippman ME, Cassidy J, Wesley M, Young RC: A randomized attempt to increase the efficacy of cytotoxic chemotherapy in metastatic breast cancer by hormonal synchronization. J Clin Oncol 1984; 2:28.

45. Rosenberg SA, Lotze MT, Mule JJ: New approaches to the immunotherapy of cancer. Ann Int Med 1989; 108:853–864.
46. White E, Lee CY, Kristal AR: Evaluation of the increase in breast cancer incidence in relation to mammography use. J Natl Cancer Inst 1990; 82:1546–1552.
47. Forrest APM, Fentiman IS: Breast cancer in the elderly; principles of management. In: Monfardini S, Fentiman IS (eds). Cancer in the Elderly (in press).
48. Ewing J: Neoplastic Diseases. 3rd Edition. WB Saunders, Philadelphia, 1934.
49. Host H, Lund E: Age as a prognostic factor in breast cancer. Cancer 1986; 57:2217–2221.
50. Sant M, Gatta G, Micheli A, Verdacchia A, et al: Survival and age at diagnosis of breast cancer in a population-based cancer registry. Br J Cancer 1991; 27:981–984.
51. Adami HO, Walker B, Meirik O, Persson I, et al: Age as a prognostic factor in breast cancer. Cancer 1985; 56:898–902.
52. Kantorowitz DA, Poulter CA, Sischy B, Paterson E, et al: Treatment of breast cancer among elderly women with segmental mastectomy or segmental mastectomy plus postoperative radiotherapy. Int J Rad Oncol Phys 1988; 15:263–270.
53. Reed MWR, Morrison JM: Wide local excision as the sole primary treatment in elderly patients with carcinoma of the breast. Br J Surg 1989; 76:898–900.
54. Taggart REB: Partial mastectomy for breast cancer. Br Med J 1978; 2:1268.
55. Greenfield S, Blanco DM, Elashjoff RM, et al: Patterns of care related to age of breast cancer patients. JAMA 1987; 257:2766–2770.
56. McCarty KS, Silva JS, Cox EB, Leight GS, et al: Relationship to age and menstrual status to estrogen receptor content in primary carcinoma of the breast. Ann Surg 1983; 197:123–127.
57. Horobin JM, Preece PE, Dewar JA, Wood RAB, et al: Long-term follow-up of elderly patients with locoregional breast cancer treated with tamoxifen alone. Br J Surg 1991; 78:213–217.
58. Gazet J-C, Markopoulos C, Ford HT, et al: Prospective randomised trial of tamoxifen versus surgery in elderly patients with breast cancer. Lancet 1988; i:679–681.
59. Robertson JFR, Todd JH, Ellis IO, et al: Comparison of mastectomy with tamoxifen for treating elderly patients with operable breast cancer. Br Med J 1988; 297:511–514.
60. Bates T, Riley DL, Houghton J, et al: Breast cancer in elderly women: a Cancer Research Campaign Trial comparing treatment with tamoxifen and optimal surgery with tamoxifen alone. Br J Surg 1991; 78:591–594.
61. Bates T, Riley D, Houghton J, Baum M: Is tamoxifen adequate treatment for breast cancer in elderly patients: is there still an issue? Surgical Research Society, London, January 1992.
62. Gaskell DJ, Forrest APM, Carteret S, Chetty U, et al: Use of primary tamoxifen therapy for elderly women with breast cancer: when and for whom is it worthwhile? Br J Surg (in press).
63. Kilonel LN, Harkin JH, Nomura AM, Chad SY: Dietary fat intake and cancer incidence among five ethnic groups in Hawaii. Cancer Res 1981; 41:3727–3728.
64. Feinleib M: Breast cancer and artificial menopause. J Natl Cancer Inst 1968; 41:315–329.
65. MacMahon B, Cole P, Brown J: Etiology of human breast cancer. J Natl Cancer Inst 1973; 50:21–42.
66. Cuzick J, Wang DY, Bulbrook RD: The prevention of breast cancer. Lancet 1986; 1:83–86.
67. Powles TJ, Hardy JR, Ashley SE, et al: A pilot trial to evaluate the acute toxicity and feasibility of tamoxifen for prevention of breast cancer. Br J Cancer 1989; 60:126–131.
68. Nayfield SG, Karp JE, Ford LG, Dorr FA, et al: Potential role of tamoxifen in prevention of breast cancer. J Natl Cancer Inst 1991; 83:1450–1459.
69. McDonald CC, Stewart HJ: Fatal myocardial infarction in the Scottish adjuvant tamoxifen trial. Br Med J 1991; 303:435–437.
70. Fornander T, Rutqvist LE, Cedermark B, et al: Adjuvant tamoxifen in early breast cancer: occurrence of new primary cancers. Lancet 1989; 1:117–119.

71. Cuzick J, Baum ML: Tamoxifen and contralateral breast cancer. Lancet 1985; 2:282.
72. Pike MC, Ross RK, Lobo RA, Key TJA, et al: LHRH agonists and the prevention of breast and ovarian cancer. Br J Cancer 1989; 60:142–148.
73. Anderson TJ, Battersby S: The involvement of oestrogen in the development and function of the normal breast: histological evidence. Proc Royal Soc Edinb 1989; 95B:23–32.
74. Henderson BE: Aging: The Quality of Life Conference. Washington, 1992.
75. Prentice R, Thompson D. Clifford C, Gorbach S, et al: Dietary fat reduction and plasma estradiol concentration in healthy postmenopausal women. J Natl Cancer Inst 1990; 82:129–134.
76. Wrensch MR, Petrakis NL, King EB, et al: Breast cancer incidence in women with abnormal cytology in nipple aspirates of breast fluid. Am J Epidemiol (in press).

Index